HIGH-GRADE GLIOMAS

CURRENT CLINICAL ONCOLOGY

Maurie Markman, MD, SERIES EDITOR

HIGH-GRADE GLIOMAS

Diagnosis and Treatment

Edited by

GENE H. BARNETT, MD

Brain Tumor Institute, Department of Neurological Surgery
Cleveland Clinic Foundation, Cleveland, OH

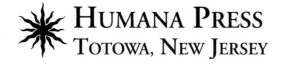
HUMANA PRESS
TOTOWA, NEW JERSEY

© 2007 Humana Press Inc.
999 Riverview Drive, Suite 208
Totowa, New Jersey 07512

humanapress.com

For additional copies, pricing for bulk purchases, and/or information about other Humana titles, contact Humana at the above address or at any of the following numbers: Tel: 973-256-1699; Fax: 973-256-8341; E-mail: orders@humanapr.com or visit our website at http://humanapr.com

Due diligence has been taken by the publishers, editors, and authors of this book to assure the accuracy of the information published and to describe generally accepted practices. The contributors herein have carefully checked to ensure that the drug selections and dosages set forth in this text are accurate and in accord with the standards accepted at the time of publication. Notwithstanding, as new research, changes in government regulations, and knowledge from clinical experience relating to drug therapy and drug reactions constantly occurs, the reader is advised to check the product information provided by the manufacturer of each drug for any change in dosages or for additional warnings and contraindications. This is of utmost importance when the recommended drug herein is a new or infrequently used drug. It is the responsibility of the treating physician to determine dosages and treatment strategies for individual patients. Further it is the responsibility of the health care provider to ascertain the Food and Drug Administration status of each drug or device used in their clinical practice. The publisher, editors, and authors are not responsible for errors or omissions or for any consequences from the application of the information presented in this book and make no warranty, express or implied, with respect to the contents in this publication.

This publication is printed on acid-free paper. ∞
ANSI Z39.48-1984 (American National Standards Institute)
Permanence of Paper for Printed Library Materials.

Cover design by Patricia F. Cleary.

Cover illustrations: Figure 1, Chapter 7; Figure 15, Chapter 10; Figure 27, Chapter 1.

Photocopy Authorization Policy:
Authorization to photocopy items for internal or personal use, or the internal or personal use of specific clients, is granted by Humana Press Inc., provided that the base fee of US $30.00 is paid directly to the Copyright Clearance Center at 222 Rosewood Drive, Danvers, MA 01923. For those organizations that have been granted a photocopy license from the CCC, a separate system of payment has been arranged and is acceptable to Humana Press Inc. The fee code for users of the Transactional Reporting Service is: [1-58829-511-7/07 $30.00].

Printed in the United States of America.   10 9 8 7 6 5 4 3 2 1

EISBN 159745-185-1
Library of Congress Cataloging-in-Publication Data
High-grade gliomas : diagnosis and treatment / edited by Gene H. Barnett.
    p. ; cm. — (Current clinical oncology)
  Includes bibliographical references and index.
  ISBN 1-58829-511-7 (alk. paper)
  1. Gliomas.   I. Barnett, Gene H. II. Series: Current clinical oncology (Totowa, N.J.)
  [DNLM: 1. Glioma—therapy. 2. Glioma—diagnosis. 3. Therapies, Investigational.   QZ 380 H638 2007]
  RC280.B7H54 2007
  616.99'481—dc22   2006024846

Preface

This is truly an exciting time in the field of neuro-oncology, particularly in the area of high-grade gliomas. The management of patients with high-grade gliomas has historically been one of the most challenging and disheartening fields in medicine, where failure is the rule and longevity is the exception. The jaded often state that despite purported advances in surgical and radiotherapeutic techniques and a myriad of clinical trials of medical therapies, the survival statistics for glioblastoma have not changed in the last three decades. The nihilism associated with these tumors is such that some practitioners still advise against treatment or even biopsy, recommending palliative care with the diagnosis based only on history and an MRI scan. If the current state-of-the-art in the diagnosis and management of high-grade gliomas was truly so bleak, there would be no reason to compile and publish a monograph on the subject. The fact is that we have recently entered an era where real progress is being made in our understanding and treatment of high-grade gliomas that is directly benefiting some patients.

We are slowly but surely chipping away at this problem. One approach has exploited correlations between particular molecular markers and therapeutic response. The first such "breakthrough" in high-grade glioma was the observation that loss of chromosomes 1p and 19q uniformly predict chemosensitivity in anaplastic oligodendrogliomas (1). Subsequent work has refined this relationship using additional markers to forecast longevity in patients with these tumors (2). More recently we have seen similar observations in glioblastoma where methylation of the methyl-guanine-methyl transferase (MGMT) gene promoter is associated with better response to temozolomide (TMZ) (3). Similarly, co-expression of the vIII mutation of epidermal growth factor receptor (EGFR) and the PTEN tumor suppressor gene predicts response to EGFR inhibitors (4).

Another approach has been large multi-center clinical trials using conventional and unconventional agents. Stupp et al have shown that radiotherapy with concurrent low dose temozolomide and subsequent high dose TMZ leads to longer survival than radiotherapy alone for newly diagnosed glioblastoma (5). Presently a large multicenter trial is comparing the use of an immuotoxin (IL13-PE39QQR) delivered by convection enhanced delivery against carmustine-impregnated biodegradable wafers in patients with operable glioblastoma at first recurrence. Yet another avenue of investigation is to use preclinical animal testing to improve response by refining traditional therapeutic delivery schedules, combining agents and investigating various modes of delivery and concentrations of agents achieved in tumor, brain and CSF.

So in this volume we present the spectrum of issues pertaining to high-grade gliomas from the basics of clinical characteristics and management to the state-of-the-art in diagnosis and therapeutics, as well as current areas of investigation that may lead to the treatments of tomorrow. We explore whether molecular diagnosis complements histology or is likely to supercede it, the most current information in imaging techniques to assist us in diagnosing and monitoring treatment, and the latest in "conventional" treatments such as surgery, radiation, and cytotoxic chemotherapy.

After decades of uniformly poor outcomes, we have entered an era where meaningful advances are being made in our understanding of the biology of high-grade gliomas that is leading to better, more rational, patient-specific treatments. I hope you find this book informative and useful.

Gene Barnett, MD, FACS

REFERENCES

1. Cairncross JG, Ueki K, Zlatescu MC, et al. Specific genetic predictors of chemotherapeutic response and survival in patients with anaplastic oligodendrogliomas. J Natl Cancer Inst 1998;90(19):1473–1479.
2. Ino Y, Betensky RA, Zlatescu MC, et al. Molecular subtypes of anaplastic oligodendroglioma: implications for patient management at diagnosis. Clin Cancer Res 2001;7(4):839–845.
3. Hegi M E, Diserens A-C, Gorlia T, et al. MGMT gene silencing and benefit from temozolomide in glioblastoma. N Engl J Med 2005;352:997–1003.
4. Mellinghoff IK, Wang MY, Vivanco I, et al. Molecular determinants of the response of glioblastomas to EGFR kinase inhibitors. N Engl J Med 2005;353:2012–2024.
5. Stupp R., Mason W P, van den Bent MJ, et al. Radiotherapy plus concomitant and adjuvant temozolomide for glioblastoma. N Engl J Med 2005;352:987–996.

Contents

DAVID A. REARDON, MD • *Neuro-Oncology Program, Department of Surgery, Duke University Medical Center, Durham, NC*

TIMOTHY P. L. ROBERTS, PhD • *Department of Medical Imaging, University of Toronto, University Health Network; and Toronto Western Research Institute, Toronto, Ontario*

PAUL M. RUGGIERI, MD • *Department of Diagnostic Radiology, The Cleveland Clinic Foundation, Cleveland, OH*

HIRAL K. SHAH, MD • *Department of Human Oncology, University of Wisconsin, Madison, WI*

P. K. SNEED, MD • *Department of Radiation Oncology, University of California, San Francisco, CA*

ALEXANDER M. SPENCE, MD • *Department of Neurology, University of Washington School of Medicine, Seattle, WA*

MICHAEL P. STEINMETZ, MD • *Department of Neurological Surgery, The Cleveland Clinic Foundation, Cleveland, OH*

GLEN H. J. STEVENS, DO, PhD • *The Brain Tumor Institute, Department of Neurology, The Cleveland Clinic Foundation, Cleveland, OH*

JOHN H. SUH, MD • *The Brain Tumor Institute, Department of Radiation Oncology, The Cleveland Clinic Foundation, Cleveland, OH*

KRISTIN SWANSON, PhD • *Department of Neuropathology, University of Washington School of Medicine, Seattle, WA*

TINA THOMAS, MD • *The Brain Tumor Institute, The Cleveland Clinic Foundation, Cleveland, OH*

STEVEN TOMS, MD, MPH • *The Brain Tumor Institute, Department of Neurological Surgery, The Cleveland Clinic Foundation, Cleveland, OH*

M. GRAÇA H. VICENTE, PhD • *Department of Chemistry, Louisiana State University, Baton Rouge, LA*

MICHAEL VOGELBAUM, MD, PhD • *The Brain Tumor Institute, Department of Neurological Surgery, The Cleveland Clinic Foundation, Cleveland, OH*

MARCUS L. WARE, MD, PhD • *Departments of Neurosurgery and Radiation Oncology, University of California, San Francisco, CA*

CAROL J. WIKSTRAND, PhD • *Neuro-Oncology Program, Department of Pathology, Duke University Medical Center, Durham, NC*

MICHAEL R. ZALUTSKY, PhD • *Department of Radiology, Neuro-Oncology Program, Duke University Medical Center, Durham, NC*

Companion CD ROM

All illustrations, both black and white and color, are contained on the accompanying CD ROM.

I CLASSIFICATION OF HIGH-GRADE GLIOMA

1 Classification of High-Grade Glioma

1 Histologic Classification of High-Grade Gliomas

Richard A. Prayson

Summary

High-grade gliomas (HGG), as a group, are the most common primary neoplasms of the central nervous system (CNS). Historically, and to a great extent currently, morphologic classification has and does dictate treatment. This chapter reviews the pathologic features and grading parameters for high-grade astrocytomas, oligodendrogliomas, mixed gliomas, and ependymomas. The histologic subtypes of glioblastoma multiforme and the affects of radiotherapy on gliomas will be discussed. The potential role for cell proliferation markers (Ki-67, MIB-1) in evaluating HGGs will be examined.

Key Words: Malignant glioma; glioma; glioblastoma multiforme; anaplastic oligodendroglioma; anaplastic ependymoma; gliosarcoma; anaplastic mixed glioma; radiation; Ki-67 antibody; cell proliferation.

INTRODUCTION

High-grade gliomas (HGGs), in particular glioblastoma multiforme (GBM), are the most common primary tumors of the central nervous system (CNS). Despite limitations, histologic classification and grading continues to be the basis on which many therapeutic decisions are made. In recent years, recognition of the association of certain genetic alterations, most notably deletions on chromosomes 1p and 19q with the oligodendroglioma phenotype and chemoresponsiveness, has had a significant impact on clinical decision making and has proven to be a significant addition to the morphologic evaluation of gliomas (1–4). This chapter will focus on the morphologic features of HGGs including grading, limitations of current grading and classification approaches, differential diagnostic considerations, and the utilization of cell proliferation markers in evaluating gliomas.

DIFFUSE FIBRILLARY ASTROCYTOMA

Diffuse or fibrillary astrocytomas account for the bulk of HGGs. Two main grading approaches are currently employed in evaluating astrocytomas. The modified Ringertz system is a three-tier approach in which tumor grade is denoted by name (5,6). Low-grade astrocytomas are marked by mild hypercellularity and atypical astrocytic cells characterized by nuclear enlargement, nuclear hyperchromasia, and nuclear pleomorphism. Rare mitotic figures may be encountered. The intermediate grade anaplastic astrocytomas (AA) are more cellular than the low-grade tumors. Nuclear pleomorphism is more evident and mitotic figures

From: *Current Clinical Oncology: High-Grade Gliomas: Diagnosis and Treatment*
Edited by: G. H. Barnett © Humana Press Inc., Totowa, NJ

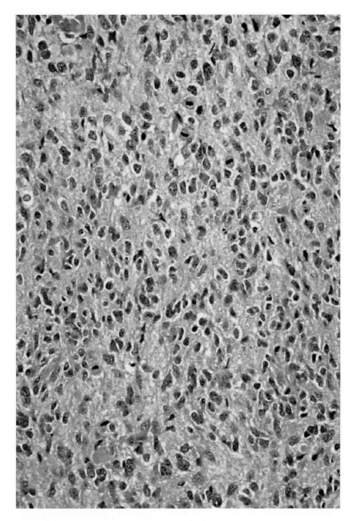

Fig. 1. AA characterized by prominent hypercellularity, mitotic activity, and nuclear atypia (nuclear enlargement, pleomorphism and hyperchromasia) (hematoxylin and eosin, original magnification ×200).

are more readily encountered. A subset of AA is marked by vascular or endothelial proliferation, which accounts for the enhancement seen radiographically in HGGs. These vascular changes are marked by a piling up or proliferation of all the normal cellular constituents of the vessel wall including endothelial cells, fibroblasts, pericytes, and smooth muscle cells. The diagnosis of high-grade GBM, in the modified Ringertz system, requires the presence of geographic necrosis; the necrosis may or may not be rimmed by a pseudopalisade of tumor cells.

The other main grading approach for astrocytomas which enjoys widespread use is the World Health Organization (WHO) system *(7)*. The WHO system is a four-tier system in which tumor grade is denoted by Roman numerals I–IV. The grade I designation is used for certain low-grade astrocytoma variant lesions such as pilocytic astrocytoma and subependy-

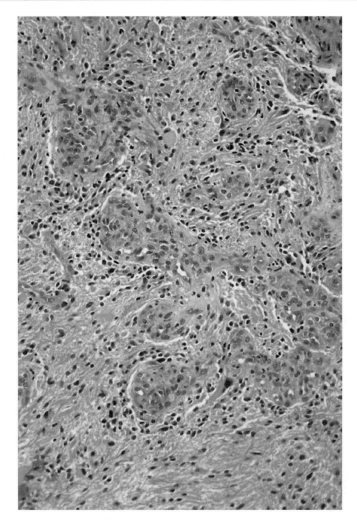

Fig. 2. Vascular proliferative changes in a GBM (hematoxylin and eosin, original magnification ×200).

mal giant cell astrocytoma. The low-grade fibrillary astrocytoma of Ringertz roughly corresponds to the WHO grade II astrocytoma. WHO grade III astrocytoma includes a subset of the Ringertz AA (those tumors which are devoid of vascular proliferative changes) (Fig. 1). The WHO grade IV astrocytoma (GBM) includes those Ringertz AA that demonstrate vascular proliferative changes (Fig. 2) and the Ringertz GBM with necrosis (Fig. 3). The main difference between the two grading approaches, with respect to fibrillary astrocytomas, lies in the relative significance attached to the vascular proliferation. In the WHO system, vascular proliferative changes in the proper background, even in the absence of necrosis, are sufficient enough to warrant a diagnosis of GBM (grade IV).

There are a variety of other findings that one may encounter in high-grade astrocytomas that do not necessarily affect tumor grade. Microcystic degeneration is a fairly common

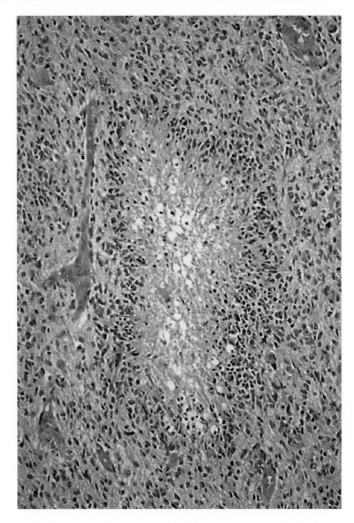

Fig. 3. A GBM marked by geographic necrosis rimmed by a pseudopalisade of tumor cells (hematoxylin and eosin, original magnification ×100).

feature of fibrillary astrocytoma. About 15% of astrocytomas may demonstrate foci of microcalcification. Particularly at the infiltrative edge of an astrocytoma, one may observe satellitosis of tumor cells around pre-existing structures, such as vessels or neurons (Fig. 4). This satellitosis phenomenon, when observed in fibrillary astrocytomas, is referred to as a secondary structure of Scherer and is often more pronounced at the infiltrating edge of high-grade astrocytomas. Focal subpial aggregation of tumor cells may be observed and occasional tumors may directly extend into the leptomeninges. In contrast to some of the astrocytoma variant lesions, Rosenthal fibers, granular bodies, perivascular chronic inflammation, and vascular sclerosis are relatively uncommon findings and their presence (particularly Rosenthal fibers and granular bodies) should prompt serious consideration before a diagnosis of GBM is made.

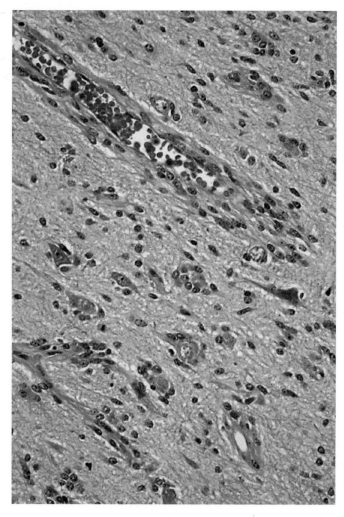

Fig. 4. Satellitosis of tumor cells around cortical neurons and vessels (secondary structures of Scherer) at the infiltrating edge of a GBM (hematoxylin and eosin, original magnification ×200).

A subset of high-grade astrocytomas may be marked by the presence of gemistocytic astrocytes. These large cells are characterized by abundant eosinophilic cytoplasm (filled with intermediate molecular weight glial filaments) and an eccentrically placed, enlarged nucleus (Fig. 5). Large numbers of these cells (comprising > 20% of the tumor in one study) in a tumor have been associated with more aggressive behavior *(8)*. These tumors are generally treated as if they are higher grade astrocytomas. Interestingly, when one evaluates such tumors with a cell proliferation marker such as Ki-67 (or MIB-1), the gemistocytic cells are generally quiescent and most of the proliferating cells are the more conventionally atypical astrocytic cells with the irregular, elongated, and hyperchromatic nuclei in the background *(9,10)*.

There are a variety of morphologic variants of GBM that have been described that are important to recognize primarily because of their resemblance to other neoplasms. In gen-

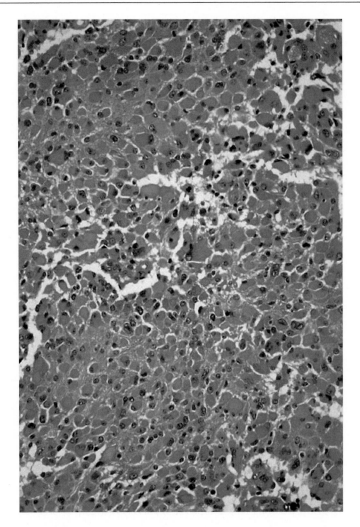

Fig. 5. Gemistocytic astrocytoma characterized by increased numbers of large astrocytic cells with abundant eosinophilic cytoplasm (hematoxylin and eosin, original magnification ×200).

eral, there is little difference in terms of treatment approaches or outcome between these morphologic variants. Gliosarcoma is one of the earliest variants recognized (Feigin tumor) *(11–14)*. The gliosarcoma consists of an admixture of recognizable glioblastomosis foci and areas resembling sarcoma (Fig. 6). Most commonly, the sarcoma component looks like a fibrosarcoma or malignant histiocytoma, although occasionally angiosarcomatous, osteosarcomatous, or chondrosarcomatous areas may be observed. When the sarcomatous component is spindled, a combination of a reticulin stain and glial fibrillary acidic protein (GFAP) immunostain may be useful in differentiating the lesion from a spindled glioblastoma mutliforme. The sarcomatous component is reticulin-rich (Fig. 7); the only reticulin usually observed in a GBM is concentrated in foci of vascular proliferation. In contrast to the glioblastoma areas, the sarcoma component is GFAP negative. In a spindled GBM,

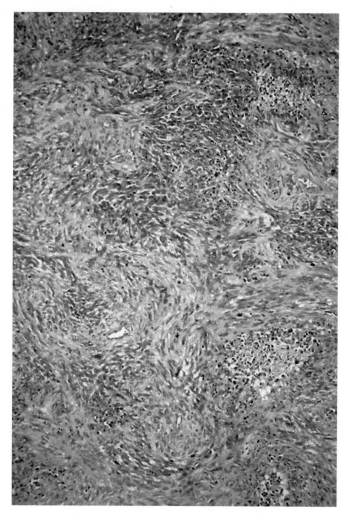

Fig. 6. Gliosarcoma characterized by a mixture of glioblastomatous and spindled cell sarcomatous patterns (hematoxylin and eosin, original magnification ×100).

many of the spindle cells will be GFAP positive and the spindled region reticulin poor. Pure sarcomas do not demonstrate GFAP immunoreactivity. Historically, these tumors were thought to arise from an initial GBM that secondarily induced a malignant transformation of neighboring mesenchymal cells, resulting in the development of the sarcomatous component. More recent genetic studies have demonstrated identical genetic alterations in the glioblastomatous and sarcomatous components, implying derivation from a common cell of origin *(15,16)*. It would seem that astrocytomas have the capability to undergo mesenchymal differentiation, a concept further supported by the occasional reports of benign appearing mesenchymal elements in astrocytomas.

Two particular variants of GBM that phenotypically resemble carcinomas include the epithelioid and small cell variants. The epithelioid variant of glioblastoma is marked by the

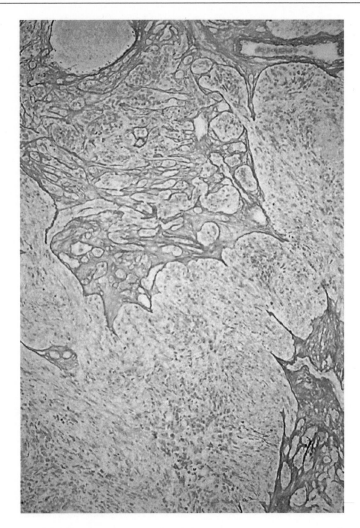

Fig. 7. A reticulin stain highlighting the reticulin rich sarcomatous component of a gliosarcoma (reticulin, original magnification ×100).

presence of discohesive cells that have distinct cytoplasmic borders, a moderate amount of cytoplasm, and a rather prominent nucleus with a large nucleolus (Fig. 8) *(17,18)*. The features of this variant, if predominant in a tumor, may cause confusion with a metastatic large cell carcinoma (or at times even melanoma). The small cell variant of glioblastoma is similarly characterized by a discohesive proliferation of cells with scant cytoplasm, resembling a metastatic small cell carcinoma (Fig. 9) *(19,20)*. In many cases, these phenotypes are admixed with more conventional appearing areas of glioblastoma and may be diagnostically straightforward. In tumors where these patterns predominate, immunohistochemistry may be employed to aid in distinguishing these tumors from metastatic carcinoma. These cells still variably stain with GFAP and do not generally stain with epithelial markers (e.g., cytokeratins, epithelial membrane antigen). Some care must be taken, however, in the

Contributors

MANMEET SINGH AHLUWALIA, MD • *Fairview Hospital, Cleveland, OH*

MANZOOR AHMED, MD • *Department of Diagnostic Radiology, The Cleveland Clinic Foundation, Cleveland, OH*

GENE H. BARNETT, MD • *The Brain Tumor Institute, Department of Neurological Surgery, The Cleveland Clinic Foundation, Cleveland, OH*

ROLF F. BARTH, MD • *Department of Pathology, The Ohio State University, Columbus, OH*

EDWARD C. BENZEL, MD • *Cleveland Clinic Spine Institute, Department of Neurological Surgery, The Cleveland Clinic Foundation, Cleveland, OH*

MITCHELL S. BERGER, MD • *Department of Neurological Surgery, University of California, San Francisco, San Francisco, CA*

DARELL D. BIGNER, MD, PhD • *Department of Pathology, Neuro-Oncology Program, Duke University Medical Center, Durham, NC*

THOMAS E. BLUE, PhD • *Department of Nuclear Engineering Program, The Ohio State University, Columbus, Ohio*

ABRAHAM BOSKOVITZ, MD • *Neuro-Oncology Program, Department of Pathology, Duke University Medical Center, Durham, NC*

NICHOLAS BUTOWSKI, MD • *Neuro-Oncology Service, Department of Neurological Surgery, UCSF School of Medicine, San Francisco, CA*

SOONMEE CHA, MD • *Department of Radiology, University of California, San Francisco, San Francisco, CA*

SUSAN CHANG, MD • *Neuro-Oncology Service, Department of Neurological Surgery, UCSF School of Medicine, San Francisco, CA*

E. ANTONIO CHIOCCA, MD, PhD • *Dardinger Center for Neuro-Oncology, Department of Neurosurgery, The Ohio State University Medical Center, James Cancer Hospital and Solove Research Center, Columbus, OH*

JEFFREY A. CODERRE, PhD • *Department of Nuclear Engineering, Massachusetts Institute of Technology, Cambridge, MA*

BRUCE H. COHEN, MD • *Department of Neurology, The Cleveland Clinic Foundation, Cleveland, OH*

EDWARD P. COHEN, MD • *Department of Neurological Surgery, Rush Medical College, Cook County Hospital and Hektoen Institute for Medical Research; and Department of Microbiology and Immunology, University of Illinois at Chicago, Chicago, IL*

GAIL DITZ, RN • *The Brain Tumor Institute, The Cleveland Clinic Foundation, Cleveland, OH*

GREGORY N. FULLER, MD, PhD • *Department of Pathology, MD Anderson Cancer Center, Houston, TX*

ROBERTA P. GLICK, MD • *Department of Neurological Surgery, Rush Medical College, Cook County Hospital and Hektoen Institute for Medical Research; and Department of Microbiology and Immunology, University of Illinois at Chicago, Chicago, IL*

ALECK HERCBERGS, MD • *Department of Radiation Oncology, The Cleveland Clinic Foundation, Cleveland, OH*

SYED RAFAT HUSAIN, PhD • *Tumor Vaccines and Biotechnology Branch, Division of Cellular and Gene Therapies, Center for Biologics Evaluation and Research, FDA, Bethesda, MD*

ANDREW A. KANNER, MD • *Department of Neurosurgery, Tel Aviv Sourasky Medical Center, Sackler Faculty of Medicine, Tel Aviv University, Tel Aviv, Israel*

ANDREA KASSNER, PhD • *Department of Medical Imaging, University of Toronto, University Health Network, Toronto, Ontario*

BHADRAKANT KAVAR, MD, ChB, FCS, FRACS • *Departments of Neurosurgery and Surgery, University of Melbourne, Royal Melbourne Hospital, Parkville, Victoria, Australia*

ANDREW H. KAYE, MB, BS, MD, FRACS • *Departments of Neurosurgery and Surgery, University of Melbourne, Royal Melbourne Hospital, Parkville, Victoria, Australia*

G. EVREN KELES, MD • *Department of Neurological Surgery, University of California, San Francisco, San Francisco, CA*

M. L. LAMFERS, PhD • *Division of Gene Therapy, Department of Medical Oncology, VU University Medical Center, Amsterdam, The Netherlands*

MACIEJ S. LESNIAK, MD • *Division of Neurological Surgery, The University of Chicago Pritzker School of Medicine, Chicago, IL*

TERRY LICHTOR, MD, PhD • *Department of Neurological Surgery, Rush Medical College, Cook County Hospital and Hektoen Institute for Medical Research; and Department of Microbiology and Immunology, University of Illinois at Chicago, Chicago, IL*

HENRY LIN, MD • *Department of Neurological Surgery, Rush Medical College, Cook County Hospital and Hektoen Institute for Medical Research; and Department of Microbiology and Immunology, University of Illinois at Chicago, Chicago, IL*

JÜRGEN LÜDERS, MD • *Neurosurgeon, Grand Rapids, MI*

KATHLEEN LUPICA, MSN, CNP • *The Brain Tumor Institute, The Cleveland Clinic Foundation, Cleveland, OH*

DAVID A. MANKOFF, MD, PhD • *Department of Radiology, University of Washington School of Medicine, Seattle, WA*

THOMAS J. MASARYK, MD • *Department of Diagnostic Radiology, The Cleveland Clinic Foundation, Cleveland, OH*

ALEXANDER MASON, MD • *Department of Neurosurgery, The Cleveland Clinic Foundation, Cleveland, OH*

MICHAEL W. MCDERMOTT, MD • *Departments of Neurosurgery and Radiation Oncology, University of California, San Francisco, CA*

MINESH P. MEHTA, MD • *Department of Human Oncology, University of Wisconsin, Madison, WI*

SHIN-ICHI MIYATAKE, MD, PhD • *Department of Neurosurgery, Osaka Medical College, Takatsuki, Osaka Prefecture, Japan*

MARK MUZI, MS • *Department of Radiology, University of Washington School of Medicine, Seattle, WA*

ALESSANDRO OLIVI, MD • *Department of Neurosurgery, Johns Hopkins University School of Medicine, Baltimore, MD*

DAVID M. PEEREBOOM, MD • *The Brain Tumor Institute, Department of Medical Oncology, The Cleveland Clinic Foundation, Cleveland, OH*

RICHARD A. PRAYSON, MD • *Department of Anatomic Pathology, The Cleveland Clinic Foundation, Cleveland, OH*

RAJ K. PURI, MD, PhD • *Tumor Vaccines and Biotechnology Branch, Division of Cellular and Gene Therapies, Center for Biologics Evaluation and Research, FDA, Bethesda, MD*

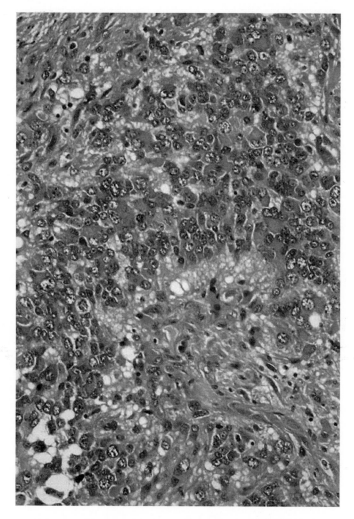

Fig. 8. Rounded cells with distinct cytoplasmic borders and prominent nucleolation in an epithelioid variant of GBM (hematoxylin and eosin, original magnification ×200).

choice of keratin antibody. Certain keratin antibodies, most notably cytokeratin AE1/3, show cross immunoreactivity and stain GBM, sometimes even more extensively than GFAP antibody does *(21)*. Lower molecular weight keratin markers, such as CAM5.2, tend to demonstrate less crossreactivity. Interestingly, the small cell variant of glioblastoma appears to be somewhat genetically homogeneous in that epidermal growth factor receptor (EGFR) amplification/overexpression is invariably present in this subset of tumors *(20)*.

The giant cell variant of GBM (monstrocellular sarcoma of Zülch) is characterized by increased numbers of large, frequently multinucleated astrocytic cells (Fig. 10) *(22)*. The cells demonstrate more atypia than the "usual" cytologic abnormality encountered in a GBM. There has been some suggestion in the literature, albeit limited, that this variant may be

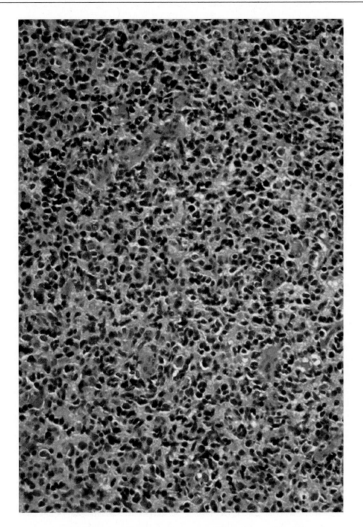

Fig. 9. Small cell variant of GBM is characterized by a proliferation of small cells resembling metastatic small cell carcinoma (hematoxylin and eosin, original magnification ×200).

somewhat more common in younger age patients and may be associated with a slightly better prognosis.

Other phenotyopic variants of high-grade astrocytoma include tumors with granular cell differentiation or spongioblastomatous pattern *(23–25)*. The presence of granular cells in an astrocytoma appears to be a marker of a higher grade lesion. The granular cells are character-ized by abundant, finely granular cytoplasm (Fig. 11). The granularity is caused by an accu-mulation of large lysosomes in the cell cytoplasm. The spongioblastomatous pattern is marked by a striking palisaded arrangement of cell nuclei with intervening fibrillary zones (Fig. 12).

Conventional treatment for high-grade astrocytomas is radiotherapy. Radiation itself can induce changes in the tissue that can mimic tumor *(26–28)*. The earliest morphologic changes associated with radiation include edema, reactive astrocytosis, and perivascular chronic

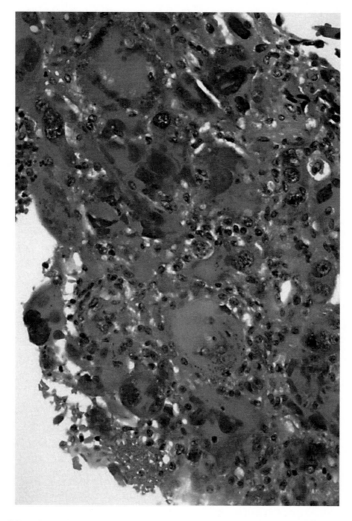

Fig. 10. Large, multinucleated cells characterize the giant cell variant of GBM (hematoxylin and eosin, original magnification ×400).

inflammation. Vascular sclerosis eventually develops with the concomitant development of necrosis (Fig. 13). In contrast to glioblastoma associated necrosis, radionecrosis is not rimmed by a palisade of astrocytic cells and it is frequently accompanied by increased numbers of macrophages (Fig. 14). Radiation can also induce significant cytologic atypia in both reactive and neoplastic astrocytes (Fig. 15), resulting (in extreme cases) in a markedly enlarged nucleus, multinucleation, and cytoplasmic vacuolation. Grading lesions that have been previously radiated can be difficult, particularly if the modified Ringertz system is being employed. Given the relative importance afforded necrosis, in the absence of a pseudopalisade of tumor cells around the necrotic focus, it is difficult to definitively distinguish between radionecrosis and tumor necrosis. In the WHO system, vascular proliferative changes can additionally be employed to upgrade a lesion to GBM. Radiation also predis-

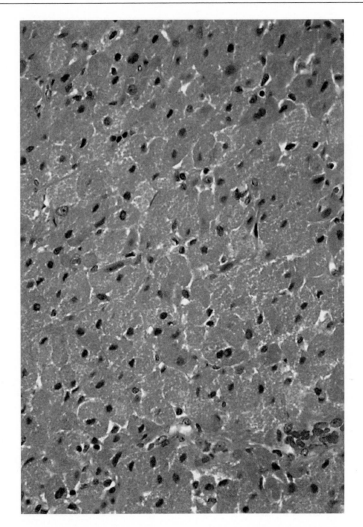

Fig. 11. A sheet of cells marked by finely granular cytoplasm in a granular cell GBM (hematoxylin and eosin, original magnification ×200).

poses one to the development of a secondary neoplasm or malignant progression in a low-grade lesion.

The concept of multifocality in astrocytomas is well accepted; as many as 10 to15% of astrocytomas may be multifocal. Multifocality is defined by the presence of two or more discrete or noncontiguous foci of tumor. Some lesions that radiographically appear to be distinct may represent a single tumor. The infiltrative nature of astrocytomas often allows them to spread far beyond what their gross and radiographic appearance would otherwise suggest. Infiltration of tumor via the commissural system to involve the contralateral side (so called "butterfly gliomas") is, unfortunately, not uncommon.

Rarely, astrocytomas may become diffusely infiltrative and involve most, if not all, of the brain. Such a lesion is referred to as gliomatosis cerebri and is associated with a particu-

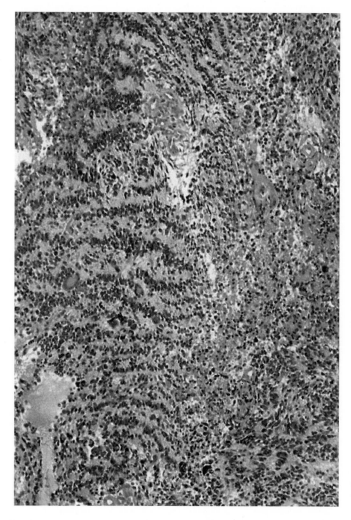

Fig. 12. A focal palisaded nuclear pattern typical of the spongioblastomatous pattern in a GBM (hematoxylin and eosin, original magnification ×100).

larly poor prognosis *(29,30)*. The diagnosis of gliomatosis cerebri requires correlation of the pathology with the radiographic findings of a diffusely infiltrative process. Often on biopsy, the gliomatosis cerebri resembles a low-grade, infiltrating astrocytoma (Fig. 16). Tumor cells are frequently spindled and may resemble microglial cells. To distinguish these cells from microglial cells, a CD68 immunostain, which highlights the microglial cells, can be used. Small foci of high-grade appearing glioma may be observed in gliomatosis.

There are a variety of astrocytoma variant tumors that are important to distinguish from fibrillary astrocytomas because of their unique clinical presentation, better prognosis, and differences in treatment approaches. Most of these tumors are low-grade lesions (WHO grade I and II tumors). Rarely, some of these neoplasms may degenerate into higher-grade

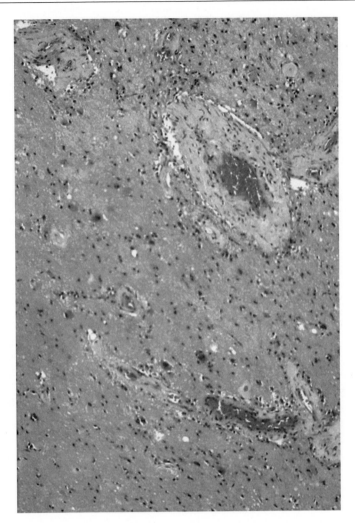

Fig. 13. Vascular sclerosis and gliosis secondary to radiation therapy (hematoxylin and eosin, original magnification ×100).

tumors. Most commonly, this occurs in pleomorphic xanthoastrocytomas. Malignant degeneration in xanthoastrocytoma (anaplastic pleomorphic xanthoastrocytomas) is a well-recognized phenomenon *(32–34)*. Criteria for distinguishing the higher-grade lesion from its lower grade counterpart are not well defined. Some of the morphologic features (such as hypercellularity, nuclear pleomorphism, and vascular proliferation) that are utilized to assign tumor grade in the fibrillary astrocytomas are regular features of the pleomorphic xanthoastrocytoma and do not have the same implication in this setting. Anaplastic tumors are marked by increased mitotic activity and/or necrosis (Figs. 17 and 18).

Malignant degeneration in pilocytic astrocytomas is an extraordinarily rare event *(35)*. Most of these cases arise in the setting of ordinary pilocytic astrocytomas that are irradiated and subsequently undergo malignant degeneration. These tumors may demonstrate areas

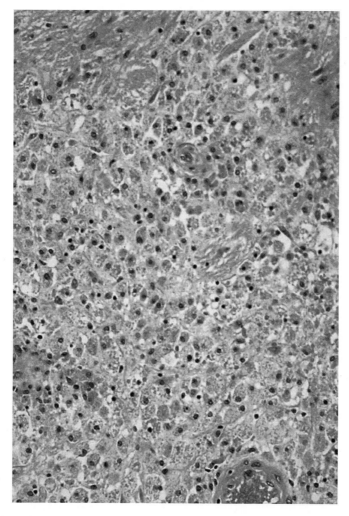

Fig. 14. A collection of macrophages in a focus of radiation-induced necrosis (hematoxylin and eosin, original magnification ×200).

that make them morphologically indistinguishable from GBM. Subependymal giant cell astrocytomas, which are probably more akin to hamartomas, are not thought to undergo malignant progression. A subset of other rare astrocytic tumors (astroblastomas and desmoplastic astrocytoma of infancy) may demonstrate aggressive morphologic features and may behave in a more aggressive fashion; however, experience is too limited in these cases to allow for the definition of precise morphologic criteria predictive of behavior *(36–39)*.

OLIGODENDROGLIOMA AND MIXED GLIOMA

Historically, the grading of oligodendrogliomas has paralleled their astrocytoma counterparts. Many of the same histologic features that are used to grade diffuse astrocytomas are

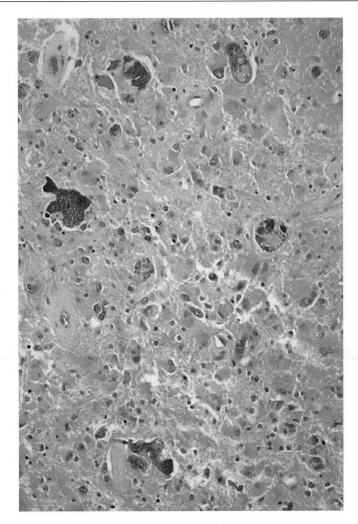

Fig. 15. Bizarre, radiation-induced atypia in a residual GBM (hematoxylin and eosin, original magnification ×200).

used to grade oligodendrogliomas; the threshold between low- and high-grade lesions is a bit different *(40–45)*. The currently favored approach to grading oligodendroglioma stratifies them into low- (WHO grade II) and high-grade anaplastic (WHO grade III) lesions *(46)*.

Low-grade oligodendrogliomas are marked by a rather monomorphic proliferation of cells with rounded nuclei and scant cytoplasm. The tumors are associated with an arcuate or "chicken wire" capillary vascular pattern and approx 80% of tumors are calcified. Like fibrillary astrocytomas, oligodendrogliomas are infiltrative tumors. Tumor cells have a propensity to satellite around pre-existing structures in the cortex (e.g., neurons, vessels) and subpial aggregation of tumor cells is common. Focal microcystic degeneration may be observed, resulting in a pattern resembling the dysembryoplastic neuroepithelial tumor or rare low-grade protoplasmic astrocytoma. A subset of tumors contains cells

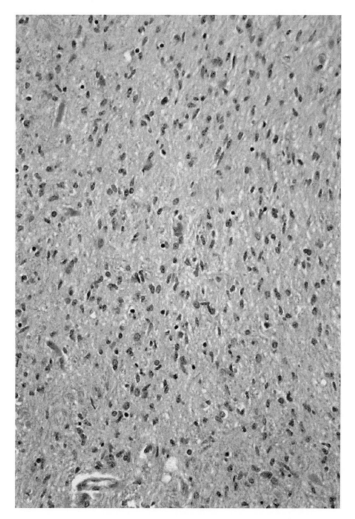

Fig. 16. Gliomatosis cerebri often resembles a low-grade astrocytoma with spindled nuclei (hematoxylin and eosin, original magnification ×200).

referred to as "minigemistocytes." The cells contain rounded oligodendrocyte nuclei with increased eosinophilic cytoplasm filled with intermediate molecular weight glial filaments (Fig. 19).

High-grade tumors are generally more cellular than low-grade tumors (Fig. 20). Nuclear pleomorphism is more prominent and in some tumors may approach the variation in nuclear size and shape that marks high-grade astrocytomas. Mitotic activity is more prevalent and often approaches and exceeds five mitotic figures/ten high power fields. Vascular proliferation and foci of necrosis may be present (Fig. 21). Some tumors resemble GBM with palisaded necrosis (Fig. 22). These tumors should not, however, be referred to as GBM; tumors of oligodendroglial lineage generally have a better prognosis and are more likely to respond to chemotherapy.

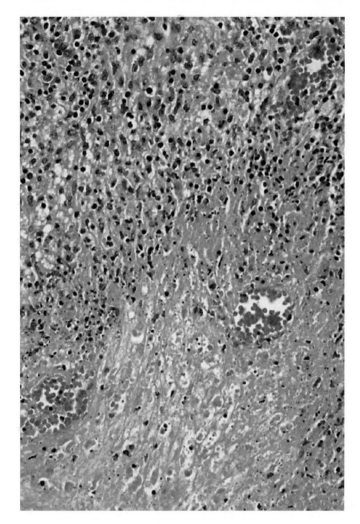

Fig. 17. Anaplastic pleomorphic xanthoastrocytoma with focus of geographic necrosis (hematoxylin and eosin, original magnification ×100).

It is not unusual, in an otherwise typical appearing oligodendroglioma, to find occasional atypical appearing astrocytic cells; admixture of astrocytoma and oligodendroglioma cells in the same tumor have been recognized since the early 1970s as a mixed glioma (oligo-astrocytoma) *(47)*. Two patterns of this tumor have been described. In one pattern, there is a diffuse admixture of cellular elements in the tumor. In the other pattern, geographically distinct areas of astrocytoma and oligodendroglioma are juxtaposed to one another in the same neoplasm (Fig. 23). Unfortunately, precise criteria regarding what percentage of a minor component needs to be present in order to designate the lesion a mixed glioma varies; the literature suggests anywhere between 20 and 35% as a guideline in this regard *(48–51)*. The diagnosis is further complicated by the lack of a reliable immunomarker for oligodendroglial cell differentiation, making distinction of cell types sometimes challeng-

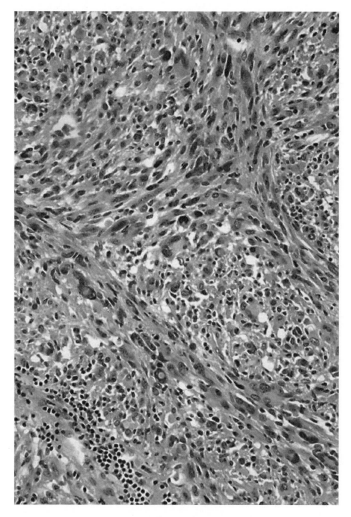

Fig. 18. Increased mitotic activity in an anaplastic pleomorphic xanthoastrocytoma (hematoxylin and eosin, original magnification ×200).

ing, particularly in the so-called diffuse pattern of the tumor. The GFAP antibody generally does not stain oligodendroglioma cells well, with the notable exception of the mini-gemistocytes. In theory, astrocytoma cells should stain with GFAP; however, in the higher grade, more poorly differentiated tumors, not all tumor cells stain. The extent of sampling also becomes an issue regarding diagnosis. One cannot comfortably make a diagnosis of mixed glioma on a small biopsy; the lesion needs to be sampled extensively enough to ensure that the designation is in fact an appropriate reflection of what the neoplasm actually is.

Given the previously enumerated problems, it is not surprising that the literature is difficult to interpret on this subset of tumors. Many studies either fail to clearly define what is meant by mixed glioma or they include mixed gliomas in studies of oligodendrogliomas.

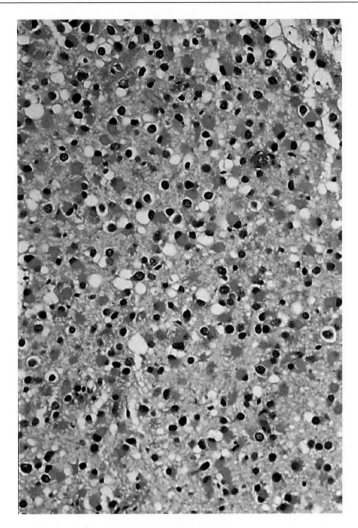

Fig. 19. Minigemistocytic oligodendroglial cells with increased cell cytoplasm in an oligodendroglioma (hematoxylin and eosin, original magnification ×200).

Assessing the behavior of these tumors has been difficult. More recently, the molecular evaluation of mixed gliomas (oligoastrocytomas) for loss on chromosomes 1p and 19q has helped to clarify this issue. Mixed gliomas which are 1p/19q deleted appear to act more like oligodendrogliomas (i.e., more likely to benefit from a course of chemotherapy and have a better prognosis), and tumors which are 1p/19q intact act more like astrocytomas *(52)*.

EPENDYMOMAS

As a group, ependymomas are the least common of the gliomas but they comprise a significant percentage of gliomas in children. The most commonly employed grading systems for

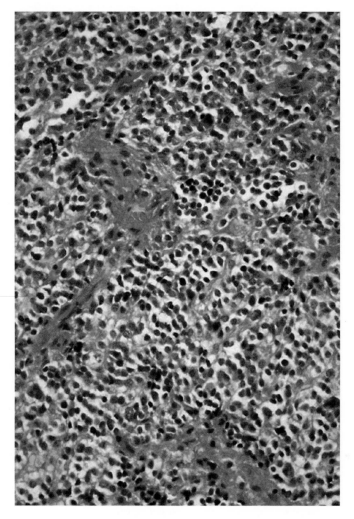

Fig. 20. Increased cellularity and nuclear pleomorphism in an anaplastic oligodendroglioma (hematoxylin and eosin, original magnification ×200).

ependymomas are two-tiered systems in which tumors are graded as low-grade (WHO grade II) and anaplastic (WHO grade III) ependymomas *(53)*. The histologic hallmark of ependymomas is the formation of true ependymal rosettes and perivascular pseudorosettes (Fig. 24). Tumors may demonstrate microcystic change, calcification, and melanin pigmentation. Similar to diffuse astrocytomas and oligodendrogliomas, anaplastic ependymomas are more cellular than low-grade tumors, more pleomorphic, and more mitotically active (Fig. 25). They may demonstrate vascular proliferative changes and/or necrosis (Fig. 26). Similar to oligodendrogliomas, the precise criteria required to distinguish an anaplastic tumor from a low-grade tumor are not well established *(54–60)*.

Many of the higher grade tumors resemble high-grade astrocytomas and the rare clear cell variant of ependymoma can mimic an oligodendroglioma. Similar to astrocytomas, ependymo-

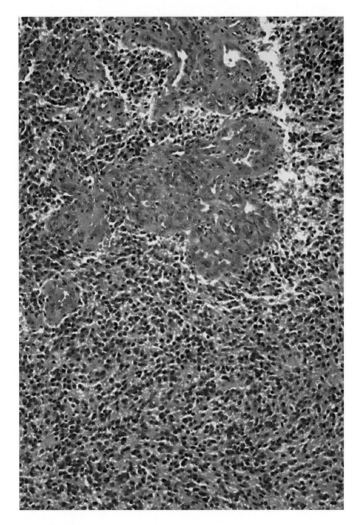

Fig. 21. Prominent vascular proliferative changes in an anaplastic oligodendroglioma (hematoxylin and eosin, original magnification ×200).

mas are GFAP and S-100 protein positive. Keratin immunoreactivity may also be observed, particularly in epithelial-type ependymomas. When the rosettes and pseudorosettes are not obvious in a high-grade tumor, or the biopsy is limited, ultrastructural examination of the neoplasm may be required to identify the tumor as ependymal. Features unique to ependymomas (vs other) HGGs include cilia, microvilli, ciliary attachments (blepharoplasts), and cell junctions (Fig. 27).

GRADING ISSUES

There are a number of limitations to currently employed, morphologic-based grading approaches in gliomas. The fact that there are continuous efforts at improving grading

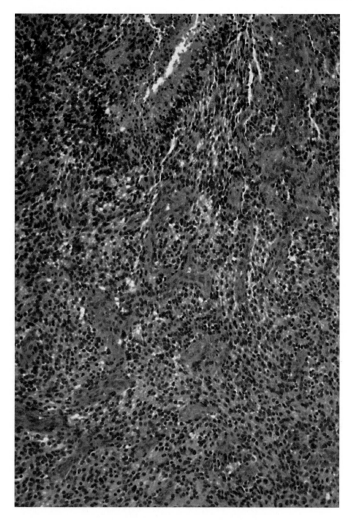

Fig. 22. Focal palisaded necrosis in an anaplastic oligodendroglioma (hematoxylin and eosin, original magnification ×200).

schemas implies recognition of the limitations of the current approaches and a lack of agreement regarding the relative importance of certain parameters in assigning grade.

Superimposed issues related to tumor heterogeneity and the implications for tumor sampling further complicate matters. HGGs are notoriously heterogeneous lesions; different areas of the tumor may have a different appearance *(61,62)*. This has significant implications with regard to surgical sampling. To ensure that the tissue sampled represents the highest grade area of the tumor underscores the importance of intraoperative correlation of the radiographic findings and communication between the surgeon and pathologist in the context of intraoperative consultation *(63)*.

Given the descriptive nature of the currently employed histologic grading systems, there is inherent interobserver variability in grading *(64–66)*. This variability extends beyond the

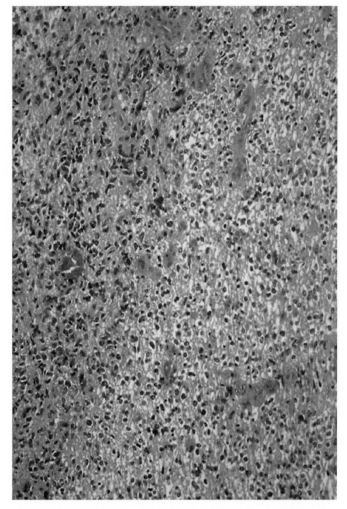

Fig. 23. Anaplastic mixed glioma (oligoastrocytoma) marked by geographically distinct areas resembling astrocytoma and oligodendroglioma (hematoxylin and eosin, original magnification×200).

grading arena and impacts the assignment of tumor type. This is particularly true in differentiating one HGG type from another and is particularly operative in the differential diagnosis of high-grade astrocytoma vs anaplastic oligodendroglioma vs malignant mixed glioma. The interobserver variability in grading underscores the intrinsic limitations of the descriptive grading systems. This can to some extent be compensated for either by experience or in a group setting, by collectively reviewing diagnoses and tumor grade assignments and refining personal criteria to conform to the group *(67)*.

CELL PROLIFERATION MARKERS

All of the aforementioned limitations to tumor grading and even to some degree assignment of tumor type has prompted numerous studies attempting to define other parameters

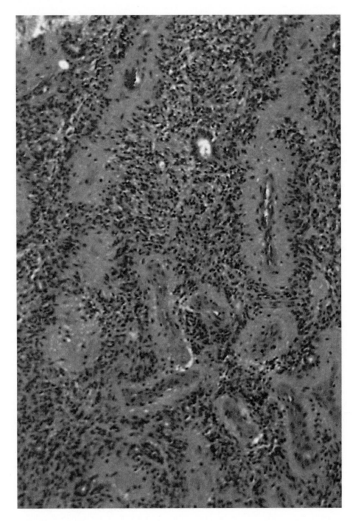

Fig. 24. Prominent perivascular pseudorosette formations in a anaplastic ependymoma (hematoxylin and eosin, original magnification ×100).

that assist in predicting behavior in a given patient and indicate optimal treatment options. The utility of certain molecular markers has already been alluded to and is the subject of another chapter.

One of the other groups of markers that has proven useful in evaluating tumors are the cell proliferation markers. There are a variety of markers (e.g., radioactive, flow cytometric, and immunohistochemically based) that have been explored in detail *(68)*. Of the currently available modalities, the most practical and effective marker is Ki-67 or MIB-1 antibody *(69–77)*. These markers stain a nuclear protein that is expressed during the proliferative phases of the cell cycle. The immunostaining has the advantage of being relatively easy to perform, easy to interpret, and relatively inexpensive. Labeling indices are determined by computing the percentage of positive staining tumor cell nuclei. Correlation between either histologic-grade or prognosis and the labeling indices have been demonstrated; high-grade

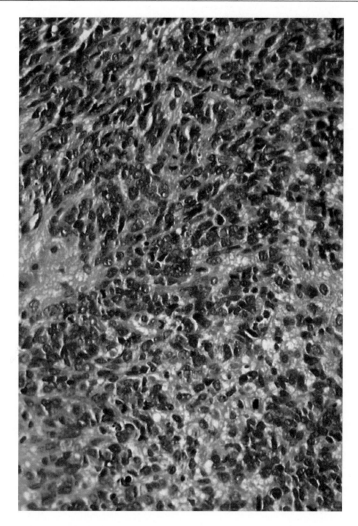

Fig. 25. Prominent hypercellularity and nuclear pleomorphism in an anaplastic ependymoma (hematoxylin and eosin, original magnification ×400).

tumors have higher labeling indices than low-grade tumors. Labeling indices are particularly useful in tumors that are histologically "on the fence" with regard to grade. A higher labeling index would be suggestive of a more proliferative lesion (more likely higher grade). A low labeling is less informative. A low index may indicate a lower grade lesion or it may be the result of sampling. Gliomas demonstrate regional heterogeneity in cell proliferation (Fig. 28A,B). A low index may be reflective of sampling and selection of an area of the tumor that is not very proliferative. Among high-grade tumors (GBM), there is no indication that labeling indices add any additional prognostic value.

The labeling index is subject to some limitations. Aside from the issue of tumor heterogeneity, indices may be affected by a variety of factors including source of antibody, staining

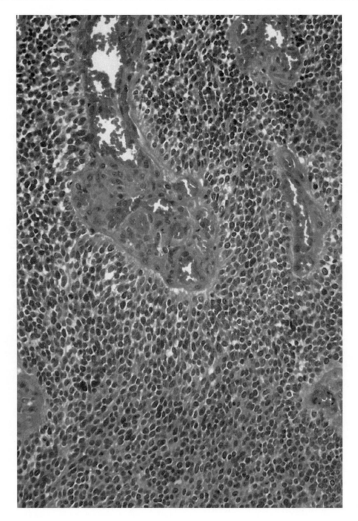

Fig. 26. Vascular proliferative changes in an anaplastic ependymoma (hematoxylin and eosin, original magnification ×100).

conditions, and interobserver variability in counting. Labeling indices may, therefore, vary somewhat from one lab to another. Because of these limitations, the establishment of precise cutoff indices with regard to grade or prognosis is not appropriate. The general value of the index is more important than the precise number generated.

CONCLUSION

In the near future, morphologic assessment of tumors will remain the basis of prognostication and treatment/management. The overall approach to evaluating gliomas, however, is becoming more multifaceted, utilizing a combination of imaging, histology, evaluation

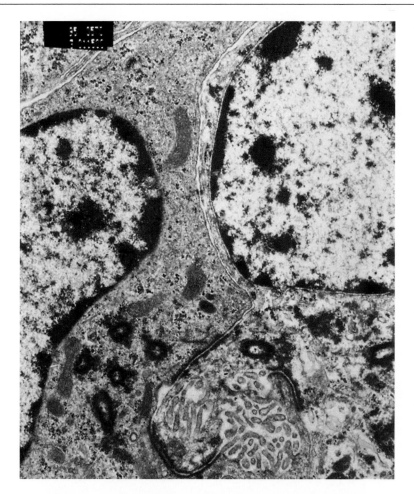

Fig. 27. Cilia and cell junctions ultrastructurally mark ependymomas and allow for their distinction from other gliomas (original magnification ×3600).

of cell proliferation, protein expression, and molecular evaluation of the tumor. The search continues for markers that predict outcome in an individual patient and predict treatment response (or non-response).

REFERENCES

1. Cairncross JC, Ueki K, Zlatescu MC, et al. Specific genetic predictors of chemotherapeutic response and survial in patients with anaplastic oliogdendrogliomas. J Natl Cancer Inst 1998;90:1473–1479.
2. Ino Y, Zlatescu MC, Sasaki H, et al. Long survival and therapeutic responses in patients with histologically disparate high-grade gliomas demonstrating chromosome 1p loss. J Neurosurg 2000;92:983–990.

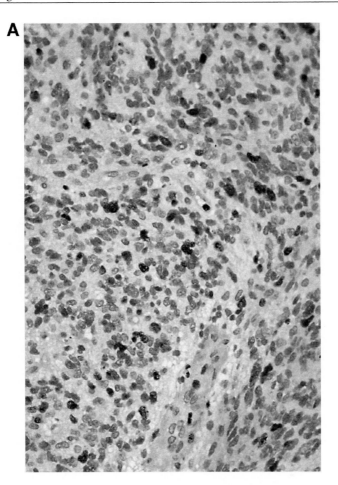

Fig. 28. (A,B) Two contiguous high power fields of a GBM stained with Ki-67 antibody. Heterogeneity in cell proliferation is readily observable in most HGGs. Nuclear staining is interpreted as positive (Ki-67, original magnification ×400). (*See* next page for Fig. 28B.)

3. Ino Y, Betensky RA, Zlatescu MC, et al. Molecular subtypes of anaplastic oligodendroglioma: Implications for patient management at diagnosis. Clin Cancer Res 2001;7:839–845.
4. Reifenberger G, Louis DN. Oligodendroglioma: Toward molecular definitions in diagnostic neuro-oncology. J Neuropathol Exp Neurol 2003;62:111–126.
5. Ringertz N. "Grading" of gliomas. Acta Pathol Microbiol Scand 1950;27:51–64.
6. Burger PC, Vogel FS, Green SB, et al. Glioblastoma multiforme and anaplastic astrocytoma: pathologic criteria and prognostic implications. Cancer 1985;56:1106–1111.
7. Cavenee WK, Furnari FB, Nagane M, et al. Diffusely infiltrating astrocytomas. In: Kleihues P, Cavenee WK, eds. Tumours of the Nervous System. Lyon, France: IARC Press, 2000:10–21.
8. Krouwer HGJ, Davis RL, Silver P, et al. Gemistocytic astrocytomas: a reappraisal. J Neurosurg 1991;74:399–406.
9. Watanabe K, Tachibana O, Yonekawa Y, et al. Role of gemistocytes in astrocytoma progression. Lab Invest 1997;76:277–284.

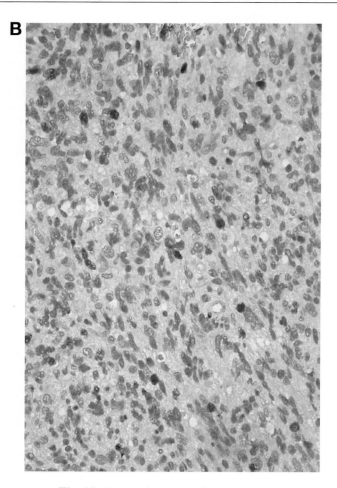

Fig. 28. *See* previous page for caption.

10. Hoshino T, Wilson CB, Ellis WG. Gemistocytic astrocytes in gliomas: an autoradiographic study. J Neuropathol Exp Neurol 1995;34:263–281.

11. Sreenan JJ, Prayson RA. Gliosarcoma: a study of 13 tumors, including p53 and CD34 immunohistochemistry. Arch Pathol Lab Med 1997;121:129–133.

12. Morantz RA, Feigin I, Ransohoff J. Clinical and pathologic study of 24 cases of gliosarcoma. J Neurosurg 1976;45:398–408.

13. Meis JM, Ho KL. Gliosarcoma: A histologic and immunohistochemical reaffirmation. Mod Pathol 1990;3:19–24.

14. Perry JR, Ang LC, Bilbao JM, et al. Clinicopathologic features of primary and post-radiation cerebral gliosarcoma. Cancer 1995;75:2910–2918.

15. Biernat W, Aguzzi A, Sure U, et al. Identical mutations of the p53 tumor suppressor gene in the gliomatous and the sarcomatous components of gliosarcomas suggest a common origin from glial cells. J Neuropathol Exp Neurol 1995;54:651–656.

16. Boerman RH, Anderl K , Herath J, et al. The glial and mesenchymal elements of gliosarcomas share similar genetic alterations. J Neuropathol Exp Neurol 1996;55:973–981.
17. Rosenblum MK, Erlandson RA, Budzilovich GN. The lipid-rich epithelioid glioblastoma. Am J Surg Pathol 1991;15:925–934.
18. Mueller W, Lass U, Herms J, et al. Clonal analysis in glioblastoma with epithelial differentiation. Brain Pathol 2001;11:39–43.
19. Burger PC. Cytologic composition of the untreated glioblastoma with implications for evaluation of needle biopsies. Cancer 1989;63:2014–2023.
20. Burger PC, Pearl DK, Aldape K, et al. Small cell architecture—a histological equivalent of EGFR amplification in glioblastoma multiforme? J Neuropathol Exp Neurol 2001;60:1099–1104.
21. Oh D, Prayson RA. Evaluation of epithelioid and keratin markers in glioblastoma multiforme. An immunohiostochemical study. Am J Clin Pathol 1999;123:917–920.
22. Katoh M, Toshimitsu A, Sugimoto S, et al. Immunohistochemical analysis of giant cell glioblastoma. Pathol Int 1995;45:275–282.
23. Kornfeld M. Granular cell glioblastoma. A malignant granular cell neoplasm of astrocytic origin. J Neuropathol Exp Neurol 1986;45:447–462.
24. Melaragno MJ, Prayson RA, Murphy MA, et al. Anaplastic astrocytoma with granular cell differentiation: case report and review of the literature. Hum Pathol 1993;24:805–808.
25. Geddes JF, Thom M, Robinson SFD, et al. Granular cell change in astrocytic tumors. Am J Surg Pathol 1996;20:55–63.
26. Cohen BH, Packer RJ. Adverse neurologic effects of chemotherapy and radiation therapy. In: Berg BO, ed. Neurological Aspects of Pediatrics. Stoneham: Butterwork, 1992:567–594.
27. Caveness WF. Experimental observations: delayed necrosis in normal monkey brain. In: Gilbert, HA, Kagen AR, eds. Radiation Damage to the Nervous System: A Delayed Therapeutic Hazard. New York, NY: Raven Press, 1992:1–38.
28. Burger PC, Mahaley Jr. MS, Dudka L, et al. The morphologic effects of radiation administered therapeutically for intracranial gliomas: a postmortem study of 25 cases. Cancer 1979;44:1256–1272.
29. Artigas J, Cervos-Navarro J, Iglesias JR, et al. Gliomatosis cerebri: clinical and histological findings. Clin Neuropathol 1985;4:135–148.
30. Elshaikh MA, Stevens GH, Peereboom DM, et al. Gliomatosis cerebri. Treatment results with radiotherapy alone. Cancer 2002;95:2027–2031.
31. Herrlinger U, Felsberg J, Küker W, et al. Gliomatosis cerebri: Molecular pathology and clinical course. Ann Neurol 2002;53:390–399.
32. Prayson RA, Morris HH. Anaplastic pleomorphic xanthoastrocytoma. Arch Pathol Lab Med 1998;122:1082–1086.
33. Macaulay RJB, Jay V, Hoffman HJ, et al. Increased mitotic activity as a negative prognostic indicator in pleomorphic xanthoastrocytoma. J Neurosurg 1993;79:761–768.
34. Giannini C, Scheithauer BW, Burger PC, et al. Pleomorphic xanthoastrocytoma. What do we really know about it. Cancer 1999;85:2033–2045.
35. Tomlinson FH, Scheithauer BW, Hayostek CJ, et al. The significance of atypia and histologic malignancy in pilocytic astrocytoma of the cerebellum: a clinicopathologic and flow cytometric study. J Child Neurol 1994;9:301–310.
36. Brat DJ, Hirose Y, Cohen KJ, et al. Astroblastoma: clinicopathologic features and chromosomal abnormalities defined by comparative genomic hybridization. Brain Pathol 2000;10:342–352.
37. Bonnin JM, Rubinstein LJ. Astroblastomas: A pathological study of 23 tumors, with a postoperative follow-up in 13 patients. Neurosurgery 1989;25:6–13.
38. VandenBerg SR. Desmoplastic infantile ganglioglioma and desmoplastic cerebral astrocytoma of infancy. Brain Pathol 1993;3:275–281.
39. Setty SN, Miller DC, Camras L, et al. Desmoplastic infantile astrocytoma with metastases at presentation. Mod Pathol 1997;10:945–995.
40. Burger PC, Rawlings CE, Cox EB, et al. Clinicopathologic correlations in the oligodendroglioma. Cancer 1987;59:1345–1352.
41. Shaw EG, Scheithauer BW, O'Fallon JR, et al. Oligodendrogliomas: the Mayo Clinic experience. J Neurosurg 1992;76:428–434.
42. Daumas-Duport C, Varlet P, Tucker M-L, et al. Oligodendrogliomas part I: patterns of growth, histological diagnosis, clinical and imaging correlations: a study of 153 cases. J Neuro Oncol 1997;34:37–59.
43. Kros JM, Troost D, van Eden CG, et al. Oligodendroglioma. A comparison of two grading systems. Cancer 1988;61:2251–2259.

44. Dehghani F, Schachenmayr W, Laun A, et al. Prognostic implication of histological, immunohistochemical and clinical features of oligodendrogliomas: a study of 89 cases. Acta Neuropathol 1998;95:493–504.

45. Mørk SJ, Halvorsen TB, Lindegaard K-F, et al. Oligodendroglioma: histologic evaluation and prognosis. J Neuropathol Exp Neurol 1986;45:65–78.

46. Reifenberger G, Kros JM, Burger PC, et al. Oligodendroglioma and anaplastic oligodendroglioma. In: Kleihues P, Cavenee WK, eds. Tumours of the Nervous System. Lyon, France: IARC Press, 2000:56–64.

47. Hart MN, Petito CK, Earle KM. Mixed gliomas. Cancer 1974;33:134–140.

48. Beckmann MJ, Prayson RA. A clinicopathologic study of 30 cases of oligoastrocytoma including p53 immunohistochemistry. Pathology 1997;29:159–164.

49. Jask—lsky D, Zawirski M, Papierz W et al. Mixed gliomas: their clinical course and results of surgery. Zentralbl Neurochir 1987;48:120–123.

50. Shaw EG, Scheithauer BW, O'Fallon JR, et al. Mixed oligoastrocytomas: a survival and prognostic factor and analysis. Neurosurgery 1994;34:577–582.

51. Reifenberger G, Kros JM, Burger PC, et al. Oligoastrocytoma and anaplastic oligoastrocytoma. In: Kleihues P, Cavenee WK, eds. Tumours of the Nervous System. Lyon, France: IARC Press, 2000:65–69.

52. Smith JS, Perry A, Borell TJ, et al. Alterations of chromosome arms 1p and 19q as predictors of survival in oligodendrogliomas, astrocytomas, and mixed oligoastrocytomas. J Clin Oncol 2000;18:636–645.

53. Wiestler OD, Schiffer D, Coons SW, et al. Ependymoma and anaplastic ependymoma. In: Kleihues P, Cavenee WK, eds. Tumours of the Nervous System. Lyon, France: IARC Press, 2000:72–77.

54. Afra D, Muller W, Slowik F, Wilcke O, Budka H, Turoczy L. Supratentorial lobar ependymomas: reports on the grading and survival periods in 80 cases, including 46 recurrences. Acta Neurochir (Wein) 1983;69:243–251.

55. Ernestus R-I, Wilcke O, Schröder R. Supratentorial ependymomas in childhood: clinicopathological findings and prognosis. Acta Neurochir (Wien) 1991;111:96–102.

56. Mørk SJ, Løken AC. Ependymoma: a follow-up study of 101 cases. Cancer 1977;40:907–915.

57. Lyons MK, Kelly PJ. Posterior fossa ependymomas: report of 30 cases and review of the literature. Neurosurgery 1991;28:659–665.

58. Rawlings III CE, Giangaspero F, Burger PC, et al. Ependymomas: a clinicopathologic study. Surg Neurol 1988;29:271–281.

59. Figarella-Branger D, Gambarelli D, Dollo C, et al. Infratentorial ependymomas of childhood: correlation between histological features, immunohistological phenotype, silver nucleolar organizer region staining values and post-operative survival in 16 cases. Acta Neuropathol (Berl) 1991;82:208–216.

60. Prayson RA. Cyclin D1 and MIB-1 immunohistochemistry in ependymomas: a study of 41 cases. Am J Clin Pathol 1998;110:629–634.

61. Paulus W, Peiffer J. Intratumoral histologic heterogeneity of gliomas: a quantitative study. Cancer 1989;64:442–447.

62. Coons SW, Johnson PC. Regional heterogeneity in the proliferative activity of human gliomas as measured by Ki-67 labeling index. J Neuropathol Exp Neurol 1993;52:609–618.

63. Brainard JA, Prayson RA, Barnett GH. Frozen section evaluation of stereotactic brain biopsies: diagnostic yield at the stereotactic target position in 188 cases. Arch Pathol Lab Med 1997;121:481–484.

64. Mittler MA, Walters BC, Stopa EG. Observer reliability in histological grading of astrocytoma stereotactic biopsies. J Neurosurg 1996;85:1091–1094.

65. Prayson RA, Agamanolis DP, Cohen ML, et al. Intraobserver reproducibility among neuropathologists and surgical pathologists in fibrillary astrocytoma grading. J Neurol Sci 2000;175:33–39.

66. Giannini C, Scheithauer BW, Weaver AL, et al. Oligodendrogliomas: Reproducibility and prognostic value of histologic diagnosis and grading. J Neuropathol Exp Neurol 2001;60:248–262.

67. Coons SW, Johnson PC, Scheithauer BW, et al. Improving diagnostic accuracy and interobserver concordance in the classification and grading of primary gliomas. Cancer 1997;79:1381–1393.

68. Prayson RA. Cell proliferation and tumors of the central nervous system, Part II: Radiolabeling, cytometric, and immunohistochemical techniques. J Neuropathol Exp Neurol 2002;61:663–672.

69. Giannini C, Scheithauer BW, Burger PC, et al. Cellular proliferation in pilocytic and diffuse astrocytomas. J Neuropathol Exp Neurol 1999;58:46–53.

70. Wakimoto H, Aoyagi M, Nakayama T, et al. Prognostic significance of Ki-67 labeling indices obtained using MIB-1 monoclonal antibody in patients with supratentorial astrocytomas. Cancer 1996;77:373–380.

71. Hsu DW, Louis DN. Efird JT, et al. Use of MIB-1 (Ki-67) immunoreactivity in differentiating grade II and grade III gliomas. J Neuropathol Exp Neurol 1997;56:857–865.

72. Montine TJ, Vandersteenhoven J, Aguzzi A, et al. Prognostic significance of Ki-67 proliferation index in supratentorial fibrillary astrocytic neoplasms. Neurosurgery 1994;34:674–679.

73. Prayson RA, Mohan DS, Song P, et al. Clinicopathologic study of forty-four histologically pure supratentorial oligodendrogliomas. Ann Diagn Pathol 2000;4:218–227.

74. Kros JM, Hop WCJ, Godschalk JJCJ, et al. Prognostic value of the proliferation-related antigen Ki-67 in oligodendrogliomas. Cancer 1996;78:1107–1113.

75. Coons SW, Johnson PC, Pearl DK. The prognostic significance of Ki-67 labeling indices for oligodendrogliomas. Neurosurgery 1997;41:878–885.

76. Prayson RA. Clinicopathologic study of 61 patients with ependymoma including MIB-1 immunohistochemistry. Ann Diagn Pathol 1999;3:11–18.

77. Schröder R, Ploner C, Ernestus R-I. The growth potential of ependymomas with varying grades of malignancy measured by the Ki-67 labeling index and mitotic index. Neurosurg Rev 1993;16:145–150.

2 Molecular Classifications

Gregory N. Fuller

Summary

The field of glioma classification is currently entering a new era with the introduction of paradigms based on molecular information. Rather than supplanting traditional morphology-based classification schemes, it is anticipated that emerging molecular biologic, genomic, transcriptomic, and proteomic data will complement and augment existing morphologic and immunophenotypic data, providing for a more accurate and refined stratification of glioma patients for directed therapies and for the resolution of several problematic issues inherent in histological classifications. Two different approaches are contributing to the improvement of glioma stratification. The first is the analysis of alterations of a limited number of genes or gene products of recently demonstrated impact on patient survival and response to therapy, such as deletion status of chromosomes 1p and 19q in oligodendroglial tumors, and $O(6)$-methylguanine-DNA methyltransferase (MGMT) promoter methylation in glioblastoma. The second is a more comprehensive analysis of the tumor genome, transcriptome, or proteome, which may in itself provide refined subclassification, or may identify specific relevant biomolecules for use in the single gene analysis approach. Both paradigms have already exerted a tangible and growing impact on glioma classification, yet it is highly likely that we have only just begun to exploit their potential contributions.

Key Words: Molecular classification; glioma; transcriptomics; genomics; proteomics; tissue microarray; MGMT; PTEN; 1p; 19q.

INTRODUCTION

The histopathologic classification of diffuse gliomas by microscopy has a long and storied history. Many different classification and grading systems of increasing precision and clinical utility have been proposed. Currently applied classifications, such as the modified Ringertz systems of Burger *(1)* and Nelson *(2)*, the St. Anne-Mayo system *(3)*, and the World Health Organization (WHO) system *(4)* are largely based on morphologic pattern recognition and relative weighting of various histologic features, with supportive input provided by immunophenotypic studies using monoclonal (MAbs) and polyclonal antibodies (PAbs) directed against various differentiation and cell proliferation makers. The clinical usefulness of these time-tested glioma classification systems cannot be overemphasized. In addition, the technical simplicity and cost efficiency of rendering a diagnosis based on the examination of a hematoxylin and eosin-stained tissue section by simple light microscopy are unparalleled. Nevertheless, morphology-based tumor stratification exhibits a number of shortcomings (Table 1). Among these are (1) subjectiveness, (2) inability to substratify patients within a given major tumor category, such as anaplastic astrocytoma (AA), and (3) inability to predict

From: *Current Clinical Oncology: High-Grade Gliomas: Diagnosis and Treatment*
Edited by: G. H. Barnett © Humana Press Inc., Totowa, NJ

Table 1
Some Shortcomings of Traditional Morphology-Based Tumor Classification Systems

- Subjective classification criteria open to variable interpretation and relative weighting by individual evaluators.
- Nonpredictive of individual patient survival within a given tumor type and grade.
- Nonpredictive of individual tumor response to particular therapeutic regimens.

Table 2
Two Current Paradigms for Molecular Classification of Gliomas

- Sequential assay of a small number of genes or gene products of known significance (e.g., 1p, 19q, 9p, 10q, *PTEN*, *P16^{INK4A}*, *TP53*, *EGFR*, *MGMT*).
- Simultaneous assay of a large number (hundreds or thousands) of genes or gene products by any one of a number of high-density, high-throughput techniques, followed by statistical analysis to identify glioma subsets and robust classifiers. Techniques include gene expression profiling, array comparative genomic hybridization and proteome profiling.

patient response or lack thereof to specific therapeutic regimens. Subjectiveness or ambiguity of interpretation is usually not an issue for gliomas that exhibit classical morphology—such as typical glioblastomas that show pleomorphism, fibrillary cytoplasmic processes, florid microvascular proliferation, and zones of tumor necrosis with pseudopalisading—or for oligodendrogliomas with monotonous, uniform cells, bland round nuclei, and prominent perinuclear halos; however, in a significant percentage of diffuse gliomas, there exists either a mixture of cells with either astrocytic or oligodendroglia features, or a large percentage of cells exhibit a combination of astrocytic and oligodendroglial features. At different times throughout the history of glioma classification, the neuropathology Zeitgeist has variously favored including such morphologically ambiguous tumors in the astrocytic camp, the oligodendroglial camp, or in a hybrid category called mixed oligoastrocytoma in which there may be topographically separate areas of astrocyte-featured cells and oligodendrocyte-featured cells, or the two populations may be intimately intermixed, or there may be a *tertium quid* variant in which all of the tumor cells display features that are intermediate between those of classical astrocytoma and classical oligodendroglioma *(5)*.

Therefore, there is a clearly defined need for a more refined, individually tailored, and less subjective glioma classification. Contemporary molecular and genomic techniques provide a wealth of possible avenues for improving current glioma stratification.

MOLECULAR CLASSIFICATION PARADIGMS

There are two paradigms for the molecular classification and substratification of diffuse gliomas that are currently enjoying widespread investigation and application (Table 2). The first is based on the assay of only a very small number of genes or gene products of known importance. The second approach employs a more global analysis of hundreds or thousands of genes using contemporary high-density, high-throughput genomic technologies. Both approaches have proven fruitful in preliminary molecular classification attempts.

Table 3
Contemporary Genomic, Transcriptomic, and Proteomic Techniques
Used for Data Acquisition for Molecular Classification Studies

DNA	RNA	Protein
Genome	Transcriptome	Proteome
Array CGH	Expression microarrays	MALDI-TOF MS
FISH + TMA	SAGE	Protein arrays
		Antibody arrays
		TMA + Ab

Abbr: Ab, monoclonal and polyclonal antibodies; CGH, comparative genomic hybridization; FISH, fluorescent *in situ* hybridization; MALDI-TOF MS, matrix-assisted laser desorption/ionization time-of-flight mass spectrometry; SAGE, serial analysis of gene expression; TMA, tissue microarray.

PATIENT STRATIFICATION BASED ON ASSAY OF A SMALL NUMBEROF MOLECULAR MARKERS

The term "molecular classification," in the most basic sense, implies the use of molecular data to effect or facilitate the reliable and reproducible stratification of patients into groups that have differing prognostic or therapeutic implications. Contemporary basic and translational molecular biological research has yielded a number of molecular marker assays with proven prognostic and/or therapeutic significance in high-grade gliomas. The most salient of these is deletion testing for markers on chromosomes 1p and 19q in oligodendrogliomas. Co-deletion of markers on both chromosomal arms is associated with better response to therapy, increased time to recurrence, and increased survival compared with morphologically similar tumors that lack this molecular signature *(6–14)*. In this instance, the assessment of only two chromosomal regions yields a clinically significant dichotomous molecular classification of oligodendroglial tumors. Assay of a few additional molecular markers, such as TP53 mutation can be used to generate an even finer molecular substratification of anaplastic oligodendrogliomas into four prognostically significant groups *(6)*. Another prominent example of molecular stratification using only a single gene assay is the assessment of epigenetic silencing of $O(6)$-methylguanine-DNA methyltransferase (MGMT) by promoter methylation in high-grade astrocytomas. Patients with tumors that exhibit MGMT gene promoter methylation survive longer after treatment with temozolomide and radiation therapy compared with patients with tumors that lack this feature *(15–17)*. Thus, MGMT promoter methylation status permits the molecular subclassification of glioblastoma patients into two different treatment response groups.

MOLECULAR STRATIFICATION BASED ON TRANSCRIPTOME PROFILING, COMPARATIVE GENOMIC HYBRIDIZATION, AND PROTEOME PROFILING

A number of contemporary high-density genomic, transcriptomic, and proteomic techniques are available that could potentially provide data useful for tumor molecular classification and novel class discovery (Table 3). In theory, quantitative information on DNA alterations, mRNA (cDNA) levels, or protein composition and quantities could be used to

Table 4
Technology-Driven Revolutions in the History of Tumor Nosology

- Light microscopy
- Electron microscopy
- Immunocytochemistry
- Genomics & Transcriptomics
- Proteomics Next!

separate gliomas into meaningful subsets for diagnostic, prognostic, and/or therapeutic purposes. Currently, transcriptome profiling *(18–26)* and array comparative genomic hybridization *(27–30)* are the dominant methodologies that have been used to generate molecular classifications of the diffuse gliomas. Initial experiments using proteomic data to subclassify gliomas have also been reported *(31)*.

Several conclusions can be drawn from the collective experience on molecular classification of gliomas using genomic and transcriptomic techniques to date: (1) molecular classification can separate tumor types and grades as well as and often better than histopathologic classification, (2) gene expression profiling can identify subgroups within histologic tumor types that are not identifiable by morphologic or immunophenotypic evaluation, and (3) nosologic groups identified by expression profiling have prognostic significance with respect to patient survival. In addition, it is clear that the analysis of hundreds or thousands of genes or gene products, although a logical starting point, is not necessary once robust classifier genes have been identified. Rather, the paradigm that is evolving is the initial quantitation of thousands of genes, followed by statistical analysis to identify small sets of only a few genes that are strong classifiers. These markers can then be used to stratify tumors for various ends, such as prognosis, susceptibility to specific therapeutic regimens, or resistance to specific therapies. Sets as small as three genes have proven as powerful as the indiscriminant evaluation of hundreds of genes in classifying gliomas *(19)*. This then raises the possibility of design of relatively simple chip sets for diagnosis that would be feasible from both technological and cost efficiency perspectives for widespread routine diagnostic application. Additionally, it may also be possible to select for robust classifier gene sets that code for expressed proteins for which antibodies could then be raised, thereby "translating" genomic classification into protein immunohistochemical classification. In contrast to high-density gene expression platforms and array comparative genomic hybridization (CGH) technology, immunohistochemistry is available in virtually all modern hospital diagnostic clinical laboratories.

CONCLUSIONS

Numerous studies by multiple institutions over the past several years have convincingly demonstrated the power and ability of molecular approaches to classify and substratify diffuse gliomas. In the words of Nutt and colleagues, "Gene expression-based classification of malignant gliomas correlates better with survival than histological classification *(25)*." At the same time, it is equally true that classical histopathological evaluation of gliomas provides much useful information and no cogent arguments for discontinuing morphologic and immunophenotypic diagnosis and classification studies have been advanced. Morphologic evaluation has the advantages of simplicity, cost effectiveness, and a long history of proven useful application. Although it is hazardous to attempt to predict the future, it seems likely that morphology will continue for some time to provide the foundation for glioma classification, with molecular analysis judiciously applied as warranted to provide more refined stratification as continued research unveils additional applications.

The history of tumor classification is replete with examples of the influence of technological advances (Table 4). The invention of the light microscope was arguably the single greatest advance in tumor nosology, introducing the modern era. Other waves of progress were provided by the transmission electron microscope for ultrastructural analysis and the introduction of immunocytochemistry for differentiation antigen identification. Currently, transcriptomic techniques (gene expression profiling) and genomic techniques (array comparative genomic hybridization and related techniques) are exerting a strong influence on the field. Proteomic technology is likely to have an increasing influence in the future as the field matures.

REFERENCES

1. Burger PC, Vogel FS, Green SB, Strike SA. Glioblastoma multiforme and anaplastic astrocytoma. Pathologic criteria and prognostic implications. Cancer 1985;56:1106–1111.
2. Nelson JS, Tsukada Y, Schoenfeld D, Fulling K, Lamarche J, Peress N. Necrosis as a prognostic criterion in malignant supratentorial astrocytic gliomas. Cancer 1983;52:550–554.
3. Daumas-Duport C, Scheithauer BW, O'Fallon J, Kelly P. Grading of astrocytomas: a simple and reproducible method. Cancer 1988;62:2152–2165.
4. Kleihues P, Cavenee WK. World Health Organization Classification of Tumors: Pathology and Genetics of Tumours of the Nervous System. Lyon, France: IARC Press, 2000.
5. Fuller GN. Central nervous system tumors. In: Parham DM, ed. Pediatric Neoplasia: Morphology and Biology. Philadelphia:Lippincott Williams & Wilkins, 1996:153–204.
6. Reifenberger G, Louis DN. Oligodendroglioma: toward molecular definitions in neuro-oncology. J Neuropathol Exp Neurol 2003;62:111–126.
7. McDonald JM, Colmam H, Perry A, Aldape K. Molecular and clinical aspects of 1p/19q loss in oligodendroglioma. In: Zhang W, Fuller GN, eds. Genomic and Molecular Neuro-Oncology. Boston:Jones and Bartlett, 2004:17–30.
8. McDonald JM, See SJ, Tremont I, et al. Prognostic impact of histology and 1p/19q status in anaplastic oligodendroglial tumors. Cancer 2005;104:1468–1477.
9. Hartmann C, Mueller W, Lass U, Kamel-Reid S, von Deimling A. Molecular genetic analysis of oligodendroglial tumors. J Neuropathol Exp Neurol 2005;64:10–14.
10. Jeuken JW, von Deimling A, Wesseling P. Molecular pathogenesis of oligodendroglial tumors. J Neurooncol 2004;70:161–181.
11. van den Bent MJ. Advances in the biology and treatment of oligodendrogliomas. Curr Opin Neurol 2004;17:675–680.
12. Cairncross JG, Ueki K, Zlatescu MC, et al. Specific genetic predictors of chemotherapeutic response and survival in patients with anaplastic oligodendrogliomas. J Natl Cancer Inst 1998;90:1473–1479.
13. Stege EM, Kros JM, de Bruin HG, et al. Successful treatment of low-grade oligodendroglial tumors with a chemotherapy regimen of procarbazine, lomustine, and vincristine. Cancer 2005;103:802–809.
14. Kitange G, Misra A, Law M, et al. Chromosomal imbalances detected by array comparative genomic hybridization in human oligodendrogliomas and mixed oligoastrocytomas. Genes Chromosomes Cancer 2005;42:68–77.
15. Hegi ME, Diserens AC, Gorlia T, et al. MGMT gene silencing and benefit from temozolomide in glioblastoma. N Engl J Med 2005;352:997–1003.
16. Stupp R, Mason WP, van den Bent MJ, et al. Radiotherapy plus concomitant and adjuvant temozolomide for glioblastoma. N Engl J Med 2005;352:987–996.
17. Hegi ME, Diserens AC, Godard S, et al. Clinical trial substantiates the predictive value of O-6-methylguanine-DNA methyltransferase promoter methylation in glioblastoma patients treated withtemozolomide. Clin Cancer Res 2004;10:1871–1874.
18. Fuller GN, Hess, KR, Rhee, CH, et al. Molecular classification of human diffuse gliomas by multidimensional scaling analysis of gene expression profiles parallels mophology-based classification, correlates with survival, and reveals clinically-relevant novel glioma subsets. Brain Pathol 2002;12:108–116.

19. Kim S, Dougherty ER, Shmulevich I, et al. Identification of combination gene sets for glioma classification. Mol Cancer Therapeut 2002;1:1229–1236.
20. Mischel PS, Cloughesy TF, Nelson SF. DNA-microarray analysis of brain cancer: molecular classification for therapy. Nat Rev Neurosci 2004;5:782–792.
21. Freije WA, Castro-Vargas FE, Fang Z, et al. Gene expression profiling of gliomas strongly predicts survival. Cancer Res 2004;64:6503–6510.
22. Godard S, Getz G, Delorenzi M, et al. Classification of human astrocytic gliomas on the basis of gene expression: a correlated group of genes with angiogenic activity emerges as a strong predictor of subtypes. Cancer Res 2003;63:6613–6625.
23. Mischel PS, Shai R, Shi T, et al. Identification of molecular subtypes of glioblastoma by gene expression profiling. Oncogene 2003;22:2361–2373.
24. Shai R, Shi T, Kremen TJ, et al. Gene expression profiling identifies molecular subtypes of gliomas. Oncogene 2003;22:4918–4923.
25. Nutt CL, Mani DR, Betensky RA, et al. Gene expression-based classification of malignant gliomas correlates better with survival than histological classification. Cancer Res 2003;63:1602–1607.
26. Caskey LS, Fuller GN, Bruner JM, et al. Toward a molecular classification of the gliomas: histopathology, molecular genetics, and gene expression profiling. Histol Histopathol 2000;15:971–981.
27. Roerig P, Nessling M, Radlwimmer B, et al. Molecular classification of human gliomas using matrix-based comparative genomic hybridization. Int J Cancer 2005;117:95–103.
28. Nigro JM, Misra A, Zhang L, et al. Integrated array-comparative genomic hybridization and expression array profilesidentify clinically relevant molecular subtypes of glioblastoma. Cancer Res 2005;65:1678–1686.
29. Jeuken JW, Sprenger SH, Boerman RH, et al. Subtyping of oligo-astrocytic tumours by comparative genomic hybridization. J Pathol 2001;194:81–87.
30. Kunwar S, Mohapatra G, Bollen A, Lamborn KR, Prados M, Feuerstein BG. Genetic subgroups of anaplastic astrocytomas correlate with patient age and survival. Cancer Res 2001;61:7683–7688.
31. Iwadate Y, Sakaida T, Hiwasa T, et al. Molecular classification and survival prediction in human gliomas based on proteome analysis. Cancer Res 2004;64:2496–2501.

II Clinical Characteristics

3 Pediatric High-Grade Glioma

Bruce H. Cohen

Summary

Brain tumors are the second-most common neoplasm in children, and the most common solid tumor. Glial tumors comprise about 40% of the primary brain tumors that occur in children. Slightly more than 50% of the glial neoplasms are low-grade tumors, and these are almost all pilocytic astrocytomas that occur in the cerebellum, optic apparatus, and diencephalon. As with adults, HGG in children may occur anywhere in the central nervous system (CNS). However, in children, there tends to be a greater percentage of tumors that are localized in the deep gray matter, cerebellum, and especially within the brainstem. Despite technological advances in neuroimaging, improvements in surgical techniques, advances in radiotherapy, and the proliferation of new anti-neoplastic agents, the prognosis for survival of high-grade glioma in children has only improved marginally over the past several decades. Although the prognosis for survival of supratentorial high-grade glioma is not as ominous in children as in adults, this survival advantage may be in part a result of stronger constitution of children as well as differences in the molecular genetic substrate of the neoplasm.

Key Words: Pediatric gliomas; brainstem HGG; supratentorial HGG.

INTRODUCTION

Brain tumors are the second-most common neoplasm in children, and the most common solid tumor. The incidence of brain tumors in children, based on an analysis of several studies, is 2 to 3 per 100,000 children per year *(1)*. Glial tumors comprise about 40% of the primary brain tumors that occur in children. Slightly more than 50% of the glial neoplasms are low-grade tumors, and these are almost all pilocytic astrocytomas that occur in the cerebellum, optic apparatus, and diencephalon. A relatively common tumor in adults, the fibrillary infiltrating astrocytomas (referred to as low-grade astrocytomas or grade II astrocytomas), is very rare in childhood. The high-grade brainstem glioma and high-grade supratentorial gliomas each account for 20% of pediatric gliomas, with the remaining 5% occurring in the cerebellum. In total, high-grade gliomas (HGG) make up about 5% of all pediatric neoplasms *(2)*. As with adults, HGG in children may occur anywhere in the central nervous system (CNS). However, in children, there tends to be a greater percentage of tumors that are localized in the deep gray matter, cerebellum, and especially within the brainstem. The HGG of the brainstem, which will be discussed separately in great detail, tend to be easy to identify with neuroimaging, and do not require biopsy for diagnosis *(3–5)*. The clinical behavior of the high-grade brainstem gliomas tends to follow a rather predictable course with early response to radiotherapy and recurrence within about 1 yr *(6,7)*. The clinical course of the supratentorial and cerebellar HGG is not as predictable in children as it is in adults. Regardless, both the genetic alterations

From: *Current Clinical Oncology: High-Grade Gliomas: Diagnosis and Treatment*
Edited by: G. H. Barnett © Humana Press Inc., Totowa, NJ

are different than in adults and the outcome is somewhat better for children than adults *(8)*. There is limited information about the genetic alterations that lead to HGG formation in childhood malignant gliomas. The molecular changes that have been found are more like those in the adult secondary glioblastoma than in the denovo pathway. However, other genetic changes suggest that the early mechanisms of tumorigenesis is different in children than in adults *(9)*.

Despite technological advances in neuroimaging, improvements in surgical techniques, advances in radiotherapy, and the proliferation of new anti-neoplastic agents, the prognosis for survival of high-grade glioma in children has only improved marginally over the past several decades. The historical data suggest that only about 20% of children survive 3 yr post-diagnosis. Although the prognosis for survival of supratentorial high-grade glioma is not as ominous in children as in adults, this survival advantage may be in part a result of stronger constitution of children as well as differences in the molecular genetic substrate of the neo-plasm *(7)*. However the infratentorial high-grade glioma, especially the intrinsic pontine glioma, remains one of the most treatment-resistant tumors, with an ultimate prognosis similar to adults with glioblastoma multiforme (GBM).

NONBRAINSTEM MALIGNANT GLIOMAS
Clinical Presentation

The clinical presentation may be quite different in infants and young children for several reasons. The skull bones do not begin to fuse until after 2 to 3 yr of life, and relatively slow-growing tumors, even if they have a malignant histology, can cause considerable macrocrania before causing increased intracranial pressure (ICP). The fact that the intracranial volume is not fixed as it is in older children and adults also explains why many infants present with nonlocalizing signs such as behavioral changes. The tumors in infants tend to be located more along the midline and therefore hydrocephalus may occur because of blockage of cerebrospi-nal fluid (CSF) at the level of the foramen of Monroe, the third ventricle, the aquaduct of Sylvius, or as a result of obstruction of the outflow tracts of the fourth ventricle. Aside from hydrocephalus, macrocrania may occur because of tumor volume alone. The clinical exami-nation of an infant or toddler may show splitting of the cranial sutures and an enlarged or bulging fontenelle without any signs of increased ICP, including absence of papilledema. Unless there are well documented head circumference measurements performed as part of the standard well-child care, the diagnosis of macrocrania may be delayed for months. When the intracranial volume does expand faster than the skull can accommodate, increased ICP can occur and manifest itself as changes in feeding patterns or vomiting. Early in the course of the illness these changes can mimic common childhood viral infections. As the pressure increases, the infant or young child may become more irritable. In extreme situations, the long-standing hydrocephalus may cause optic atrophy and optic pallor without any evidence of papilledema. As with older children and adults, focal neurologic signs and seizures may occur *(2,10)*.

The presentation in children out of the infant and toddler stage is similar to adults. In a study that was published as computer tomography (CT) was becoming first available noted that the mean duration of symptoms prior to diagnosis for children with GBM was 13 wk *(11)*. Head-ache is the earliest and most common symptom, occurring in almost 60% of children. Vom-iting occurs in 40% and seizures in 30%. Eight percent of children have more than one symptom at the time of diagnosis and 69% have symptoms for less than 3 mo. The neurologic examination is abnormal in 94% of children at the time of diagnosis *(2)*.

Treatment Considerations

As in adults with malignant glioma, there is difficulty in developing treatment trials and interpreting results; the problem, however, is considerably more difficult in children because, as rare as these tumors are in adults, there are far fewer pediatric patients to study.

Role of Surgery

Some debate remains around the use of aggressive surgery as part of the overall treatment for HGG. However, there are data to suggest that, in those tumors amenable to safe surgical resection, the overall long-term survival may be dramatically improved in those children in which a gross-total resection is accomplished. As with adult gliomas, aggressive surgery is not possible for those tumors that involve eloquent volumes of cortex, deep gray matter structures, central structures, cerebellar nuclei, and peduncles and brainstem. The most important study to suggest a role for aggressive resection involved 131 children with anaplastic astrocytomas and GBM. The distribution of location was supratentorial in 63%, deep/midline in 28%, and posterior fossa in 8%. In this study, children were treated with surgical resection followed by either radiotherapy followed by eight cycles of chemotherapy (vincristine, CCNU, and prednisone) or two cycles of 8-in-1 chemotherapy followed by radiotherapy, then an additional cycles of 8-in-1 chemotherapy. In this study, those children that underwent a gross-total or near-total resection (defined as greater than 90% resection but less than total) fared much better than those children that had a sub-total resection (defined as less than 90% resection) or biopsy. The 5-yr progression-free survival (PFS) was $35 \pm 7\%$ for the >90% resection group vs $17 \pm 4\%$ for the group with < 90% resection. For the subset of children with anaplastic astrocytomas, the 5-yr PFS was $44 \pm 11\%$ and $22 \pm 6\%$ respectively and for the children with GBM, the 5-yr PFS was $26 \pm 9\%$ and $4 \pm 3\%$ respectively *(12,13)*.

Role of Radiotherapy

The role of radiotherapy in the treatment of malignant gliomas of childhood is well established. Radiotherapy has become a standard treatment in all but very young children (defined by different authors as less than 3 yr to less than 6 yr of age). In one historical report, children with anaplastic astrocytoma treated with surgery and radiotherapy had a 29% 5-yr survival and a 26% 10-yr survival *(14)*. In another report of children with malignant gliomas treated with radiotherapy between they years 1957 and 1980, the dose of radiotherapy did correlate with outcome; those that were treated with 54–60 Gy had a 60% 5-yr survival vs those treated with 35–50 Gy. Another observation was that those with midline tumors fared poorly when compared with hemispheric tumors; 0% vs 44% 5-yr survivals respectively. The patients with grade III gliomas (anaplastic astrocytoma) had survivals of 74% at 1 yr, 56% at 2 yr, 36% at 5 yr, and 32% at 10 yr, suggesting a slightly better outcome in children vs adults with anaplastic astrocytoma. In this same study, the children with GBM had survivals of 44% at 1 yr, 26% at 2 yr, 4% at 5 yr, and there were no survivors at 10 yr, which is similar to the overall survival as observed in adults with this disease *(15)*. In another study of 50 children, 13 with GBM, 29 with anaplastic astrocytomas and 8 with other malignant gliomas, the median time to tumor progression was 31 wk, with a median survival of 98 wk, and a 3-yr survival of 32%. The 5-yr survival is not reported in this series, as only 8 patients remained censored at the time of publication *(16)*. Other studies showed a 5 to 10% 5-yr overall survival *(17)* and a 24% 1-yr overall survival *(18)* in similarly treated patients.

For most malignant gliomas, fractionated radiotherapy is the most accepted method of treatment. Involved-field radiation has been conventionally delivered by standard opposing fields, although in the past decade the use of conformal fields has become more accepted. Because many of these tumors disseminate early in their course, a staging evaluation (imaging of the entire neuroaxis with a contrast-enhanced magnetic resonance imaging [MRI] and CSF sampling) is required for all tumors located in the posterior fossa or that involves CSF pathways. In those circumstances where leptomeningeal spread of tumor is identified, consideration for craniospinal irradiation is recommended. There are some groups that recommend craniospinal irradiation irrespective of the staging evaluation if the tumor is located in the cerebellar hemispheres or involves CSF pathways. Obviously, irradiating the spine will impact on the ability to administer high quantities of cytotoxic chemotherapy, as the bone marrow of the vertebrae are essential in hemopoetic activity in children. Regardless, the biggest problem with high-grade gliomas, irrespective of location, is local disease recurrence (19).

Role of Chemotherapy

As with adults, there are hundreds of studies reporting the efficacy (and lack of efficacy) of many different chemotherapeutic agents in treating this disease. Conventional dose studies have been performed with the nitorsoureas (BCNU and CCNU), the platinum agents (cisplatin and carboplatin), vincrisitine, etoposide (VP-16), cyclophosphamide and ifosfamide, procarbazine, topotecan, and others. High-dose chemotherapy using combination chemotherapy with BCNU, carboplatin, etoposide, thiotepa and others followed by either autologous bone marrow rescue and more recently autologous stem cell rescue has been used to treat high-grade glioma as well.

The role of chemotherapy was first explored (and established) in a randomized trial of 58 children conducted by the Children's Cancer Group. Patients were randomized and treated with maximal surgical resection and involved-field radiotherapy with or without eight cycles of chemotherapy (CCNU, vincristine and prednisone). The 5-yr PFS was 18% in the radiotherapy group and 46% in the radiotherapy plus chemotherapy group (event-free survival, $p = 0.026$; overall survival, $p = 0.067$). The overall 3-yr survival was 19% in those children with GBM and 60% in those with anaplastic astrocytoma (20).

The use of pre-irradiation chemotherapy was explored in a later Children's Cancer Group study where the radiation + chemotherapy arm (CCNU, vincristine and prednisone) of the prior study was compared to two cycles of pre-radiation 8-in-1 chemotherapy followed by radiotherapy and then eight additional cycles of 8-in-1 chemotherapy. There was no difference in outcome between the two treatment arms of this study (21).

The role of high-dose chemotherapy followed by autologous bone marrow rescue (AuBMR) was explored in eleven children with GBM. The children were treated with myeloablative doses of BCNU, thiotepa, and etoposide, followed by AuBMR, and then were treated with 54Gy radiotherapy in standard fractions. There were 3 survivors (27%) at 2.9, 3.9, and 5.1 yr after treatment. One of these children developed non-Hodgkin's lymphoma 3.5 yr after treatment, 2 died of toxicity, and 6 died of their primary disease (22). In another trial conducted at relapse, the use of a high-dose thiotepa and etoposide regimen followed by AuBMR resulted in a 30% long-term disease control rate, although the children that did well had complete or near-complete surgical resections prior to treatment (23). A more recent report utilized high-dose induction chemotherapy in 21 children with high-grade gliomas (10 with glioblastoma, 9 with anaplastic astrocytoma, 2 with anaplastic oligodendroglioma). The location of these tumors was supratentorial in 17, spinal in 2, and posterior fossa in 2. Eighteen patients had residual disease after surgery. The induction therapy consisted of two courses of cisplatin (30 mg/m^2) plus etoposide (150 mg/m^2) × 3 d and vincristine (1.4 mg/m^2), cyclophosphamide (1.5 gm/m^2) and methotrexate (8 gm/m^2) followed by thiotepa (300 mg/m^2 × 3 doses), with harvesting of the peripheral stem cells after the first cisplatin and etoposide course. Following this induction, children were treated with involved-field irradiation and then were maintained on conventional doses of CCNU and vincristine. At a median of 57 mo, the overall survival was 43% and the progression-free survival was 46% *(24)*.

In adults, temozolomide has become part of the standard approach to the treatment of GBM and often used in the initial treatment of anaplastic astrocytomas and other glial neoplasms *(25)*. The efficacy of temozolomide in the setting of recurrent high-grade astrocytoma in childhood was explored in a multicenter, phase II trial. Patients were stratified on the basis of tumor location: supratentorial and cerebellar biopsy-proven grade III or IV astrocytoma (Arm A, *n* = 25) or diffuse, intrinsic brainstem glioma (Arm B, *n* = 18). Children were treated with 5 d of temozolomide at a dose of 200 mg/m^2/d and repeated every 28 d or when the bone marrow recovered. The response rate was 12% (95% confidence interval [CI] 2–31%) for patients in Arm A and 6% (95% CI 0–27%) in Arm B. Of the three responders in arm A, the duration of response was 7, 8, and 24+ mo, with a median survival of 4.7 mo. Of the children with brainstem tumors, there were no early responders but a partial response was seen in one patient after seven cycles. There were 3 additional patients with stable disease for 4, 6, and 28+ mo. If stable disease is taken into consideration the partial response and stable disease response rate was 22% (95% CI 6–48%) *(26)*. In a more recent study of 15 children with recurrent HGG, (including 7 with oligodendroglioma features) treated with temozolomide at a dose of 200 mg/m^2/d × 5 d, in 28 d cycles, the reported overall response rate was 20%, with a median progression-free survival of 2.0 mo (range 3 wk to 34+ mo) and a progression-free survival rate of 20% at 6 mo *(27)*.

MALIGNANT BRAINSTEM GLIOMAS
Clinical Considerations

Brainstem tumors account for 10 to 20% of all childhood brain tumors *(28)*. Before the introduction of the MRI, the certainty of correctly diagnosing a brainstem glioma was often in question. Even with CT, the technical limitations resulted in poor sensitivity to distinguish the myriad of tumors and other pathology in the posterior fossa. Not only was distinguishing the more malignant diffuse pontine glioma from the less aggressive focal pontine glioma uncertain, other diseases such as acute disseminated encephalomyelitis (ADEM) affecting the brainstem (also known as brainstem encephalitis) could mimic the clinical presentation and CT radiographic appearance of the diffuse pontine glioma. Therefore, the natural history of many of the brainstem tumors could not be defined until the late 1980s, and the validity of retrospective studies are questionable, because the current and more accurate methods of correct diagnosis could not be certain *(3–5)*. This discussion will focus on the diagnosis and treatment of the intrinsic pontine glioma and the intermediate grade gliomas in this region.

Clinical Presentation

The clinical presentation will depend on the exact location of the tumor within the brainstem, the rate of growth, and whether or not the flow of CSF is disturbed. In general, there is often involvement of individual or multiple cranial nerves, long-tract signs and disturbances of coordination. Bulbar symptoms, including swallowing and speech difficulties, are very common. If CSF flow is disrupted, headache and vomiting may occur, along with limitation of upgaze and alteration of motor tone. Exophytic lesions and those involving the cervicomedullary junction may not cause cranial nerve dysfunction early in the course of the illness, but tend to present with unsteadiness, nausea, and vomiting. Symptoms may develop over the course of days, or may stretch out for months or years. In general, gliomas of the posterior midbrain and tectal plate will present with macrocrania and symptoms of hydrocephalus. Depending on the extent of the lesion, impairment of upgaze and pupils that do not react to light (but will react to near accommodation) may also be present *(29)*.

General Neuroimaging Considerations

MRI generally allows for a rapid and usually accurate diagnosis. Because of the widespread availability of CT in emergency departments, some patients will come to diagnosis by way of CT, although this technique is generally inferior to MRI in terms of sensitivity and specificity. The CT appearance of the diffuse pontine glioma typically is a low-density lesion in the brainstem with associated compression and obliteration of the surrounding cisterns. The fourth ventricle is often distorted and displaced posteriorly, and obstructive hydrocephalus is common. There is little, if any, enhancement, even with HGG. Less frequently, the lower-grade gliomas affecting the brainstem are isodense or hyperdense and contain cystic areas. Exophytic portions of the tumor are only moderately well delineated on CT. If the diagnosis of a brainstem glioma is suspected by CT, the diagnosis should be confirmed with an MRI *(3–5)*.

The presence and extent of infiltrating brain stem gliomas is best seen with MRI. The higher-grade infiltrating gliomas are usually seen as masses with decreased signal intensities on T_1-weighted images and increased signal intensity lesions on T_2-weighted images. The tumors typically involve and expand the entire pons, and will often extend into the higher brainstem regions and beyond, as well as caudally into the medulla and upper cervical spinal cord. These tumors tend not to enhance with contrast agents, or do so only minimally. In some cases the tumor seems surprisingly demarcated and localized to one brain stem site, which is often associated with a less aggressive tumor *(3–5)*. Because the higher grade gliomas can disseminate early in the course of the disease, many centers are performing complete spinal cord MRIs with and without contrast at the time of diagnosis to investigate for leptomeningeal spread *(8,10–12,30–32)*.

Pathology Correlation By Means of Neuroimaging

The standard management of most brain tumors is deferred until after tissue has been obtained for pathologic examination. Although a biopsy can be safely performed on most brainstem tumors, their remains a risk and it is doubtful as to whether there is any benefit to the biopsy procedure given the excellent predictive value of the MRI. The principal prognostic factors found for patients with gliomas have been the location of the tumor and its histology; however, there is excellent correlation between the location and appearance of the tumor on MRI and the clinical course, obviating the need for pathologic examination. Several investigators have developed a proxy pathologic-pathophysiologic paradigm for brainstem gliomas based on the MRI appearance of the tumor.

The diffuse infiltrating pontine glioma has an aggressive course, even when the histology may suggest the tumor is a low-grade glioma in those patients that do undergo biopsy, suggesting a sampling effect. In general, infiltrating tumors in the upper portion of the brainstem, particularly those of the diencephalon and upper midbrain, tend to be lower grade and have longer survival following radiotherapy, when compared with the survival in patients with intrinsic pontine gliomas, but like the intrinsic pontine gliomas are not amenable to resection. In addition, there is no evidence to suggest improved survival with surgery for those with diffuse infiltrating tumors. Patients with cervicomedullary tumors, which may be intrinsic or

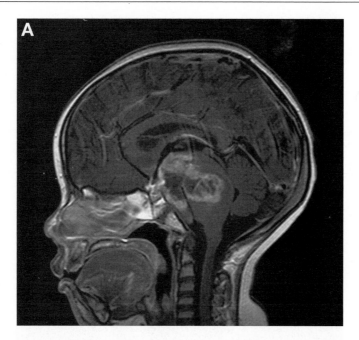

Fig. 1. These images show the typical MRI appearance of a patient with a diffuse pontine glioma. (**A**) Sagittal T1 with gadolinium. *(Continued on next page.)*

exophytic, tend to have a benign histology, usually that of a pilocytic astrocytoma; some can be cured with surgery alone although the routine use of surgery has been recently questioned. The focal brainstem and exophytic pontine gliomas have a variable degree of aggressiveness and debulking surgery followed by radiotherapy may lead to a longer survival, although the risk of worsening the neurologic function should be considered *(33–37)*.

Brainstem Malignant Glioma Subtypes

DIFFUSE INFILTRATING PONTINE GLIOMA

This tumor may occur at any age but is most common between 5 to 10 yr of age, and is distinctly uncommon before 2 yr of age *(38)*. The typical presentation of this tumor is a triad of cranial nerve palsies, ataxia, and cerebrospinal tract dysfunction. Most often the VIth and VIIth cranial nerves are involved (sometimes unilaterally), and the motor and cerebellar signs often involve contralateral limbs. Symptoms may be present for several weeks but some patients come to medical attention within hours of their first complaint. On occasion, signs and symptoms of hydrocephalus (headache, irritability, and limited upgaze) may be the factor that brings the patient to medical attention. The MRI (Fig. 1) appearance and clinical course for these tumors is quite typical and there is seldom a question of diagnosis. These tumors are hypointense on T1 weighted images and hyperintense on T2 weighted images. They may involve the entire pons and appear to expand the entire body of the affected portion of the brainstem. There may be patchy and variable enhancement of the mass, but often there is no enhancement. At times the tumor appears to wrap around the basilar artery. These tumors may have exophytic components, and may also invade through the cerebellar peduncles or extend up into the midbrain or down into the pons *(3–5,36)*. The routine evaluation of patients with

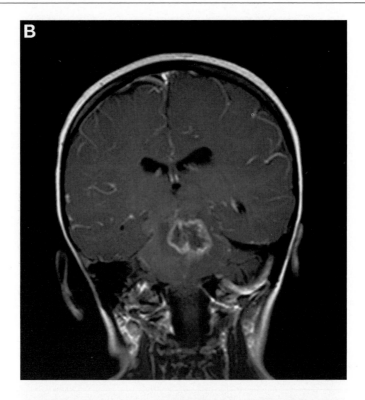

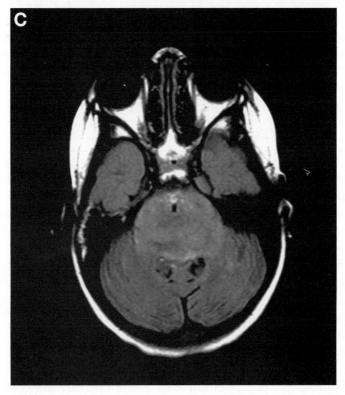

Fig. 1. *(Continued from previous page.)* **(B)** coronal T1 with gadolinium, **(C)** axial fluid-attenuated inversion recovery (FLAIR) image.

these tumors should include a complete spinal MRI to evaluate for leptomeningeal spread of tumor (LMS), which is not an uncommon finding *(32,33)*.

The initial neurologic symptoms often respond partially with the use of dexamethasone or another corticosteroid, although the improvement in function is temporary. The dose of steroids is not standardized and should be the minimal dose necessary to control symptoms. Children may require steroid therapy for weeks to months, therefore monitoring of blood pressure and blood sugar is recommended. Although not routinely practiced, the use of prophylactic antibiotic therapy (usually trimethoprim + sulfamethoxazole or pentamidine) may be considered for prevention of pneumocystis pneumonia. The risk of gastric ulceration needs to be considered, and although the use of proton pump inhibitors, H2-blockers, or buffering agents has not been proven to decrease the risk of ulceration, they are commonly used.

Approximately one-third of patients will present with symptomatic hydrocephalus, and either a shunting procedure or a third ventriculostomy should be considered. Asymptomatic or presymptomatic hydrocephalus is quite common and these children will need close monitoring during the initiation of therapy, as symptoms of progressive hydrocephalus can often mimic the side-effects of treatment *(2,33,39)*. The standard treatment for these tumors is focal radiotherapy with 1- to 2-cm margins around the tumor, usually at a dose of 4500 to 5500 cGy delivered daily in fractions of 180 to 200 cGy. There is a survival advantage to those children treated with more than 5000 cGy *(40)*. Most children have a clinical improvement and radiographic response following treatment. Even as the steroids are tapered, the neurological examination and MRI will improve, and occasionally return to normal. However, the median time to progression is about 6 mo, with the overall duration of survival in the range of 9 to 13 mo; approx 10% of patients are alive in a relapse-free state 18 mo after diagnosis *(2,6, 40)*.

Several treatment trials explored the use of hyperfractionated radiotherapy, using twice-daily (or thrice-daily) smaller radiation fractions (typically using 100 cGy doses in a bid regimen). The use of higher total treatment dosages may result in improved tumor control and survival rates. This technique also would take advantage of the fact that healthy brain tissue is better able to tolerate higher total dosages of radiotherapy if the individual dose fractions are smaller. Finally, the rapidly dividing tumor cells would not be able to repair DNA breaks during the time between dose fractions, whereas normal tissue (the relatively nonprofilerating neurons, glial, and endothelial cells of the brain) would be relatively spared the damaging effects of this treatment. The Children's Cancer Group treated 66 children with 7800 cGy of hyperfractionated radiotherapy in 100 cGy bid fractions. This treatment was well tolerated. Unfortunately the 1-yr survival rate of 35% and 3-yr survival rate of 11% was no different than historical controls *(41)*. The Pediatric Oncology Group conducted a similar study of 136 children treated with either 6600 cGy, 7020 cGy, or 7560 cGy in 110 cGy bid fractions, and had similar disappointing results. The 1-yr survival was 47% and the 2-yr survival was 6%, with the median time to progression of 6.5 mo *(42)*. In yet another study, the total treatment doses of 64.8, 66, 72, and 78 Gy were given using a similar bid fraction scheme. The response rate using hyperfractionated radiotherapy ranged from 62 to 77% but did not result in improvement in time to disease progression or impact on ultimate survival *(43,44)*. Because none of these studies altered the outcome of this disease, at this time the standard radiotherapy treatment consists of daily (5 d/wk) fractions of 180 to 200 cGy with a total treatment dose of about 5400 cGy. Because of the high risk of radiation necrosis, there is not a role for stereotactic radiosurgery, such as would be delivered by the Gamma Knife or Linac-based radiosurgical method.

Chemotherapy

Numerous trials of chemotherapy, used either in an adjuvant or neo-adjuvant setting have not demonstrated benefit. Most of the earlier trials involved single or multiple agents in a phase II setting. More recent studies have involved the use of neo-adjuvant chemotherapy or concurrent chemotherapy and/or radiation sensitizers with irradiation. Although results from some of these trials were initially encouraging, the final results have been uniformly disappointing as well *(44,45,47–50)*.

Etoposide (VP-16) was used to treat 12 patients at the time of tumor progression, and demonstrated a remarkable 50% response rate, which was durable for a median of 8 mo. The dosing of etoposide was a conventional regimen (50 mg/m^2/d × 21 d with 14 d of rest between cycles). All patients had received prior radiotherapy at diagnosis *(51)*. Subsequent studies using various agents have failed to show consistent results and to date there is no standard relapse therapy given to patients with this tumor.

The Children's Cancer Group conducted a randomized trial of two different arms of intensive pre-irradiation chemotherapy followed by hyperfactionated radiotherapy. Children were randomly assigned to receive three courses of carboplatin, etoposide, and vincristine (arm A, $n = 32$), or cisplatin, etoposide, cyclophosphamide, and vincristine (arm B, $n = 31$). Granulocyte colony-stimulating factor was used in both arms. Following chemotherapy, both groups received 7200 cGy of radiation in 100 cGy bid fractions. The radiographic response rate to the chemotherapy was $10 \pm 5\%$ in arm A and $18 \pm 9\%$ in arm B. Event-free survival was $17 \pm 5\%$ at 1 yr and $6 \pm 3\%$ at 2 yr. Although those children that responded to the chemotherapy had a longer survival, the authors concluded that neither chemotherapy regimen meaningfully improved response rate, event-free survival, or overall survival *(52)*.

In a study using standard dose radiotherapy (54–60 Gy in 1.5–1.8 Gy/d daily fractions) and high-dose tamoxifen (200 mg/m^2/d) the median survival was 10.3 mo, with a 1-yr survival rate of $37.0 \pm 9.5\%$, which the authors conclude did not improve the prognosis for this tumor *(53)*.

The most intensive chemotherapy regimen has employed high-dose chemotherapy with autologous bone marrow rescue, which failed to improve survival for children with this tumor *(54)*.

Effective therapy for the intrinsic pontine glioma has remained one of the most elusive in neurooncology. Most investigators conclude that the standard approach to treating these tumors begins with staging of the tumor and if contained to the pons, treating with standard dose radiotherapy delivered in a single daily fraction to the tumor plus a 1- to 2-cm margin. Leptomeningeal dissemination is present in one-third of children at diagnosis and if identified at diagnosis, or at any time in the illness, radiotherapy can be used with a palliative attempt to treat the involved areas. Although there is no evidence that neoadjunctive or adjunctive chemotherapy prolongs the time to relapse, the use of low-dose etoposide or experimental agents may be considered at relapse. The survival in patients with this particular tumor has not improved in the last several decades despite escalating both radiation and cytotoxic chemotherapy dosing to the maximum tolerated levels. Further advances will likely require a unique chemotherapeutic agent or biological agent.

Dorsal Exophytic Brainstem Tumors

Dorsal exophytic brainstem gliomas are a distinct subgroup of neoplasms that account for 20% of all brainstem tumors. They generally have a relatively benign histology and slow growth characteristics, and do not carry the near universal dismal prognosis seen in the intrinsic pontine gliomas. However, some do have higher grade histology, but do not share the same dismal prognosis of the intrinsic pontine glioma.

These tumors may present in early infancy and generally appear before puberty. They most often grow out of the floor of the fourth ventricle and into the ventricle itself, as opposed to invading the brainstem. The tumor may obstruct the flow of CSF. The MRI appearance is hypointense on T1 and hyperintense on T2, but unlike the more malignant intrinsic pontine glioma, these tumors have sharp borders and enhance intensely with contrast. And unlike many other brainstem tumors, they are sometimes amenable to surgical excision with a positive outlook *(55)*.

Symptoms can be insidious, and patients may have a mild set of symptoms for months or years before the diagnosis is made. The initial symptoms may be caused by intermittent obstruction of CSF flow. Occasional vomiting and failure to thrive without overt neurologic signs may result in prolonged evaluations by specialists without correct diagnosis. Because of the location, the child may have only mild or intermittent cranial nerve paresis, and may not have any pyramidal tract findings unless the tumor is invasive. Symptoms will vary by age, with failure to thrive and chronic vomiting seen in infants, whereas older patients present with a combination of headache, vomiting, and ataxia *(4)*.

The treatment for these tumors is primarily surgical, although a complete surgical excision is usually not feasible because there is not a plane between the tumor and brainstem. In addition, the tumor can invade a large area of the brainstem surface, in which case only the exophytic component can be removed. CSF flow may be re-established with successful debulking, but if this is not possible a ventriculo-peritoneal shunt or third ventriculostomy will be necessary.

These tumors most often have a low-grade glial histology and tend to be grade I or grade II astrocytomas. However, higher grade astrocytomas and gangliogliomas have been reported and therefore surgical consideration needs to be considered with each patient. The small percentage of tumors that recur typically remain histologically benign and are amenable to repeat tumor excision. Following a surgical excision, even if there is remaining tumor, it is reasonable to withhold radiotherapy or other treatments in favor of expectant observation with interval MR imaging and examinations *(55–57)*.

Radiation therapy has been generally reserved for patients with either HGG or progression that is not amenable to repeat surgery. For those patients with high-grade neoplasms, it is recommended that surveillance MRI of the spine be performed to properly stage the patient's disease. Unless there is evidence of tumor spread, involved-field radiotherapy using standard dose and dose-fractions is recommended *(55–57)*.

Brainstem Tumors and Neurofibromatosis Type I

Gliomas are far more common in persons with neurofibromatosis type 1 (NF-1) than in the general population. Although most of these tumors occur along the visual pathway (i.e., optic nerves, optic chiasm with or without hypothalamic involvement, and extending into the optic tracks) and most of these are low-grade gliomas, some gliomas may occur in the brainstem and have higher grade histology *(58)*. It is both difficult and important to distinguish true neoplasm from the *focal areas of signal intensity* that are commonly found in children with NF1. These *focal areas of signal intensity*, which are bright on both FLAIR and T2 weighted images, are common in the deep gray masses, the brainstem and cerebellum, and may have some mass effect. These MRI abnormalities are often found on surveillance scanning or on scanning performed for clinical problems unrelated to brainstem function. In most instances, observation with repeated examinations and repeated imaging is all that is necessary. However, if the child does have progressive neurologic signs related to the area of involvement, surgical biopsy for confirmation and either chemotherapy, radiotherapy, or both would be indicated for malignant pathology. Children with NF1 and intrinsic brainstem masses have a better prognosis than the typical child with a pontine glioma *(58–61)*.

Malignant Glioma of the Spinal Cord

As with adults, malignant gliomas of the spinal cord are rare. The natural history is not well defined but these tend to be as aggressive as their corresponding tumors in the brain. The standard treatment involves confirmation by biopsy and surgical resection if possible. Following staging with brain and spine MRI, standard dose radiotherapy is considered the standard of care. In a Children's Cancer Group study, 18 children with malignant glioma of the spinal cord were treated with maximal surgical resection, followed by 2 cycles of 8-in-1 chemotherapy, standard involved-field radiotherapy, and then 8 additional cycles of 8-in-1 chemotherapy. The histology of these tumors included 4 GBM, 8 anaplastic astrocytomas, 1 mixed malignant gliomas, and 5 with discordant malignant glioma pathology. The surgical results included six with gross-total or near-total resections, four with partial or subtotal resections, and three with biopsy only. Leptomeningeal spread of tumor was identified in six of these children at the time of diagnosis. The 5-yr PFS as $46 \pm 14\%$. Seven of 13 of the children (54%) were alive at a median of 76 mo (51–93 months) from the end of treatment *(62)*.

CONCLUSIONS

As with adults, the successful treatment of malignant gliomas in children remains elusive. Aggressive attempts at surgical resection and radiotherapy are the backbone of treatment, with chemotherapy as a helpful adjunct in the nonbrainstem high-grade gliomas. There is a survival advantage for those patients that do undergo successful gross-total or near-total resections of their tumors, and there does seem to be a survival advantage if chemotherapy is added to radiotherapy as opposed to radiotherapy alone. For the intrinsic pontine glioma standard irradiation offers the most tolerable treatment, and more intense therapy has not been shown to be helpful. Treatment using high-dose chemotherapy with bone marrow or stem cell rescue has not resulted in any long-term benefit in terms of duration of survival in any of these patients. As with adult gliomas, insights into the molecular mechanisms of tumor pathogenesis and treatments designed to alter these mechanisms may result in better treatments.

REFERENCES

1. Leviton, A. Principles of Epidemiology. In: Cohen ME, Duffner PK, eds. Brain Tumors in Children. Principles of Diagnosis and Treatment 2nd Edition. Raven Press:New York, 1994:27–49.
2. Bruce H. Cohen and James Garvin: Brain Tumors. In: Rudolph, Hoffman, Rudolph, eds.Roudolph's Pediatrics, 21st Edition., Appleton & Lange:Stamford, 2002.
3. Fischbein NJ, Prados MD, Wara W, Russo C, Edwards MSB, Barkovich AJ. Radiologic classification of brain stem tumors: correlation of magnetic resonance imaging appearance and clinical outcome. Pediatr Neurosurg 1996;24:9–23.
4. Zimmerman, RA. Neuroimaging of pediatric brain stem diseases other than brain stem glioma. Pediatr Neurosurg 1996;25:83–92.
5. Packer RJ, Zimmerman RA, Luerssen TG, Sutton LN, Bilaniuk LT, Bruce DA, Schut L. Brainstem gliomas of childhood: magnetic resonance imaging. Neurology 1985;35:397–401.
6. Panitch ES, Berg BO. Brainstem tumors of childhood and adolescence. Am J Dis Child 1970;119:465–467.
7. Albright AL, Guthkelch AN, Packer RJ, et al. Prognostic factors in pediatric brain-stem Gliomas. J Neurosurg 1986;65:751–755.
8. Packer RJ. Brain Tumors in Children (Neurological Review). Arch Neurol 1999;56:421–425.

9. Rickert CH, Sträter R, Kaatsch P et al. Pediatric high-grade astrocytomas show chromosomal imbalances distinct from adult cases. Am J Pathol 2001;158:1525–1532.

10. Principles of Clinical Diagnosis. In :Cohen ME, Duffner PK, eds. Brain Tumors in Children. Principles of Diagnosis and Treatment. Raven Press: New York, 1984:9–21.

11. Dohrmann GJ, Farwell JR, Flannery JY. Glioblastoma multiforme in children. J Neurosurg 1976;44: 442–448.

12. Wisoff JH, Boyett JM, Berger MS, et al. Current neurosurgical management and the impact of the extent of resection in the treatment of malignant gliomas of childhood: a report of the Children's Cancer Group trial no. CCG-945. J Neruosurg 1998;89(1):52–59.

13. Finlay JL, Wisoff JH. The impact of extent of resection in the management of malignant gliomas of childhood. Shild Nerv Sys 1999;15(11–12):786–788.

14. Bloom HJ, Glees J, Bell J, Ashley SE, Gorman C. The treatment and long-term prognosis of children with intracranial tumors: a study of 610 cases, 1950–1981.[erratum appears in]. Int J Radiat Oncol Biol Phys 1990;18(4):723–45; erratum, Int J Radiat Oncol Biol Phys 1990;19(3):829.

15. Marchese MJ. Chang CH. Malignant astrocytic gliomas in children. Cancer 1990;65(12):2771–2778

16. Dropcho EJ, Wisoff JH, Walker RW, Allen JC. Supratentorial malignant gliomas in childhood: a review of fifty cases. Ann Neurol 1987;22(3):355–364.

17. Bloom HJ. Intracranial tumors: response and resistance to therapeutic endeavors, 1970–1980. Int J Radiat Oncol Biol Phys 1982;8(7):1083–1113

18. Sheline GE. Radiation therapy of brain tumors. Cancer 1977;39(2):873–81.

19. Packer RJ, Vezina G, Nicholson HS, Chadduck WM. Childhood and Adolescent Gliomas. In: Berger MS, Wilson CD, eds. The Gliomas. Philadelphia:Saunders, 1999;689–701.

20. Sposto R, Ertel IM, Jenkin RDT, et al. The effectiveness of chemotherapy for treatment of high-grade astrocytoma in children: results of a randomize trial. J Neurooncol 1989;7:165–171.

21. Finlay J, Boyett J, Yates A, et al. Randomized phase III trial in childhood high-grade astrocytomas comparing vincristine, lomustine and prednisone with eight-drug-in-one-day regimen. J Clin Oncol 1995;13:112–123.

22. Grovas AC, Boyett JM, Lindsley K, Rosenblum M, Yates AJ, Finlay JL. Regimen-related toxicity of myeloablative chemotherapy with BCNU, thiotepa, and etoposide followed by autologous stem cell rescue for children with newly diagnosed glioblastoma multiforme: report from the Children's Cancer Group. Med Pediatr Oncol 1999;33(2):83–87.

23. Finlay JL, Goldman S, Wong MC, et al. Pilot study of high-dose thiotepa and etoposide with autologous bone marrow rescue in children and young adults with recurrent CNS tumors. J Clin Oncol 1996;14:2495–2503.

24. Massimino M, Gandola L, Luksch R, et al. Sequential chemotherapy, high-dose thiotepa, circulating progenitor cell rescue, and radiotherapy for childhood high-grade glioma. Neuro Oncol 2005;7(1):41–48.

25. Stupp R, Mason WP, van den Bent MJ, et al. European Organization for Research and Treatment of Cancer Brain Tumor and Radiotherapy Groups. National Cancer Institute of Canada Clinical Trials Group. Radiotherapy plus concomitant and adjuvant temozolomide for glioblastoma. N Engl J Med 2005;352(10):987–996

26. Lashford LS, Thiesse P, Jouvet A, et al. Temozolomide in malignant gliomas of childhood: A United Kingdom Children's Cancer Study Group and French Society for Pediatric Oncology Intragroup Study. J Clin Oncol 2002;20:4684–4691.

27. Verschuur AC, Grill J, Lelouch-Tubiana A, Couanet D, Kalifa C, Vassal G. Temozolomide in paediatric high-grade glioma: a key for combination therapy? Br J Cancer 2004;91:425–429.

28. Farwell JR, Dohrmann GJ, Flannery JT. Central nervous system tumors in children. Cancer 1977;40:3123–3132.

29. Brain Stem Tumors. In: Cohen ME, Duffner PK, eds. Brain Tumors in Children. Principles of Diagnosis and Treatment, 2nd Edition. New York:Raven Press, 1994:241–262.

30. Donahue B, Allen J, Siffert J, Rosovsky M, Pinto R. Patterns of recurrence in brain stem gliomas: evidence for craniospinal dissemination. Int J Radiat Oncol Biol Phys 1998;40(3):677–680.

31. Packer RJ, Allen J, Nielsen S, Petito C, Deck M, Jereb B. Brainstem glioma: clinical manifestations of meningeal gliomatosis. Ann Neuro 1983;14:177–182.

32. Motoyama Y, Ogi S, Nabeshima S. Pontine glioblastoma multiforme initially presenting with leptomeningeal gliomatosis. Neurol Med Chir 2002;42(7):309–313.

33. Packer RJ. Brain tumors in children. Arch Neurol 1999;56(4):421–425.

34. Cartmill M, Punt J. Brain stem gliomas, the role of biopsy. Br J Neurosurg 1997;11:177.

35. Albright AL. Diffuse brainstem tumors. When is a biopsy necessary? Pediatric Neurosurg 1996;24:252–255.

36. Albright AL, Packer RJ, Zimmerman R, et al. Magnetic resonance scans should replace biopsies for the diagnosis of diffuse brain stem Gliomas: a report from the Children's Cancer Group. Neurosurgery 1993;33:1026–1030.
37. Epstein F. McCleary EL. Intrinsic brain-stem tumors of childhood: surgical indications J Neurosurg 1986;64:11–15.
38. Cohen BH, Packer RJ, Siegel KR, et al. Brain tumors in children under two years: Treatment, survival and long-term prognosis. Pediatr Neurosurg 1993;19(4):171–179.
39. Bruce H. Cohen and James Garvin: Brain Tumors. In: Rudolph, Hoffman, Rudolph, eds. Roudolph's Pediatrics, 21th Edition. Stamford: Appleton & Lange, 2002.
40. Packer,RJ, Nicholson SH, Venzina FL, Johnson DL. Brainstem gliomas. Neurosurg Clini N Am 1992;3: 863–880.
41. Packer RJ, Boyett JM, Zimmerman RA, et al. Outcome of children with brain stem gliomas after treatment with 7800 cGy of hyperfractionated radiotheapy. Cancer 1994;74:1827–1834.
42. Freeman CR, Krischer J, Sanford RA, et al. Hyperfractionated radiotherapy in brainstem tumor: results of a Pediatric Oncology Group Study. Int J Radiat Oncol Biol Phys 1998;15:311–318.
43. Packer RJ, Boyett JM, Zimmerman RA et al. Hyperfractionated radiation therapy (72 Gy) for children with brain stem gliomas: A Children's Cancer Group phase I/II trial. Cancer 1993;72:1414–1421.
44. Packer RJ, Boyett JM, Zimmerman RA, et al. Brain stem gliomas of childhood: outcome after treatment with 7800 cGy or hyperfractionated radiotherapy: a Children's Cancer Group phase I/II trial. Cancer 1994;74: 1827–1834.
45. Jennings MT, Freeman ML, Murray MJ. Strategies in the treatment of diffuse pontine gliomas: the therapeutic role of hyperfractionated radiotherapy and chemotherapy. J Neurooncol 1996;28:207–222.
46. Lashford LS, Thiesse P, Jouvet A, et al. Temozolomide in malignant gliomas of childhood: A United Kingdom Children's Cancer Study Group and French Society for Pediatric Oncology Intergroup Study. J Clin Oncol 2002;20(24):4684–4691.
47. Freeman CR, Kepner J, Kun LE, et al. A detrimental effect of a combined chemotherapy-radiotherapy approach in children with diffuse intrinsic brain stem gliomas?. Int J Rad Oncol Biol Phys 2000;47(3):561–564.
48. Allen J, Siffert J, Donahue B, et al. A phase I/II study of carboplatin combined with hyperfractionated radiotherapy for brainstem gliomas. Cancer 1999;86(6):1064–1069.
49. Kaplan AM, Albright AL, Zimmerman RA, et al. Brainstem gliomas in children. A Children's Cancer Group review of 119 cases. Pediatr Neurosurg 1996;24(4):185–192.
50. Marcus, K., Dutton, S., Barnes, P., et al. A phase I trial of etandizole and hyperfractionated radiotherapy in children with diffuse brainstem glioma. Intern J Radiat Oncol Biol Physics 2003;55:1182–1185.
51. Chamberlain MC. Recurrent brainstem gliomas treated with oral VP-16. J Neurooncol 1993;15(2):133–139.
52. Jennings MT, Sposto R, Boyett JM, et al. Preradiation chemotherapy in primary high-risk brainstem tumors: phase II study CCG-9941 of the Children's Cancer Group. J Clin Oncol 2002;20:3431–3437.
53. Broniscer A, Leite C, Lanchote V, Machado T, Cristofani L, and the Brainstem Glioma Cooperative Group. Radiation therapy and high-dose tamoxifen in the treatment of patients with diffuse brainstem gliomas: results of a Brazilian cooperative study. J Clin Oncol 2000;18:1246–1253.
54. Dunkel IJ, Finlay JL. High-dose chemotherapy with autologous stem cell rescue for brain tumors. Crit Rev Oncol Hematol 2002;41(2):197–204.
55. Pollack IF, Hoffman HJ, Jumphreys RP, Becker L. The longterm outcome after surgical treatment of dorsally exophytic brain-stem gliomas. J Neurosurg 1993;78:859–863.
56. Pollack IF, Pang D, Albright AL. The long-term outcome in children with late onset aqueduct stenosis resulting from benign intrinsic tectal tumors. J Neurosurg 1994;80:681–688.
57. Hoffman HJ. Dorsally exophyic brain stem tumors and midbrain tumors. Pediatr Neurosurg 1996;24:256–262.
58. Hughes RAC. Neurological complications of neurofibromatosis 1. In: Huson SM, Hughes RAC, eds. The neurofibromatoses. A pathogenetic and clinical overview. London:Chapman & Hall Medical, 1994;204–222.
59. Bilaniuk LT, Molloy PT, Zimmerman RA, et al. Neurofibromatosis type 1: brain stem tumours. Neuroradiology 1997;39(9):642–653.
60. Pollack IF, Shultz B, Mulvihill JJ. The management of brainstem gliomas in patients with neurofibromatosis 1. Neurology 1996;46:1652–1660.
61. Rosser T, Packer RJ. Intracranial neoplasms in children with neurofibromatosis. J Child Neurol 2002;17:630–637.
62. Allen JC, Aviner S, Yates AJ, et al. Treatment of high-grade spinal cord astrocytoma of childhood with "8-in-1" chemotherapy and radiotherapy: a pilot study of CCG-945. Children's Cancer Group. J Neurosurg 1998; 88(2):215–220.

4 Adult High-Grade Glioma

Nicholas Butowski and Susan Chang

Summary

Why adults develop high-grade gliomas (HGG) is still unknown. These aggressive tumors may present in a number of ways, depending on such factors as growth rate and anatomic location. Whereas standard histopathological and epidemiological studies have helped us categorize patients with HGG into risk groups, treatment results for most patients are still unsatisfactory. An improved epidemiological understanding of brain tumors in conjunction with continued advances in the use of molecular markers will hopefully lead to better treatment and prevention strategies. This chapter serves as an introduction into the epidemiology of HGG and their associated risk factors. We also present the neurological signs and symptoms that a glioma may cause, and the prognostic factors used for estimating survival.

Key Words: Glioblastoma; brain tumor; glioma; epidemiology.

INTRODUCTION

This chapter is an introduction to the clinical characteristics of adult high-grade glioma (HGG). Included within the designation of high-grade or malignant gliomas are anaplastic astrocytoma (AA), glioblastoma multiforme (GBM), anaplastic oligodendroglioma (AO), anaplastic oligoastrocytoma (AOA), and anaplastic ependymoma. The discussion below reviews relevant epidemiologic data and risk factors for developing HGG. Also reviewed are the general and focal neurological signs and symptoms that a glioma may cause and the prognostic factors used for estimating survival.

EPIDEMIOLOGY

HGG are the most common primary central nervous system (CNS) neoplasms. They also continue to be among the top ten causes of cancer-related deaths despite a relatively low incidence when compared with other cancers. According to the American Cancer Society, an estimated 17,000 new cases of primary malignant brain tumor were diagnosed in 2002 in the United States (9600 in males and 7400 in females) *(1)*. This represents 1.3% of all cancers diagnosed in 2002; however, an estimated 13,100 deaths in 2002 were attributed to primary malignant brain tumors, approx 2% of cancer-related deaths in the US *(1)*.

The incidence rate of primary malignant brain tumor is 6.4 cases/100,000 person-yr. This rate is higher in males (7.6/100,000 person-yr) than females (5.4/100,000 person-yr) *(2)*. The global incidence rate of primary malignant brain tumor is 3.6/100,000 person-yr in males and 2.5/100,000 person-yr in females. The incidence rates are higher in more developed countries

From: *Current Clinical Oncology: High-Grade Gliomas: Diagnosis and Treatment*
Edited by: G. H. Barnett © Humana Press Inc., Totowa, NJ

(males: 5.9/ 100,000 person-yr; females: 4.1/100,000 person-yr) than in less developed countries (males: 2.8/100,000 person-yr; females: 2.0/100,000 person-yr). The prevalence rate for primary malignant brain tumors is 29.5/100,000 persons. It is estimated that in the United States more than 81,000 persons are living with a diagnosis of primary malignant brain tumor *(3)*.

Recently, some have questioned whether brain tumor incidence is increasing. Review and comparison across time periods or across studies is difficult because of such problems as diagnostic discrepancies and ascertainment bias in registry data. Nonetheless, after extensive review, this apparent increase is thought to be to the result of many factors including better diagnostic procedures, better access to medical care, and better care for the elderly, all leading to greater detection rather than an actual increased incidence *(4,5)*. Nevertheless, more uniform and unbiased diagnosis and registration methods must become accepted and employed before this issue is truly resolved.

Age, Gender, Ethnicity, and Geography

Whereas a malignant glioma can occur at any age, the average age of onset for glioblastoma is 62 yr *(2)*. In general, gliomas affect males 40% more frequently than females *(6)*. According to a recent study, this greater incidence of glioblastoma in males becomes evident around the age of menarche, is greatest around the age of menopause, and then decreases, suggesting a possible protective effect provided by female hormones *(7)*, though such a protective effect is merely speculation.

Glioma incidence data is subject to variations in diagnostic and reporting techniques amongst different ethnicities or geographic regions. As stated previously, brain-tumor incidence tends to be higher in countries with more developed medical care; however, this is not always the case. For example, the incidence rate for malignant brain tumors in Japan is less than half of that in Northern Europe *(5)*. In the United States, gliomas are more common in Caucasians than in African Americans, non-white Hispanics, Chinese, Japanese, and Filipinos *(5)*. These dissimilarities are hard to attribute exclusively to differences in access to health care or diagnostic practices. Conceivably, incidence is affected by genetics in a manner that has yet to be exposed. Chen et al. showed that among adults with astrocytic glioma of any grade, tumors from Caucasians had different spectra of genetic abnormalities when compared with non-Caucasian patients *(8)*. Such discoveries warrant further research into the possible implications of differences in genetics amongst races playing a significant role in tumorogenesis.

Risk Factors

Research into the etiology and possible contributing causes of gliomas is ongoing, but is hindered by many factors including the relative rarity of the disease and rapid death of patients with aggressive subtypes. As such, studies to date have revealed little with regard to specific causal factors. High-dose therapeutic ionizing radiation to the head, administered for benign conditions or for cancer treatment, has been shown to increase the risk of glioma as well as meningioma and nerve sheath tumors *(9)*.

Other established risk factors include the hereditary genetic syndromes listed in Table 1. These syndromes explain less than 5% of glioma cases. Outside of these known genetic syndromes, information on familial aggregation is indefinite at best. There does seem to be a slightly increased incidence of glioma in first-degree relatives, and a gender predominance

Table 1
Hereditable Genetic Syndromes

Syndrome	Gene affected	CNS lesion	Chromosome
Li-Fraumeni syndrome	p53	Malignant glioma	17q
Neurofibromatosis 1	NF1	Glioma of optic pathway/brainstem	17q11
Neurofibromatosis 2	NF2	Acoustic neuroma, meningioma	22q12
Tuberous sclerosis	TSC1, TSC 2	Subependymal giant cell astrocytoma, cortical tuber	9q34, 16p13.3
Von-Hippel-Lindau	VHL	Hemangioblastoma of cerebellum/spine	3p25
Turcot's syndrome	APC	Glioblastoma multiforme, medulloblastoma	5q21
Retinoblastoma	RB1	Pineoblastoma	13q14
Gorlin's Syndrome	PTCH	Medulloblastoma	9q22.3
Lhermitte-Duclos/ Cowden	PTEN	gangliocytoma of cerebellum	10q23.2

with malignant gliomas being more common in males than females; however, a well-defined mode of inheritance is not readily evident. Several "glioma families" have been followed over time, but the pattern of inheritance is indistinct as tumors seem to skip generations, have variable times of onset and, in parent-child pairs, the child is often diagnosed before the parent *(10)*. Various segregation analyses of familial glioma favor an autosomal recessive mode of inheritance, but a multifactorial model was not rejected and deserves further analysis *(11)*. Additionally, other segregation analyses favor a polygenic model. Armed with this information, investigators have initiated studies of genetic polymorphisms that, when coupled with certain environmental exposures, may lead to brain tumors. Unfortunately, several studies of genetic alterations involved in oxidative metabolism, DNA stability and repair, and immune response have led to conflicting reports *(5)*. Clearly, more precise explanations of the etiologic and therapeutic relevance of this information continue to be hindered by low incidence of disease, and await further studies.

Numerous noninherited risk factors also have been examined in relation to brain tumors. For example, there have been several studies suggesting a possible role of the immune system in tumorogenesis. For instance, people who received polio vaccines contaminated with the SV40 virus have been shown to be at increased risk of developing glioma, though other studies have failed to support this claim *(5)*. Viral antigens from JC virus and human herpes virus 6 have been detected in brain tumor subtypes, but their possible etiologic role is unclear *(12,13)*. Nucleic acids and proteins from human cytomegalovirus (hCMV) have also been found in HGG *(14)*. Intriguingly, other studies have indicated that prior infection with vermicelli zoster may decrease glioma risk. Likewise, there appears to be an inverse association of allergic diseases (e.g., asthma, eczema, general allergy) with glioma, further suggesting an immunologic role in the formation of glioma *(5)*. Of course, more study is needed to elaborate the potential role of viruses, allergic diseases, and allergy medicines in brain tumor development.

Another area of concern discussed in the popular media is that of a possible risk from exposure to electromagnetic fields through power lines. To date, the overwhelming amount of evidence does not support any such relationship *(15,16)*. However, there continues to be anecdotal concern over such matters fueled by increased exposure to radio frequency involved in the increased use of handheld phones and wireless radio devices. Again, numerous studies fail to indicate a causal relationship *(17,18)*. In fact, a recent case-control study found no relationship between brain cancer mortality and radiofrequency exposure *(19)*. Of course, the effects of long-term exposure remain to be determined. Another area of popular concern is the possible association between head trauma and brain tumor risk. To date, no correlation between head trauma and glioma has been supported. In fact, a recent study comparing adult patients with glioma and a history of head injury requiring medical attention with controlled patients failed to support an association during an average of eight years of follow up *(20)*. However, there was a slight increased risk in the first year following the injury that the authors attributed to increased detection. This leaves a measure of uneasiness about unequivocally denying an association between head trauma and brain-tumor development.

Studies of diet, vitamins, alcohol, tobacco, and environmental exposures have revealed little information about the cause of glioma. Nitrate exposure from cured meats likely does not influence brain-tumor development *(5)*. However, reliable assessment of true exposure to nitrates is difficult, mainly because of widespread potential exposure through tobacco smoke and cosmetics, not to mention the endogenous digestive exposure. Although tobacco is a nearly ubiquitous environmental source of carcinogens, studies have not supported a role in developing a brain tumor *(21)*. Alcohol consumption does not seem to increase one's risk of developing a glioma, and may actually decrease risk *(22)*. Lastly, little to no significant association with increased brain-tumor risk has been found with exposure to pesticides, synthetic rubber, or agents known to be carcinogens, including vinyl chloride and petrochemicals *(5)*.

CLINICAL PRESENTATION

Symptoms or signs of brain tumors are produced by the tumor mass, the adjacent edema, or the infiltration and destruction of normal tissue. However, these symptoms and signs and are best appreciated by considering the tumor location and growth rate. For example, rapidly growing tumors located in eloquent cortex or along the ventricular system may manifest after only a small amount of growth. Those in less eloquent areas of the brain may manifest only after substantial growth. Moreover, no specific sign or symptom is pathognomonic for a brain tumor.

Brain tumors can cause either "generalized" or "focal" neurological dysfunction. Included within the "generalized" grouping are those signs and symptoms related to increased intracranial pressure (ICP) and seizures. Increases in ICP may result from cerebral edema (damage to brain tissue from tumor infiltration), vasogenic edema (produced by leakage of the blood-brain barrier), obstruction of cerebrospinal fluid (CSF) flow, or obstruction of venous flow. Under these conditions, the patient may develop headache, nausea, vomiting, lassitude, and visual abnormalities like papilledema or diplopia. An acute rise in ICP (as caused by blockage of CSF pathways or hemorrhage into the tumor) may cause a sudden onset of these symptoms accompanied by a significant change in level of alertness. If elevations in ICP go untreated, patients may develop herniation. There are three general types of herniation: tentorial, tonsillar, and subfalcine.

Tentorial herniation involves displacement of the uncus over the edge of the tentorium cerebelli, with resulting compression of the third cranial nerve producing an ipsilaterally dilated pupil. As displacement continues, the midbrain is pushed away from the displaced hemisphere, resulting in the contralateral cerebral peduncle being pressed up against the tentorium. The injury to the cerebral peduncle, also known as Kernohan's notch, results in hemiparesis on the same side of the body as the tumor; this is often referred to as a false localizing sign. If untreated, further downward and medial displacement of the hemisephere through the tentorial opening compresses the posterior cerebral artery, resulting in an infarct of the occipital lobe with consequent contralateral homonymous hemianopsia.

Tonsillar herniation entails downward displacement of the cerebellar tonsils through the foramen magnum, with consequent compression of the brainstem and cervical spine. Patients may complain of neck stiffness or pain and tilt their head to one side to help reduce discomfort. If untreated, the patient may develop respiratory or cardiac abnormalities.

Subfalcine herniation, also known as cingulate herniation, occurs when the medial part of the hemisphere is pushed beneath the edge of the falx cerebri. This action generally results in damage to or ischemia of the cingulate lobe and medial motor cortex and therefore manifests itself with contralateral lower-limb weakness and urinary incontinence.

Headache occurs in approx 50% of patients with brain tumors (23). The headaches usually are not severe and are classically more noticeable in the morning, tend to improve later in the day, and worsen with coughing, straining, or another activity that may increase ICP. A unilateral headache indicates the side of the lesion approx 80% of the time. Headaches can occur in brain-tumor patients without an increase in ICP, and are subsequently thought to be a result of traction on pain-sensitive structures such as the meninges or blood vessels. Of course, headache is a nonspecific symptom occurring in most people as the result of many causes other than a brain tumor. As such, one should always consider other possible reasons why a patient may experience a headache. Furthermore, remember that the most distinguishing feature of a brain-tumor headache is its association with other neurological signs such as personality changes, motor deficits, or seizures.

The incidence of seizures at presentation of a brain tumor varies with histological subtype, ranging from 90% in patients with low-grade gliomas to 35% of patients with GBM (24). Seizures may occur during the clinical course in approx 30% of patients with any sort of brain tumor, which is why many patients are prophylactically treated with anti-seizure medicine. However, randomized controlled studies have demonstrated that prophylactic anticonvulsants are unlikely to be useful in brain-tumor patients who have not had a seizure (25). Whether and what type of seizure a tumor will produce depend on the location and growth rate of the tumor. Seizures are more frequent when the tumor is cortical and slow growing (26). Several commonly used anticonvulsants (e.g., Dilantin, Tegretol, and phenobarbital) induce hepatic enzymes and thus may lower the blood levels of a variety of medicines used as palliative or chemotherapeutic agents. This point must be considered when designing and evaluating the efficacy and toxicity of treatment regimens. As with headaches, other etiologies need to be considered in the evaluation of a patient with new-onset seizures; nevertheless, timely imaging should be performed to rule out a focal lesion like a tumor.

Within the "focal" group of signs and symptoms are those neurological deficits caused by the anatomic location of the tumor. These focal findings are generally gradual in onset and progressive, in contrast with acute occurrences such as those seen with vascular events. A site-specific discussion of signs and symptoms follows, but a few general principles can be easily recalled: supratentorial tumors may produce motor or sensory deficits, visual field deficits, dysphasia, or a combination of these; cognitive or personality changes of considerable variety can be seen in patients with frontal lobe involvement, gliomatosis, or meningeal dissemination; and infratentorial tumors or posterior fossa tumors generally produce multiple cranial nerve deficits, cerebellar dysfunction, or long tract signs.

Tumors within the frontal lobe often cause progressive cognitive decline, emotional liability, and contralateral grasp reflexes. If the left inferior frontal gyrus is involved, the patient may experience productive aphasia. Focal motor seizures or contralateral motor weakness may result from involvement of the precentral gyrus. Lastly, anosmia may result from pressure on the olfactory nerve.

In the temporal lobes, left-sided involvement may lead to receptive aphasia whereas right-sided lesions may disturb the perception of musical notes or quality of speech. Uncal involvement may manifest itself with olfactory or gustatory seizures; these events may be accompanied by lip smacking or licking movements and impairment of consciousness, without actual loss of consciousness. For instance, a patient may experience an aura of déjajvu or jamais vu followed by or accompanied by odd smells or lip smacking. More generalized involvement may lead to emotional changes, behavioral difficulties, and auditory hallucinations. Lastly, involvement of the temporal optic radiations may result in crossed upper quadrantonopsia.

Tumors of the parietal region may cause contralateral dysfunction of sensation or sensory seizures. Sensory loss manifests itself with postural instability and impaired appreciation of size, shape, or texture. Involvement of the optic radiations passing through this region can cause contralateral lower quadrantonopsia. If the left supramarginal gyrus is affected, the patient may experience ideational apraxia. Tumor infiltration into the left angular gyrus can result in alexia, agraphia, right–left confusion, and finger agnosia, or a combination thereof. Nondominant (usually right-sided) involvement often manifests itself with anoagnosia (neglect or denial of an affected limb) or constructional apraxia.

Tumors of the occipital lobe generally produce crossed homonymous hemianopsia or visual hallucinations. Involvement of the left occipital lobe can result in visual agnosia for objects and/or colors. Bilateral damage results in cortical blindness. Several other visual syndromes can occur from occipital lobe defects including Balint's syndrome (a triad of optic ataxia, an inability to move the hand to an object by using vision; ocular apraxia, an inability to voluntarily control the gaze; and simultanagnosia,an inability to recognize more than one object shown at the same time)—and Anton's syndrome (a form of cortical blindness in which the patient denies the visual impairment).

In the case of cerebellar lesions, if the vermis is affected, the patient will experience truncal ataxia. If the hemispheres are affected the patient will experience appendicular ataxia (incoordination of the limbs usually accompanied by hypotonia). Vertical nystagmus can also be observed with cerebellar involvement.

Tumors affecting the brainstem generally manifest themselves with cranial nerve palsies, nystagmus, and long tract signs (pyramidal or sensory). Tumors affecting the pituitary-hypothalamic axis may produce signs and symptoms of excess or deficiency of pituitary hormones in any combination.

Ependymomas, followed by astrocytomas, are the most frequent gliomas of the spinal cord in adult patients. Primary spinal tumors cause signs and symptoms that generally arise from nerve-root compression before parenchymal destruction. As such, patients generally present with radicular pain; conversely, patients can present with deficits resulting from central syringomyelia, which leads to destruction of lower motor neurons and results in segmental muscle weakness and diminished reflexes. The onset of symptoms may be gradual or acute and is generally asymmetric in nature. Of course, the exact set of symptoms depends on which cord level is affected. In general, cervical lesions affect the arms, shoulders, and neck regions. Thoracic lesions affect the abdominal muscles and region. Lumbosacral lesions may affect the lower extremities, pelvic region, and bladder. Cauda equina lesions also affect the lower extremities, bladder, and bowel.

RADIOLOGICAL ASSESSMENT

When a brain tumor is suspected, the initial step in evaluation is brain imaging with computer tomography (CT) or magnetic resonance imaging (MRI), with gadolinium administration (*see* Chapters 5 and 6 for details). These studies will assist in determining the location and size of the lesion in addition to the extent of mass effect and degree of cerebral edema. MRI is generally the preferred study, as it is superior to CT in a number of ways: (1) MRI resolution and sensitivity are higher, (2) there is less chance of artifact in the posterior fossa or pituitary fossa, and (3) MRI provides a more accurate three-dimensional reconstruction of the tumor, which can better guide surgical resection or biopsy. CT does remain superior for demonstrating acute hemorrhage.

PROGNOSTIC FACTORS AND CLINICAL OUTCOME

The overall survival for patients with malignant glioma has not improved much over the past 30 yr. From 1975 to 1995, patients younger than 65 with primary malignant brain cancer made moderate improvements in survival, but older patients made no such advances *(5)*. Glioblastoma remains the histological subtype with the poorest survival, with a mean survival of less than 1 yr and less than 3% of patients with glioblastoma multiformesurviving 5 yr after diagnosis *(27)*. The mean survival for AA is only slightly better, at 2 to 5 yr *(28)*. Increased mitotic activity and or increased MIB-1 labeling (staining for cell division) correlate with reduced survival in glioblastoma multiforme patients and across histologic subtypes of HGG *(29,30)*.

Among HGG, correct histological identification can be complicated because of the high degree of variability in tissue appearance and collection. The process is also prone to a degree of subjectivity with a fair degree of inter-observer variability. Such challenges may lead to errors in identification and subsequentl errors in prognostic estimation. In an attempt to help remedy this situation, gene-expression based classification is gaining favor and may greatly assist in appropriately estimating prognosis and guiding clinically relevant treatment. In fact, a recent study demonstrated that gene-expression profiling, when coupled with class prediction methodology, classified diagnostically challenging malignant glioma in a manner that better correlated with clinical outcome as compared with histopathologic identification *(31)*. Nevertheless, further studies and reproducible results are needed before this technique is widely utilized, especially considering the increasing evidence that a sequential accumulation of independent genetic alterations is essential for tumor development.

There is also limited but increasing data on the prognostic value of molecular markers. Studies among patients with AO demonstrate that certain chromosomal abnormalities do correlate with survival; specifically, studies have shown that loss of chromosome arms 1p and 19q is associated with chemosensitivity and improved overall survival *(32)*. Similarly, patients with glioblastoma multiforme (without features of an oligodendroglioma) with a 1p and 19q deletion also have a significantly longer survival than patients with glioblastoma multiforme that do not have these deletions *(33)*. In patients with AA, Smith et al. demonstrated that loss of the pTEN tumor suppressor gene is associated with poor survival *(34)*. Additionally, epi-

Table 2
Karnofsky Performance Score

Score	Function
100	Normal, no evidence of disease
90	Able to perform normal activity with only minor symptoms
80	Normal activity with effort, some symptoms
70	Able to care for self but unable to do normal activities
60	Requires occasional assistance, cares for most needs
50	Requires considerable assistance
40	Disabled, requires special assistance
30	Severely disabled
20	Very ill, requires active supportive treatment
10	Moribund

dermal growth factor receptor (EGFR and p53 expression have been studied in glioblastoma multiformepatients with the finding that EGFR overexpression (particularly when combined with normal p53 expression) may correlate with poorer survival in patients aged less than 55 *(35)*. Overexpression of MDM2, a p53 inhibitor, has also been found to significantly correlate with short-term survival in glioblastoma multiformepatients. Deletions or mutations in the p14ARF gene, responsible for activation of p53, have been discovered in 70% of glioblastoma multiforme, but the prognostic value is still under scrutiny *(36)*. As glioma appears to be a polygenic disease, further study is ongoing into the prognostic value of molecular signatures to understand how they may guide effective therapy.

Many other factors other than histology have been investigated for their association with survival in malignant glioma patients. Age continues to be strong a prognostic indicator, although the age range associated with more-favorable outcome varies between studies *(37)*. In general, an age less than 45 yr is associated with increased survival *(5)*. Stratifying patients into risk groups based on age is likely to lead to better prognostic information. For example, a recent retrospective study employing recursive partitioning of 832 glioblastoma patients who were enrolled into prospective clinical trials at the time of initial diagnosis established 3 risk groups based on age: ≤40, 40 to 65, and ≥65 *(38)*. Based on the commonly accepted belief that functional status also predicts longer survival *(39)*, this study maintained that the 40 to 65 age group be subdivided by Karnofsky Performance Score (KPS) into >80 or <80, with the <80 group behaving similarly to the age ≥65 group. KPS is summarized in Table 2. Mental status has also been shown to be a prognostic factor. In fact, a recent publication reports that baseline mini-mental status score correlates more strongly with time to progression and survival than performance status *(40)*.

Tumor location, size, and extent of resection are variables that have also been studied in relation to predicting survival. Multivariate analyses have not shown tumor location or size to be significant prognostic factors *(40)*. The benefit of extent of resection continues to be unresolved, though most of the neuro-oncology literature testifies to the benefit of extensive resection especially when compared with biopsy alone *(41)*. It must be noted, though, that these studies are retrospective in nature and subject to selection bias. They state that patients with surgically resectable tumors have a better survival rate than those with nonrersectable tumors; this is not the same as stating that prognosis is improved by extensive resection. Nonetheless, in the absence of randomized clinical trials and prospectively collected data, this question will remain unanswered.

Of special note is that the poor survival associated with malignant glioma has important implications for designing and conducting clinical trials aimed at determining etiology or treatment. For example, incidence based studies must often rely on information from family members or caretakers because of difficulties in identifying and interviewing patients before a rapid death; obviously, such indirect information gathering can lead to erroneous information. Additionally, patients in phase II and III trials of experimental treatments need to be compared with appropriate historical control groups that take into account prognostic markers and afford for stratification into similar groups.

THE FUTURE

An understanding of the epidemiologic, molecular, and genetic events regulating HGG is growing. Standard histopathology and epidemiologystudies to date have helped us group patients into risk groups, which aide physicians in determining prognosis and treatment. Nonetheless, treatment results for most patients are still unsatisfactory, likely because of the genetic and epidemiological heterogeneity amongs brain tumors. We need a better understanding of how epidemiological and genetic mechanisms influence the development of brain tumors and the clinical course of patients with HGG. Continued advances in the use of genetic or molecular markers in conjunction with standard histopathological identification can lead to a more accurate tumor classification system that will allow improved assessment of prognosis and more standardized future studies and resulting data. Moreover, we are hopeful that with an improved genetic and epidemiological understanding of brain tumors we may be able to prevent them or create better treatment strategies.

REFERENCES

1. Cancer Facts and Figures 2002. Atlanta, Georgia:American Cancer Society, Inc., 2002.
2. Central Brain Tumor Registry of the United States, 1995–1999. (Accessed July 1, 2004; available at http://www.cbtrus.org.)
3. Davis FG, Kupelian V, Freels S, McCarthy B, Surawicz T. Prevalence estimates for primary brain tumors in the United States by behavior and major histology groups. Neuro-oncology 2001;3:152–158.
4. Legler JM, Ries LA, Smith MA, et al. Cancer surveillance series [corrected]: brain and other central nervous system cancers: recent trends in incidence and mortality. J Natl Cancer Inst 1999;91:1382–1390.
5. Wrensch M, Minn Y, Chew T, Bondy M, Berger MS. Epidemiology of primary brain tumors: current concepts and review of the literature. Neuro-oncology 2002;4:278–299.
6. Surawicz TS, McCarthy BJ, Kupelian V, Jukich PJ, Bruner JM, Davis FG. Descriptive epidemiology of primary brain and CNS tumors: results from the Central Brain Tumor Registry of the United States, 1990–1994. Neuro-oncology 1999;1:14–25.
7. McKinley BP, Michalek AM, Fenstermaker RA, Plunkett RJ. The impact of age and sex on the incidence of glial tumors in New York state from 1976 to 1995. J Neurosurg 2000;93:932–939.
8. Chen P, Aldape K, Wiencke JK, et al. Ethnicity delineates different genetic pathways in malignant glioma. Cancer Res 2001;61:3949–3954.
9. Gurney JG, Kadan-Lottick N. Brain and other central nervous system tumors: rates, trends, and epidemiology. Curr Opin Oncol 2001;13:160–166.
10. Osborne RH, Houben MP, Tijssen CC, Coebergh JW, van Duijn CM. The genetic epidemiology of glioma. Neurology 2001;57:1751–1755.
11. Malmer B, Iselius L, Holmberg E, Collins A, Henriksson R, Gronberg H. Genetic epidemiology of glioma. Br J Cancer 2001;84:429–434.

12. Inskip PD, Linet MS, Heineman EF. Etiology of brain tumors in adults. Epidemiol Rev 1995;17:382–414.
13. Cuomo L, Trivedi P, Cardillo MR, et al. Human herpesvirus 6 infection in neoplastic and normal brain tissue. J Med Virol 2001;63:45–51.
14. Cobbs CS, Harkins L, Samanta M, et al. Human cytomegalovirus infection and expression in human malignant glioma. Cancer Res 2002;62:3347–3350.
15. Wrensch M, Yost M, Miike R, Lee G, Touchstone J. Adult glioma in relation to residential power frequency electromagnetic field exposures in the San Francisco Bay area. Epidemiology 1999;10:523–527.
16. Gurney JG, van Wijngaarden E. Extremely low frequency electromagnetic fields (EMF) and brain cancer in adults and children: review and comment. Neuro-oncology 1999; 1:212–220.
17. Elwood JM. A critical review of epidemiologic studies of radiofrequency exposure and human cancers. Environ Health Perspect 1999;107(1):155–168.
18. Jauchem JR. A literature review of medical side effects from radio-frequency energy in the human environment: involving cancer, tumors, and problems of the central nervous system. J Microw Power Electromagn Energy 2003;38:103–123.
19. Inskip PD, Tarone RE, Hatch EE, et al. Cellular-telephone use and brain tumors. N Engl J Med 2001;344: 79–86.
20. Inskip PD, Mellemkjaer L, Gridley G, Olsen JH. Incidence of intracranial tumors following hospitalization for head injuries (Denmark). Cancer Causes Control 1998;9:109–116.
21. Minn Y, Wrensch M, Bondy ML. Epidemiology of primary brain tumors. In: Prados M, ed. Brain Cancer. Hamilton, Ontario: B.C. Decker, 2002:1–15.
22. Wrensch M, Bondy ML, Wiencke J, Yost M. Environmental risk factors for primary malignant brain tumors: a review. J Neurooncol 1993;17:47–64.
23. DeAngelis LM. Brain tumors. N Engl J Med 2001;344:114–123.
24. Vecht CJ, Wagner GL, Wilms EB. Treating seizures in patients with brain tumors: Drug interactions between antiepileptic and chemotherapeutic agents. Semin Oncol 2003;30:49–52.
25. Forsyth PA, Weaver S, Fulton D, et al. Prophylactic anticonvulsants in patients with brain tumour. Can J Neurol Sci 2003;30:106–112.
26. Behin A, Hoang-Xuan K, Carpentier AF, Delattre JY. Primary brain tumours in adults. Lancet 2003;361:323–331.
27. Central Brain Tumor Registry of the United States, 2002. (Accessed July 1, 2004, at http://www.cbtrus. org.)
28. Prados MD, Seiferheld W, Sandler HM, et al. Phase III randomized study of radiotherapy plus procarbazine, lomustine, and vincristine with or without BUdR for treatment of anaplastic astrocytoma: final report of RTOG 9404. Int J Radiat Oncol Biol Phys 2004;58:1147–1152.
29. Reavey-Cantwell JF, Haroun RI, Zahurak M, et al. The prognostic value of tumor markers in patients with glioblastoma multiforme: analysis of 32 patients and review of the literature. J Neurooncol 2001;55: 195–204.
30. Korshunov A, Golanov A, Sycheva R. Immunohistochemical markers for prognosis of cerebral glioblastomas. J Neurooncol 2002;58:217–236.
31. Nutt CL, Mani DR, Betensky RA, et al. Gene expression-based classification of malignant gliomas correlates better with survival than histological classification. Cancer Res 2003;63:1602–1607.
32. Smith JS, Perry A, Borell TJ, et al. Alterations of chromosome arms 1p and 19q as predictors of survival in oligodendrogliomas, astrocytomas, and mixed oligoastrocytomas. J Clin Oncol 2000;18:636–645.
33. Senger D, Cairncross JG, Forsyth PA. Long-term survivors of glioblastoma: statistical aberration or important unrecognized molecular subtype? Cancer J 2003;9:214–221.
34. Smith JS, Tachibana I, Passe SM, et al. PTEN mutation, EGFR amplification, and outcome in patients with anaplastic astrocytoma and glioblastoma multiforme. J Natl Cancer Inst 2001;93:1246–1256.
35. Simmons ML, Lamborn KR, Takahashi M, et al. Analysis of complex relationships between age, p53, epidermal growth factor receptor, and survival in glioblastoma patients. Cancer Res 2001;61:1122–1128.
36. Shiraishi T, Tabuchi K. Genetic alterations of human brain tumors as molecular prognostic factors. Neuropathology 2003;23:95–108.
37. Curran WJ, Jr., Scott CB, Horton J, et al. Recursive partitioning analysis of prognostic factors in three Radiation Therapy Oncology Group malignant glioma trials. J Natl Cancer Inst 1993;85:704–710.
38. Lamborn KR, Chang SM, Prados MD. Prognostic factors for survival of patients with glioblastoma: recursive partitioning analysis. Neuro-oncology 2004;6:227–235.

39. Scott JN, Rewcastle NB, Brasher PM, et al. Which glioblastoma multiforme patient will become a long-term survivor? A population-based study. Ann Neurol 1999;46:183–188.

40. Buckner JC. Factors influencing survival in high-grade gliomas. Semin Oncol 2003;30:10–14.

41. Schiff D, Shaffrey ME. Role of resection for newly diagnosed malignant gliomas. Expert Rev Anticancer Ther 2003; 3:621–630.

III Diagnostic Tools for High-Grade Glioma

5 Computerized Tomography

Manzoor Ahmed and Thomas J. Masaryk

Summary

MRI is undoubtedly at the forefront of brain tumor imaging. It is the imaging study of choice, not only for diagnosis but also as a preferred modality for characterization and treatment planning of brain tumors. CT is superior in detecting calcification, hemorrhage, and in evaluating bone changes related to tumors. Patients with pacemakers or metallic devices, as well as critically ill or unstable patients, represent some of the specific areas in which CT is the diagnostic modality of choice. The arrival of multichannel, spiral CT has rejuvenated its role because of the high speed scanning which facilitates sophisticated multiplanar three-dimensional (3D) imaging as well as dynamic imaging (i.e., CT-perfusion [CTP] and CT angiography [CTA]). These advanced techniques are extremely useful in preoperative localization, intraoperative navigation, and radiation therapy targeting.

Key Words: Computed tomography; spiral CT; MDCT.

INTRODUCTION

MRI is undoubtedly at the forefront of brain tumor imaging. It is the imaging study of choice, not only for diagnosis but also as a preferred modality for characterization and treatment planning of brain tumors. Although computed tomography (CT) appears somewhat antique in the context of diagnosing central nervous system (CNS) neoplasms, it continues to play a significant role in patient management. CT is superior in detecting calcification, hemorrhage, and in evaluating bone changes related to tumors. Patients with pacemakers or metallic devices, as well as critically ill or unstable patients, represent some of the specific areas in which CT is the diagnostic modality of choice. As a result of its speed and accessibility, CT is used in immediate postoperative evaluation. The arrival of multichannel, spiral CT has rejuvenated its role because of the high speed scanning which facilitates sophisticated multiplanar three-dimensional (3D) imaging as well as dynamic imaging (i.e., CT-perfusion [CTP] and CT angiography [CTA]). These advanced techniques are extremely useful in preoperative local-ization, intraoperative navigation, and radiation therapy targeting.

STATE OF THE ART: CT IMAGING OF BRAIN TUMORS

Multidetector CT

Multislice or multidetector CT (MDCT) *(1,2)* denotes the ability of a scanner to acquire more than one slice simultaneously. To be capable of doing so, the detector system must be composed of more than a single row of detectors. The MDCT era started in 1992 with a dual slice scanner. State of the art scanners currently have 16 rows of detectors, but 32, 40, and

From: *Current Clinical Oncology: High-Grade Gliomas: Diagnosis and Treatment*
Edited by: G. H. Barnett © Humana Press Inc., Totowa, NJ

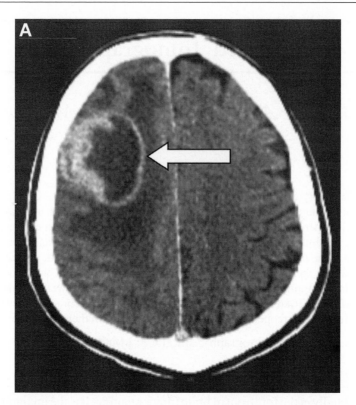

Fig. 1. Multiplanar reformation (MPR). Simultaneous orthogonal display in **(A)** axial, **(B)** coronal, and **(C)** sagittal planes. Typical necrotic GBM (*arrows*) with thick nodular rim enhancement is better localized on this 3D display, involving the middle and superior frontal gyri.

64-slice systems will soon be used in clinical practice. In addition to the number of detectors, the rotational speed has increased from 1.0 to about 0.375 s/rotation. The advantages of MDCT can be summarized by the acronym **RSVP: R**esolution-improved spatial resolution along the z-axis ("acquisition of thin slices"), **S**peed-reduced time for scanning a given portion of the body, **V**olume-increased length of the body that can be traversed for a given set of scan parameters, and **P**ower-efficient usage of X-ray tube power.

Multiplanar Reformation and 3D Reconstruction

MDCT can acquire isotropic data sets which enables anatomic evaluation in an infinite number of planes and projections while maintaining image resolution and quality *(3)*. Multiplanar reformation (MPR) means simultaneous display of orthogonal or oblique sagittal, axial, and coronal reconstructions (Fig. 1). It is extremely useful in localizing a lesion, particularly if there is more than one lesion. Maximum intensity projection (MIP) is another post processing technique in which single layer of brightest voxels along a line (or projection) at a specified angle (orthogonal or oblique) is displayed. A major drawback is that it lacks depth information (i.e., displays only the density of objects and not spatial information). This technique suits post-contrast studies as the post-processed images display highlights the contrast enhanced structures with partial suppression of the background (e.g., vessels.) Shaded surface display (SSD), combines depth information as well as tissue density based on preset thresh-

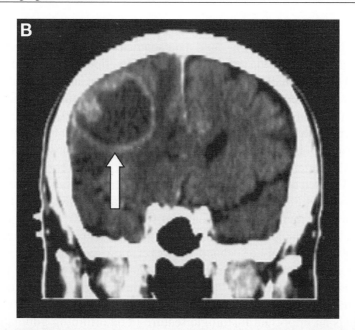

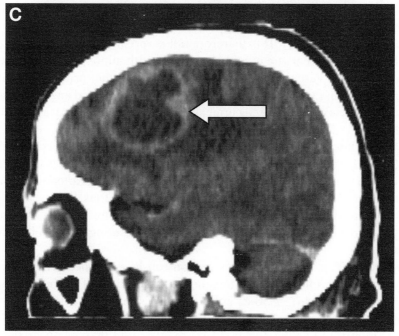

olds; the first layer of voxels within defined density thresholds is used for display, leading to the visualization of the surface of all structures that fulfill the threshold conditions. Depth information is preserved but the attenuation information is scaled proportionately. Volume rendering (VR) utilizes all the information in the volume data set, groups of voxels are selected within a series defined threshold densities, each color coded with appropriate depth shading/ opacity. This is considered one of the best 3D techniques, particularly for intraoperative navigation.

CT Angiography and Perfusion

Intracranial CTA is performed via rapid data acquisition cued to the arrival of an arterial bolus of contrast administered via intravenous power injection. High-resolution axial images are then acquired longitudinally (i.e., in the direction of flow), and then evaluated using MIP or volume rendered post processing with thresholds set for contrast enhanced vessels.

CTP is another dynamic imaging technique, also performed after bolus contrast administration, in which a pixel-by-pixel time–density curve is created by rapid data acquisition over a stationary area of interest *(4)*. Considering the linear relationship between the density changes and contrast agent concentration, as well as the lack of confounding sensitivity to flow artifacts, CT-based quantifications potentially offer a more accurate representation of the tissue microvasculature than similar magnetic resonance (MR) perfusion (MRP) imaging studies. However, there is limited data currently available regarding CT perfusion imaging in brain tumor imaging. Compared with MRP, the major limitation of CTP is that a limited volume of brain can be scanned. However, new techniques are being developed to overcome this limitation (e.g., table toggle technique) *(5)*. CTP has the potential to play a significant role in brain tumor imaging; the rationale is as follows: Vajkoczy and Menger described endothelial proliferation as a common feature of glioma vasculature *(6)*. Endothelial proliferation is an important histologic feature in determining glioma grade, with the other features being nuclear atypia, mitoses, and necrosis. The diameter of normal cerebral capillaries has a limited range of 3 to 5 µm, whereas gliomas contain tortuous, hyperplastic vessels 3 to 40 µm in diameter. It is therefore not surprising that regional cerebral blood volume (rCBV) measurements are reliably correlated with tumor grade and histologic findings of increased tumor vascularity. Malignant tumors, whether primary tumors or metastases, are commonly characterized by neovascularity and increased angiogenic activity *(7)*. The neovasculature has also increased permeability because of the local alteration in blood–brain barrier (BBB) *(8)*.

Cerebral blood flow (CBF) is the flow (mL/min/100 g) through a given vascular network in the brain. CBV is the volume of blood (mL/100 g) within the vessels. Mean transit time (MTT) is the mean transit time of all blood elements entering at the arterial input and leaving at the venous output of the vascular network. Time to peak (TTP) is the time to peak enhancement. In addition to these parameters which are related to flow dynamics, microvascular permeability is also assessed in perfusion imaging by measuring permeability surface (PS) area product *(9)*.

With multislice CT, a 2- to 3-cm-thick section can be examined. The region (slice) of interest has to be selected for perfusion imaging (e.g., a portion of the brain tumor, surgical cavity or post radiation field). A 50-cc bolus of contrast material is injected at a high rate (usually 8 mL/s) using a power injector and large bore (18 gage) intravenous line; tissue attenuation is monitored as the contrast first reaches and then perfuses the brain with one image/s acquired during wash-in and wash-out. Semiautomatic post-processing is used to create scaled, color maps of TTP or MTT, CBF, and CBV in less than 1 min *(10)*. Two mathematical approaches are used to calculate these parameters *(11)*: (1)the maximum slope model requires a rapid, tight bolus to calculate the slope of time attenuation curve which is used to approximate CBF and (2) the deconvolution analysis model calculates regional MTT by deconvolving the time-attenuation curve *(12)*. The latter method requires an arterial input function to deconvolve the curve *(13–15)* and theoretically provides absolute values for CBF and CBV. Nevertheless, there are variables (e.g., choice of input function, recirculation correction) which may limit the accuracy of these values *(16)*.

CBV and PS are the most meaningful parameters in evaluation of any type of tumors. CBF, TTP, and MTT are more of value in vascular-occlusive diseases. The major application for microvascular assessment using dynamic contrast-enhanced CT is differentiation of the most malignant region of tumor before conducting stereotactic biopsy. This may be particularly valuable in previously treated lesions in an effort to differentiate radiation necrosis, post-surgical scar tissue, and recurrent tumor. Additionally, tumor can be graded based on its blood volume and permeability. There is limited available data on CTP in brain tumor imaging. Data from MRP studies of brain tumors can be used as a means of extrapolating meaningful conclusions as well as predicting the role of CTP in future. Increased CBV and PS (or other parameters of permeability such as k-trans) are reliable indicators of high-grade brain tumors *(17)*. However, differentiation between high-grade and low-grade tumors needs a threshold or cut-off value *(18)*, therefore interpretation becomes difficult in borderline cases. Lam et al. *(19)* showed a maximum CBV value of 2.95 ± 2.127 mlL100 g for low-grade tumors compared with 9.48 ± 4.520 mL/100 g in high-grade tumors. In human gliomas, estimates of permeability have been shown to be predictive of the pathologic grade and correlate with the mitotic activity of a tumor *(20)*. Additional studies suggest rCBV is a more accurate predictor of tumor grade than permeability co-efficient in three-tiered glioma classification system *(21,22)*.

Differentiating radiation necrosis from the recurrent brain tumor can be very challenging. Sugahara et al. *(23)* showed the utility of MRP imaging. In their study, enhancing lesions with a normalized rCBV ratio >2.6 or <0.6 suggested tumor recurrence or non-neoplastic contrast-enhancing tissue, respectively. CTP holds enormous potential for this purpose (Fig. 2, A–C).

Preoperative Planning and Intraoperative Navigation

State of the art, neuronavigation procedures involve the use of high resolution CT or MRI data acquisition with fiducial markers or stereotactic frames data transfer, presurgical viewing and planning, and intraoperative registration and navigation *(24)*. The three main objectives of resection are: (1) accurate localization, (2) complete or controlled removal and, (3) sparing of normal brain function. Surgical navigation allows real-time localization in the operative field of corresponding CT or MRI images utilizing mechanical, sonic, or infrared surgical pointing devices once data sets have been registered utilizing the fiducial markers and the Cartesian volume of the image data set. There are three different measures of accuracy in surgical navigation systems *(25)*: (1) mechanical accuracy (i.e., how well the system knows its own position in space), (2) registration accuracy (i.e., alignment of the cursor, representing the tip of the pointer, anatomically and accurately positioned in the image) and, (3) application accuracy indicates how reliably the pointer tip in physical space corresponds to its anatomical position of the cursor in the CT or MR image. Frame based stereotactic systems possess the best mechanical and registration accuracy and are capable of localizing very small tumors. However, a major drawback is the limited physical access and approach afforded by the frame at the time of surgery. Frameless navigation is much more flexible with no restrictions on microsurgical techniques *(25)*.

The main problem of the navigation system based on preoperative scanning is the inability to predict intraoperative spatial distortion produced by mass effect and brain shift following craniotomy and durotomy. One solution to this problem is to perform intraoperative imaging using intraoperative MRI or CT. Intraoperative CT consists of a mobile gantry and matched operating table that can be directly docked to the gantry. Anesthesia and surgery are performed on the same table *(26)*. There has been improved efficiency and better work flow in both

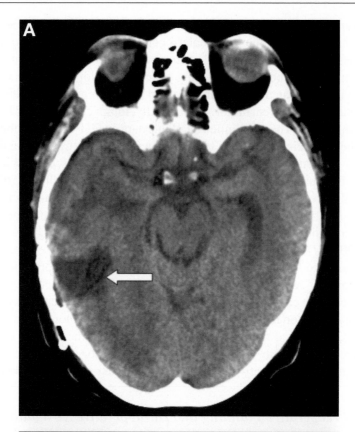

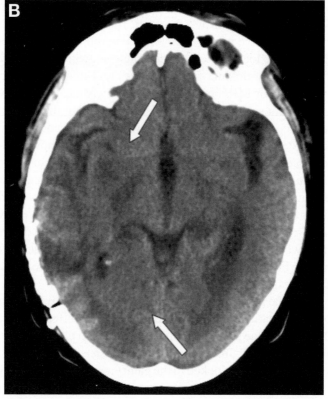

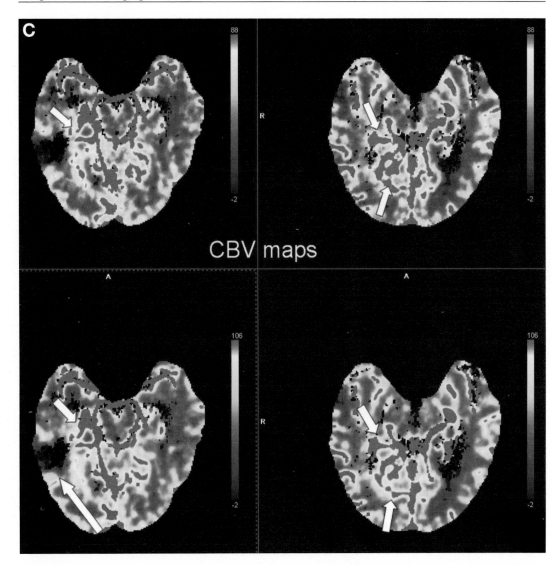

Fig. 2. Recurrent HGG detected on CT perfusion. (**A**, *arrow*) Noncontrast CT images show: a focal surgical defect in the right temporal lobe. (**B**, *arrow*) Note nonfocal and nonspecific surrounding region of low attenuation coefficient in the right temporal and occipital lobes. (**C**) Recurrent HGG detected on CT perfusion. Multiple CBV map images demonstrate asymmetric focal region of increased blood volume (*arrows*) (based on qualitative assessment). Biopsy of this region showed recurrent HGG.

microsurgery and endoscopic surgery as a result of the introduction of intraoperative CT with fewer repeat surgeries *(25,26)*.

GENERAL CT CHARACTERISTICS OF GLIOMAS

CT imaging features of high grade gliomas are nonspecific. There is an overlap of imaging features between low- and high-grade gliomas (HGG).

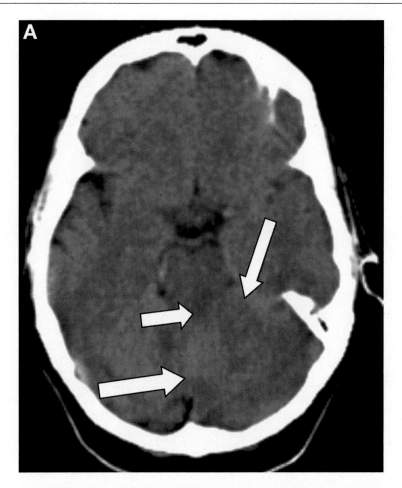

Fig. 3. (A) Infratentorial GBM. Noncontrast CTshowing subtle heterogenous density with mass effect (effacement of left perimesencephalic cistern) *(short arrow)* in the left cerebellar hemisphere. **(B)** Axial T2 and **(C)** post-contrast T1 MR images demonstrate large area of signal abnormality with minimal focal enhancement *(arrows)*. (Parts **B** and **C** are on page 81.)

Location

HGG can occur anywhere in the brain (Fig. 3), but are most commonly lobar in the supratentorial compartment *(27)*. Multicentric tumors (Figs. 4 and 5) are those with neither macroscopic nor microscopic connection whereas those with such a continuity are termed multifocal *(28,29)*. The multifocal subtype tends to disseminate more frequently through leptomeningeal space *(30,31)*.

Attenuation Coefficient ("Density")

HGG have variable densities on CT (Fig. 6), usually isodense to moderately hyperdense to gray matter (the isocenter of the mass may appear denser because of the surrounding vasogenic edema). A small or atypically hypodense mass may not be visible on nonenhanced CT study, masked by the presence of the surrounding, low-density, vasogenic edema (Fig. 7). Such cases can be occasionally mistaken for subacute infarcts unless contrast is administered. X-ray attenuation coefficient has no significant relationship to grading of gliomas.

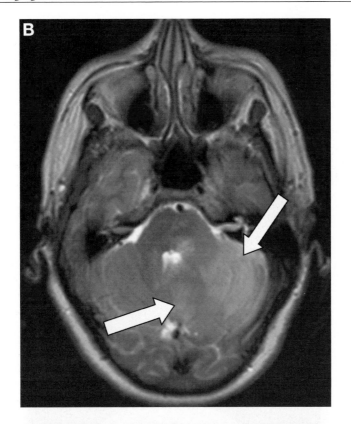

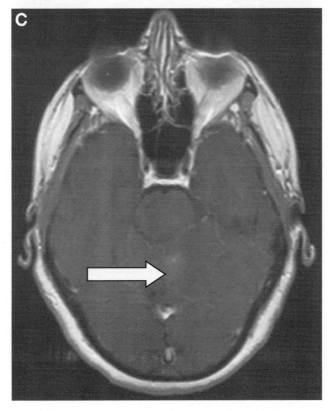

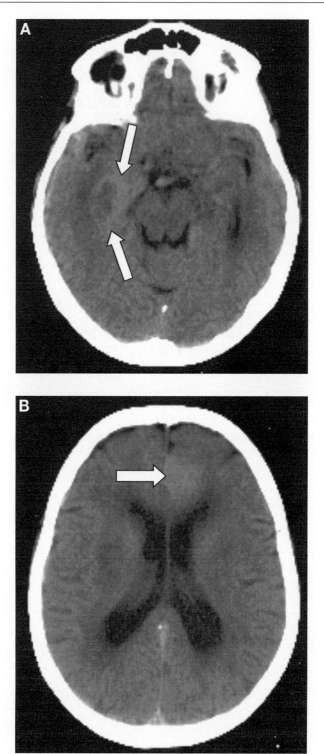

Fig. 4. (A,B) Ulticentric GBM. Enhanced CTdemonstrates focal hyperdense superficial masses (*arrows*) in the **(A)** right temporal lobes and **(B)** left mesial frontal, the former appears necrotic. There is minimal enhancement compared to pre contrast images(not shown).This appearance is difficult to distinguish from intracranial lymphoma except that lymphoma typically shows intense homogenous enhancement.

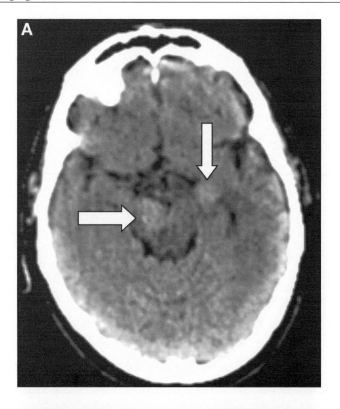

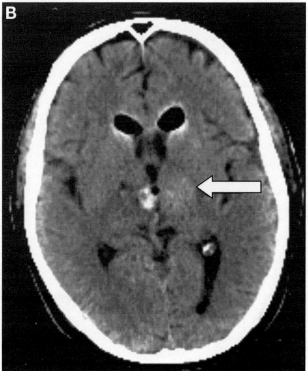

Fig. 5. Multicentric AA. **(A,B)** Noncontrast CT imagesshowing focal hyperdense masses (*arrows*) in the right cerebral peduncle, left mesial temporal lobe, and left thalamus. Note post-operative changes in **B**.

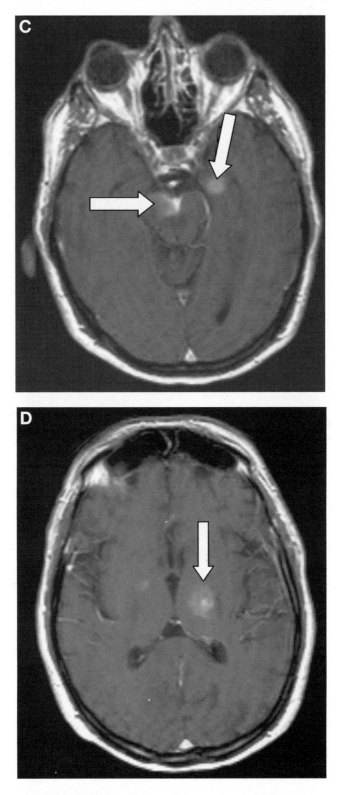

Fig. 5. *(continued from page 83)* **(C,D)** Focal enhancing masses (*arrows*) demonstrated on corresponding post contrast axial T1 weighted MR images.

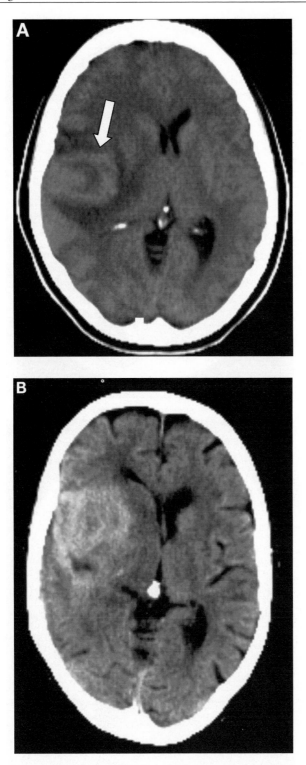

Fig. 6. Focal superficial GBM, two different patients. (**A**) Noncontrast CT image shows a mixed density right fronto-temporal mass (*arrow*) with mild surrounding vasogenic edema. (**B**) Example of extensive hyperdense cortical and subcortical mass in the right frontotemporal operculum with mass effect and midline shift.Note lack of significant vasogenic edema in **B**, an unusual finding in GBM.

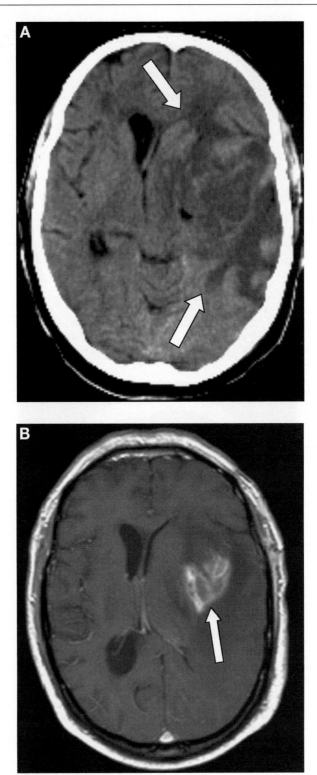

Fig. 7. (A) GBM Mmasked by vasogenic edema. Large area of vasogenic edema in the left cerebral hemisphere including the basal ganglia (arrows), demonstrated on this noncontrast CT image. No focal mass evident. **(B)** Post-contrast T1 MR image shows enhancing necrotic mass (arrow).

Hemorrhage

Hemorrhage, depicted as an area of high attenuation coefficient, is more commonly seen in advanced grade gliomas (World Health Organization [WHO] grade III–IV), particularly glioblastoma, but it is not a pathognomonic feature; 12% of symptomatic hematomas can be caused by low-grade gliomas) *(32)*. Thus, it is important to remember that any atypical cerebral hematomas (e.g., hematoma with disproportionate edema) will need follow up to rule-out underlying tumor. Relationship of hemorrhage to the grade of a tumor can be explained by the endothelial proliferation, a common histologic feature of HGG.

Calcifications

Low-grade gliomas are more likely to be calcified (Fig. 8). Nevertheless, a small percentage of HGG also shows calcifications *(33)*. One of the hypothesis regarding calcified HGG is their transformation from low-grade to high-grade, the former responsible for the presence of calcification; it is thus regarded as a positive prognostic factor in HGG and may be suggestive of an oligodendroglial origin *(33)*.

Vasogenic Edema

Vasogenic edema is an indirect indicator of the aggressive growth of a brain tumor, mainly responsible for the secondary mass effect. Focal region of vasogenic edema may be the only finding on unenhanced CT in cases of HGG or intracranial metastases. White matter edema produced by HGG, particularly GBM, can be quite extensive (Fig. 7) and actually represents a tumor plus edema *(34)*.

Contrast Enhancement

Contrast enhancement on CT imaging has a high sensitivity and specificity for HGG (about 87 and 79%, respectively) *(33)*. About 20% of low-grade gliomas will also show enhancement *(33)*. Likewise, a substantial number of nonenhancing brain tumors can turn out to be HGG, particularly anaplastic astrocytomas (AA) *(35)* (Fig. 9). Overall, enhancement on CT imaging is a negative prognostic factor, irrespective of the glioma grade *(33)*. Furthermore, Yamada et al. *(36)* showed contrast enhanced area (CEA) of >4 cm and heterogenous enhancement as negative prognostic factors while CEA <4cm and homogenous enhancement indicated better prognosis.

HISTOLOGY SPECIFIC CT CHARACTERISTICS

Gliomas can be simply divided into astrocytomas, oligodendrogliomas, ependymomas, and mixed gliomas. Astrocytic tumors can be further divided into two macroscopic categories: indolent, circumscribed (grade I), or diffuse/ malignant (grades II–IV). Histologic grading of each of subtype of glioma is critical for assessing prognosis and planning therapy. This grading system, which is now well recognized *(37)*, relies upon recognition of four parameters: nuclear atypia, mitoses, endothelial proliferation, and necrosis. The presence of two or more of the above described features places the tumor in the high grade category *(38)*. CT-imaging based differentiation of various histologic sub-types of gliomas is limited. For the sake of completion, we discuss below the CT imaging features of different histologic cell types with an emphasis on imaging–pathologic correlation.

Anaplastic Astrocytoma

Anaplastic astrocytomas (AA) are infiltrating tumors with biologic behavior and average age of diagnosis intermediate between simple astrocytomas (grade I and II) and GBM (grade

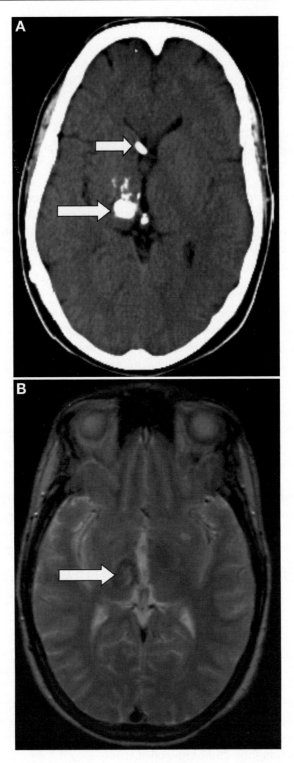

Fig. 8. Calcified glioma. **(A)** Unenhanced CT demonstrates focal coarse calcification (*long arrow*) in the right thalamus with out significant vasogenic edema. Biopsy compatible with low-grade oligoden-droglioma. Note shunt catheter tip (*short arrow*). **(B)** Axial T2 weighted MR image shows correspond-ing area of susceptibility related to calcification (*arrow*).

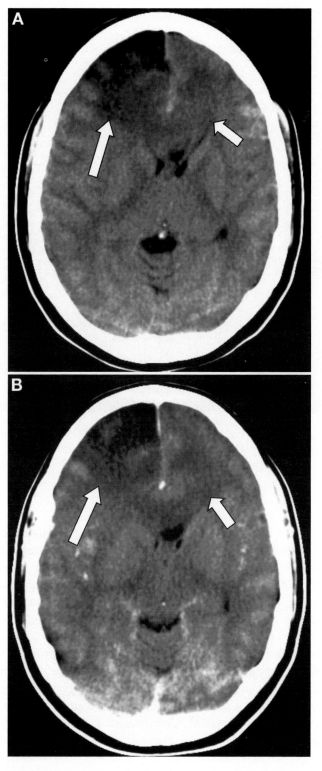

Fig. 9. AOA. **(A)** Pre- and **(B)** post-contrast CT. Right frontal lobe low density mass (*long arrows*) with cortical and subcortical involvement mimicking an acute or subacute infarct. There is no significant enhancement. Note contralateral extension into mesial frontal lobe (*short arrows*).

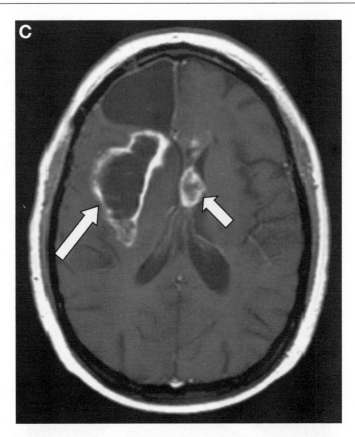

Fig. 9. *(Continued from page 89.)* Follow up post contrast axial T1 MR image showing rim enhancing necrotic mass *(long arrows)* along with leptomeningeal recurrence *(short arrow)*.

IV). AA represent about one-quarter of all gliomas *(39)*. Although they can originate as primary tumors, significant numbers of AA are thought to have transformed from benign tumors, particularly the diffuse infiltrative astrocytomas (grade I and II) *(40)*. They can potentially progress to GBM. The gemistocytic astrocytomas—having increased eosinophilic cytoplasm—have an increased tendency for malignant transformation and, although generally low-grade gliomas, may show enough malignant features to be diagnosed as AA *(40)*.

Because of their infiltrative growth, AA may have indistinct margins which are often reflected as ill-defined, inhomogenous lesions on CT. Because of its high cellularity, the attenuation usually ranges from intermediate to high in relation to the normal brain (Fig. 5). Alternatively, as cystic change or necrosis and hemorrhage are uncommon, AA are generally more homogenous compared with GBM. Calcification is rarely seen unless there has been transformation from a lower grade glioma. Post-contrast CT studies usually show limited to moderate patchy/heterogenous enhancement *(35,44)*. AA may show leptomeningeal dissemination (including the ependymal surface) *(41)*. Differentiation from GBM is generally very difficult, particularly on CT (Fig. 10). Marked vasogenic edema, mass effect, hemorrhage and necrosis favor GBM.

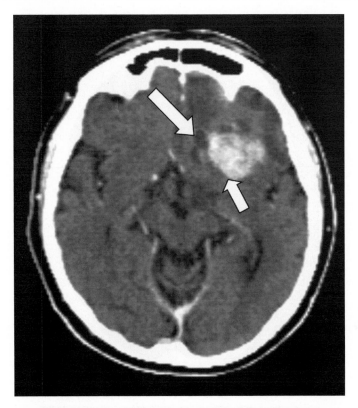

Fig. 10. Focal AA, GBM -like features. Contrast enhanced CT image showing left frontal lobe complex mass with large portion of enhancement. Note small areas of cystic degeneration (*large arrow*), the mass is also abutting the corpus callosum (*short arrow*).

Glioblastoma Multiforme

GBM is the most common primary intracranial tumor and constitutes more than half of all glial tumors *(42)*. GBM correspond to WHO grade IV with the most aggressive behavior and poor differentiation. Like AA, some are also hypothesized to transform from lower grade gliomas, whereas others may arise *de novo*.

The cerebral hemispheres are the most common location; typically in the centrum semi-ovale with a tendency to cross midline along the white matter tracts in the "butterfly" pattern (Fig. 11). They can involve basal ganglia, and are rarely found in the posterior fossa (Fig. 3). Primary intraventricular glioblastomas have been rarely reported. The majority of GBM are solitary lesions; multifocal or multicentric GBM occur in about 3% of cases *(28)* (Fig. 4).

The typical appearance of GBM on nonenhanced CT is a mixed density complex mass with disproportionate surrounding vasogenic edema, usually involves corpus callosum (Fig. 11). The marked heterogeneity on either CT or MRI corresponds to the pathologic hallmark findings of necrosis and hemorrhage as well as marked cellular pleomorphism, which at times makes the determination of histologic origin of some GBM very difficult. Central necrosis is an imaging hallmark of GBM (Fig. 1). Hemorrhage, seen in about 20% of GBM , can be easily identified on CT *(43)*. Vasogenic edema is a prominent imaging feature of GBM and commonly extends along the white matter tracts. One of the common management related ques-

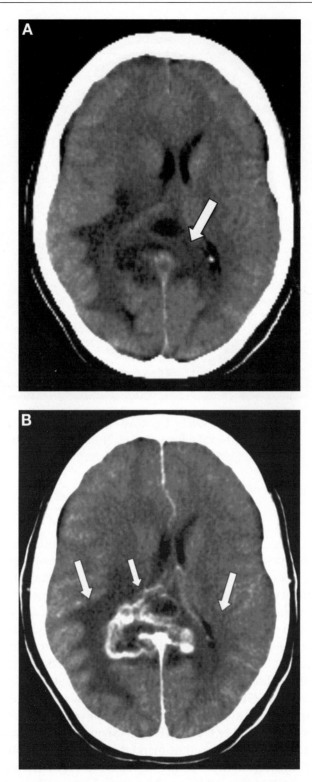

Fig. 11. GBM of corpus callosum. **(A)** Pre- and **(B)** post-contrast CT images showing diffuse vasogenic edema with complex enhancing mass (*short arrows*) originating in the splenium of corpus callosum. Somewhat semi-butterfly appearance of the vasogenic edema with asymmetry towards the right side (*long arrows*).

tions concerns the delineation of tumor vs edema. This is often not accurately answered in cases of GBM (even by MRI) as the extensive vasogenic edema seen on imaging in such cases may actually represent a combination of an infiltrating tumor and an accompanying edema. Perfusion imaging has shown some utility to delineate the extent of the tumor and identify the most suspicious area for biopsy *(23,44)*.

GBM typically shows heterogenous rim enhancement with irregular thick and nodular margins (Fig. 1) corresponding to the prominent endothelial proliferation seen on pathology, with a poor BBB and more aggregate around the necrotic center. The enhancing tumor around the necrotic center also probably explains the "pseudopalisading" pattern of neoplastic cell aggregation around necrosis, as previously described in *(27)*. These large areas of necrosis reflect aggressive tumor growth that subsequently outstrips vascular supply; they are associated with poor prognosis *(45)*. As a result of the infiltrative nature of AA, GBM, and other HGG, histologic margins of the tumor are poorly delineated on post contrast CT.

The most common dissemination route is direct extension along white matter tracts, including spread across the commissures. Other routes include subependymal (portends poor prognosis) and neuroaxial spread via the CSF. As a result of the beam-hardening artifact created by the skull in CT (particularly at the basal cisterns), MRI is the diagnostic study of choice for evaluating dissemination.

Anaplastic Oligodendroglioma /Oligoastrocytoma

The term anaplastic oligodendroglioma (AO) (WHO grade III) is used when there are focal or diffuse histologic features of malignancy. Typically these tumors involve cortex and subcortical white matter. About one-half of oligodendrogliomas are anaplastic *(46)*. Mixed tumors, such as anaplastic oligoastrocytoma (AOA) (Fig. 9), have a relatively poor prognosis *(47)*.

AO are indistinguishable from oligodendroglioma (WHO II) on CT or MRI. On a CT, a typical finding is a well defined mixed density superficial frontal lobe mass with calcifications, which may be nodular, clumped, or even gyriform *(48,49)* (Fig. 8). The involved cortex is expanded, cystic degeneration is common, and hemorrhage or necrosis may also be seen *(50)*. The lesions may expand, remodel, or erode the calvarium. About 50% of all oligodendrogliomas show enhancement, usually heterogenous. AO are more likely to enhance than low-grade oligodendrogliomas *(50)* (Fig. 9C). A new focus of enhancement is suggestive of malignant transformation *(51)*.

Gliomatosis Cerebri

Gliomatosis cerebri represents diffuse, cortical glial cell proliferation with preservation of brain cytoarchitecture so that a focal mass is not grossly appreciable *(52,53)*. Generally, gliomatosis cerebri is restricted to cases with contigous involvement of at least two lobes; less commonly with extension into deep nuclear structures, brainstem, and cerebellum *(54)*. Primary leptomeningeal gliomatosis is considered a sub-type of gliomatosis cerebri *(55,56)*. The term gliomatosis though sounds like a sub-type of glioma, but its cell of origin is controversial and considered unknown *(55)*. Regardless, gliomatosis cerebri is still considered a HGG (WHO grade III) because of its grim prognosis, although the histological features more closely mimic low grade lesions *(57,58)*.

Diagnosis of gliomatosis cerebri may be difficult on CT imaging in the absence of a focal mass lesion with no appreciable abnormality in some cases. The reason for subtely of findings on CT and sometimes MRI is probably related to the infiltrative nondestructive nature of the gliomatosis cerebri as it infiltrates along the vessels and white matter tracts. On a CT there are

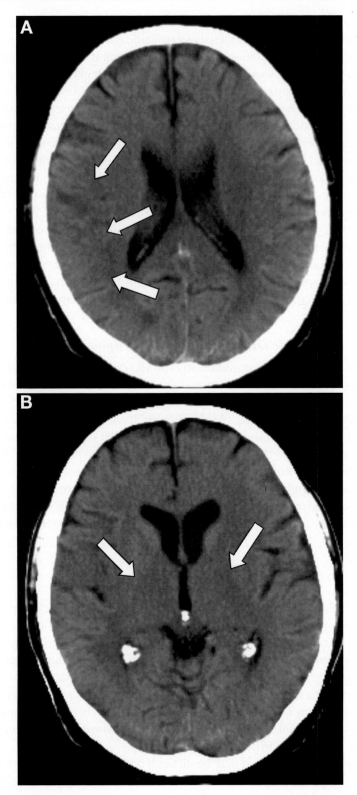

Fig. 12. Gliomatosis cerebri. (**A,B**) Noncontrast CT, (**C**) axial FLAIR, and (**D**) post contrast T1 MR images. (**A**, *arrows*) There is subtle loss of gray-white matter differentiation and *(continued on next page)*

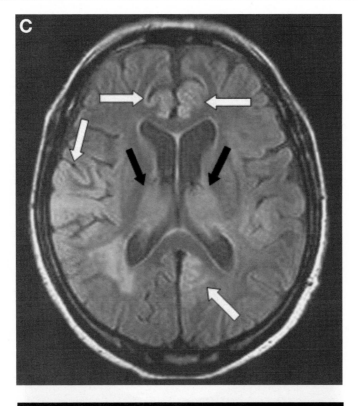

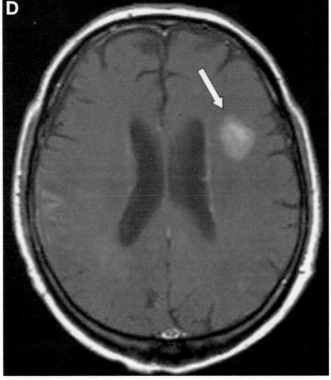

(**B**, *arrows*) bilateral thalamic diffuse lucency resulting in loss of interface between posterior limbs of internal capsules and lateral thalami. Corresponding (more obvious) increased signal evident on MRI (*arrows*).

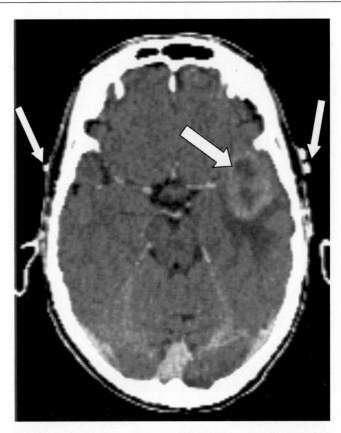

Fig. 13. GS as a recurrent high grade glioma. Fifty-four-year-old female with about 6 mo history of gross total resection of left temporal lobe GBM followed by adjuvant radiotherapy. Post-contrast CT image shows a recurrent rim enhancing necrotic left temporal lobe mass at the site of previous mass. Imaging features are similar to a GBM. Note fiducial markers (*arrows*) for stereotactic localization.

usually diffuse, ill defined, iso- to hypodense multifocal regions with subtle cortical thickening, sulcal effacement, and loss of gray-white matter demarcation (as both gray and white matter are involved) (Fig.12 A,B). Deep gray matter structures can be involved (Fig. 12 B,C). Contrast enhancement is uncommon, but if present is usually very subtle unless the process is quite advanced *(59)*. The enhancement pattern is either linear or patchy *(60)* (Fig. 12D).

The extent of disease is evaluated much better on MRI (particularly T2-weighted and FLAIR MR images) than on CT scans *(60)*.

Gliosarcoma

Gliosarcomas (GS) actually represent a subtype of GBM in which a sarcomatous component is present. GS are typically present along the periphery, abutting the dura *(61)*. Like glioblastoma, they correspond to WHO grade IV. Extracranial metastases are more commonly seen than GBM *(61)*. GS may appear in previously irradiated regions of the brain *(62,63)* (Fig. 13).

On CT, GS tends to present as a sharply defined, round or lobulated, hyperdense solid mass with relatively homogeneous contrast enhancement and peri-tumoral edema. They have a tendency to invade adjacent dural reflections *(64,65)*. The hyperdensity is attributed to sarcomatous component as it is highly vascular and cellular. The lesions are often well demarcated from surrounding tissue, leading to complete removal and prolonged survival despite high malignancy *(66)*. Nevertheless, aggressive tumor regrowth occurs often after incomplete resection with prognosis almost similar to GBM *(61,67,68)*. Typically, the hyperdense mass abutting the dura mimics a meningioma; both in imaging and surgery. However, compared with meningioma, they are more heterogenous, have a smaller dural based attachment, and there is usually a significant amount of parenchymal edema. Some cases of GS have imaging features like GBM, having a large necrotic center with irregular enhancement *(69)* (Fig. 13).

Malignant Brain Stem Glioma

Brain stem gliomas are a heterogenous group of, typically, pediatric brain tumors. Adult brainstem gliomas are rare *(70)*. Focal, more benign subtypes (i.e., tectal, focal tegmental, dorsal exophytic, cervicomedullary) are usually pilocytic gliomas while diffuse (intrinsic) pontine gliomas are of the fibrillary type with a higher WHO grade and poor prognosis *(71)*. Diffuse pontine gliomas have a somewhat better prognosis in children with NF1 whereas the prognosis is worse for NF1 adults *(72)*.

On noncontrast CT, diffuse pontine gliomas are usually seen as a low-attenuation ill defined mass expanding the pons (Fig.14A). Abnormal signal intensity with expanded configuration of pons, exophytic growth into the basal cisterns, and occasional encasement of basilar artery are better appreciated on MRI (Fig.14B). Calcification is rarely seen. Hydrocephalus is uncommon even in large infiltrative tumors, seen in only about 10% of cases at presentation (unlike focal tumors such as tectal glioma) *(73)*. Enhancement is variable in pontine gliomas and indicates poor prognosis particularly in adults *(70)*. CSF dissemination occurs in up to 50% of cases *(74)*.

Anaplastic Ependymoma

Ependymomas generate considerable controversy with regard to their rational clinical management. Malignant histologic features seen in ependymomas are related to prognosis, but not as strongly as seen with astrocytomas *(75,76)*. According to WHO grading, ependymal tumors have been divided into subependymomas (grade I), ependymomas (grade II), and anaplastic ependymomas (grade III) *(77)*. Besides the typical histologic features of ependymomas which includes glial (perivascular "pseudorossettes") and epithelial (ependymal "true rosette" pattern) components, anaplastic ependymomas (AE) show endothelial proliferation, mitoses, necrosis, and loss of typical cellular architecture *(78,79)*.

Tominaga et al. *(78)* reported CT imaging features in seven cases of anaplastic ependymomas. All had both cystic and solid components with CT detectable, calcific fragments. Increasing endothelial proliferation facilitates contrast enhancement. As these features are similar to subepyndemoma and ependymoma (grade I and II), distinction between them is difficult on the basis of imaging findings (Fig. 15).

Anaplastic Pleomorphic Xanthoastrocytoma

Anaplastic pleomorphic xanthoastrocytoma (PXA) is a benign supratentorial astrocytoma which occurs almost exclusively in young patients. They are classified as WHO grade II. Histologically, pleomorphism is the hallmark of PXA in addition to other characteristic features. Anaplastic PXA is rare *(80)*. PXA may need a long follow up as malignant transformation has been seen after many years *(81)*.

Imaging features of PXA are either a cyst with an enhancing mural nodule or, less commonly, a solid tumor *(82–84)*. Calcification may be present (Fig. 16). The mural nodule is

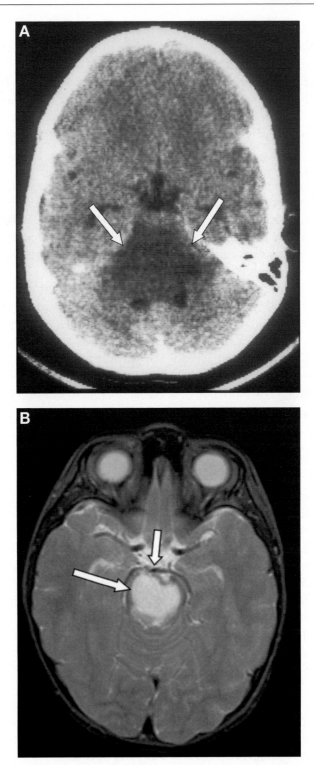

Fig. 14. Diffuse pontine glioma (DPG). Noncontrast CT image displaying a large area of lucency in the posterior fossa (*arrows*) representing expansion of brainstem by infiltrative mass. Axial T2 weighted MRI of another patient showing hyperintense expansile mass (*long arrow*), early stage as basilar artery is intact and not yet involved (*short arrow*).

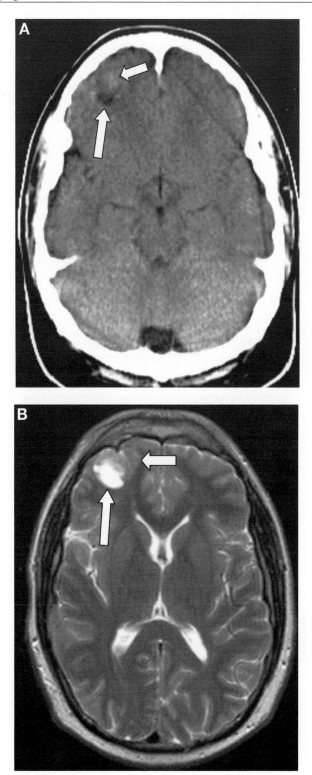

Fig. 15. Anaplastic ependymoma. Noncontrast CT and axial T2 MR images. Focal region of mixed density in the right frontal lobe (*long arrow*) with punctate calcifications (*short arrow*). Note lack of vasogenic edema.MRI demonstrates well defined solid (*short arrow*) and cystic (*long arrow*) portions of the mass.

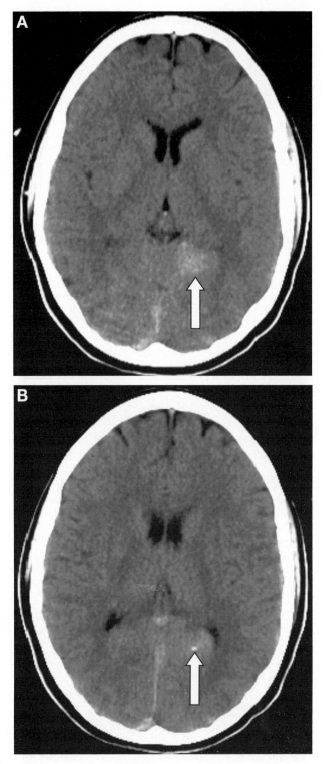

Fig. 16. Pleomorphic xanthoastrocytoma. (**A,B**) Noncontrast CT images. (**A**, *long arrows*) Focal periventricular left occipital hyperdensity with (**B**, *short arrows*) punctuate calcifications. The lesion was removed but later on had a recurrent tumor at the same location (not shown). Biopsy showed anaplastic pleomorphic xanthoastrocytoma.

usually attached to the leptomeninges as the tumor usually has a peripheral location *(83)*. On unenhanced CT, the mural nodule or solid tumor has variable density. Angiography may show a hypervascular tumor with supply from meningeal arteries *(85)*. It is because of these imaging features that PXA can be confused with meningioma. Anaplastic PXA presents as a recurrent tumor with leptomeningeal dissemination.

Astroblastoma (Anaplastic)

A rare glial neoplasm, occurring in young patients. The cell of origin is debatable as they share features of astrocytoma and ependymoma. Based on histologic features, they can be low grade or high grade *(86)*.

Typical CT features (irrespective of the grade) are a mixed solid and cystic lobulated mass; the solid portion has a characteristic "bubbly" appearance (better seen on MRI). Punctate calcifications may be seen. Solid component shows heterogenous enhancement whereas there is usually rim enhancement of the cystic portion. Astroblastomas lack significant peritumoral edema *(87)*.

SUMMARY

Computed tomography continues to play a significant role in the management of HGG. CT is superior in detecting calcification, hemorrhage and in evaluating bone changes related to tumors. Patients with pacemakers or metallic devices as well as critically ill or unstable patients represent some of the specific areas in which CT is the diagnostic modality of choice. CT is also study of choice for assessment of immediate post-operative complications. The arrival of multichannel, spiral CT has facilitated sophisticated 3D as well as dynamic imaging. These advanced techniques are useful in preoperative localization, intraoperative navigation, radiation therapy targeting and differentiation of recurrent tumor from post therapy changes.

REFERENCES

1. Chawla S. Advances in multidetector computed tomography: applications in neuroradiology J Comput Assist Tomogr 2004;28 Suppl:S12–S16.
2. Kalra MK, Maher MM, D'Souza R, Saini S. Multidetector Computed Tomography Technology: Current Status and Emerging Developments J Comput Assist Tomogr 2004;28:S2–S6.
3. Tomandl BF, Kostner NC, Schempershofe M, et al. CT angiography of intracranial aneurysms: a focus on postprocessing Radiographics 2004;24:637–655.
4. Tomandl BF, Klotz E, Handschu R, et al. Comprehensive imaging of ischemic stroke with multisection CT Radiographics 2003;23:565–592.
5. Roberts HC, Roberts TP, Smith WS, Lee TJ, Fischbein NJ, Dillon WP. Multisection dynamic CT perfusion for acute cerebral ischemia: the "toggling-table" technique. AJNR Am J Neuroradiol 2001;22:1077–1080.
6. Vajkoczy P, Menger MD. Vascular microenvironment in gliomas. J Neurooncol 2000;50:99–108.
7. Folkman J. The role of angiogenesis in tumor growth. Semin Cancer Biol 1992;3:65–71.
8. Jain RK, Gerlowski LE. Extravascular transport in normal and tumor tissues. Crit Rev Oncol Hematol 1986;5:115–170.
9. Roberts HC, Roberts TP, Ley S, Dillon WP, Brasch RC. Quantitative estimation of microvascular permeability in human brain tumors: correlation of dynamic Gd-DTPA-enhanced MR imaging with histopathologic grading. Acad Radiol 2002;9 Suppl 1:S151–S155.
10. Klotz E, Konig M. Perfusion measurements of the brain: using dynamic CT for the quantitative assessment of cerebral ischemia in acute stroke. Eur J Radiol 1999;30:170–184.
11. Cook AJ PSSDLZ. Comparison of contrast injection protocols in CT brain perfusion using two calculation algorithms. Radiology 221(P), 480. 2001. Ref Type: Abstract.
12. Axel L. Cerebral blood flow determination by rapid-sequence computed tomography: theoretical analysis. Radiology 1980;137:679–686.

13. Nabavi DG, Cenic A, Craen RA, et al. CT assessment of cerebral perfusion: experimental validation and initial clinical experience. Radiology 1999;213:141–149.

14. Wintermark M, Maeder P, Thiran JP, Schnyder P, Meuli R. Quantitative assessment of regional cerebral blood flows by perfusion CT studies at low injection rates: a critical review of the underlying theoretical models. Eur Radiol 2001;11:1220–1230.

15. Eastwood JD, Engelter ST, MacFall JF, Delong DM, Provenzale JM. Quantitative assessment of the time course of infarct signal intensity on diffusion-weighted images. AJNR Am J Neuroradiol 2003;24:680–687.

16. Wintermark M, Thiran JP, Maeder P, Schnyder P, Meuli R. Simultaneous measurement of regional cerebral blood flow by perfusion CT and stable xenon CT: a validation study. AJNR Am J Neuroradiol 2001;22:905–914.

17. Law M, Yang S, Wang H, et al. Glioma grading: sensitivity, specificity, and predictive values of perfusion MR imaging and proton MR spectroscopic imaging compared with conventional MR imaging. AJNR Am J Neuroradiol 2003;24:1989–1998.

18. Shin JH, Lee HK, Kwun BD, et al. Using relative cerebral blood flow and volume to evaluate the histopathologic grade of cerebral gliomas: preliminary results. AJR Am J Roentgenol 2002;179:783–789.

19. Lam WW, Chan KW, Wong WL, Poon WS, Metreweli C. Pre-operative grading of intracranial glioma. Acta Radiol 2001;42:548–554.

20. Roberts HC, Roberts TP, Bollen AW, Ley S, Brasch RC, Dillon WP. Correlation of microvascular permeability derived from dynamic contrast-enhanced MR imaging with histologic grade and tumor labeling index: a study in human brain tumors. Acad Radiol 2001;8:384–391.

21. Law M, Yang S, Babb JS, et al. Comparison of cerebral blood volume and vascular permeability from dynamic susceptibility contrast-enhanced perfusion MR imaging with glioma grade. AJNR Am J Neuroradiol 2004;25:746–755.

22. Provenzale JM, Wang GR, Brenner T, Petrella JR, Sorensen AG. Comparison of permeability in high-grade and low-grade brain tumors using dynamic susceptibility contrast MR imaging. AJR Am J Roentgenol 2002;178:711–716.

23. Sugahara T, Korogi Y, Tomiguchi S, et al. Posttherapeutic intraaxial brain tumor: the value of perfusion-sensitive contrast-enhanced MR imaging for differentiating tumor recurrence from nonneoplastic contrast-enhancing tissue AJNR Am J Neuroradiol 2000;21:901–909.

24. Haberland N, Ebmeier K, Hliscs R, et al. Neuronavigation in surgery of intracranial and spinal tumors. J Cancer Res Clin Oncol 2000;126:529–541.

25. Grunert P, Muller-Forell W, Darabi K, et al. Basic principles and clinical applications of neuronavigation and intraoperative computed tomography. Comput Aided Surg 1998;3:166–173.

26. Matula C, Rossler K, Reddy M, Schindler E, Koos WT. Intraoperative computed tomography guided neuronavigation: concepts, efficiency, and work flow. Comput Aided Surg 1998;3:174–182.

27. Rees JH, Smirniotopoulos JG, Jones RV, Wong K. Glioblastoma multiforme: radiologic-pathologic correlation. Radiographics 1996;16:1413–1438.

28. Barnard RO, Geddes JF. The incidence of multifocal cerebral gliomas. A histologic study of large hemisphere sections. Cancer 1987;60:1519–1531.

29. Van Tassel P, Lee YY, Bruner JM. Synchronous and metachronous malignant gliomas: CT findings. AJNR Am J Neuroradiol 1988;9:725–732.

30. Kyritsis AP, Levin VA, Yung WK, Leeds NE. Imaging patterns of multifocal gliomas. Eur J Radiol 1993;16:163–170.

31. Rao KC, Levine H, Itani A, Sajor E, Robinson W. CT findings in multicentric glioblastoma: diagnostic-pathologic correlation. J Comput Tomogr 1980;4:187–192.

32. Licata B, Turazzi S. Bleeding cerebral neoplasms with symptomatic hematoma. J Neurosurg Sci 2003;47:201–210.

33. Lote K, Egeland T, Hager B, Skullerud K, Hirschberg H. Prognostic significance of CT contrast enhancement within histological subgroups of intracranial glioma. J Neurooncol 1998;40:161–170.

34. Earnest F, Kelly PJ, Scheithauer BW, et al. Cerebral astrocytomas: histopathologic correlation of MR and CT contrast enhancement with stereotactic biopsy. Radiology 1988;166:823–827.

35. Ginsberg LE, Fuller GN, Hashmi M, Leeds NE, Schomer DF. The significance of lack of MR contrast enhancement of supratentorial brain tumors in adults: histopathological evaluation of a series. Surg Neurol 1998;49:436–440.

36. Yamada S, Takai Y, Nemoto K, et al. Prognostic significance of CT scan in malignant glioma. Tohoku J Exp Med 1993;170:35–43.

37. Daumas-Duport C, Scheithauer B, O'Fallon J, Kelly P. Grading of astrocytomas. A simple and reproducible method. Cancer 1988;62:2152–2165.

38. Wang HC, Ho YS. Clinicopathological evaluation of 78 astrocytomas in Taiwan with emphasis on a simple grading system. J Neurooncol 1992;13:265–276.
39. Davis FG, Kupelian V, Freels S, McCarthy B, Surawicz T. Prevalence estimates for primary brain tumors in the United States by behavior and major histology groups. Neuro -oncol 2001;3:152–158.
40. Peraud A, Ansari H, Bise K, Reulen HJ. Clinical outcome of supratentorial astrocytoma WHO grade II. Acta Neurochir (Wien) 1998;140:1213–1222.
41. Grabb PA, Albright AL, Pang D. Dissemination of supratentorial malignant gliomas via the cerebrospinal fluid in children. Neurosurgery 1992;30:64–71.
42. Ricci PE. Imaging of adult brain tumors. Neuroimaging Clin N Am 1999;9:651–669.
43. Kondziolka D, Bernstein M, Resch L, et al. Significance of hemorrhage into brain tumors: clinicopathological study. J Neurosurg 1987;67:852–857.
44. Wong JC, Provenzale JM, Petrella JR. Perfusion MR imaging of brain neoplasms. AJR Am J Roentgenol 2000;174:1147–1157.
45. Barker FG, Davis RL, Chang SM, Prados MD. Necrosis as a prognostic factor in glioblastoma multiforme. Cancer 1996;77:1161–1166.
46. Lee YY, Van Tassel P. Intracranial oligodendrogliomas: imaging findings in 35 untreated cases. AJR Am J Roentgenol 1989;152:361–369.
47. Tamura M, Zama A, Kurihara H, et al. Clinicohistological study of oligodendroglioma and oligoastrocytoma. Brain Tumor Pathol 1997;14:35–39.
48. Vonofakos D, Marcu H, Hacker H. Oligodendrogliomas: CT patterns with emphasis on features indicating malignancy. J Comput Assist Tomogr 1979;3:783–788.
49. Tice H, Barnes PD, Goumnerova L, Scott RM, Tarbell NJ. Pediatric and adolescent oligodendrogliomas. AJNR Am J Neuroradiol 1993;14:1293–1300.
50. Lee YY, Van Tassel P. Intracranial oligodendrogliomas: imaging findings in 35 untreated cases. AJR Am J Roentgenol 1989;152:361–369.
51. Lebrun C, Fontaine D, Ramaioli A, et al. Long-term outcome of oligodendrogliomas. Neurology 2004;62: 1783–1787.
52. Artigas J, Cervos-Navarro J, Iglesias JR, Ebhardt G. Gliomatosis cerebri: clinical and histological findings. Clin Neuropathol 1985;4:135–148.
53. Ross IB, Robitaille Y, Villemure JG, Tampieri D. Diagnosis and management of gliomatosis cerebri: recent trends. Surg Neurol 1991;36:431–440.
54. Carpio-O'Donovan R, Korah I, Salazar A, Melancon D. Gliomatosis cerebri. Radiology 1996;198:831–835
55. Kleihues P, Louis DN, Scheithauer BW, et al. The WHO classification of tumors of the nervous system. J Neuropathol Exp Neurol 2002;61:215–225.
56. Leproux F, Melanson D, Mercier C, Michaud J, Ethier R. Leptomeningeal gliomatosis: MR findings. J Comput Assist Tomogr 1993;17:317–320.
57. Yamada SM, Hayashi Y, Takahashi H, Teramoto A, Matsumoto K, Yamada S. Histological and genetic diagnosis of gliomatosis cerebri: case report. J Neurooncol 2001;52:237–240.
58. Elshaikh MA, Stevens GH, Peereboom DM, et al. Gliomatosis cerebri: treatment results with radiotherapy alone. Cancer 2002;95:2027–2031.
59. Ross IB, Robitaille Y, Villemure JG, Tampieri D. Diagnosis and management of gliomatosis cerebri: recent trends. Surg Neurol 1991;36:431–440.
60. Shin YM, Chang KH, Han MH, et al. Gliomatosis cerebri: comparison of MR and CT features. AJR Am J Roentgenol 1993;161:859–862.
61. Morantz RA, Feigin I, Ransohoff J, III. Clinical and pathological study of 24 cases of gliosarcoma. J Neurosurg 1976;45:398–408.
62. Perry JR, Ang LC, Bilbao JM, Muller PJ. Clinicopathologic features of primary and postirradiation cerebral gliosarcoma. Cancer 1995;75:2910–2918.
63. Lach M, Wallace CJ, Krcek J, Curry B. Radiation-associated gliosarcoma. Can Assoc Radiol J 1996;47: 209–212.
64. Jack CR, Jr., Bhansali DT, Chason JL, et al. Angiographic features of gliosarcoma. AJNR Am J Neuroradiol 1987;8:117–122.
65. Cerame MA, Guthikonda M, Kohli CM. Extraneural metastases in gliosarcoma: a case report and review of the literature. Neurosurgery 1985;17:413–418.
66. Maiuri F, Stella L, Benvenuti D, Giamundo A, Pettinato G. Cerebral gliosarcomas: correlation of computed tomographic findings, surgical aspect, pathological features, and prognosis. Neurosurgery 1990;26:261–267.
67. Lee YY, Castillo M, Nauert C, Moser RP. Computed tomography of gliosarcoma. AJNR Am J Neuroradiol 1985;6:527–531.

68. Morantz RA, Feigin I, Ransohoff J, III. Clinical and pathological study of 24 cases of gliosarcoma. J Neurosurg 1976;45:398–408.
69. Maiuri F, Stella L, Benvenuti D, Giamundo A, Pettinato G. Cerebral gliosarcomas: correlation of computed tomographic findings, surgical aspect, pathological features, and prognosis. Neurosurgery 1990;26:261–267.
70. Guillamo JS, Monjour A, Taillandier L, et al. Brainstem gliomas in adults: prognostic factors and classification. Brain 2001;124:2528–2539.
71. Fisher PG, Breiter SN, Carson BS, et al. A clinicopathologic reappraisal of brain stem tumor classification. Identification of pilocystic astrocytoma and fibrillary astrocytoma as distinct entities. Cancer 2000;89:1569–1576.
72. Guillamo JS, Creange A, Kalifa C, et al. Prognostic factors of CNS tumours in Neurofibromatosis 1 (NF1): a retrospective study of 104 patients. Brain 2003;126:152–160.
73. Raffel C, Hudgins R, Edwards MS. Symptomatic hydrocephalus: initial findings in brainstem gliomas not detected on computed tomographic scans. Pediatrics 1988;82:733–737.
74. Donahue B, Allen J, Siffert J, Rosovsky M, Pinto R. Patterns of recurrence in brain stem gliomas: evidence for craniospinal dissemination. Int J Radiat Oncol Biol Phys 1998;40:677–680.
75. Schiffer D, Chio A, Giordana MT, et al. Histologic prognostic factors in ependymoma. Childs Nerv Syst 1991;7:177–182.
76. Gerszten PC, Pollack IF, Martinez AJ, Lo KH, Janosky J, Albright AL. Intracranial ependymomas of childhood. Lack of correlation of histopathology and clinical outcome. Pathol Res Pract 1996;192:515–522
77. Ernestus RI, Schroder R, Stutzer H, Klug N. The clinical and prognostic relevance of grading in intracranial ependymomas. Br J Neurosurg 1997;11:421–428.
78. Tominaga T, Kayama T, Kumabe T, Sonoda Y, Yoshimoto T. Anaplastic ependymomas: clinical features and tumour suppressor gene p53 analysis. Acta Neurochir (Wien) 1995;135:163–170.
79. Talan-Hranilovic J, Lambasa S, Kogler A. Anaplastic ependymoma in children—increasing incidence? Neurol Croat 1991;41:51–55.
80. Lubansu A, Rorive S, David P, et al. Cerebral anaplastic pleomorphic xanthoastrocytoma with meningeal dissemination at first presentation. Childs Nerv Syst 2004;20:119–122.
81. van Roost D, Kristof R, Zentner J, Wolf HK, Schramm J. Clinical, radiological, and therapeutic features of pleomorphic xanthoastrocytoma: report of three patients and review of the literature. J Neurol Neurosurg Psychiatry 1996;60:690–692.
82. Luh GY, Bird CR. Imaging of brain tumors in the pediatric population. Neuroimaging Clin N Am 1999;9:691–716.
83. Tonn JC, Paulus W, Warmuth-Metz M, Schachenmayr W, Sorensen N, Roosen K. Pleomorphic xanthoastrocytoma: report of six cases with special consideration of diagnostic and therapeutic pitfalls. Surg Neurol 1997;47:162–169.
84. Tien RD, Cardenas CA, Rajagopalan S. Pleomorphic xanthoastrocytoma of the brain: MR findings in six patients. AJR Am J Roentgenol 1992;159:1287–1290.
85. Maleki M, Robitaille Y, Bertrand G. Atypical xanthoastrocytoma presenting as a meningioma. Surg Neurol 1983;20:235–238.
86. Brat DJ, Hirose Y, Cohen KJ, Feuerstein BG, Burger PC. Astroblastoma: clinicopathologic features and chromosomal abnormalities defined by comparative genomic hybridization. Brain Pathol 2000;10:342–352.
87. Port JD, Brat DJ, Burger PC, Pomper MG. Astroblastoma: radiologic-pathologic correlation and distinction from ependymoma. AJNR Am J Neuroradiol 2002;23:243–247.

6 Magnetic Resonance Imaging

Paul M. Ruggieri

Summary

Magnetic resonance (MR) is clearly the accepted imaging standard for the preliminary evaluation, peri-operative management, and routine longitudinal follow-up of patients with high-grade gliomas (HGG). The purpose of this chapter is to review the imaging characteristics of HGG using
conventional MR imaging techniques. Whereas the newer techniques of MR diffusion, perfusion,
diffusion tensor imaging, and MR spectroscopy will be included as part of this discussion of the high
grade neoplasms, the detailed concepts of such studies will be discussed elsewhere in this text.

Key Words: MR imaging; anaplastic astrocytoma; glioblastoma multiforme; gliosarcoma;
gliomatosis cerebri; oligodendroglioma.

INTRODUCTION

Magnetic resonance (MR) is clearly the accepted imaging standard for the preliminary
evaluation, peri-operative management, and routine longitudinal follow-up of patients with
high-grade gliomas (HGG). The purpose of this chapter is to review the imaging characteristics
of HGG using conventional MR imaging techniques. Whereas the newer techniques of MR
diffusion, perfusion, diffusion tensor imaging, and MR spectroscopy will be included as part
of this discussion of the high grade neoplasms, the detailed concepts of such studies will be
discussed elsewhere in this text.

In general terms, high-grade glial neoplasms are conventionally thought of as infiltrative
parenchymal masses that are hyperintense on FLAIR fluid-attenuated inversion recovery
(FLAIR) and T2-weighted images, hypointense on unenhanced T1-weighted images, may or
may not extend into the corpus callosum, are surrounded by extensive vasogenic edema, and
prominently enhance following gadolinium administration. It must be pointed out that this
description is clearly just a generalization as many high-grade neoplasms clearly do not follow
these "rules" and some of these characteristics may even be seen in low-grade neoplasms. The
most common and obvious contradiction is the pilocytic astrocytoma in children and young
adults. This is clearly a low-grade neoplasm although MR imaging demonstrates a solid soft
tissue nodule that enhances strikingly following gadolinium administration. Conversely, many
HGG do not enhance at all with gadolinium *(1)*. Such contradictions would suggest that
isolated MR imaging characteristics frequently do not permit a clear distinction between the
different primary glial neoplasms or the histologic grades of these masses. Earlier studies
demonstrated sensitivities for MRI alone ranging from 55 to 83% for grading of gliomas *(2–
7)*. One of these studies suggested mass effect and necrosis as the most reliable predictors of

From: *Current Clinical Oncology: High-Grade Gliomas: Diagnosis and Treatment*
Edited by: G. H. Barnett © Humana Press Inc., Totowa, NJ

tumor grade but these generalizations are frequently contradicted. Whereas enhancement is thought to be common in higher grade masses, all such masses do not enhance and, in one study, nearly 20% of glioblastomas did not enhance *(6,8)*. It is likely safe to state that a prominently enhancing parenchymal mass in an adult is unlikely to be a low-grade neoplasm. In practice, the primary job of imaging in the preliminary evaluation of such patients is to characterize the extent of disease and the impact on the adjacent normal brain. Limited conventional MRI features in conjunction with demographic data and the clinical presentation can help to distinguish the different neoplasms and to identify the more aggressive masses. It is still becoming increasingly common to employ specialized studies such as diffusion, perfusion, and MR spectroscopy if conventional evaluation fails to make these distinctions in patients with conflicting clinical and imaging data. Alternatively, such studies can be utilized in the follow-up of gliomas to differentiate tumor recurrence, malignant degeneration, and the sequelae of therapy if conventional MRI fails to do so.

ANAPLASTIC ASTROCYTOMA

Anaplastic astrocytomas (AA) are histologically classified as World Health Organization (WHO) grade III neoplasms. Analagous to infiltrative astrocytomas, these tumors have infiltrative margins on histology. On the other hand, they contain areas of pleomorphism and high cellularity and may demonstrate areas of necrosis and cyst formation like their higher grade counterparts. Up to 75% of AA are felt to arise from lower grade gliomas whereas the anaplastic group may also dedifferentiate into glioblastomas over time *(9)*. The age of presentation also tends to be intermediate between these two groups, typically discovered during the fourth to fifth decades of life in patients presenting with seizures, focal neurologic deficits, or signs of increased intracranial pressure (ICP) *(10)*. In view of the above, it should not be surprising that AA tend to have imaging findings that are intermediate between the infiltrative astrocytomas and glioblastomas.

The AA can be quite variable in location but nearly all are supratentorial and most are centered in the deep white matter and may secondarily involve the deep gray-matter structures. These masses generally have poorly defined margins and are somewhat heterogeneous in signal intensity characteristics on all MR pulse sequences, most evident on the FLAIR and T2-weighted images (Fig. 1). The amount of surrounding vasogenic edema is quite variable but more commonly relatively mild and frequently indistinguishable from the margins of the nonenhancing component of the mass. Consequently, it is difficult to determine the true extent of neoplastic cell invasion when planning complete resection by MRI. FLAIR and T2-weighted images certainly demonstrate the extent of parenchymal involvement better than the T1-weighted images but tumor cells can extend into parenchyma that is normal in signal intensity on all pulse sequences. Of the two, the FLAIR images generally make it easier to appreciate the MRI abnormality because the darkened cerebrospinal fluid (CSF) makes involvement along the pial and ependymal surfaces of the brain more obvious and resetting the gray scale makes the subcortical involvement more apparent. The T1-weighted images are generally more useful for assessing mass effect and location of the mass. The unenhanced T1-weighted images may also show small foci of mild hyperintensity related to dystrophic calcification (shortened T1-relaxation time resulting from the impact on water molecules by the calcium along the margins of the crystalline matrix) that could be misleading when assessing gadolinium enhancement. Small foci of hemorrhage that may arise *de novo* or may be related to a recent stereotactic biopsy procedure are commonly more obviously hyperintense on the T1-weighted images. The parenchyma that enhances with gadolinium represents the

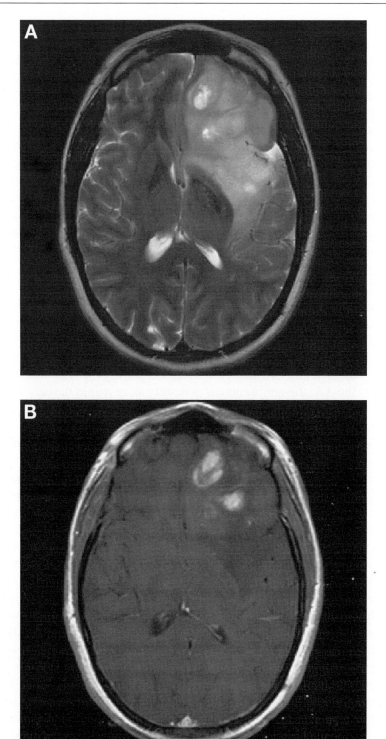

Fig. 1. Anaplastic astrocytoma: (**A**) Axial T2-weighted image demonstrating large infiltrative mass in the left frontal lobe that is heterogeneously hyperintense, presumably representing the heterogeneity of the histology. (**B**) Large irregular nodular foci and small ill-defined patchy foci of enhancement are detected in the inferior left frontal lobe on this gadolinium-enhanced T1-weighted spin echo images.

area with the most extensive breakdown in the blood–brain barrier (BBB) and generally indicates the more aggressive component of the mass but clearly does not reflect the true extent of the mass. The enhancement within the masses is generally patchy or heterogeneous in nature. Ring enhancement is atypical as this is generally seen in glioblastomas with central necrosis. On the other hand, some AA may not enhance at all. One prior study demonstrated that nearly 40% of nonenhancing masses were found to be AA (8). The associated mass effect is contingent on size, location, and surrounding edema but is usually moderate in degree. Evidence of prior hemorrhage is relatively infrequent in contrast to glioblastomas. It is also important to remember that AA generally spread in a contiguous fashion along normal white-matter tracts but may also disseminate in the CSF along the pial and ependymal surfaces if the mass is contiguous with the ventricles or the outer surface of the brain. This is most sensitively demonstrated on gadolinium-enhanced T1 images as linear and/or nodular enhancement along the ependymal or pial surfaces of the brain and/or spinal cord or as confluent masses of varying sizes in the basilar cisterns, over the cerebral convexities, or within the spinal canal.

GLIOBLASTOMA MULTIFORME

Glioblastoma multiforme is classified as a WHO grade IV neoplasm and is among the most common primary intracranial neoplasms. Glioblastomas account for the majority of glial tumors, over half of astrocytic tumors, and up to 20% of all intracranial tumors (1,11). Although uncommon in the pediatric population, glioblastomas make up more than half of primary intracranial neoplasms in adults with a peak incidence during the sixth and seventh decades of life. Similar to the AA, the glioblastomas generally arise within the cerebral hemispheres and symptoms at presentation usually include headache, seizures, focal neurologic deficit, change in personality, and/or signs of increased intracranial pressure.

Histologically, these masses are characterized as infiltrative masses with high cellularity, cellular pleomorphism, and increased mitotic index. These tumors are characteristically very heterogeneous with evidence of microvascular and endothelial proliferation, tumoral hemor-rhage, and variably sized foci of tissue necrosis (12,13). Imaging characteristics reflect the histopathologic findings as these masses are generally quite heterogeneous in appearance on MR and computed tomography (CT). Hemorrhage may be seen in up to 20% of masses and evidence of necrosis is conventionally thought of as the "imaging hallmark" of glioblastomas (14–16). Dystrophic calcification is quite uncommon, likely due to the relatively aggressive nature of the mass.

MRI demonstrates an infiltrative, intra-axial, soft tissue mass within the cerebral hemi-spheres that is heterogeneous in signal intensity on all pulse sequences. Although glioblasto-mas are quite cellular, the soft tissue components are generally heterogeneously hyperintense on the FLAIR and T2-weighted images. There is generally a large amount of surrounding vasogenic edema resulting from the proliferation of abnormal blood vessels within the mass and transudation of fluid into the interstitium through the leaky endothelium. There may also be neoplastic cells within the edematous tissue that is indistinguishable from the edema alone (17–19). In either case, this will appear as surrounding prominent hyperintensity on T2 and FLAIR and less obvious hypointensity on T1-weighted MR images. As the corpus callosum is made up of densely packed white matter that is generally resistant to the spread of vasogenic edema, FLAIR and T2 signal abnormalities that are contiguous with the mass and extend into the corpus callosum can generally be thought of as contiguous spread of neoplasm rather than extension of vasogenic edema regardless of whether there is enhancement with gadolinium in this region of the corpus callosum or not (Fig. 2).

The vascularity and necrosis in these masses explains the presence of prior hemorrhage that may be seen in these masses. Acute hemorrhage will appear as a focus of hypointensity on T1- and T2-weighted images, subacute hemorrhage will appear hyperintense on both sequences, and remote hemorrhage may be seen as mild hyperintensity on T1 or, more likely, irregular or linear foci of hypointensity on the T2-weighted images. Turbo- or fast-spin echo acquisitions are now used routinely for conventional MRI. Unfortunately, these pulse sequences inadvertently suppress the signal loss because of local field inhomogeneities caused by the iron deposition at the site of remote hemorrhage. If there is a suspicion of prior hemorrhage, it is necessary to perform a T2*-weighted gradient echo acquisition with a relatively long echo time in addition to conventional MR pulse sequences to more sensitively evaluate for the presence of prior hemorrhage. Such sequences will accentuate foci of prior hemorrhage as irregular foci of hypointensity resulting from a localized tissue gradient (hemorrhage adjacent to normal brain tissue) causing loss of signal in the tissues.

Contrast enhancement in these masses is usually quite prominent and heterogeneous in nature. The enhancement is generally more prominent peripherally as a thick, irregular rim surrounding a central area of necrosis that may occupy up to 80% of the volume of the overall mass (20). Although not uniformly present, glioblastomas classically demonstrate multi-loculated enhancement, comparable to that seen with abscess cavities. Abscess cavities would be more likely to have a thinner, more uniform rim that is hypointense on T2-weighted sequences in contrast with glioblastomas. The central cavities of abscesses are also more apt to have restricted diffusion on diffusion-weighted sequences than a glioblastoma (21,22). If these imaging findings and the clinical presentation still present a dilemma, alternative specialized studies could be employed for further preoperative evaluation.

The overwhelming majority of glioblastomas are solitary, supratentorial, intra-axial masses that spread within the parenchyma along white-matter tracts. In less than 5% of cases, these masses may be multifocal or multicentric. Such masses are thought to arise simultaneously at several sites if the masses are clearly separated by normal appearing white matter on all pulse sequences and are not contiguous with a pial or ependymal surface. Even more commonly than AA, glioblastomas may disseminate within the CSF space along the leptomeninges, ependymal surfaces of the ventricles, and pial surfaces of the brain and/or spinal cord to cause cranial nerve symptoms, hydrocephalus, radiculopathies, and myelopathy. It is possible to identify larger deposits of neoplasm that have spread within the CSF as hyperintense to isointense nodules of tissue on FLAIR images or hypointense to isointense masses on T1-weighted images. Gadolinium enhanced T1-weighted imaging is a far more sensitive means of evaluation for leptomeningeal spread of neoplasm and will be recognized as linear or nodular enhancement along the leptomeninges or pial or ependymal surfaces. Early signs on MRI may be unexplained new hydrocephalus without evidence of infection, new linear enhancement along the ependymal surfaces of the ventricles, or enhancement along the cranial nerves in the basilar cisterns (commonly cranial nerves III, V, VII, and VIII).

GLIOSARCOMA

Gliosarcomas are rare glioblastomas that contain an anaplastic glial component comparable to a glioblastoma, as well as, a mesenchymal component (23). Most commonly, the mesenchymal component is a malignant fibrous histiocytoma or fibrosarcoma but other alternatives include sarcomatous derivatives of smooth muscle, striated muscle, cartilage, and bone (24–26). These masses present during the fifth to seventh decades of life and are thought to arise from vascular constituents of glioblastomas. Gliosarcomas have also been reported

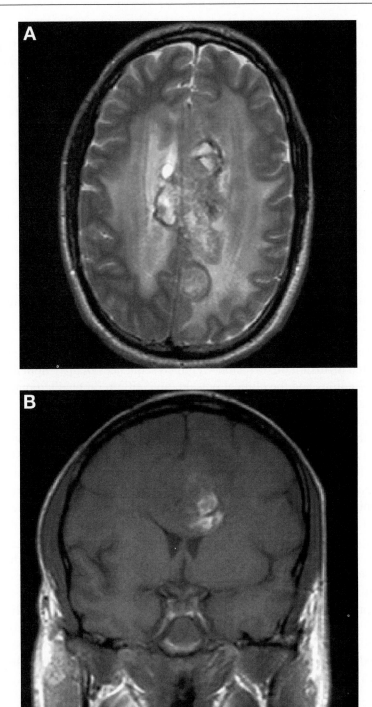

Fig. 2. Glioblastoma multiforme: **(A)** Axial TSE T2 image demonstrates a large heterogeneous soft tissue mass that extends to either side of midline. There is extensive confluent surrounding hyperintensity in the white matter of both cerebral hemispheres that likely represents a combination of edema and infiltrative neoplasm. **(B)** The mass clearly involves both mesial frontal lobes and the patchy hyperintensity within the mesial left frontal lobe suggests recent hemorrhage.

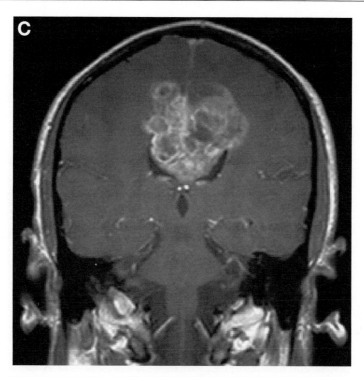

Fig. 2. *(continued from previous page)* **(C)** Following gadolinium administration, there is prominent, heterogeneous and multiloculated enhancement that involves both frontal lobes and the intervening body of the corpus callosum, typical for a glioblastoma.

following radiation therapy for pituitary adenomas, leukemia and lymphoma, presumably from vascular or astrocytic elements of a preexistent mass *(27–29)*. Such secondary masses arise after a relatively long latent period ranging from 1 to 12 yr after the therapy, appear within the irradiated parenchyma, and are different than the original mass *(29,30)*. In contrast with most primary intracranial masses, it is relatively common for the gliosarcomas to metastasize to sites outside of the central nervous system (CNS) *(24,31,32)*.

These masses are generally supratentorial and most commonly temporal in location. The masses are frequently relatively peripheral and may abut the dural surface similar to meningiomas but are still clearly intra-axial in location. Similar to the glioblastomas, the gliosarcomas are somewhat heterogeneous in signal intensity characteristics on MRI as a result of hemorrhage and necrosis within the masses. On the other hand, the gliosarcomas are discrepant as the underlying soft tissue component is still relatively hypointense on T2-weighted images, likely because of the high cellularity and high vascularity of the masses. Surrounding edema is frequent and the enhancement may be uniform or ring-like but very prominent following gadolinium administration *(33)*.

GLIOMATOSIS CEREBRI

Gliomatosis cerebri (GC) is defined as a generalized infiltration of parenchyma by neoplastic glial cells involving at least two, and more commonly three lobes of the brain *(34,35)*. The

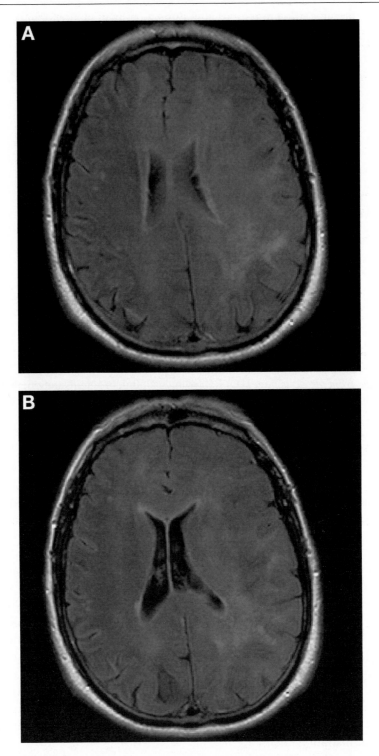

Fig. 3. Gliomatosis cerebri: **(A–C)** Axial turbo spin echo FLAIR images of the brain demonstrates diffuse subtle hyperintensity involving the white matter of nearly the entire left cerebral hemisphere and contiguous extension across midline through the corpus callosum into the right cerebral hemisphere. There is relatively mild mass effect in proportion to the size of the mass and the architecture of the hemispheres is largely maintained.

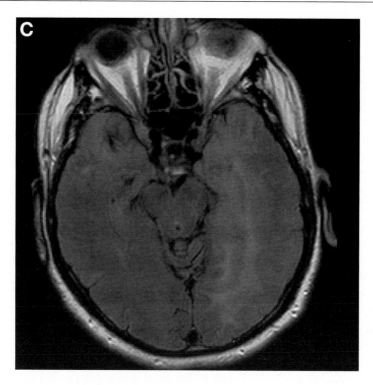

Fig. 3C. *(Continued from previous page.)*

involved areas should all be contiguous in contrast to a multifocal or multicentric glioma in which the multiple lesions appear completely separate. Beyond this, the overall architecture of the brain parenchyma is generally preserved on imaging and gross pathology. Although gliomatosis may present any time from the first decade to the sixth decade, it usually presents during the second through fourth decades without a predilection for sex. The clinical presentation may be nonspecific and usually insidious over a period of months to years, including a change in personality, dementia, hydrocephalus, and signs of increased intracranial pressure (ICP) prior to the onset of focal neurologic symptoms *(36,37)*.

Parenchymal involvement is usually supratentorial and predominantly involves the white matter with secondary involvement of deep and superficial gray matter and may also include the brainstem and cerebellum. On rare occasions, gliomatosis may present as a diffuse leptomeningeal process, indistinguishable from leptomeningeal metastases from distant primaries *(38,39)*. The "more common" parenchymal variety is typically recognized as a poorly defined, confluent and frequently mildly hyperintense process on the FLAIR and T2-weighted MR images that may be somewhat heterogeneous. The involved tissue is mildly increased in volume yet the overall structure of the tissue is still relatively well maintained (Fig. 3). The tissue may be isointense to mildly hypointense on T1-weighted images or hypointense and mildly heterogeneous on the T1-weighted gradient echo volume acquisitions typically used for preoperative three-dimensional (3D) localization. There is usually no enhancement with gadolinium on the T1-weighted images but may be present late in the disease process and described as linear or patchy in nature when it is present *(40)*.

OLIGODENDROGLIOMA

Oligodendrogliomas are considerably less common than glioblastomas and other astrocytomas and have a bimodal age distribution at presentation: the smaller initial peak occurs during the latter part of the first decade whereas the more common age of presentation is during the third to fifth decades of life *(41)*. These masses almost invariably arise supratentorially and are most commonly found in the frontal white matter and less commonly in the temporal and parietal white matter *(42)*. A few reports have also documented primary posterior fossa masses in children which are thought to be more aggressive *(43)*. Oligodendrogliogliomas may also rarely arise within the spinal cord *(44)*.

The histology of oligodendrogliomas can be widely variable and different criteria have been proposed for characterizing the histologic grading of these masses for prognostic purposes and therapeutic decisions *(45–50)*. As there is no one reliable criterion, each of these systems implements a combination of criteria to grade these masses. Among these proposals, only one of these systems includes an imaging criterion in the grading system—contrast enhancement *(49)*. Regardless of which criteria are used for histologic grading, the WHO recognizes only two categories: oligodendrogliomas and anaplastic oligodendrogliomas— the latter of which we are most interested in for this discussion. Molecular studies of oligodendrogliomas suggest that vascular endothelial growth factor receptors are highly expressed in the anaplastic oligodendrogliomas. This would imply that portions of oligodendrogliomas that degenerate to higher grade masses may then express these receptors and induce neovascularity and central necrosis *(51)*. These factors would argue the importance of enhancement, tumor heterogeneity and necrosis as important imaging criteria for more aggressive oligodendrogliomas. Cytogenetic studies are also generally utilized in predicting response to therapy: loss of chromosome 1p is associated with increased chemosensitivity; loss of 1p and 19q associated with higher chemosensitivity and longer survival; and the deletion of p16 on chromosome 9p in anaplastic oligodendrogliomas is associated with reduced survival *(52,53)*. Unfortunately, there are no real imaging correlates for these genetic characteristics.

Conventional MRI characteristics are somewhat nonspecific. The oligodendrogliomas present as confluent and relatively well-defined foci of hyperintensity on FLAIR and T2 with predominant involvement of the subcortical white matter and secondary involvement of the overlying cortical gray matter. Whereas a very high percentage of these masses are reportedly calcified on histology, up to 60% are calcified on CT *(54,55)*. The calcifications are typically large, dense, and globular on CT but can be easily missed altogether (even in retrospect) on MRI and do not clearly correlate with the histologic grade of the mass. Likewise, these masses may also contain cysts or foci of prior hemorrhage in 20% of cases but are not clearly predictive of tumor grade or the uniformity of histology. In some cases, the patients may present because of acute parenchymal hemorrhage within the mass but this is relatively rare. Surrounding edema is reported in 60% of cases and more commonly seen with higher grade neoplasms but may be difficult to distinguish from the underlying mass on FLAIR and T2. The signal intensity on T1-weighted images may be hypointense or mixed hypo- and hyperintense, perhaps because of prior hemorrhage and/or dystrophic calcification. Enhancement with gadolinium is also quite variable but more commonly seen with the higher grade neoplasms. When present, the gadolinium enhancement is subtle and patchy or honeycomb-like in nature *(54,56)*. Leptomeningeal metastases may also be seen in the setting of anaplastic oligodendrogliomas causing more extensive diffuse enhancement of the leptomeninges *(57)*.

It is relatively common for oligodendrogliomas to be mixed with components of an astrocytoma of varying degrees of malignancy. Anaplastic oligodendrogliomas may also degenerate into glioblastomas. Unfortunately, there are no good imaging criteria to preoperatively distinguish a mixed oligoastrocytoma from a pure oligodendroglioma. Degeneration into a glioblastoma may be distinguishable on preoperative imaging studies, the criteria for which are listed above.

DIFFUSION

MR diffusion imaging initially gained popularity and is now routinely used in the evaluation of patients with acute strokes *(58–61)*. In MR diffusion imaging, strong magnetic gradients are applied in each of three orthogonal directions to imaging sequences in equal but opposing directions. These gradients establish gradients across the individual imaging voxels and diffusing protons within these voxels cause a loss of phase coherence over time that accounts for signal loss within those voxels. The signal loss is proportional to the distance the diffusing protons moved over that time period. Protons whose diffusion is "restricted" by physical barriers or because they are bound to macromolecules will not change their net phases. Apparent diffusion coefficients (ADCs) can be calculated by ratios of intravoxel signal intensities taken from at least two sequences with differing gradient strengths. In the case of an acute stroke, the ischemic injury results in cytotoxic edema and influx of Na^+ and water from the extracellular space to the intracellular compartment. The brownian motion of water that would normally take place in the extracellular compartment is then restricted in the cells by the cell membranes. Conversely, protons within the CSF of the ventricles will move in a relatively unrestricted fashion, lose proportionately more signal, and have high apparent diffusion coefficients.

Preliminary implementations of diffusion imaging were limited by artifact from physiologic motion (normal brain pulsation) and long imaging times. The routine use of echoplanar imaging (EPI) reduces the problem of physiologic motion dramatically and makes the overall acquisition time very short (typically on the order of 1.5 min) so gross patient motion is rarely a problem. The residual practical problems in this acquisition largely relate to local field inhomogeneities caused by the air/soft tissue interface at the skull base. This results in signal loss and geometric distortion in the inferior frontal lobes, temporal lobes, and the posterior fossa. Such problems are further aggravated by artifact from metal in dental work and ventriculostomies or anywhere in the region of the skull base with higher field strength magnets (e.g., 3.0 Tesla). The dilemma is that artifact could potentially be misinterpreted as restricted diffusion. This can be minimized with stronger and faster gradients in the MR machines, multishot echo-planar acquisitions, and more recently, parallel acquisition techniques using phased array head coils. Parallel acquisition techniques also have the potential to improve the spatial resolution of the voxels in these images which is currently on the order of $4 \times 2 \times 5$ mm with conventional coils and EPI.

This concept has been applied to a number of other situations to complement conventional MRI sequences for improved specificity. It has been argued that solid intracranial neoplasms will cause a reduction in the apparent diffusion coefficient whereas surrounding edema, cyst formation and necrosis will increase the calculated apparent diffusion coefficient. The restricted diffusion in solid neoplasms has been attributed to an increase in cellularity and the corresponding reduction in the extracellular fluid space in contrast to normal brain tissue *(62–66)*. Although a statistically significant correlation has been demonstrated between lower ADC values, higher cellularity, and higher-grade neoplasms in large groups, ADC values have not been proven useful to make these distinctions in individual patients. Interestingly, some of these same investigators attempted to correlate the increased cellularity of these tumors with the degree of T2 hypointensity (presumed to indicate high cellularity in conventional MRI such as is commonly seen in primary CNS lymphoma) and failed to demonstrate consistent results. Investigators have also attempted to characterize different primary gliomas by their ADC values, but these studies have utilized different techniques with variable hardware and software in small groups of patients making this data of limited clinical utility. Moreover, the nature of the pathology in question is exceedingly variable within an individual patient, making it difficult to effectively measure even with a consistent technique *(63)*. This would likely contribute to the overlap in ADC values previously measured in gliomas, metastases, and meningiomas.

Another hope was that diffusion could help to preoperatively characterize the peripheral T2 and FLAIR hyperintensity to distinguish a solitary metastasis from a primary glioma. The peripheral T2 hyperintensity in the white matter surrounding metastases should be vasogenic edema within the extracellular fluid space whereas the peripheral hyperintensity surrounding gliomas should be infiltrating neoplastic cells. Once again, investigators found no significant difference in diffusion characteristics of this tissue. The white matter surrounding gliomas likely contains edema and infiltrating tumor cells which have canceling effects on the diffusion study and could be quite variable between different patients and possibly even within a single patient. In the end, diffusion studies are more likely to complement conventional MRI studies rather than provide a new physiologic contrast that is clearly better than conventional sequences in the evaluation of patients with gliomas. For example, diffusion sequences could serve to identify the most densely cellular component of a primary glioma as a guide for localizing a biopsy site. The diffusion sequences may also serve as an additional indicator of malignant degeneration of a known lower grade neoplasm beyond more conventional parameters such as new gadolinium enhancement and/or worsening mass effect (Fig. 4).

Alterations in the histology and quantity of fluid in the intracellular and extracellular spaces have also been implemented to distinguish chemo- and/or radiation therapy-induced necrosis from recurrent neoplasm in the routine follow-up of patients with HGG *(67,68)*. Tissue containing radiation-induced necrosis should have a marked paucity of cells and recurrence of a HGG within the parenchyma should contain more densely packed cells. Although the histology is quite discrepant, the appearance of these two entities on conventional MRI may be indistinguishable owing to physical proximity to the site of the original tumor, surrounding vasogenic edema, localized mass effect, and the breakdown in the blood–brain barrier (BBB) causing gadolinium enhancement. In practice, the distinctions have often relied upon clinical suspicion, short-term follow-up conventional MRI, positron emission tomography (PET), single photon emission computed tomography (SPECT), and, ultimately, surgical biopsy. One recent study compared two small groups of patients with WHO grade III and IV gliomas who had recurrence of the primary neoplasm vs therapy-induced necrosis *(68)*. They were able to demonstrate significantly lower ADC values in those patients with recurrence than in those patients with therapy induced necrosis, presumably related to higher cellularity in the recurrence group *(66,69)*. These differences were more significant when the data were normalized to regions of interest in the opposite normal hemisphere in the same patients by generating ADC ratios. This data set a threshold of 1.62, above which suggested treatment induced necrosis while values below this were only found in patients with tumor recurrence.

DIFFUSION TENSOR IMAGING

The principle of diffusion imaging can also be implemented to perform diffusion tensor imaging (DTI) and reproduce directional maps of the cerebral white matter. Instead of apply-

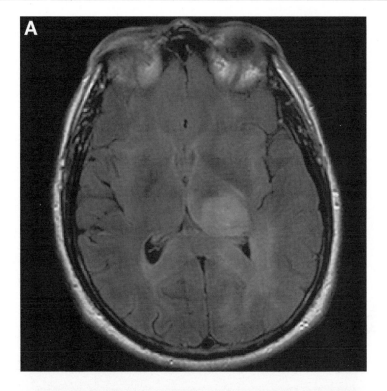

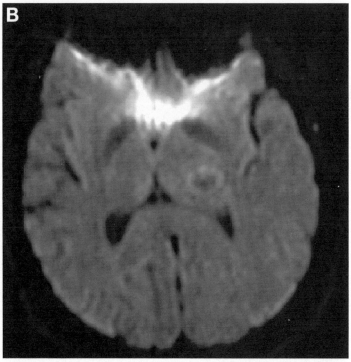

Fig. 4. Gliomatosis cerebri: **(A)** FLAIR image through the thalamus in the same patient as Fig. 3 demonstrates a more confluent mass with more prominent mass effect, distinctly different from the diffuse infiltrative process elsewhere. **(B,C)** Axial diffusion trace image and correlative ADC map demonstrate restricted in the periphery of this focus suggesting restricted diffusion. Note the striking

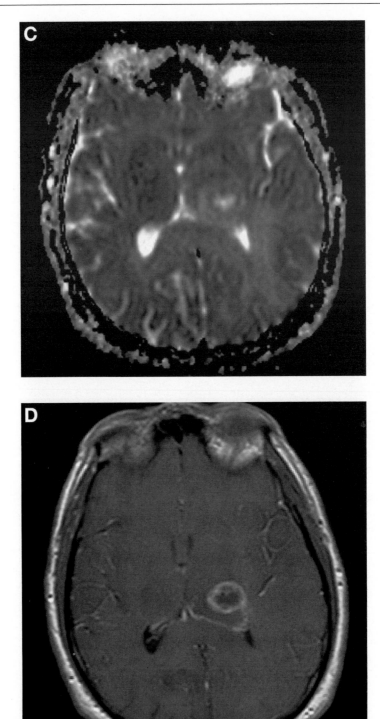

Fig. 4. *(continued from opposite page)* signal loss and geometric distortion in the inferior frontal poles resulting from the local field inhomogeneity of the brain/skull base interface. **(D)** There is prominent enhancement of this rim of tissue following gadolinium administration but there was no enhancement elsewhere. Biopsy of this focus revealed glioblastoma.

ing the strong diffusion gradients in each of the conventional three orthogonal directions, these same gradients and various combinations of these gradients are applied in a minimum of six directions in the same echo-planar sequences (70,71). The diffusion in white matter is clearly dependent on the orientation of the white matter bundle. Specifically, white matter diffusion is greatest along the longitudinal axis of the myelin sheaths and neuronal axons and minimal perpendicular to their longitudinal axes as a result of the physical barriers of the membranes. As a result, such measurements can be used to demonstrate the orientation of white matter tracts in vivo. The diffusion measurements in each of the six directions are used to generate a 3 × 3 diffusion tensor matrix. Diagonalization of these data generate ellipsoids for each imaging voxel whose major, minor and intermediate axes define the orientation of the white matter in the voxel (72,73). These axes are characterized as eigenvectors to indicate the direction of these axes and eigen values to reflect the maximal diffusivity in these directions. The eigen value for the major eigen vector of each voxel indicates the maximal diffusivity or primary orientation of the white matter in a specific imaging voxel. Diffusion anisotropy is a measure of the deviation of the ellipsoid from a sphere. In the case of a sphere, the fractional anisotropy (FA) is equal to zero and there is equal diffusion in all directions. The converse would be a fractional anisotropy of 1.0 in which the diffusion is essentially all along one direction as might be expected in a highly organized white matter tract. Maps can be generated and displayed in a variety of fashions, the most common of which are color FA maps. By convention, red indicates a right/left direction, green indicates an anterior/posterior direction, and blue indicates a cephalo-caudad direction. The intensity of the color is directly proportionately to the FA in each voxel. If a region of interest (ROI) is chosen in a specific white matter bundle, a region-growing algorithm can be applied to demonstrate the three-dimensional course of the white matter tract in a process called tractography (74–78). Alternatively, ROIs can be chosen on the diffusion maps to quantify the direction and magnitude of the diffusion in the white matter using fractional anisotropy and mean diffusivity (average eigen values for the three vectors defining the ellipsoids).

Not surprisingly, DTI has also been implemented in a variety of intracranial pathologies, including patients with HGG (71,79–82). The results of studies implemented for diagnostic purposes have demonstrated somewhat mixed results. Mean diffusivity (MD) was not found to be diagnostic for distinguishing low- and high-grade gliomas. Whereas the MD of low-grade gliomas (LGG) was somewhat higher than HGG, the differences were not statistically significant. It is also not possible to distinguish edema from infiltrative neoplasm along the margins of LGG and HGG with DTI (83). The mean diffusivity of the T2-hyperintensity in the white matter surrounding parenchymal metastases was found to be significantly greater than in the hyperintensity surrounding primary gliomas (80). In another study of HGG, normal white matter had higher FA and lower MD than the underlying mass and surrounding edema. Similarly, the gadolinium-enhancing rim of the masses had higher FA and lower MD than the nonenhancing center. When comparing solitary and multifocal primary masses, the MD was lower and the FA was higher in the enhancing components of multifocal gliomas than in solitary gliomas (79). The surrounding T2-hyperintensity was similarly discrepant in multifocal disease, perhaps to infiltrating, nonenhancing neoplasm in the white matter.

DTI studies have also been implemented in preoperative planning of patients with HGG (Fig. 5). When planning surgery in these patients, the goal is obviously to maximize the extent of resection of the mass without compromising eloquent structures. DTI has been used to locate major white matter tracts (e.g., corticospinal tracts) and determine if these tracts are simply displaced and normal, edematous, infiltrated by tumor, or frankly destroyed (71,82).

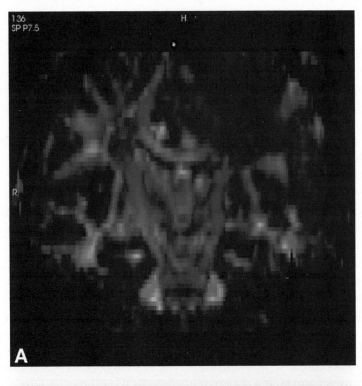

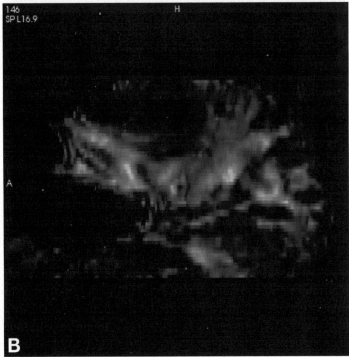

Fig. 5. Hig-grade glioma: **(A,B)** Coronal and sagittal planar reconstructions of colorized fractional anisotropy maps demonstrating complete disruption of the normal white matter tracts in the region of the large infiltrative left frontal mass and mild displacement of the corticospinal tracts (blue) dorsally.

Four different categories have been described to characterize these tracts on DTI, including: (1) bulk displacement of the tract causing abnormal location and direction and normal or slightly reduced FA; (2) edematous tract with a normal location and direction and reduced FA; (3) tract infiltrated by tumor causing a change in direction of the tract and reduced FA; and (4) complete disruption of the tract by infiltrating neoplasm causing markedly reduced FA. In practice, it may be somewhat more difficult to implement these distinct classifications, as there will likely be combinations of these findings in large white matter tracts.

PERFUSION

MR perfusion (MRP) imaging has also been utilized in the diagnosis and management of HGG. Conventional MRI provides qualitative information about the degree of breakdown in the BBB. Gadolinium enhancement within a mass is more commonly seen with HGG than low-grade masses but this is clearly not uniform as alluded to above. Angiogenesis is an important factor in the growth and malignant transformation of gliomas but does not necessarily correlate with the presence of enhancement on MRI. Perfusion imaging provides the capability of calculating parameters such as cerebral blood flow (CBF) and cerebral blood volume (CBV) as quantifiable measures of the extent and nature of blood vessels supplying gliomas. It has been argued that the angiogenesis found in higher grade gliomas is more sensitively detected in MRP studies as areas of increased cerebral blood flow and cerebral blood volume (Fig. 6). Such studies have been performed with PET and SPECT in the past with relatively high specificity for malignancy but these studies have also been hampered by low spatial resolution, reduced sensitivity for low-grade intra-axial masses, and limited availability *(84–87)*. Alternatively, MRP can be performed at the same time as the routine follow-up MRI of patients with HGG with minimal additional time and cost and with good correlation to PET-derived values *(6,88–91)*. MRP studies themselves have also been found to directly correlate with histologic grade and individual histologic features of malignancy *(92–94)*.

MRP imaging can be performed by one of two different methods. Arterial spin labeling applies an inversion or tagging radiofrequency pulse to the inflowing blood outside the volume of interest, waits for an appropriate transit time to flow into the volume and exchange free water within the tissue, image the volume, and subtract a control image. A modification of the Kety method is utilized to calculate perfusion parameters of the tumors *(95,96)*. Clinical experience with this method is relatively limited and MRP imaging is far more commonly performed with dynamic susceptibility-weighted contrast-enhanced MRI *(7,92,97,98)*. This technique implements a rapid intravenous bolus of gadolinium and relies on high-intravascular concentration of the contrast to cause local field inhomogeneities surrounding the perfusing vessels. Tissue perfusion is measured by monitoring the degree of signal loss over time on a voxel-by-voxel basis on sequential T2*-weighted echo-planar images. The echo-planar acquisition permits coverage of the entire head and very high temporal resolution. Because all patients with HGG will receive gadolinium as part of the routine diagnostic study anyway, this study is performed immediately prior to the contrast-enhanced T1 imaging and adds minimal time to the exam.

Both arterial-spin labeling and first pass bolus methods of MRP can be implemented in a clinical setting and can differentiate low- and high-grade neoplasms based on the discrepancies of blood flow to these neoplasms *(97)*. Arterial spin labeling is noninvasive, permits repeated measurements, is not impacted by a disruption of the BBB, and provides perfusion parameters with minimal post-processing. Absolute values of perfusion are also possible with arterial spin labeling, making it easier to compare different patients and to longitudinally

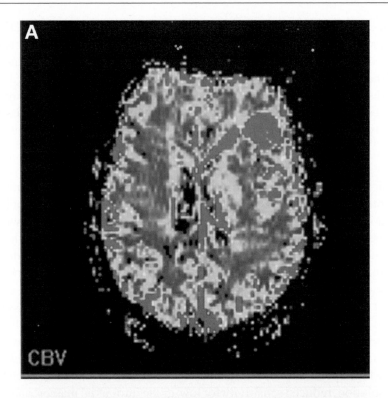

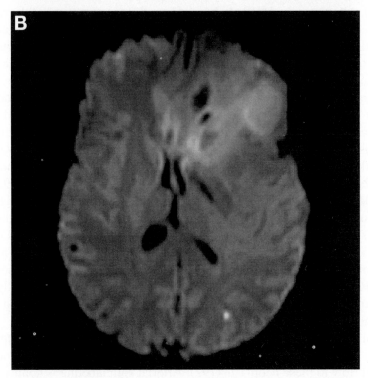

Fig. 6. High-grade glioma: **(A)** Localized elevation in the CBV in the left inferior frontal gyrus (red) suggesting a more aggressive component of the mass for biopsy. **(B,C)** Corresponding focus of mildly restricted diffusion on the diffusion trace image and the ADC map.

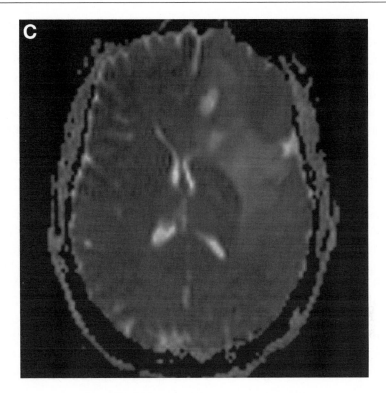

Fig. 6C. *(Continued from opposite page.)*

follow individual patients during the course of therapy. On the other hand, it is still possible to provide information about tumor grading without absolute measurements and such measurements must still be corrected for age and the individual. Accurate measurements are contingent on the relaxation time of the tissues, vascular transit time to the tissues, and equilibrium magnetization of the blood. The spin labeling technique is limited by signal-to-noise in older individuals because reduced cardiac output prolongs inflow from the labeling volume to the volume of interest. The differential blood flow to gray and white matter also has an impact on transit time (200–400 ms in gray matter and 700–1000 ms in white matter). These factors would suggest more reliable results for masses located within the gray matter or more highly vascularized masses in white matter. By contrast, the first pass bolus methods produce images with higher signal-to-noise, permit data from a larger volume of interest, and allow easier calculation of parameters beyond CBF flow such as relative CBV, permeability, and oxygen extraction fraction. This latter method assumes no contrast extravasation into the extracellular fluid space and therefore demands an initial injection of gadolinium to reduce the impact of this systematic error. First pass bolus methods also demand the user to choose an appropriate arterial input function for calculation of the perfusion parameters. Depending on the location, size, heterogeneity, and vascularity of the mass, a single large vessel (e.g., ipsilateral middle cerebral artery) may not provide a uniform reference point for measurements throughout the mass.

Clinical studies support the use of MRP studies to improve the sensitivity and specificity of MRI in the grading of gliomas *(6,7,89,93,94,97–100)*. In one study, MRI factors such as signal intensity heterogeneity, gadolinium enhancement, mass effect, border definition, amount of edema, hemorrhage, necrosis, and involvement of the corpus callosum were used as indicators of tumor grade *(7)*. The sensitivity, specificity, positive predictive value, and negative predictive value for HGG with MRI were calculated as 72.5, 65, 86.1, and 44.1%. To minimize the misclassification of neoplasms, a threshold of 1.75 for rCBV was utilized in first pass bolus perfusion studies and demonstrated corresponding values of 95, 57.5, 87, and 79.3%. A threshold of 2.97 produced the same sensitivity as MRI whereas the specificity, positive predictive value, and negative predictive values were 87.5, 94.6, and 52.5%. This and other studies found mean rCBV values of 5.18 and 2.14, 3.64 and 1.11, 5.07 and 1.44, and 5.84 and 1.26 for HGG and LGG respectively *(6,7,94,101)*. On the other hand, there was no statistically significant difference between AA and glioblastomas with MRP studies.

MRP studies have also been utilized to differentiate a solitary metastasis from a primary, HGG *(98)*. No differences could be identified between these two entities if the rCBV was compared within the central, gadolinium-enhancing foci on the T1-weighted images, but statistically significant differences could be appreciated in the surrounding hyperintensity on the FLAIR and T2-weighted sequences. In particular, the mean rCBV immediately adjacent to and peripheral to the gadolinium-enhancing foci of metastases and HGG were found to be 0.39 ± 0.19 and 1.31 ± 0.97, and 0.66 ± 0.17 and 1.06 ± 0.66, respectively. The higher perfusion surrounding the gliomas was attributed to nonenhancing tumor infiltration that dissipates with increasing distance from the enhancing focus while the reduced perfusion surrounding the metastases likely relates to vasogenic edema compressing the local microvasculature.

Although neoplasms are characterized by increased vascularity, radiation and chemotherapy generally compromise the microvasculature so that treated neoplasms will have reduced vascularity. It has therefore been suggested that MRP studies can be used like nuclear medicine studies to distinguish treatment effects from recurrent or residual neoplasm *(102,103)*. Good correlation between PET, SPECT, and MRP otherwise would support this but few well-controlled studies have been performed to date.

SPECTROSCOPY

MR spectroscopy (MRS) is becoming more commonplace in the routine evaluation of patients with intracranial masses as the software becomes more widely available and user-friendly on MR machines. Proton MRS can be practically implemented on any 1.5T MR system with clinically useful exam times, signal-to-noise, and spatial resolution. Higher field systems (e.g., 3.0 Tesla [T]) provide the theoretical advantages of improved signal to noise, shorter exam times, and improved spectral resolution (peak separation). The actual improvements in signal-to-noise are closer to 20–50% resulting from greater line width at 3.0T as a result of greater field inhomogeneities and shorter T2 and T2* relaxation times *(104,105)*. Certainly, most studies are performed at 1.5T. The most practical considerations affecting the visibility of metabolites in MR spectra are the relaxation times of the metabolites and the sequence parameters. In single voxel techniques, chemical-shift imaging, or 3D multivoxel techniques, the primary choice in parameters with conventional MRS software is between short and long echo times. Long echo time acquisitions produce spectra that include-acetylaspartate (NAA), choline (Cho), creatine/phosphocreatine (Cre), and possibly lactate (Lac) peaks. Short echo time acquisitions include these same metabolites as well as myo-inositol (Ins), glutamate and glutamine (Glx), and possibly alanine (Ala), glucose (Gc), scyllo-inositol/taurine (scyIns/Tau), and proteins/lipids *(106–111)*.

NAA is present in relatively large quantities in the brain (8–10 mM) and therefore is the largest peak in normal spectra (at 2.02 ppm). A number of different roles have been proposed for NAA although its exact significance is unclear. Although it is generally felt to be neuron specific, it can also be found in immature oligodendrocytes and astrocyte progenitor cells (112). Reduced NAA is found early in development and with any process that causes a decline in the number of neurons, an impairment in neuronal metabolism, or replacement of normal neurons. Although the reasons are unclear, there is normally a progressive increase in NAA in the cerebral gray matter from ventral to dorsal and from the cerebral hemispheres to the spinal cord (111).

The Cho peak at 3.2ppm primarily represents phospho-/glycerophospho-/phosphatidyl-choline. An elevation in brain total Cho is therefore felt to reflect increased membrane turnover as would be seen with cell proliferation related to gliosis, primary neoplasm, or normal myelination. Conversely, Cho can rise with increased membrane breakdown such as with demyelinating and dysmyelinating disorders. Regional variation in the brain is the reverse of that described for NAA.

Cre consists of two peaks located at 3.04 ppm and 3.94 ppm. These peaks reflect a combination of creatine and phosphocreatine and hence, an indication of the energy stores in the brain. Not surprisingly, there is relatively high concentration of creatine in the brain with a progressive increase from white matter, to gray matter and the cerebellum (111). The amount of Cre is relatively constant in each tissue type in normal brain and is frequently used as an internal standard. In pathologic tissue, this generalization is not that reliable, particularly in areas of necrosis (113).

Lac is generally present in only minute amounts (<0.5 mM) in the brain and undetectable in normal spectra (114). The lactate peak can be visualized in any condition that results in anaerobic glycolysis such as energy metabolism disorders, hypoxia, stroke, neoplasms, or siezures. It can also be present in macrophages and therefore may be seen with acute inflammation. Lastly, lactate will also accumulate if there is poor washout from the tissue as with cysts, necrotic foci, or infarcts. When present, it is recognized as a doublet with 0.2 ppm peak splitting, centered at 1.32 ppm, and inverted below the baseline at long TEs (e.g., 135 ms) but projected above the baseline at short (e.g., 20 ms) and very long (e.g., 272 ms) TEs.

The Ins peak is found at 3.56 ppm. Whereas Ins accounts for the majority of this peak, myoinositol-monophosphate and glycine also contribute to it. Myoinositol is not present in neurons and may be glia-specific as variations are linked to myelin formation and breakdown (111,115,116). This would not be surprising as it is a component of membrane phospholipids. It is suggested that Ins is important in osmotic regulation of the brain, serves as an energy reserve, and as a reserve pool for inositol diphosphate—a second messenger.

Glutamate (Glu) and glutamine (Gln) and GABA (γ–aminobutyric acid) are generally inseparable at 1.5T and result in a complex peak (Glx) between 2.1 and 2.5 ppm. Glu is an excitatory amino acid found in neurons. Beyond this, Glu participates in the regulation of ammonia, fatty acid synthesis, and the Kreb's cycle. Gln also has a role in ammonia regulation but is restricted to cerebral astrocytes. GABA is a product of Glu and functions as an inhibitory neurotransmitter.

Ala (1.5ppm) is a nonessential amino acid with no known function that is often hidden in the lactate peak regardless of the echo time in the acquisition. Tau is another amino acid that serves as an excitatory neurotransmitter as well as in brain growth and osmoregulation (12). Tau resonates between 3.26 and 4.0 ppm and likely combines with scyIns (an isomer of Ins) at 3.35 ppm to produce a small peak at 3.3 ppm that may be hidden by the adjacent Cho peak.

The lipids produce metabolite peaks at 0.9 ppm (methyl protons of lipids and macromolecules), 1.3 ppm (methylene protons of neutral lipids and lactate), and 2.0 ppm (lipid and cytosolic protein macromolecules) *(117,118)*. The chemical moieties in proteins also contribute to these peaks and peripherally positioned voxels may reflect contamination from the overlying subcutaneous fat. Otherwise, the lipid peaks may be accentuated in the setting of a necrotic focus, HGG and meningiomas, myelin breakdown, and certain inborn errors of metabolism.

Much has been written about proton MRS in the evaluation of intracranial neoplasms in vivo *(119–129)*. Although the conclusions from these studies are somewhat variable, this is clearly in part related to the inconsistency of the MRS techniques and post-processing as well as volume-averaging artifact from the placement of variably sized voxels. Nevertheless, these studies all seem to support the generalizations that neoplasms are characterized by a low NAA/Cre ratio, an elevated Cho/Cre ratio, and in some cases elevated lactate (Fig. 7). The NAA is reduced as the mass replaces normal neurons and/or the tumor cells produce lesser amounts of NAA than normal neurons. Cre may be reduced if energy stores are reduced from the high metabolic demand of the tumor. The Cho is thought to be high because of increased membrane turnover imposed by more rapid cell growth and proliferation in the tumor. The Cho tends to be more prominently elevated in more aggressive solid neoplasms and is thought to be an indicator of cellularity but it does not necessarily correlate directly with tumor grade. Although it has been suggested that Lac tends to be more common in more malignant or necrotic masses, this is clearly controversial *(121,126,128–130)*. These discrepancies may also be in part technical although Lac can definitely be seen on MRS in benign masses such as pilocytic astrocytomas and its presence hinges on the level of glycolytic activity, efficiency of electron transport in the tumor cells, and washout from the tissue *(129,131)*. Elevated lipid levels may be complimentary to Lac—if not more helpful—in distinguishing more malignant masses *(118,120,128,131)*.

Although it is possible to quantify metabolites with MRS, most clinical studies rely on metabolite ratios and are compared to age-matched controls and, in the case of intracranial neoplasms, contralateral normal brain parenchyma. As suggested above, more aggressive neoplasms tend to have higher Cho/Cre ratios and lower NAA/Cre ratios. A linear correlation has been demonstrated between Cho/Cre and the cell proliferation index for Ki-67 positive cells which would imply that Cho may be a predictor of tumor grade by MRS but more likely just relates to cellularity *(132,133)*. A recent study comparing LGG and HGG with ROC analysis to assess the performance of multivoxel proton MRS identified thresholds comparable to other studies of 1.08 for Cho/Cre, 0.75 for Cho/NAA *(2,7,122,134–136)*. Such cutoffs yielded relatively high sensitivities (97.5 and 96.7%) but low specificities (12.5 and 10.0%) for distinguishing high and LGG. It is important to state that there have been variable results in showing statistically significant difference in these ratios when comparing AA with glioblastomas. The presence of necrosis on the imaging study and lipid and lactate on MRS still cannot necessarily make this distinction.

Distinguishing oligodendrogliomas from astrocytomas is perhaps of greater clinical significance given the response to chemotherapy of some oligodendrogliomas and mixed oligoastrocytomas. Both of these groups typically have reduced NAA and elevated choline levels. Short echo time MRS acquisitions can be used to evaluate for increased levels of Glx that have been reported in low- and high-grade oligodendrogliomas *(137–139)* . These same short echo time MRS studies could be used to identify myoinositol and alanine as markers for oligodendrogliomas *(139–142)*. One dilemma would be that Glx and myoinositol both reso-

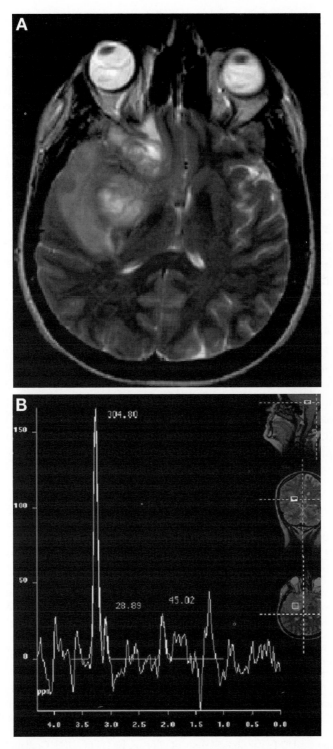

Fig. 7. High-grade glioma: **(A)** Axial T2 image demonstrates an infiltrative mass of heterogeneous hyperintensity in the inferior right frontal and temporal lobes. **(B)** A single voxel taken from a multivoxel MR proton spectroscopy study at 1.5T with a long echo time (TE 135 ms) which demonstrates a markedly elevated choline peak (304.89), elevated choline/creatine ratio (approx 10/1), and NAA (45.02) reduced nearly to the level of background noise.

nate at 3.55 ppm. The distinction between the high- and low-grade neoplasms would depend on the presence of elevated lipids and lactate and reduced myoinositol levels in the higher grade neoplasms.

MRS has also been used in an attempt to differentiate metastases from HGG. No significant differences in the spectra have been consistently identified when comparing the mass lesions themselves. As shown with MRP, it is possible to distinguish these masses when data are obtained from the parenchyma surrounding the central gadolinium-enhancing focus. The Cho/Cre ratio in the peritumoral parenchyma is significantly higher with gliomas than with metastases (2.28 ±1.24 vs 0.76 ± 0.23) as the T2-hyperintensity surrounding gliomas also contains infiltrating tumor cells. The parenchyma surrounding metastases may show a global diminution of metabolites due to the dilution effect of vasogenic edema. There is no significant difference in the NAA/Cre ratios when comparing the two groups in this region.

Lastly, MRS can be used to distinguish between other entities such as treatment induced necrosis and recurrent neoplasm. One small study used ROC analysis to demonstrate good reliability of MRS when readers assumed recurrent tumor was characterized by normal-to-high Cho and readily visible Cre while radiation necrosis contained voxels with markedly reduced Cho and Cre (143). Other studies similarly concluded that an elevated Cho/Cre ratio could be used to identify recurrent tumor in these patients while other investigators contradicted this (144,145). Cho can actually be elevated in early radiation- induced lesions due to demyelination and reactive astrocytosis. Elevated Cho/Cre may also be evident in late severe radiation necrosis and may be accompanied by Lac. Serial MRS studies would show a progressive decline in NAA/Cre and NAA/Cho and a relatively stable Cho/Cre with radiation necrosis. A study with brachytherapy suggested an easier alternative is to use the patient's irradiated normal tissue as a control instead of the brains of healthy volunteers (146). With these internal references, NAA/Cho, NAA/Cre and Cho/Cre approached 1.0 in radiation necrosis. In this study, elevated lipids were only present with radiation necrosis following therapy.

REFERENCES

1. Ricci PE. Imaging of adult brain tumors. Neuroimaging Clin No Am 1999;9:651–669.
2. Moller-Hartmann W, Herminghaus S, Krings T, et al. Clinical application of proton magnetic resonance spectroscopy in the diagnosis of intracranial mass lesions. Neuroradiology 2003;44:371–381.
3. Dean BL, Drayer BP, Bird CR. Gliomas: classification with MR imaging. Radiology 1990;174:411–415.
4. Watanabe M, Tanaka R, Takeda N. Magnetic resonance imaging and histopathology of cerebral gliomas. Neuroradiology 1992;34:463–469.
5. Kondziolka D, Lunsford LD, Martinez AJ. Unreliability of contemporary neurodiagnostic imaging in evaluating suspected adult supratentorial (low grade) astrocytoma. J Neurosurg 1993;79:533–536.
6. Knopp EA, Cha S, Johnson G, et al. Glial neoplasms: dynamic contrast-enhanced T2*-weighted MR imaging. Radiology 1999;211:791–798.
7. Law M, Yang S, Wang H, et al. Glioma grading: sensitivity, specificity and predictive values of perfusion MR imaging and proton MR spectroscopic imaging compared with conventional MR imaging. AJNR Am J Neuroradiol 2003;24:1989–1998.
8. Ginsberg LE, Fuller GN, Hashmi M, et al. The significance of lack of MR contrast enhancement of supratentorial brain tumors in adults: histopathological evaluation of a series. Surg Neurol 1998;49:436–440.
9. Smirniotopoulos JG. The new WHO classification of brain tumors. Neuroimaging Clin No Am 1999;9:595–613.
10. McKeran RO, Thomas DGT. The clinical study of gliomas. In:Thomas DG, Graham D I, eds. Brain tumors: Scientific Basis, Clinical Investigation, and Current Therapy. London: Butterworth, 1980:194–230.
11. Russel D, Rubinstein L. Tumors of central nervous system origin. In: Rubinstein LJ, ed. Pathology of Tumors of the Nervous System. Baltimore, MD:Williams and Wilkins, 1989:
12. Paulus W, Pfeifer J. Intratumoral histologic heterogeneity of gliomas. Cancer 1989;64:442–447.
13. Vandenberg, ST. Current concepts of astrocytic tumors. J Neuropathol Exp Neurol 1992;51:644–657.

14. Kondziolka D, Bernstein M, Resch ., et al. Significance of hemorrhage into brain tumors: clinicopathological study. J Neurosurg 1987;67:852–857.

15. Burger PC, Heinz ER, Shibata T, et al. Topographic anatomy and CT correlations in the untreated glioblastomas multiforme. J Neurosurg 1988;68:698–704.

16. Lilja A, Bertstrom K, Spannare B, et al. Reliability of CT in assessing histopathological features of malignant supratentorial gliomas. J Comput Assist Tomogr 1981;5:625.

17. Earnest F IV, Kelly PJ, Scheithauer BW, et al. Cerebral astrocytomas: histopathologic correlation of MR and CT contrast enhancement with stereotactic biopsy. Radiology 1988;166:823–827.

18. Atlas SW. Adult supratentorial tumors. Seminars in Roentgenol 1990;25:130–154.

19. Tovi M, Lolja A, Erickson A. MR imaging in cerebral gliomas: tissue component analysis in correlation with histopathology of whole-brain specimens. Acta Radiol 1994;35:495–505.

20. Drevelegas A, Karkavelas G. High grade gliomas. In: Drevelegas A., ed. Imaging of Brain Tumors with Histological Correlations. Berlin:Springer-Verlag, 2002:109–136.

21. Hartmann M, Jansen O, Heiland S, et al. Restricted diffusion within ring ehnancement is not pathognomonic for brain abscess. AJNR Am J Neuroradiol 2001;22:1738–1742.

22. Desprechins B, Stannik T, Koerts G, et al. Use of diffusion-weighted MR imaging in the differential diagnosis between intracerebral necrotic tumors and cerebral abscesses. AJNR Am J Neuroradiol 1999;20:1252–1257.

23. Feigin IM, Gross SW. Sarcoma arising in glioblastoma of the brain. Am J Pathol 1955;31:633–665.

24. Morantz RA, Feigin I, Ransohoff J. Clinical and pathological study of 24 cases of gliosarcoma. J Neurosurg 1976;45:398–408.

25. Lee YY, Castillo M, Nauert C, Moser RP. Computed tomography of gliosarcoma. AJNR Am J Neuroradiol 1985;6:527–531.

26. Meis JM, Martz KL, Nelson JS. Mixed glioblastoma multiforme and sarcoma. A clinicopathologic study of 26 radiation therapy oncology group cases. Cancer 1991;67:2342–2349.

27. Beute BJ, Fobben GS, Hubschman O, et al. Cerebellar gliosarcoma: report of a probable radiation-ionduced neoplasm. AJNR Am J Neuroradiol 1991;12:554–556.

28. Averback P. Mixed intracranial sarcomas: rare forms and a new association with previous radiation therapy. Ann Neurol 1998;4:229–233.

29. Kaschten B, Flandroy P, Reznil M, et al. Radiation induced gliosarcoma. J Neurosurg 1995;83:154–162.

30. Marcus G, Levin DF, Rutherford GS. Malignant gliomaa following radiation therapy for unrelated primary tumor. Cancer 1986;58:886–894.

31. Cerame MA, Buthikonda M, Kohli CN. Extraneural metastases in gliosarcoma. A case report and review of the literature. Neurosurgery 1985;17:413–418.

32. Maiuri F, Stella I, Benvenuti D, et al. Cerebral gliosarcomas: correlation of computed tomographic findings, surgical aspect, pathological features and prognosis. Neurosurgery 1990;26:261–267.

33. Lieberman KA, Fuller CE, Caruso RD. Postradiation gliosarcoma with osteosarcomatous components. Neuroradiology 2001;43:555–558.

34. Ross IB, Robitaille Y, Villemure JG, Tampieri D. Diagnosis and management of gliomatosis cerebri: recent trends. Surg Neurol 1991;36:431–440.

35. Artigas J, Cervis-Navaro J, Iglesias JR, et al. Gliomatosis cerebri: clinical and gistological findings. Clin Neuropathol 1985;4:135–148.

36. Couch JR, Weiss SA. Gliomatosis cerebri: report of four cases and review of the literature. Neurology 1976; 24:504–511.

37. Dickson DW, Horoupian DS, Thal LJ, et al. Gliomatosis cerebri presenting with hydrocephalus and dementia. AJNR Am J Neuroradiol 1988;9:200–202.

38. Rippe DJ, Boyko OB Fuller GN, et al. Gadopentetate-dimeglumine-enhanced MR imaging of gliomatosis cerebral: appearance mimicking leptomeningeal tumor dissemination. AJNR Am J Neuroradiol 1990;11: 800–801.

39. Leproux F, Melanson D, Mercier C, et al. Leptomeningeal gliomatosis: MR findings. J Comput Assist Tomogr 1993;17:317–320.

40. Shin YM, Chang KH, Han MH, et al. Gliomatosis cerebri: comparison of MR and CT features. AJR Am J Roentgenol 1993;161:859–862.

41. Wilkinson IMS, Anderson JF, Holmes AE. Oligodendroglioma: an analysis of 42 cases. J Neurol Neurosurg Psychiatry 1987;50:304–312.

42. Chin HW, Hazel JJ, Kim TH, et al. Oligodendrogliomas I A clinical study of cerebral oligodendrogliomas. Cancer 1980;45:1458–1466.

43. Packer RJ, Sutton LN, Rorke LB, et al. Oligodendroglioma of the posterior fossa in childhood. Cancer 1985;56:195–199.

44. Pagni CA, Canavero S, Gaidolfi E. Intramedullary "holocord" oligodendroglioma: case report. Acta Neurochir 1991;113:96–99.

45. Ringertz N. Grading of gliomas. APMIS 1950;27:51–64.

46. Smith MT, Ludwig CL, Godfrey AD, et al. Grading of oligodendrogliomas. Cancer 1983;52:2107–2114.

47. Shaw EG, Scheithauer BW, O-Fallon JR, et al. Oligodendrogliomas: the Many Clinic experience. J Neurosurg 1992;76:428–434.

48. Burger PC, Scheithauer BW. Central nervous system. Atlas of tumor pathology. Washington, DC: Armed Forces Institute of Pathology, 1994:107–120.

49. Daumas-Duport C, Tucker ML, Kolles H. Oligodendrogliomas. Part II: A new grading system based on morpholoical and imaging criteria. J Neurooncol 1997;34:61–78.

50. Shibata T, Burger PC, Kleihaus P. Ki-67 immunoperoxidase stain as a marker for the histologic grading of nervous system tumors. Acta Neurochir Suppl 1988;43:103–106.

51. Chan ASY, Leung SY, Wong MP, et al. Expression of vascular endothelial growh factor and its receptors in the anaplastic progression of astrocytoma, oligodendroglioma, and ependymoma. Am J Surg Pathol 1998;22:816–826.

52. Cairncross JG, Ueki K, Zlatescu MC, et al. Specific genetic predictors of chemotherapeutic response and survival in patients anaplastic oligodendrogliomas. J Natl Cancer Inst 1998;90:1473–1479.

53. Paleologos NA, Carincross J. Treatment of oligodendroglioma: an update. Neurooncology 1999;1:61–68.

54. Lee YY, Van Tassel P. Intracranial oligodendrogliomas: imaging findings in 35 untreated cases. AJR Am J Roentgenol 1989;152:361–369.

55. Segall HD, Destian S, Nelson MD, et al. CT and MR imaging in malignant gliomas. In:Apuzzo M.I.J., ed. Malignant cerebral glioma. Park Ridge, IL: AANS Publications Committee, 1990:63–77.

56. Couldwell WT, DeMattia JA, Hinton DR. Oligodendroglioma. In:Kaye A.H., Law E.R., eds. Brain Tumors: an encyclopedic approach. London: Churchill Livingstone, 2001:525–540.

57. Burger PC. Classification, grading and patterns of spread of malignant gliomas. In: Apuzzo MLJ, ed. Malignant Cerebral Glioma. Park Ridge, IL: AANS Publications Committee, 1990:3–17.

58. Hajnal JV, Doran M, Hall AS, et al. MR imaging of anisotropically restricted diffusion of water in the nervous system: technical, anatomic and pathologic considerations. J Comput Assist Tomogr 1991;15:1–18.

59. Le Bihan D, Breton E, Lallemand D, et al. MR imaging of intravoxel incoherent motions: application to diffusion and perfusion in neurologic disorders. Radiology 1986;161:401–408.

60. Chien D, Kwong KK, Gress DR, et al. MR diffusion imaging of cerebral infarction in humans. AJNR Am J Neuroradiol 1992;13:1097–1102.

61. Warach S, Chien D, Li W, et al. Fast magnetic resonance diffusion-wieghted imaging of acute human stroke. Neurology 1992;42:1717–1723.

62. Brunberg JA, Chenevert TL, McKeever PE, et al. In vivo MR determination of water diffusion coefficients and diffusion anisotropy: correlation with stgructural alteration in gliomas of the cerebral hemispheres. AJNR Am J Neuroradiol 1995;16:361–371.

63. Sugahara T, Korogi Y, Kochi M, et al. Usefulness of diffusion-weighted MRI with echo-planar technique in the evaluation of cellularity in gliomas. Magn Reson Med 1999;9:53–60.

64. Stadnik TW, Chaskis C, Michotte A, et al. Diffusion-weighted MR imaging of intracerebral masses: comparison with conventional MR imaging and histologic findings. AJNR Am J Neuroradiol 2001;22:969–976.

65. Castillo M, Smith JK, Kwock L, et al. Apparent diffusion coefficients in the evaluation of high-grade cerebral gliomas. AJNR Am J Neuroradiol 2001;22:60–64.

66. Kono K, Inoue Y, Nakayama K, et al. The role of diffusion-weighted imaging in patients with brain tumors. AJNR Am J Neuroradiol 2001;22:1081–1088.

67. Tsui EY, Chan JH, Ramsey RG, et al. Late temporal lobe necrosis in patients with nasopharyngeal carcinoma: evaluation with combined multi-section diffusion weighted and perfusion weighted MR imaging. Eur J Radiol 2001;39:138.

68. Hein PA, Eskey CJ, Dunn JF, et al. Diffusion-weighted imaging in the follow-up of treated high-grade gliomas: tumor recurrence versus radiation injury. AJNR Am J Neuroradiol 2004;25:201–209.

69. Guo AC, Cummings TJ, Dash RC, et al. Lymphomas and high-grade astrocytomas: comparison of water diffusibility and histologic characteristics. Radiology 2002;224:177–183.

70. Wakana S, Jiang H, Nagae-Poetscher LM, et al. Fiber tract-based atlas of human white matter anatomy. Radiology 2003;230:77–87.

71. Jellison BJ, Field AS, Medow J, et al. Diffusion tensor imaging of cerebral white matter: a pictorial review of physics, fiber tract anatomy, and tumor imaging patterns. AJNR Am J Neuroradiol 2004;25:356–369.

72. Moseley ME, Cohen Y, Kucharczyk J, et al. Diffusion-weighted MR imaging of anisotropic water diffusion in cat central nervous system. Radiology 1990;176:439–446.

73. Basser PJ, Matiello J, Le Bihan D. MR diffusion tensor spectroscopy and imaging. Biophys J 1994;66: 259–267.
74. Jones DK, Simmons A, Williams SC, et al. Non-invasive assessment of axonal fiber connectivity in the human brain via diffusion tensor MRI. Magn Reson Med 1999;42:37–41.
75. Contouro TE, Lori NF, Cull TS, et al. Tracking neuronal fiber pathways in the living human brain. Proc Natl Acad Sci U S A 1999;96:10422–10427.
76. Mori S, Crain BJ, Chacko BP, et al. Three dimensional tracking of axonal projections in the brain by magnetic resonance imaging. Ann Neurol 1999;45:265–269.
77. Basser PJ, Pajevic S, Pierpaoli C, et al. In vitro fiber tractography using DT-MRI data. Magn Reson Med 2000;44:625–632.
78. Jones DK, Simmons A, Williams SC, et al. Non–invasive assessment of axonal fiber connectivity in the human brain via diffusion tensor MRI. Neuroimage 2000;12:184–195.
79. Sinha S, Bastin ME, Whittle IR, et al. Diffusion tensor MR imaging of high-grade cerebral gliomas. AJNR Am J Neuroradiol 2002;23:520–527.
80. Lu S, Ahn D, Johnson G, et al. Diffusion-tensor MR imaging of intracranial neoplasia and associated peritumoral edema: intrroduction of the tumor infiltration index. Radiology 2004;232:221–228.
81. Nimsky C. Ganslandt O, Hastreiter P, et al. Intraoperative diffusion-tensor MR imaging: shiftging of white matter tracts during neurosurgical procedures-initial experience. Radiology 2005;234:218–225.
82. Witwer BP, Moftakhar R, Hasan KM, et al. Diffusion-tensor imaging of white matter tracts in patients with cerebral neoplasm. J Neurosurg 2002;97:568–575.
83. Tropine A, Vucurevic G, Delani P, et al. Contribution of diffusion tensor imaging to delineation of gliomas and glioblastomas. J Magn Reson Imaging 2004;20:905–912.
84. Lammertsma A, Wise R, Jones T. In vivo measurements of regional cerebral blood flow and blood volume in patients with brain tumours using positron emission tomography. Acta Neurochir 1983;69:5–13.
85. Black K, Emerick T, Hoh C, et al. Thallium-201 SPECT and positron emission tomography equal predictors of glioma grade and recurrence. Neurol Res 1994;16:93–96.
86. Kaplan WD, Takvorian T, Morris JH, et al. Thallium-201 brain tumor imaging: a comparative study with pathologic correlation. J Nucl Med 1990;28:47–52.
87. Kim KT, Black KL, Marciano D, et al. Thallium-201 SPECT imaing of brain tumors: methods and results. J Nucl Med 1990;31:965–969.
88. Uematsu H, Maeda M, Sadato N, et al. Blood volume of gliomas determined by double-echo dynamic perfusion-weighted MR imaging: a preliminary study. AJNR Am J Neuroradiol 2001;22:1915–1919.
89. Lev M, Rosen B. Clinical applications of intracranial perfusion MR imaging. Neuroimaging Clin No Am 1999;9:309–331.
90. Le Bas J, Kremer S, Graand S, et al. NMR perfusion imaging: applications to the study of brain tumor angiogenesis. Bull Acad Nat Med 2000;184:557–567.
91. Ostergaard L, Johannsen P, Host-Poulson P, et al. Cerebral blood flow measurements by magnetic resonance imaging bolus tracking: comparison with [(15)O]H2O positron emission tomography in humans. J Cereb Blood Flow Metab 1998;18:935–940.
92. Roberts JC, Roberts TPL. Brasch RC, et al. Quantitative measurement of microvascular permeability in human brain tumors achieved using dynamic contrast-enhanced MR imaging: correlation with histologic grade. AJNR Am J Neuroradiol 2000;21:891–899.
93. Roberts H, Roberts T, Bollen A, et al. Correlation of microvascular permeability derived from dynamic contrast-enhanced MR imaging with histologic grade and tumor labeling index: a study in human brain tumors. Acad Radiol 2001;8:384–391.
94. Aronen H, Gazit I, Louis D, et al. Cerebral blood volume maps of gliomas: comparison with tumor grade and histologic findings. Radiology 1994;191:41–51.
95. Silva A, Kim S, Garwood M. Imaging blood flow in brain tumors using arterial spin labeling. Magn Reson Med 2000;44:169–173.
96. Gaa J, Warach S, Wen P, et al. Noninvasive perfusion imaging of human brain tumors with EPISTAR. Eur Radiol 1996;6:518–522.
97. Warmuth C, Gunther M, Zimmer C. Quantification of blood flow in brain tumors: comparison of arterial spin labeling and dynamic susceptibility-weighted contrast-enhanced MR imaging. Radiology 2003;228:523–532.
98. Law M, Cha S, Knopp EA, et al. High-grade gliomas and solitary metastases: differentiation by using perfusion and proton spectroscopic MR imaging. Radiology 2002;222:715–721.
99. Roberts H, Roberts TPL, Brasch RC, et al. Quantitative measurement of microvascular permeability in human brain tumors achieved using dynamic contrast-enhanced MR imaging: correlation with histologic grade. AJNR Am J Neuroradiol 2000;21:891–899.

100. Wong ET, Jackson EF, Hess KR, et al. Correlation between dynamic MRI and outcome in patients with malignant gliomas. Neurology 1998;50:777–781.

101. Sugahara T, Korogi Y, Kochi M, et al. Correlation of MR imaging-determined cerebral blood volume maps with histologic and angiographic determination of vascularity of gliomas. AJR Am J Roentgenol 1998;171:1479–1486.

102. Wenz F, Rempp K, Hess T, et al. Effect of radiation on blood volume in low-grade astrocytomas and normal brain tissue: quantification with dynamic susceptibility contrast MR imaging. AJR Am J Roentgenol 1996;166:187–193.

103. Pardo FS, Aronen JJ, Kennedy D, et al. Functional cerebral imaging in the evaluation and radiotherapeutic treatment planning of patients with malignant glioma. Int J Radiat Oncol Biol Phys 1994;30:663–669.

104. Barker PB, Hearshen DO. Boska MD. Single-voxel proton MRS of the human brain at 1.5T and 3.0T. Magn Reson Med 2001;45:765–769.

105. Gonen O, Gruber S, Belinda S, et al. Multivixel 3D proton spectroscopy in the brain at 1.5 versus 3.0T: signal-to-noise ratio and resolution comparison. AJNR Am J Neuroradiol 2001;22:1727–1731.

106. Birken DL, Oldendorf WH. N-acetyl-L-aspartic acid: a leterature reviw of a compound prominent in 1H spectroscopic studies of brain. Neurosci Biobehav Rev 1989;13:23–31.

107. Ross BD. Biochemical considerations in 1H spectroscopy. Glutamate and glutamine; myo-inositol and related metabolites. NMR Biomed 1991;4:59–53.

108. Howe FA, Maxwell RJ, Saunders DE, et al. Proton spectroscopy in vivo. Magn Reson Q 1993;9:31–59.

109. Vion-Dury J, Meyerhoff DJ, Cozzone PJ, et al. What might be the impact on neurology of the analysis of brain metabolism by in vivo magnetic resonance spectroscopy? J Neurol 1994;241:354–371.

110. Castillo M, Kwock L, Mukherji SK. Clinical applications in proton MR spectroscopy. AJNR Am J Neuroradiol 1996;17:1–15.

111. Pouwels PJW, Frahm J. Regional metabolite concentrations in human brain determined by quantitative localized proton MRS. Magn Reson Med 1998;39:53–60.

112. Urenjak J, Williams SR, Gadian DG, et al. Specific expression of N-acetylaspartate in neurons, oligodendro-cyte-type-2 astrocyte progenitors, and immature oligodendrocytes in vitro. J Neurochem 1992;59:55–61.

113. Lowry OH, Berger SJ, Chi M-Y, et al. Diversity of metabolic patterns in human brain tumors-I. High energy phosphate compounds and basic composition. J Neurochem 1977;29:959–977.

7

Magnetic Resonance Spectroscopy

G. Evren Keles, Soonmee Cha, and Mitchel S. Berger

Summary

Magnetic resonance imaging (MRI) is the current standard neuroimaging modality for patients with high-grade gliomas (HGG). A valuable addition to the morphologic information obtained from MRI is magnetic resonance spectroscopy (MRS), which provides information regarding the metabolic status of the brain and tumor. In the clinical setting, MRS can be obtained during the same session as the MRI examination, therefore providing both morphological and metabolic imaging with minimal additional time.

Key Words: MRI; MRS; adjuvant therapy planning.

INTRODUCTION

Magnetic resonance imaging (MRI) is the current standard neuroimaging modality for patients with high-grade gliomas (HGG). A valuable addition to the morphologic information obtained from MRI is magnetic resonance spectroscopy (MRS), which provides information regarding the metabolic status of the brain and tumor. In the clinical setting, MRS can be obtained during the same session as the MRI examination, therefore providing both morphological and metabolic imaging with minimal additional time. As the literature regarding the use of MRS for patients with gliomas has increased substantially over the last decade, MRS has become an essential part of the clinical management of patients with HGG. Metabolic data obtained from MRS provides information that is useful at various stages of HGG management including diagnosis, treatment planning, and evaluation of response to therapy. This chapter outlines the basic principles of MRS, how various metabolites are altered in HGG, and the use of MRS in the multidisciplinary management of patients harboring these tumors.

BACKGROUND

By using the same basic principles as in MRI, MRS techniques provide metabolic assessments by quantifying the levels of important intracellular compounds. In order to acquire 1H (proton) MR spectra of these compounds, water resonance is suppressed and the area excited by radiofrequency pulse is limited to within the skull to prevent signal contamination from subcutaneous lipids. Spectra from regions of interest (ROI) may be obtained as either a single spectrum from each region (i.e., single-voxel MRS) or as a multidimensional array of spectra (i.e., magnetic resonance spectroscopic imaging [MRSI]) that is also known as chemical shift imaging (CSI) (1). Single-voxel techniques provide a single spectrum from a defined volume of tissue, and lack spatial resolution, whereas excitation and recording of a multidimensional

From: *Current Clinical Oncology: High-Grade Gliomas: Diagnosis and Treatment*
Edited by: G. H. Barnett © Humana Press Inc., Totowa, NJ

array of spectra from hundreds of smaller contiguous voxels provide significant increase in spatial resolution. MRSI, the most common method for acquiring spectra in multiple voxels, is important for HGG as these tumors are histologically heterogeneous even within the regions appearing uniform on anatomical imaging, and, tumor cells are often present beyond the area depicted on MRI *(2,3)*.

For HGG that constitute the topic of this chapter, metabolites of interest which can be evaluated with MRS include *N*-acetylaspartate (NAA), choline (Cho), creatine (Cre), lactate (Lac) and lipids. Analysis of proton MRS data entailed selection of a population of normal voxels (typically contralateral to the lesion), based on the absence of disease as seen on T2-weighted and contrast-enhanced T1-weighted images. The Cho and NAA levels in all voxels were then normalized using the mean of the corresponding metabolite levels observed in the normal voxels, generating a unitless measure of metabolite concentrations, which could be compared across examinations with minimal errors from differences in coil loading. Alteration in their respective levels constitutes the basis of metabolic imaging of HGG. In addition, there are other metabolites such as glutathione and alanine, which may have increased levels in meningiomas *(4,5)*, and *myo*-inositol levels are known to be higher in lower grade gliomas *(6)*. NAA, which is localized in viable neurons and absent in other central nervous system (CNS) cells, is important for the regulation of neuronal protein and neurotransmitter synthesis, and myelin production *(7,8)*. NAA is decreased in gliomas when compared with normal brain tissue. However, postradiation neuronal dysfunction may also result in decreased NAA levels *(9)*. Cho and its derivatives that form the Cho peak are involved in membrane phospholipid metabolism. Cho levels are elevated in regions of hypercellularity and increased membrane turnover. In HGG, histologic heterogeneity and presence of necrotic areas may result in highly variable levels of Cho within the tumor *(10)*. The Cre peak, which includes phosphocreatine, is indicative of cellular bioenergetic processes, and is usually reduced in HGG *(11,12)*. Lac levels, which indicate anaerobic metabolization of glucose, may represent cellular breakdown, and are very low in normal brain tissue. Although nonspecific, increased Lac levels are often seen in HGG *(11,12)*.

USE OF MAGNETIC RESONANCE SPECTROSCOPY IN THE CLINICAL SETTING

Metabolic data obtained from MRS provides information that is useful at various stages of HGG management including diagnosis, treatment planning, and evaluation of response to therapy.

Preoperative Evaluation and Surgical Planning

Over the past 15 yr, MRS techniques have been used to help differentiate tumor from normal brain in patients suspected of harboring HGG, to predict histological grade, and for surgical planning. Increased Cho levels and decreased NAA levels when compared with normal brain are general characteristics of gliomas. However, these alterations may also be observed in conditions where membrane turnover is increased and mature neuron populations are decreased.

Although histological diagnosis is the undisputable standard for the diagnosis and grading of gliomas, there has been interest in using MRS to correlate metabolite levels with histological grade *(13,14)*. In general, further variation from normal metabolite peaks is considered to correlate with histologically higher grades *(15)* (Fig. 1). The reports in the literature are controversial, however, and despite some promising reports, the quality of evidence is limited to retrospective case series as there is no prospective report in the literature where histological grade was predicted based on information obtained from MRS data *(8,16–20)*. An increased Cho level, in addition to higher Lac/Lip ratios, have been suggested in several of the earlier single-voxel studies despite histologic heterogeneity of gliomas within the same grade, as well as variability among various areas of individual lesions *(17–19)*. Although parts of the same tumor may suggest different histologic grades, the overall diagnoses were based on the portion with the highest histologic grade. Including later studies that provided a multidimensional array of spectra from the ROI, a consistent finding has been high resonance in the spectral region of Cho and/or a low-NAA resonance which results in an increased Cho/NAA ratio *(1,6,8,19,20)*.

In a patient population consisting of 49 gliomas, Li et al. *(10)* showed that the tumor burden measured with either the volumes of the metabolic abnormalities or the metabolic levels in the most abnormal voxels was correlated with the degree of malignancy of the tumor. The volumes of elevated Cho and decreased NAA were helpful for distinguishing low-grade from high-grade lesions, and, volume of abnormal Lac was correlated with the existence of necrosis and with the volume of contrast-enhancing lesions in high-grade lesions. The differences in the volume of abnormal Lac/Lip were also statistically significant between patients in each grade *(10)*.

In another study performed on 100 biopsy samples from 44 patients with gliomas obtained during open resections, the authors observed a difference among the four histological classes, and a subsequent pairwise comparison of data revealed differences between the Cho/NAA index (CNI) of the nontumorous samples and those of grades II, III and IV. No differences were found in the pairwise comparison of CNIs of the three grades of tumor or when the CNIs of the grade II tumors were contrasted with those of grades III and IV tumors combined *(21)*.

Although extent of resection is one of the predictors of outcome for HGG, stereotactic biopsy remains to be an option at the initial management of a subset of patients with HGG *(22)*. For those patients undergoing stereotactic biopsies, in addition to MRI data, which is generally used to determine the locations to be biopsied within the tumor, information obtained from MRS is helpful in determining the areas that are more likely to represent tumor histology and might be helpful in selecting the best biopsy sites. In a study correlating metabolite levels measured by preoperative MRSI with histologic findings of biopsies obtained during image-guided resections from the same locations, the authors showed that if the metabolic abnormality consisted of increased Cho (2 standard deviations above normal levels) and decreased NAA (2 standard deviations below normal levels), histologic findings of the biopsy specimen invariably was positive for tumor *(2)*. In this study, even when the increase in Cho levels was less than 2 standard deviations (SD) above normal, the histologic findings were consistent with tumor in 85% of the cases as long as Cho was greater than NAA *(2)*. In another study that correlated MRSI data with subsequent histologic analysis of biopsied tumor samples, all areas of confirmed tumor demonstrated significantly increased choline levels and a mean Cho/NAA ratio that was at least greater than 4 SD above the mean found in normal tissue *(23)*.

Knowing the extent of the disease is essential in planning and effectively conducting resective surgery on a HGG. In a study, which included 34 patients with anaplastic astrocytomas and glioblastoma multiforme, MRSI data was compared with information obtained from MRI *(3)*. For both grades, although T2 estimated the region at risk of microscopic disease as being as much as 50% greater than by MRSI, metabolically active tumor still extended outside the T2 region in 88% of patients by as many as 28 mm. In addition, T1 suggested a lesser volume and different location of active disease compared to MRSI *(3)*.

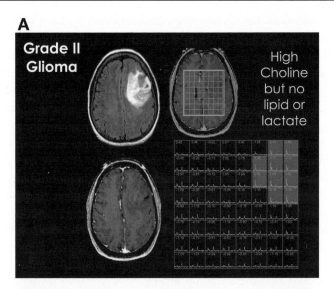

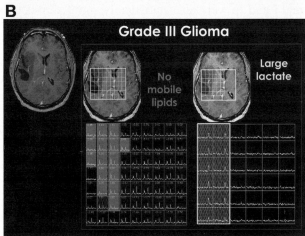

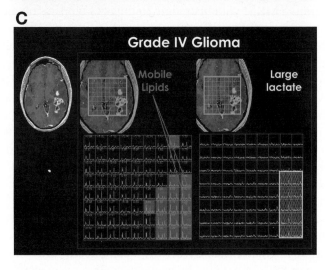

Fig. 1. MRS images depicting the metabolic characteristics of **(A)** grade II, **(B)** grade III, and **(C)** grade IV astrocytomas.

McKnight et al. *(21)* compared MRSI data with histology results from biopsies obtained during surgery to evaluate the sensitivity and specificity of the Cho to NAA index (CNI), which is used to distinguish tumor from nontumorous tissue within the T2 hyperintense and contrast enhancing lesions. The authors reported that samples containing tumor were distinguished from those containing a mixture of normal, edematous, gliotic, and necrotic tissue with 90% sensitivity and 86% specificity by using a CNI threshold of 2.5 *(21)*. Recently, in a study performed on pre-radiotherapy patients with glioblastoma who had already undergone surgery, a significantly shorter median survival time was observed for patients with a large volume of CNI2 than for patients with a small CNI2 volume (12.0 and 17.1 mo, respectively, $p = 0.002$), emphasizing the importance of volume of the postresection metabolic abnormality in predicting survival for patients with HGG *(24)*. The authors' finding in patients who will undergo radiotherapy is in accordance with the prognostic importance of tumor extent in patients with glioblastoma who will undergo chemotherapy *(25)*.

Intraoperative frameless neuronavigation systems are important tools in the current neurosurgical treatment of brain tumors. The data set used is usually based on a preoperatively obtained MR scan which provides structural information about the tumor and surrounding brain tissue. Incorporation of MRSI data to these systems has the potential of enabling the surgeon to observe the extent of the metabolic abnormality and the spatial extent of the tumor. Another surgical implication is, despite its lesser availability, the ability to obtain real-time MRS data with the second and third generation intraoperative MRI systems *(26)*.

Adjuvant Therapy Planning

The role of MRSI in planning adjuvant therapies is mainly based on its ability to determine the extent of metabolic abnormality which is often beyond the morphologic boundaries observed on conventional MR scans. For HGG, areas of potential use include planning of radiotherapy, gamma-knife radiosurgery, and brachytherapy. Increasing use of adjuvant therapeutic modalities that aim focal delivery at residual tumor make the need for accurate delineation of tumor extent more important.

Postoperative radiotherapy is an essential part of the management of HGG. The standard approach of defining target volume based on the contrast enhancing area with an added margin does not take into account the fact that enhancement may not always correlate with histologic malignancy. Presence of active disease has been shown outside the enhancing region, in the T2-hyperintense areas and beyond *(3,27)*. To assess the potential effect of MRSI on the target volumes used for radiation therapy planning for HGG, Pirzkall et al. *(3)* evaluated 34 patients with HGG by comparing areas of MRI based signal abnormalities with NAA and Cho levels obtained by three-demensional (3D) MRSI. Their data showed that metabolically active tumor may extend outside the T2 region, and, T1-weighted MRI suggested a lesser volume and different location of active disease compared to MRSI. The authors concluded that the use of MRSI to define target volumes for radiotherapy planning would increase the volume receiving a boost dose of radiation and change its location, in addition to reducing the volume receiving a standard dose *(3)*. In another study, the registration and display of MRS data within radiotherapy planning software has been shown to be feasible and reproducible *(28)*.

The prognostic value of MRSI in planning gamma-knife radiosurgery was evaluated by Graves et al. *(29)* in a retrospective analysis on 36 recurrent malignant gliomas. In this study, those patients who had a gamma-knife treatment volume determined by MRI contrast enhancement with no suspected tumor pattern detected by MRSI outside the contrast enhancement had a significantly better outcome than those patients who had MRSI suspected disease extending outside the MRI derived treatment volume *(29)*. Specifically, for patients harboring a glioblastoma, those patients with regions containing tumor-suggestive spectra outside the gamma-knife target had a significant increase in contrast-enhancing volume, a decrease in time to progression, and a reduction in survival time when compared with patients exhibiting spectral abnormalities restricted to the gamma-knife target *(29)*. At our institution we are currently incorporating MRSI data to define treatment volumes for gamma-knife radiosurgery *(30)*.

Evaluation of Response to Therapy

In order to evaluate response to therapy, MRSI data obtained from sequential examinations need to be directly correlated. It has been shown that accuracy of registration can be achieved within one to two pixels, and following translations and rotations to align the coordinate system from one examination to the other, the images and spectral data may be matched voxel by voxel *(31)*. In addition to the increasing use of MRSI as part of the standard multimodality management and follow-up of patients with HGG, MRSI data is also considered for the evaluation of experimental therapeutic modalities such as immunogene therapy using replication-incompetent viruses and convection enhanced delivery of immunotoxins *(32,33)*.

Although MRI is the standard imaging modality in evaluating response to therapy, the distinction between radiotherapy-induced necrosis and progressive tumor is not always clear. In a study planned to assess the use of serial 3D MRSI to analyze the dose-dependence of changes in metabolite ratios and time variation of individual metabolites in non-tumorous white matter, Lee et al. *(34)* reported a statistically significant rise in the Cho/NAA ratio 2 to 6 mo after therapy in regions receiving >25 Gy, changes in the Cho/Cr ratio that were only significant 2 mo after therapy, a general trend toward increased Cho/Cr at higher doses, and no significant dose-dependence in the Cr levels.

In one of the earlier studies using serial MRSI, Wald et al. *(35)* evaluated patients with glioblastoma after brachytherapy, and observed a significant reduction in Cho levels after therapy, as well as an increase in Cho levels for patients who demonstrated subsequent progression with increased Cho in regions that previously appeared either normal or necrotic. Since then, the ability to distinguish recurrent tumor from radiation effects based on Cho/NAA, normalized Cho, normalized NAA, and normalized Lac has been studied by several groups *(36–40)*. Their common finding was higher Cho and lower NAA in recurrent tumor compared with adjacent enhancing tissue that had no histologic evidence of tumor. In addition, a global decrease in peak amplitudes is consistent with radiation injury without neoplasm. As spectral changes following radiation therapy have been shown to be transient (i.e., often appearing tumor-like within the first 2 to 4 mo after therapy and returning to a relatively normal pattern after 8 mo) both the spectral patterns and their temporal characteristics need to be evaluated to differentiate radiation effects from recurrent tumor *(9)*.

CONCLUSION

MRS is an important adjunct in the management of patients with HGG. Its clinical use includes depiction of metabolically abnormal tissue to guide surgery and planning of adjuvant therapies, as well as evaluation of response to therapy. In the neurosurgical setting, the metabolic information obtained from MRS, combined with various pre- and intraoperative imaging techniques such as perfusion MRI *(41)*, diffusion tensor imaging *(42,43)*, and intraoperative MRI *(26)* enable the surgeon to better understand the extent of the disease and its relationship with various intracranial structures.

REFERENCES

1. Vigneron DB, Nelson SJ, Murphy-Boesch J, Kelley DA, Kessler HB, Brown TR, Taylor JS. Chemical shift imaging of human brain: axial, sagittal, and coronal P-31 metabolite images. Radiology 1990;177(3):643–649.
2. Dowling C, Bollen AW, Noworolski SM, et al. Preoperative proton MR spectroscopic imaging of brain tumors: correlation with histopathologic analysis of resection specimens. AJNR Am J Neuroradiol 2001;22(4): 604–612.
3. Pirzkall A, McKnight TR, Graves EE, et al. MR-spectroscopy guided target delineation for high-grade gliomas. Int J Radiat Oncol Biol Phys 2001;50(4):915–928.
4. Opstad KS, Provencher SW, Bell BA, Griffiths JR, Howe FA. Detection of elevated glutathione in meningiomas by quantitative in vivo 1H MRS. Magn Reson Med 2003;49(4):632–637.
5. Tate AR, Majos C, Moreno A, Howe FA, Griffiths JR, Arus C. Automated classification of short echo time in in vivo 1H brain tumor spectra: a multicenter study. Magn Reson Med 2003;49(1):29–36.
6. Castillo M, Smith JK, Kwock L: Correlation of myo-inositol levels and grading of cerebral astrocytomas. AJNR Am J Neuroradiol 2000;21(9):1645–1649.
7. Meyerand ME, Pipas JM, Mamourian A, Tosteson TD, Dunn JF. Classification of biopsy-confirmed brain tumors using single-voxel MR spectroscopy. AJNR Am J Neuroradiol 1999;20(1):117–123.
8. Negendank WG, Sauter R, Brown TR, et al. Proton magnetic resonance spectroscopy in patients with glial tumors: a multicenter study. J Neurosurg 1996;84(3):449–458.
9. Esteve F, Rubin C, Grand S, Kolodie H, Le Bas JF. Transient metabolic changes observed with proton MR spectroscopy in normal human brain after radiation therapy. Int J Radiat Oncol Biol Phys 1998;40(2):279–286.
10. Li X, Lu Y, Pirzkall A, McKnight T, Nelson SJ. Analysis of the spatial characteristics of metabolic abnormalities in newly diagnosed glioma patients. J Magn Reson Imaging 2002;16(3):229–237.
11. Howe FA, Barton SJ, Cudlip SA, et al. Metabolic profiles of human brain tumors using quantitative in vivo 1H magnetic resonance spectroscopy. Magn Reson Med 2003;49(2):223–232.
12. Majos C, Alonso J, Aguilera C, et al. Proton magnetic resonance spectroscopy ((1)H MRS) of human brain tumours: assessment of differences between tumour types and its applicability in brain tumour categorization. Eur Radiol. 2003;13(3):582–591.
13. Furuya S, Naruse S, Ide M, et al. Evaluation of metabolic heterogeneity in brain tumors using 1H-chemical shift imaging method. NMR Biomed 1997;10(1):25–30.
14. Preul MC, Caramanos Z, Collins DL, et al. Accurate, noninvasive diagnosis of human brain tumors by using proton magnetic resonance spectroscopy. Nat Med 1996;2(3):323–325.
15. Hunter JV, Wang ZJ. MR spectroscopy in pediatric neuroradiology. Magn Reson Imaging Clin N Am 2001; 9(1):165–189.
16. Arnold DL, Shoubridge EA, Villemure JG, Feindel W. Proton and phosphorus magnetic resonance spectroscopy of human astrocytomas in vivo. Preliminary observations on tumor grading. NMR Biomed 1990;3(4): 184–189.
17. Bruhn H, Frahm J, Gyngell ML, et al. Noninvasive differentiation of tumors with use of localized H-1 MR spectroscopy in vivo: initial experience in patients with cerebral tumors. Radiology 1989;172(2):541–548.
18. Poptani H, Gupta RK, Roy R, Pandey R, Jain VK, Chhabra DK. Characterization of intracranial mass lesions with in vivo proton MR spectroscopy. AJNR Am J Neuroradiol 1995;16(8):1593–1603.
19. Shimizu H, Kumabe T, Tominaga T, et al. Noninvasive evaluation of malignancy of brain tumors with proton MR spectroscopy. AJNR Am J Neuroradiol 1996;17(4):737–747.
20. Taylor JS, Langston JW, Reddick WE, et al. Clinical value of proton magnetic resonance spectroscopy for differentiating recurrent or residual brain tumor from delayed cerebral necrosis. Int J Radiat Oncol Biol Phys 1996;36(5):1251–1261.
21. McKnight TR, von dem Bussche MH, Vigneron DB, et al. Histopathological validation of a three-dimensional magnetic resonance spectroscopy index as a predictor of tumor presence. J Neurosurg 2002;97(4): 794–802.
22. Keles GE, Anderson B, Berger MS. The effect of extent of resection on time to tumor progression and survival in patients with glioblastoma multiforme of the cerebral hemisphere. Surg Neurol 1999;52(4):371–379.
23. Vigneron D, Bollen A, McDermott M, et al. Three-dimensional magnetic resonance spectroscopic imaging of histologically confirmed brain tumors. Magn Reson Imaging 2001;19(1):89–101.
24. Oh J, Henry RG, Pirzkall A, et al. Survival analysis in patients with glioblastoma multiforme: predictive value of choline-to-N-acetylaspartate index, apparent diffusion coefficient, and relative cerebral blood volume. J Magn Reson Imaging 2004;19(5):546–554.

25. Keles GE, Lamborn KR, Chang SM, Prados MD, Berger MS. Volume of residual disease as a predictor of outcome in adult patients with recurrent supratentorial glioblastomas multiforme who are undergoing chemotherapy. J Neurosurg 2004;100(1):41–46.

26. Keles GE. Intracranial neuronavigation with intraoperative magnetic resonance imaging. Curr Opin Neurol. 2004;17(4):497–500.

27. Kelly PJ, Daumas-Duport C, Kispert DB, Kall BA, Scheithauer BW, Illig JJ. Imaging-based stereotaxic serial biopsies in untreated intracranial glial neoplasms. J Neurosurg 1987;66(6):865–874.

28. Graves EE, Pirzkall A, Nelson SJ, Larson D, Verhey L. Registration of magnetic resonance spectroscopic imaging to computed tomography for radiotherapy treatment planning. Med Phys 2001;28(12):2489–2496.

29. Graves EE, Nelson SJ, Vigneron DB, et al. A preliminary study of the prognostic value of proton magnetic resonance spectroscopic imaging in gamma knife radiosurgery of recurrent malignant gliomas. Neurosurgery 2000;46(2):319–26.

30. McDermott MW, Chang SM, Keles GE, et al. Gamma knife radiosurgery for primary brain tumors. In: Germano IM, ed. LINAC and Gamma Knife Radiosurgery. Park Ridge, IL:American Association of Neurological Surgeons, 2000;189–202.

31. Nelson SJ, McKnight TR, Henry RG. Characterization of untreated gliomas by magnetic resonance spectroscopic imaging. Neuroimaging Clin N Am 2002;12(4):599–613.

32. Kunwar S. Convection enhanced delivery of IL13-PE38QQR for treatment of recurrent malignant glioma: presentation of interim findings from ongoing phase 1 studies. Acta Neurochir Suppl 2003;88:105–111.

33. Ren H, Boulikas T, Lundstrom K, Soling A, Warnke PC, Rainov NG. Immunogene therapy of recurrent glioblastoma multiforme with a liposomally encapsulated replication-incompetent Semliki forest virus vector carrying the human interleukin-12 gene—a phase I/II clinical protocol. J Neurooncol 2003;64(1-2):147–154.

34. Lee MC, Pirzkall A, McKnight TR, Nelson SJ. 1H-MRSI of radiation effects in normal-appearing white matter: dose-dependence and impact on automated spectral classification. J Magn Reson Imaging 2004;19(4):379–388.

35. Wald LL, Nelson SJ, Day MR, et al. Serial proton magnetic resonance spectroscopy imaging of glioblastoma multiforme after brachytherapy. J Neurosurg 1997;87(4):525–534.

36. Chan YL, Yeung DK, Leung SF, Cao G. Proton magnetic resonance spectroscopy of late delayed radiation-induced injury of the brain. J Magn Reson Imaging 1999;10(2):130–137.

37. Kamada K, Houkin K, Abe H, Sawamura Y, Kashiwaba T. Differentiation of cerebral radiation necrosis from tumor recurrence by proton magnetic resonance spectroscopy. Neurol Med Chir (Tokyo) 1997;37(3):250–256.

38. Preul MC, Leblanc R, Caramanos Z, Kasrai R, Narayanan S, Arnold DL. Magnetic resonance spectroscopy guided brain tumor resection: differentiation between recurrent glioma and radiation change in two diagnostically difficult cases. Can J Neurol Sci 1998;25(1):13–22.

39. Rabinov JD, Lee PL, Barker FG, et al. In vivo 3-T MR spectroscopy in the distinction of recurrent glioma versus radiation effects: initial experience. Radiology 2002;225(3):871–879.

40. Rock JP, Hearshen D, Scarpace L, et al. Correlations between magnetic resonance spectroscopy and image-guided histopathology, with special attention to radiation necrosis. Neurosurgery 2002;51(4):912–919.

41. Cha S. Perfusion MR Imaging of Brain Tumors. Top Magn Reson Imaging 2004;15(5):279–289.

42. Berman JI, Berger MS, Mukherjee P, Henry RG. Diffusion-tensor imaging-guided tracking of fibers of the pyramidal tract combined with intraoperative cortical stimulation mapping in patients with gliomas. J Neurosurg 2004;101(1):66–72.

43. Henry RG, Berman JI, Nagarajan SS, Mukherjee P, Berger MS. Subcortical pathways serving cortical language sites: initial experience with diffusion tensor imaging fiber tracking combined with intraoperative language mapping. Neuroimage 2004;21(2):616–622.

8 Imaging Tumor Biology

Physiological and Molecular Insights

Timothy P. L. Roberts and Andrea Kassner

Summary

Anatomic medical imaging offers the ability to detect and delineate brain tumors. In addition, emerging techniques (in particular MRI variants) offer insight into aspects of tumor physiology and metabolism, thus allowing characterization of tumor dysfunction, in principle, at a metabolic, cellular, and vascular level. This chapter will present advances in faster and higher resolution magnetic resonance spectroscopic imaging (MRSI) as a probe of abnormal metabolism; diffusion weighted imaging (DWI) as a measure of tumor cellularity, and the related technique of diffusion tensor imaging (DTI) as a measure of structural organization; and, imaging of tumor perfusion and vascular permeability, as a measure of vascularity and as an approach to the study of angiogenesis.

Key Words: MRI; MRSI; DWI; DTI.

1. INTRODUCTION

Anatomic medical imaging offers the ability to detect and delineate brain tumors for example using T2-weighted or T1-weighted post-gadolinium magnetic resonance imaging (MRI). In addition, emerging techniques (in particular MRI variants) offer insight into aspects of tumor physiology and metabolism, thus allowing characterization of tumor dysfunction, in principle, at a metabolic, cellular, and vascular level. This chapter will present advances in (1) faster and higher resolution magnetic resonance spectroscopic imaging (MRSI) as a probe of abnormal metabolism; (2) diffusion weighted imaging (DWI) as a measure of tumor cellularity, and the related technique of diffusion tensor imaging (DTI) as a measure of structural organization; and, (3) imaging of tumor perfusion and vascular permeability, as a measure of vascularity and as an approach to the study of angiogenesis. Multispectral or combinatorial approaches harnessing multiple physiological specificities will also be introduced. These physiologically specific imaging techniques will be developed in the context of tumor grading as well as in the monitoring of cytotoxic and tumoristatic therapies. In particular, the role of imaging as a marker of biological activity of anti-angiogenic therapies will be discussed as a potential means of elucidating the biologically effective dose and as an early indicator of responsiveness. Furthermore, the role of advanced imaging techniques in guiding surgical approaches will be presented synergistically with reference to identification of eloquent cortex (with functional magnetic resonance imaging, [fMRI], and magnetic source imaging, [MSI]) and subcortical white matter (with diffusion tensor imaging, [DTI]). Together these advances offer increasingly specific opportunities for diagnosis, characterization, treatment planning

From: *Current Clinical Oncology: High-Grade Gliomas: Diagnosis and Treatment*
Edited by: G. H. Barnett © Humana Press Inc., Totowa, NJ

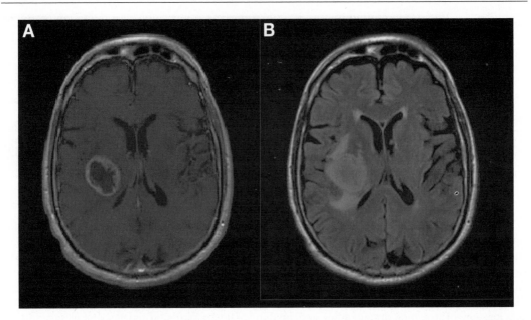

Fig. 1. Gliblastoma multiforme (GBM) on conventional MRI. (**A***t*) T1-weighted axial acquisition after administration of 0.1 mmol/kg Gd-based contrast agent clearly delineates tumor "rim enhancement." (**B**) FLAIR (CSF-suppressed, T2-weighted) image at the same level demonstrates peritumoral edema (hyperintensity).

and therapy monitoring of brain tumors. Beyond physiology, however, it is clear that underlying biochemical changes associated with neuro-oncology demand attention. Preliminary insights into the newly emerging field(s) of molecular imaging, based on optical fluorescence, nuclear medicine and indeed novel MRI will also be introduced with a vision of ultimately uniting molecular/biochemical processes and physiological descriptions at the cellular and vascular level into a comprehensive view of brain tumor characterization.

PHYSIOLOGICALLY SPECIFIC IMAGING

Conventional Magnetic Resonance Imaging

Conventional MRI, particularly T2-weighted and fluid attenuation inversion recovery (FLAIR) techniques and T1-weighted sequences with gadolinium enhancement, have proven highly useful in the radiological definition and localization of intracranial tumors with high spatial (anatomic) resolution, as well as providing the distinction between intra-axial (e.g., glioma) and extra-axial (e.g., meningioma) lesions (Fig. 1). However, powerful as they have proven, the physiological insights they shed are limited in specificity and are thus augmented by the emerging technologies discussed below.

Magnetic Resonance Spectroscopy and Spectroscopic Imaging

Abnormal tumor metabolism, with elevated cell membrane turnover and depleted neuronal viability may have characteristic signatures visible in the proton-MR spectrum. MRS and its imaging counterpart, MRSI, allow elucidation of the relative regional concentration of certain key metabolic products. Interest typically focuses on the relative levels of free choline-containing compounds, including phosphocholine and glycerophosphocholoine (designated Cho),

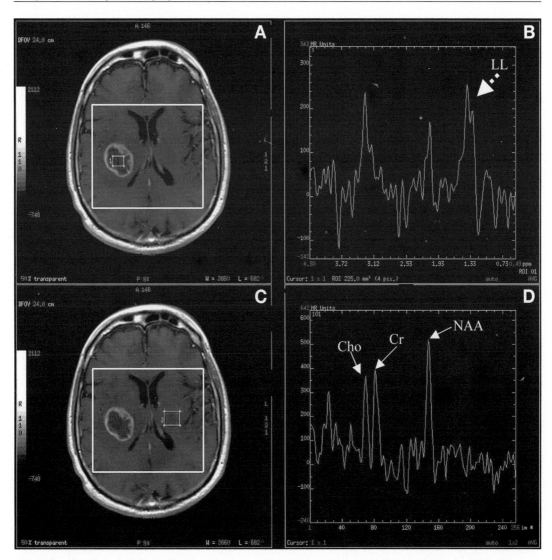

Fig. 2. ROI selection and the corresponding MR spectra **(A,B)** tumor (GBM) and **(C,D)** in healthy tissue. Whereas the healthy tissue shows clear Cho, Cr, and NAA resonances (with an NAA:Cho ratio of approx 1.2), the tumor shows markedly reduced NAA, elevated Cho (NAA:Cho ratio of approx 0.5) and the presence of a large resonance at 1.2–1.4 ppm corresponding to "lipid and lactate (LL)." All spectra are acquired at 1.5T at TE = 144 ms using a PRESS sequence. Spectra represented in the right hand panels are derived from the region described by the green box in the corresponding images.

which may be elevated by excessive membrane synthesis and turnover; creatine and phosphocreatine (designated Cr), associated with cellular energetics; *N*-acetyl aspartate (NAA, a signature of viable neurons); and lactate and free lipids (commonly combined as "lipid and lactate" because of their overlapping spectral resonances) *(1)* (Fig. 2).

In MRSI, also known as CSI, individual spectra are obtained for each voxel of a two-dimension (2D) or three-dimensional (3D) grid covering the lesion and/or healthy control tissue. As such regional variation in metabolite concentration can be investigated (Fig. 3). The

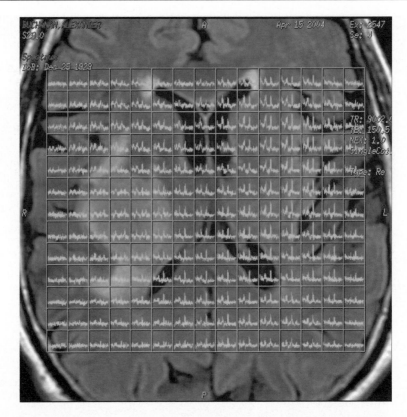

Fig. 3. A grid of "voxels" spanning the axial brain slice each reveals local distribution of key metabolites, Cho, Cr, NAA and the abnormal presence of lipids and/or lactate. Overlaid on the T2-weighted FLAIR MRI one can readily appreciate the decreased peak height of the NAA resonance in the vicinity of the tumor in contradistinction to the contralateral hemisphere. One can also recognize the limited spatial resolution of the spectroscopic technique, suggesting its utility as an adjunct or complement to conventional imaging.

fundamental limitation of this powerful advance is the increased length of scans, resulting in clinical adoption of rather low matrix or grid sizes—a typical 16 × 16 2D grid acquisition might have a scan duration of approx 4 min.

Based on multivoxel approaches, or MRSI, it is thus possible to achieve an assessment of regional variations in the metabolite concentrations, by observing the relative magnitude of the distinct "peaks" or "resonances" at each spatial site. Quantitative approaches typically assess either the peak height or area under the peak and frequently control for systematic variations by normalization (ratio forming) to either an external reference or an internal marker (commonly the local Cr resonance, which is relatively invariant, or the contralateral metabolite level—giving a quantitative estimation of depletion or elevation). Because such quantitative information is obtained over a grid of voxels it is possible to synthesize "metabolite maps" where the intensity of each voxel is determined by the local metabolite level (either resonance peak or area). Because these maps are derivable only at the low resolution of the MRSI exam, they are commonly overlaid on high resolution "anatomic" MRI scans (Fig. 4).

Although there is general consensus that higher grade tumors tend to be associated with elevated Cho, decreased NAA, and the presence of lipid/lactate resonances, most studies find

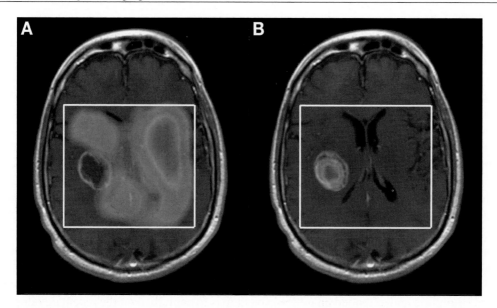

Fig. 4. Parametric metabolite map of **(A)** *N*-acetyl aspartate (NAA) and **(B)** "lipid and lactate" distribution overlaid on contrast enhanced MRI, delineating a right hemispheric grade IV GBM. NAA is depleted in the region of the tumor, where lipid and lactate are clearly elevated (hotter colors = yellow, red).

considerable overlap between tumors of different histological grades *(1,2)*. This tends to support the role of MRSI as an adjunct to other physiologically-specific methods in non-invasive prediction of tumor grade. However, the utility of MRSI, or the definition of the "metabolic lesion" may in fact extend beyond diagnosis and may be an important contributor to effective treatment planning. By sensitive detection of metabolic signatures of abnormality (e.g., elevated Cho and decreased NAA) beyond the margins of the radiologic appearance of the tumor, it is speculated that the presence infiltrative tumor cells in otherwise normal appearing parenchyma can be identified. In a study of MRSI prior to gamma-knife treatment of the tumor, Graves et al. demonstrated that evidence of metabolic abnormality extending beyond the contrast enhancing margin of the tumor (used to define the radiotherapy target) was associated with poor treatment response *(3)*. In a follow-up study Graves et al. demonstrated evidence for tumor recurrence in regions of metabolic abnormality not included in the gamma-knife target zone *(4)*. These studies suggest an important role for MRSI in defining the extent of metabolic abnormality and in planning treatment, either radiotherapy or surgical.

Beyond diagnosis and treatment planning, Li et al. assessed the prognostic utility of MRSI in predicting survival in patients with malignant gliomas *(5)*. In addition to age and degree of contrast enhancement, they found that poor outcome was predicted by elevated Cho (either referred to Cr or to NAA), elevated lipid and lactate and low values of NNA/Cr.

Because the utility of spatial metabolic interrogation holds significant potential promise, approaches to increase the speed of acquisition are being pursued to enable higher spatial resolution and 3D acquisitions to be achievable in clinically practical scan times. Two fundamental strategies are of special interest: multi-echo acquisitions (modeled on multi-echo imaging, fast-spin echo, and echo-planar imaging) and parallel acquisitions using multiple receive RF coils and the principles of sensitivity encoding (SENSE) *(6)*. Both are enhanced by the ongoing trend towards the use of higher magnetic field strength MR scanners (especially 3 Tesla [T] compared with the previous standard 1.5T). Multi-echo spectroscopic techniques (such as turbo spectroscopic imaging, TSI, and PEPSI) rely on the acquisition of multiple echoes after each RF excitation pulse *(7–9)*. These echoes are required to build up the image matrix and thus collecting 2, 3, 5 or more per excitation pulse has a commensurate reduction in overall scan time. Unfortunately these approaches introduce two potential confounds. First, each echo of the echo train is necessarily acquired at a different echo time (TE) and is thus differently T2-weighted. Furthermore, in order to achieve reasonably short echo-train durations, individual echo acquisitions must be constrained in time. This has a consequence in terms of the spectral resolution of the resultant spectra (spectral resolution is related by the Fourier transform to the inverse of the echo duration; thus a 100 ms echo acquisition would yield 10 Hz spectral resolution). An interesting added benefit of 3T vs 1.5T is that not only is overall signal-to-noise ratio increased, but also spectral separation (in Hz) between metabolites is increased, potentially making 10 Hz resolution "metabolically acceptable" at 3T where it would fail to resolve similar metabolite resonances at lower field strengths *(10)*. A second strategy to reduce acquisition times for MRSI and consequently enable higher spatial resolution and extended anatomic coverage is to capitalize on the recent development of parallel imaging approaches, using multiple RF receiver coils and the principles of SENSE *(6)*. By exploiting multiple receive elements, a reduction in the number of phase encoding steps can be achieved with commensurate reduction in scan time. Because MRSI is characterized by one additional dimension per phase encoding than analogous MRI (in which no spectral information is obtained), it potentially stands to benefit even more from such acceleration, with "speed-up" factors of 4 or more being achievable *(11)*. In combination with turbo-spin echo approaches, overall acceleration factors of 7 to 9 have been demonstrated, drastically reducing MRSI acquisition times and opening the door for higher resolution and 3D application in realistic scan times *(7)*.

Diffusion Weighted Imaging and Diffusion Tensor Imaging

Diffusion weighted magnetic resonance imaging (DWI) is a widely adopted technique in the field of cerebral ischemia. By exploiting its high sensitivity to the mobility of water molecules, images can be obtained which clearly delineate diffusion "restriction, or hindrance" as well as "elevation, or even, facilitation." Interpretations of the underlying causes of these observed changes vary, but a prevailing consensus considers dense cell packing a predictor of reduced diffusion, whereas vasogenic edema is associated with considerably elevated diffusion, when compared with normal tissues. This generalization is confounded further by the anisotropic diffusion of white matter (in which diffusion is different parallel and perpendicular to fiber bundles) (Fig. 5).

In general, findings on DWI of intra-axial tumors have shown considerable heterogeneity and thereby little diagnostic utility. Cystic or necrotic regions are typically associated with elevated ADC because dense cellularity may lead to reduced apparent diffusion coefficient (ADC) values. Nonetheless, Sugahara et al. were able to demonstrate a significant correlation between the minimum ADC value in HGG and the histologically determined cell density (from light microscopic analysis of cell nucleus count) *(12)*. Selecting the minimum ADC value as the dependent variable ameliorates the variation associated with intra-tumoral heterogeneity. However, within the population of HGG they studied, the minimum ADC value observed ranged from 0.82 to 2.46×10^{-3} mm^2/s, indicating the inter-tumor variability. Despite this variance, the minimum ADC value was nonetheless found to be significantly different from

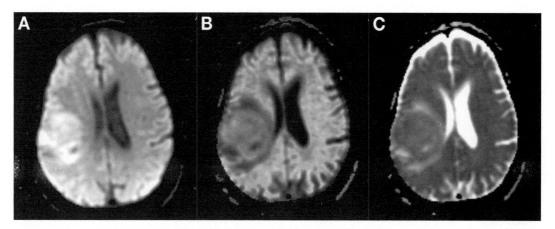

Fig. 5. GBM. (**A**) Diffusion weighted image; (**B**) exponential diffusion weighted image (T2-normalized), and (**C**) synthesized map of apparent diffusion coefficient (ADC) showing heterogeneous iso-, hypo-, and hyper-intensity (elevated diffusion) in the necrotic core and more uniform hyperintensity in the peritumoral edema.

a population of low-grade gliomas (LGG) (associated with higher values of minimum ADC). Thus, the property of water diffusion in tumors appears to relate to underlying cellularity and may be a useful constituent property in the physiological characterization of the tumor.

Although the ADC reflects the mean diffusivity, a variant of DWI allows description of the directional dependence of water diffusion. That is, in certain environments (e.g., white matter) there may be a preferred direction of diffusion (e.g., along the fiber), with considerably reduced diffusivity in other directions (e.g., across the fiber). Directional sensitivity can be incorporated into the DWI experiment by appropriate application of magnetic field gradient pulses. By performing several different DWI acquisitions, each with different directional encoding of diffusion, a description of the directional dependence of diffusion can be elucidated. This technique, known as diffusion tensor imaging (DTI) effectively leads to a voxel wise description of water diffusion in terms of both directional preference and diffusion magnitude. Whereas equal diffusivity in all spatial directions is termed isotropic diffusion, directional preference is described as "anisotropic diffusion" and can be quantified by a variety of metrics, of which the "fractional anisotropy" (FA) is most widely encountered. In regions of high anisotropy, FA takes a higher value; in regions of isotropic diffusion, FA equals zero. Figure 6 illustrates a map of fractional anisotropy, overlaid on an anatomic image. White matter regions are clearly depicted by high FA values, except in the region of tumor invasion (right, posterior). Based on such pixel-wise maps of fractional anisotropy and pixel-wise determination of the preferred direction of diffusion (known as the principal eigenvector), it is possible from any start point to trace a path of preferred diffusion, which is assumed to reflect the path of white matter fibers forming the fiber tracts. A variety of algorithms have been proposed for this, with fiber assignment by continuous tracking (FACT) being the currently most widely implemented *(13,14)*.

The clinical appreciation of DTI (and quantitative white matter fiber assessment) is emerging in two distinct areas: first, in the distinction between infiltrative tumors (causing a loss of anisotropy) vs lesions where fibers are anatomically distorted or shifted, but in which anisotropy is nonetheless preserved *(15)*. Second, the identification of peritumoral white matter fiber

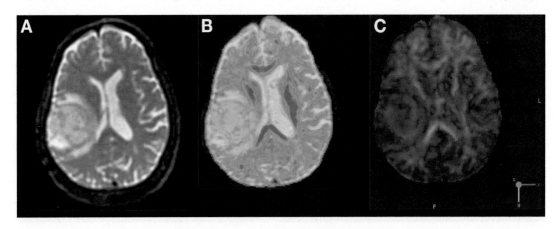

Fig. 6. Disturbance of white matter fiber integrity by invasive GBM. (**A**) T2-weighted echo planar image demonstrates large right hemispheric parietal mass. (**B**) Overlaid fractional anisotropy map demonstrates both the anatomic distortion of fibers (in the more anterior portion of the right hemisphere periventricular white matter) and its infiltration and loss of anisotropy (in the more posterior portion), where fractional anisotropy is quantitatively reduced (represented as a departure from red towards green/yellow on overlay. (**C**) colored map of principal eigenvector (pixel-wise preferred diffusion direction).

tracts is a potentially valuable adjunct to the presurgical planning and intraoperative guidance of resective procedures *(16,17)*.

Dynamic Contrast Enhanced-Magnetic Resonance Imaging

If dynamic MRI is performed in concert with bolus injection of gadolinium-based contrast media, it is possible to track the bolus as it passes through the tissues of the brain. In the context of tumor imaging, it is not only the first pass (perfusion-related) transit of the contrast agent which is of interest, but also progressive enhancement revealed over the course of the next 3 to 5 min. Conceptually, initial enhancement will reflect the vascular fractional volume of the tissue (a tissue with 5% vascular volume will initially enhance 5% as much as a reference blood vessel containing 100% blood); any progressive enhancement, however, will relate to the extravasation of contrast medium from the intravascular to the interstitial space. Given the lack of such extravasation in the healthy brain (where contrast media cannot cross the intact blood–brain barrier [BBB]), such hyperpermeability can be viewed as an indicator of pathologic compromise of BBB integrity. Kinetic modeling of the dynamic signal intensity vs time curves from tissue and a reference blood vessel (e.g., the sagittal sinus) allows interpretation of the dynamic data in terms of fBV and microvascular permeability, directly *(18–20)*. Because this analysis can be performed on a pixel-by-pixel basis, it is possible to generate parameter maps or pseudo-images, where image intensity relates to the physiological parameter of interest (fBV or Kps) (Fig. 7).

Studies have demonstrated the superior distinction between tumors of various grade by the adoption of such measures of microvascular permeability (Fig. 8), over consideration of relative blood volume alone *(19)*. However, assessment of microvascular permeability is not only useful for grading tumors, but should also be taken in context of emerging evidence that microvascular permeability elevation may be an indicator of the process of angiogenesis and thus may be a sensitive marker of the process of anti-angiogenesis via new generations of

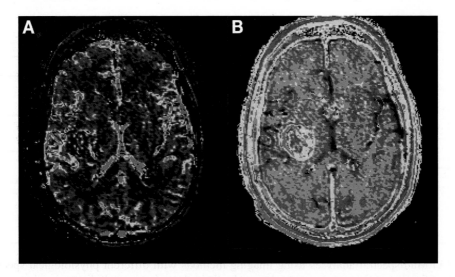

Fig. 7. Characterization of the microvasculature in a grade IV GBM. Dynamic contrast enhanced MRI can be modeled to yield pixel-wise estimates of **(A)** fractional blood volume and **(B)** microvascular permeability in this axial slice through a patient with a right parietal lesion. In this example, while fBV does not show marked tumor delineation, a rim of hyperintensity on the Kps map clearly identifies a peripheral zone of tumor characterized by high microvascular permeability.

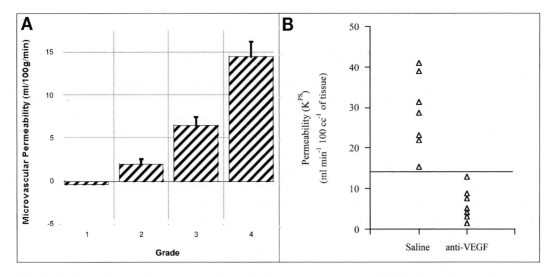

Fig. 8. (A) In patients with glioma, estimates of microvascular permeability showed a significant correlation with tumor grade ($r = 0.7$) (20). **(B)** In an experimental rodent model of human glioma (U87), a significant reduction in microvascular permeability was observed in the group undergoing treatment with Avastin™, a monoclonal antibody to vascular endothelial growth factor (21).

pharmaceutical, such as Avastin™ (Genentech Inc., South San Francisco, CA) (21). Such agents which may indirectly reduce tumor growth rate rather than killing tumor cells directly demand an effective indicator of biological efficacy, such as quantitative assessment of microvascular permeability reduction, as traditional endpoints may no longer be appropriate.

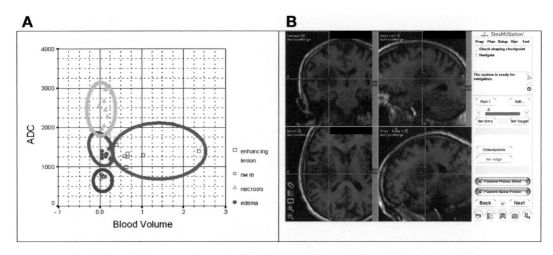

Fig. 9. (A) Multispectral analyses using imaging methods with different physiological specificities allow identification of tissue types and subtypes by their clustering in multidimensional space. In this example tissues can be distinguished based on their location in a 2D plane, the axes of which are defined by the apparent diffusion coefficient and fractional blood volume. Other axes from which this 2D projection was obtained include microvascular permeability and metabolic abnormality (defined as the ratio of Cho/NAA). **(B)** Gold standard assessments of tissue classification were obtained by invasive tissue sampling (resection/biopsy) guided by intraoperative neuronavigation *(47)*.

3. MULTISPECTRAL ANALYSES AND MULTIMODAL INTEGRATION

Whereas the above described emerging imaging technologies offer tantalizing glimpses of physiological specificity and clear clinical utility, a comprehensive tissue characterization may require description at the metabolic, cellular, and vascular level. Consequently, much effort is being devoted to the appropriate combination of results from such physiologically specific imaging approaches in methods described variously as "cluster analysis," "factor analysis," or "multispectral approaches." These offer the possibility of identifying features or "physiological phenotypes" that distinguish tissues, characterize heterogeneity within lesions, and yield the most specificity in determining prognosis and treatment response. Figure 9 illustrates an example of multispectral image analysis in which different tissues types, overlapping in one physiological dimension, can be separated by their clustering pattern in the appropriate multidimensional space (in this example a 2D space defined by apparent diffusion coefficient and fractional blood volume). Gold standard tissue classification, based on radiologic assessment, is augmented by image guided biopsy and resection procedures in which the site of tissue sampling is identified on 3D anatomic MRI at the time of the surgical procedure via a neuronavigational workstation.

Taken together, the currently available techniques of spectroscopic imaging, DWI and perfusion/permeability imaging offer an increased level of physiological specificity for the characterization of brain tumors, offering utility at the diagnostic and prognostic levels as well as offering biologically-specific indicators for the stratification, selection, targeting, and monitoring of therapy. However, emerging pharmaceutical approaches and oncologic understanding suggest the importance of the consideration of brain tumors not only at the physiological level, but also at the subcellular and genetic levels. Newly emerging is the field of molecular imaging, offering yet further specificity and promising to be an imaging partner to the rapid developments and understanding in cancer biology at the cellular, molecular, and genetic level. The remainder of this chapter will introduce the general principles and outlook for the field of molecular imaging as it applies to basic and clinical science.

MOLECULAR IMAGING

Molecular imaging (MI) is emerging as a new tool and enables the in vivo characterization and measurement of biological processes at the cellular and molecular level *(22)*. The aims of this field are to noninvasively characterize and quantify molecular changes associated with disease instead of imaging the resulting morphological changes. For example, molecular changes in cancer occur several years before a mass becomes visible. Molecular imaging therefore provides the potential for earlier characterization of disease, better understanding of the biology and evaluation of treatment response.

Imaging and quantifying biological processes in vivo is very challenging and requires the following key elements: (1) specific and sensitive site-targeted probes, (2) amplification strategies to enhance the signal of the probe, and (3) imaging systems with high spatial resolution and sensitivity including optical, nuclear, and MRI *(22)*.

Imaging Targets and Amplification Strategies

Potential molecular imaging targets include DNA and mRNA sequences or proteins. Imaging DNA sequences in cells is challenging because the number of copies per cell is very small and the DNA is supercoiled and hidden deep within the cell nucleus. Imaging the message of a gene via mRNA or, preferably, a protein is therefore much more feasible *(23)* as it uses natural biochemical flows of genetic information via transcription of the DNA into mRNA and translation of the mRNA into the protein (Fig. 10). Proteins can be targeted by their structure or their function. Proteins are either localized intracellularly, on the cell membrane, or secreted into the extracellular space and can be detected at any of these locations. Finally, the whole cell can be labeled, either by means of specific markers on the cell membrane or by uptake of the probe into the cell.

Once a target is found, a substance (ligand) that binds to it has to be identified. Ligands must have the ability to reach the target at sufficient concentration and sufficient length of time to be detectable in vivo. However, rapid excretion, nonspecific binding, metabolism, and delivery barriers hinder this process and must be overcome. Furthermore, any unbound ligands have to be eliminated in order to minimize background noise—a critical issue for in vivo MI. To date, a number of chemical and biological amplification strategies have been developed to facilitate molecular imaging at the protein level *(22)*.

Imaging Systems for Molecular Imaging

Molecular information can be obtained with some but not all of the available imaging modalities (Fig. 11). The most commonly used modalities are optical, nuclear, and MRI. Although optical methods are very powerful and allow imaging of molecular processes in an inexpensive way, their clinical application is limited because the optical imaging is surface weighted and has limited penetration depth and resolution. However, niche applications for clinical use may emerge when coupled with endoscopic technology such as catheter based lenses. For clinical purposes, techniques of nuclear medicine (positron emission tomography [PET] and single photon emission computed tomography [SPECT]) and MRI are the most promising modalities.

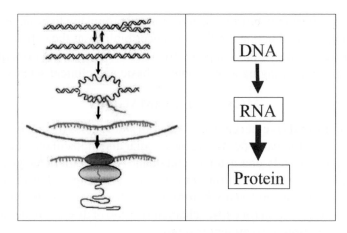

Fig. 10. Potential molecular imaging targets can be at the DNA, RNA, or protein level.

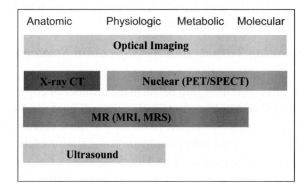

Fig. 11. Current imaging modalities used for anatomical, physiological, and molecular imaging.

Optical Imaging

Optical imaging exploits absorption, emission, scattering, and fluorescent techniques but it is fluorescence and luminescence that are particularly useful for in vivo studies *(24)*. Fluorescence is a physical process and requires electromagnetic stimulation (use of an external light source). A fluorochrome is activated by a specific excitation wavelength to emit light at a lower wavelength. Tissue penetration of photons is maximized in the near-infrared (NIR) spectrum; therefore, NIR fluorochromes are frequently used. Amplification of the signal is usually obtained by accumulation or by activation of smart, or biochemically-activated, probes. In order to externally image and follow the natural course or impediment of tumor progression, the use of green fluorescent protein (GFP)—originally extracted from the jellyfish (*Aequorea victoria*)—has proven to be very useful *(25)*. However, a major drawback of GFP is the fact that its emission wavelength (510 nm) is close to the autofluorescence of many tissues which causes significant background signals *(25,26)*. This is one of the reasons that GFP with redshifted emission have been engineered *(27)*. More recently, a new red fluorescent protein that emits light at 583 nm has been isolated from tropical corals *(28)*. Luminescence, on the other hand, does not require a light source but arises from the conversion of chemical energy

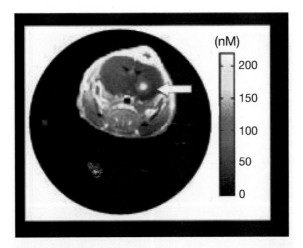

Fig. 12. Fluorescence imaging: enzyme activity in a 9L glioma model in a live mouse. The image is superimposed onto an MRI image. Reproduced with permission from ref. *25*.

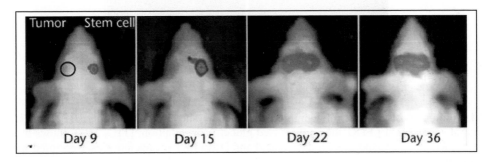

Fig. 13. Bioluminescence imaging: migration of luciferase-labeled neural progenitor cells across the brain midline attracted by a contralaterally implanted glioma. Reproduced with from ref. *25*.

to light. Luminescence occurring in living organisms is referred to as bioluminescence. It is an energy (i.e., ATP-) dependent biological process, where light is generated by oxidation of luciferin by luciferase, the former being the substrate and the latter being the catalyzing enzyme. Cells expressing the luciferase gene luminesce upon the addition of luciferin, a process that is less harmful for cells than the electromagnetic stimulation used to detect GFP. Although the light produced is extremely weak, a light-tight chamber allows imaging of the bioluminescence *(28,29)*. An excellent overview of in vivo optical imaging is provided by Frostig *(30)*. In general, optical imaging approaches using fluorescent proteins and bioluminescence are prevalent in biological imaging and are commonly used to track cells (including stem and tumor cells) and to act as gene reporters in a wide variety of systems *(31,32)*. Figure 12 shows an example of fluorescence imaging using a cathepsin B-activatable probe in a 9L glioma model. Figure 13 shows an example of bioluminescence.

Nuclear Imaging

Nuclear imaging techniques including PET and SPECT use radiolabeled tracers to image interactions of biological processes in vivo. These techniques have a lower spatial resolution

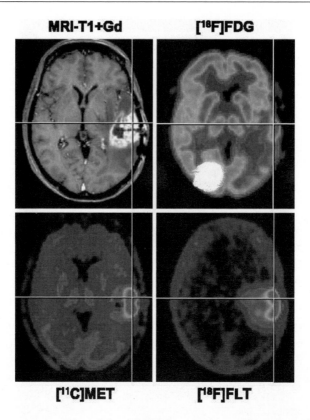

MRI-T1+Gd   **[¹⁸F]FDG**

[¹¹C]MET   **[¹⁸F]FLT**

Fig. 14. Glioma: Post-contrast T1-weighted MRI image shows alteration of BBB and extent of peritumoral edema. [18F] FDG shows increased glucose consumption, [11C] MET shows increased activity of membrane transporters for amino acid and [18F] FLT for nucleosides. Reprinted with permission from ref. *33*.

than MRI (typically several mm for PET compared with approx 1 mm for MRI), but are inherently quantitative and highly sensitive. Picomolar concentration of isotopes can be detected with no depth limit but with only little anatomical information, making combinations with CT or MRI very useful. The newly commercialized combination of PET and CT is becoming widespread in the clinical setting, allowing anatomic registration of functional PET data, as well as attenuation correction for improved quantitative interpretation of the PET data. PET and SPECT are currently the most advanced methods to image molecular events in patients, and indeed several molecular imaging probes are already under evaluation in clinical trials.

For PET, positron-emitting isotopes are produced in a cyclotron. They are used to label small molecules, recognized by enzymes, receptors, or other targets. Depending on the radiotracer used, various molecular processes can be visualized, most of them relating to increased cell proliferation in tumors. 18F-fluorodeoxyglucose (FDG), a glucose analog, is the most widely used tracer molecule for PET imaging to detect metabolic active tumors. Cancer cells have high uptake and metabolism rate of glucose and, hence, FDG. This up-regulation is an early event during malignant transformation and, importantly, precedes anatomical changes. This is therefore of potential value in early diagnosis and staging of cancer. However, because some tumors show hypo- or isometabolism in 18F FDG PET, more specific radiotracers

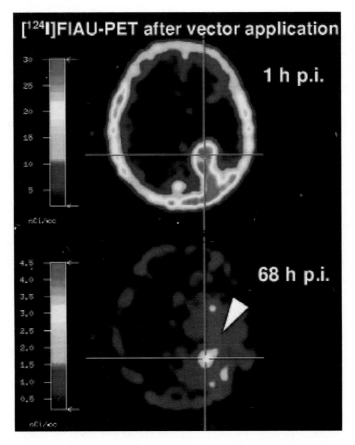

Fig. 15. Extent of vector-mediated gene expression in [^{124}I] FIAU-PET 1 h and 68 h post-injection. Tumor showed signs of necrosis after 68 h post-injection. Reprinted with from ref. *35*.

are required such as methyl-[11C]-L-Methionine (MET) and 3'-deoxy-3'-[18F] fluoro-L-thymidine (FLT) to image increased activity of membrane transporters for amino acid and nucleosides, respectively *(33)*. An example of increased cell proliferation in a glioma using multitracer PET imaging is shown in Fig. 14.

PET has also been applied to study multidrug resistance, apoptosis (programmed cell death), and gene expression. To study gene expression with PET, the herpes simplex virus type 1 thymidine kinase (HSV-1-tk) has been used as a marker gene *(34)*. HSV-1-tk isotopes analogs are phosphorylated by the viral kinase and then trapped within the cell. The accumulation of activity is therefore an indicator of HSV-1-tk presence and thus successful transfection. In clinical gene therapy trials for recurrent glioblastomas, transduction of HSV-1-tk gene with subsequent prodrug activation by ganciclovir was found to be safe. PET with I-124-labeled 2'-fluoro-2'-deoxy-1b-D-arabino-furanosyl-5-iodo-uracil ([^{124}I]-FIAU)—a specific marker substrate for gene expression of HSV-1-tk—was used to identify the location, magnitude, and extent of vector-mediated HSV-1-tk gene expression in a phase I/II clinical trial of gene therapy for recurrent glioblastoma in five patients. The extent of HSV-1-tk gene expression seemed to predict the therapeutic response *(35)*. Figure 15 shows FIAU PET in a glioma before and after vector application.

SPECT utilizes gamma-emitting isotopes, which are usually cheaper and have a longer half-live than positron-emitting isotopes used for PET imaging. The resolution of PET is still superior, but new developments in image requisition and software are trying to improve the resolution. With SPECT, several isotopes can be imaged simultaneously, providing multiparameter measurements. SPECT has been used to track molecules or cells such as radio-labeled annexin-V to image apoptosis or tumor-specific peptides in vivo *(36)*. Preliminary reports show that SPECT imaging might play a role as a surrogate marker after chemotherapy as well.

Magnetic Resonance Imaging

MRI is emerging as a particularly advantageous modality for MI because of its high spatial resolution (when compared with PET and SPECT), very good sample penetration (when compared with optical imaging methods), it's widespread clinical availability, and lack of ionizing radiation. A tremendous drawback, however, is its low sensitivity compared with these other methods, which necessitates the development of powerful amplification strategies. MR contrast agents that could serve as potential bases for molecular imaging probes are in clinical use but specific derivatives for molecular imaging have not yet been approved *(23)*. In general, MR contrast agents are designed to shorten the relaxation times of the tissue of interest and therefore increase the relaxation rates *(37)*. There are two major classes of MR contrast agents; paramagnetic contrast agents which are designed to predominantly affect T1 and thus tend to provide increased MR signal and superparamagnetic agents and agents designed to predominantly shorten T2 and T2* relaxation times and thereby decrease signal on appropriately weighted MR imaging sequences. In both cases, the potency of a contrast agent is commonly expressed as relaxivity and is typically measured relative to the paramagnetic or superparamagnetic ion concentration, such as gadolinium or iron (with units of mmol/s). For targeted contrast agents, however, the relaxivity per particle is more useful for comparing the contrast agent effect per binding site. In current development, there are two main strategies for MRI-suitable contrast media for molecular imaging; those based on iron oxide and those using nanoparticles or emulsions which incorporate gadolinium ions. These will be briefly elaborated explained below.

Molecular Imaging With Iron Oxides

Ultrasmall superparamagnetic iron oxides (USPIO) are potent MRI contrast agents. The iron produces strong local disruptions in the magnetic field which leads to increased T2* relaxation. This increased relaxation causes decreased image intensity in areas with iron oxide accumulation (also known as susceptibility artifacts). Because of the extremely large change in MRI signal induced by superparamagnetic particles, they offer a potential solution to the problem of MR insensitivity, and have been developed for a wide variety of contrast agent applications, including imaging vasculature, bowel, liver, spleen, lymphatics, tumors, and stem cell therapy *(38–40)*. In particular, dextran-coated USPIO particles with a 15- to –25-nm diameter have a very long circulating half-life and are preferentially taken up by macrophages and the reticuloendothelial system (RES) in the body. This uptake allows them to be employed for passive targeted imaging of pathological inflammatory processes, such as unstable atherosclerotic plaques *(41)*. Another passive targeted imaging study by Stiskal et al. compared two candidate iron oxide particles for the sensitive detection of radiation induced liver injury in an experimental model. Results showed readily visualizable damage to the RES system *(42)*. Dextran-coated USPIOs are also employed for single cell imaging *(43)*. Although MR resolutions are rarely comparable with cell dimensions, these complexes distort the magnetic field

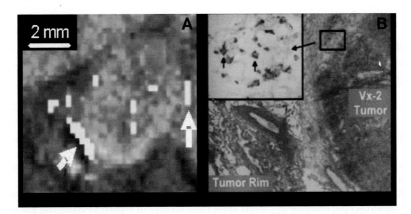

Fig. 16. (A) T1-weighted image showing vx-2 tumor. Yellow overlay indicates signal enhancement (along periphery proximate to tumor/blood vessel interfaces) 120 min post injection. **(B)** Corresponding histology of tumor with H+E as well as αvβ3 staining. Black arrows show formation of small angiogenic vessels along periphery near tumor/blood vessel interface. Reprinted with permission from ref. *46.*

far beyond their boundaries of the cell, thus massively amplifying signal on T2*-weighted images. However, for significant signal change, many USPIO particles need to be within an imaging voxel. Recently, a paper by Shapiro et al. demonstrated that single micrometer-sized iron oxide particles (MPIOs) could be detected in individual cells *(44)*. This should open numerous future possibilities for cellular imaging using MRI.

Molecular Imaging With Paramagnetic Nanoparticles

Nanoparticles can be formulated to carry paramagnetic gadolinium ions and targeted to a number of important biochemical epitopes, such as αvβ3-integrin—an important marker of angiogenesis (new vessel formation) and an essential component of tumor growth and spread. The αvβ3-integrin plays a critical role in smooth muscle cell migration and cellular adhesion, both of which are required for the formation of new blood vessels. The integrin is expressed on the luminal surface of activated endothelial cells but not on mature quiescent cells *(45)*. In a recent paper by Winter et al., the utility of αvβ3-integrin targeted nanoparticles for the detection and characterization of angiogenesis associated with tumor growth was demonstrated in a Vx-2 tumor model (Fig. 16) *(46)*.

SUMMARY

In summary, techniques of physiologically specific imaging offer characterization of tumors at a metabolic, cellular, and vascular level. In current clinical practice these techniques offer utility for diagnosis, prognosis, treatment selection and planning, as well as therapy monitoring. However, the field of cancer biology is advancing rapidly and demands on imaging are increasing commensurately, such that a requirement for not only imaging physiology but also imaging in vivo biochemical processes is apparent. The emerging technologies, described as "molecular imaging" offer a promising and powerful array of tools to visualize disease processes and therapeutic responses at the sub-cellular and molecular level. Although still in their infancy, molecular imaging techniques are evolving rapidly and progressing towards the clinic. It seems likely that the resulting capabilities of this technological evolution will shape the field of diagnostic and therapeutic neuro-oncology for years to come.

ACKNOWLEDGMENTS

The authors would like to thank Prof Abhijit Guha, Toronto Western Hospital, Prof Mitchel Berger, University of California San Francisco and Patrick Winter and colleagues at Washington University, St. Louis for helpful discussions relating to the present work.

REFERENCES

1. Nelson SJ. Multivoxel magnetic resonance spectroscopy of brain tumors. Mol Cancer Ther 2003;2:497–507.
2. Li X, Lu Y, Pirzkall A, McKnight T, Nelson SJ. Analysis of the spatial characteristics of metabolic abnormalities in newly diagnosed glioma patients. J Magn Reson Imaging 2002;16:229–237.
3. Graves EE, Nelson SJ, Vigneron DB, et al. A preliminary study of the prognostic value of proton magnetic resonance spectroscopic imaging in gamma knife radiosurgery of recurrent malignant gliomas. Neurosurgery 2000;46:319–328.
4. Graves EE, Nelson SJ, Vigneron DB, et al. Serial proton MR spectroscopic imaging of recurrent malignant gliomas after gamma knife radiosurgery. AJNR Am J Neuroradiol 2001;22:613–624.
5. Li X, Jin H, Lu Y, Oh J, Chang S, Nelson SJ. Identification of MRI and 1H MRSI parameters that may predict survival for patients with malignant gliomas. NMR Biomed. 2004;17:10–20.
6. Pruessmann KP, Weiger M, Boesiger P. SENSE: sensitivity encoding for fast MRI. Magn Reson Med 1999; 42:952–962.
7. Dydak U, Pruessmann KP, Weiger M, Tsao J, Meier D, Boesiger P. Parallel spectroscopic imaging with spin-echo trains. Magn Reson Med 2003;50:196–200
8. Posse S, DeCarli C, Le Bihan D. Three-dimensional echo-planar MR spectroscopic imaging at short echo times in the human brain. Radiology 1994;192(3):733–738.
9. Tyszka JM, Mamelak AN. Volumetric echo-planar spectroscopic imaging. Magn Reson Med 2001;46: 219–227.
10. Dydak U. Advanced MR spectroscopic imaging techniques. In: Proceedings of 42nd Annual Meeting. Seattle, WA: American Society for Neuroradiology, 2004; p. 48d.
11. Dydak U, Weiger M, Pruessmann KP, Meier, Boesiger P. Sensitivity-encoded spectroscopic imaging. Magn Reson Med 2001;46:713–722.
12. Sugahara T, Korogi Y, Kochi M, et al. Usefulness of diffusion-weighted MRI with echo-planar technique in the evaluation of cellularity in gliomas. J Magn Reson Imaging 1999;9:53–60.
13. Mori S, Crain BJ, Chacko VP, van Zijl PC. Three-dimensional tracking of axonal projections in the brain by magnetic resonance imaging. Ann Neurol 1999;45(2):265–269.
14. Mori S, Kaufmann WE, Davatzikos C, et al. Imaging cortical association tracts in the human brain using diffusion tensor based axonal tracking. Magn Reson Med 2002;47:215–223.
15. Field AS, Alexander AL, Wu Y-C, Hasan KM, Witwer B, Badie B. Diffusion tensor eigenvector directional color imaging patterns in the evaluation of cerebral white matter tracts altered by tumor. J Magn Reson Imaging 2004;20:555–562.
16. Berman JI, Berger MS, Mukherjee P, Henry RG. Diffusion-tensor imaging-guided tracking of fibers of the pyramidal tract combined with intraoperative cortical stimulation mapping in patients with gliomas. J Neurosurg 2004;101(1):66–72.
17. Keles GE, Berger MS. Advances in neurosurgical technique in the current management of brain tumors. Semin Oncol 2004;31(5):659–665.
18. Shames DM, Kuwatsuru R, Vexler V, Muhler A, Brasch RC. Measurement of capillary permeability to macromolecules by dynamic magnetic resonance imaging: a quantitative noninvasive technique. Magn Reson Med 1993;29:616–622.
19. Roberts HC, Roberts TPL, Brasch RC, Dillon WP. Quantitative estimation of microvascular permeability in human brain tumors: correlation with histopathological grade. AJNR Am J Neuroradiol 2000;21(5): 891–899.
20. Roberts HC, Roberts TPL, Bollen AW, Ley S, Brasch RC, Dillon WP. Correlation of microvascular permeability derived from dynamic contrast-enhanced MR imaging with histologic grade and tumor labeling index: a study in human brain tumors. Acad Radiol 2001;8(5):384–391.
21. Gossmann A, Helbich TH, Kuriyama N et al. Dynamic contrast-enhanced magnetic resonance imaging as a surrogate marker of tumor response to anti-angiogenic therapy in a xenograft model of glioblastoma multiforme. J Magn Reson Imaging 2002;15(3):233–240.
22. Weissleder R, Mahmood U. Mol Imag Radiol. 2000;219:316–333.

23. Grimm J. Molecular imaging—new horizons for radiology. Medical Solutions 2003;1:74–79.
24. Dzik-Jurasz. Molecular imaging in vivo: an introduction. Br J Radiol 2003;76:S98–S109.
25. Weissleder R, Ntziachristos V. Shedding light onto live molecular targets. Nat Med 2003;9:123–128.
26. Tsien RY. The green fluorescent protein. Annu Rev Biochem 1998;67:509–544.
27. Heim R, Tsien RY. Engineering green fluorescent protein for improved brightness, longer wavelengths and fluorescence resonance energy transfer. Curr Biol 1996;6:178–182.
28. Contag CH, Spilman SD, Contag PR, et al. Visualizing gene expression in living mammals using a bioluminescent reporter. Photochem Photobiol 1997;66(4):523–531.
28. Matz MV, Fradkov AF, Labas YA, et al. Fluorescent proteins from nonbioluminescent Anthozoa species. Nat Biotechnol 1999;17 :969–973.
29. Contag PR, Olumu IN, Stevenson DK, Contag CH. Bioluminescent indicators in living mammals. Nat Med 1998;4:245–247.
30. Frostig R. In-vivo optical imaging of brain function. In: Frostig R, ed. CRC Press, 2002.
31. Contag CH, Ross BD. It's not just about anatomy: in vivo bioluminescence imaging as an eyepiece into biology. J Magn Reson Imaging 2002;16:378–387.
32. Contag CH, Bachmann MH. Advances in in-vivo bioluminescence imaging of gene expression. Ann Rev Biomed Eng 2002;4:235–260.
33. Jacobs AH, Dittmar C, Winkeler A, Garlip G, Heiss WD. Molecular imaging of gliomas. Mol Imaging 2002;1:309–335.
34. Satio Y, Price RW, Rottenberg DA, et al. Quantitive autoradiographic mapping of herpes simplex virus encephalitis with a radiolabeled antiviral drug. Science 1982;217:1151–1153.
35. Jacobs A, Voges J, Reszka R, et al. Positron-emission tomography of vector-mediated gene therapy for gliomas. Lancet 2001;358:727–729.
36. Van de Wiele C, Lahorte C, Vermeersch H, et al. Quantitative Tumor Apoptosis Imaging Using Technetium-99m–HYNIC Annexin V Single Photon Emission Computed Tomography. J Clin Oncol 2003;21:3483–3487.
37. Weisskoff RM, Caravan P. MR contrast agent basics. In: Lardo A, Fayad Z, Chronos NAF, Fuster V, eds. Cardiovascular Magnetic Resonance: Established and Emerging Applications. New York: Martin Dunitz, 2003;17–38.
38. Wang YX, Hussain SM, krestin GP. Superparamagnetic iron oxide contrast agents. Eur J Radiol 2001;11:2319–2331.
39. Weinmann HJ, Ebert W, Misselwitz B, Schmitt-Willich H. Tissue-specific MR contrast agents. Eur J Radiol 2003;46:33–44.
40. Bulte JW, Duncan ID, Frank JA. In vivo magnetic resonance tracking of magnetically labeled cells after transplantation. J Cereb Blood Flow Metab 2002;22:899–907.
41. Schmitz SA, Taupitz M, Wagner S, Wolf KJ, Beyersdorff D, Hamm B. Magnetic resonance imaging of atherosclerotic plaques using superparamagnetic iron oxide particles. J Magn Reson Imaging 2001;14:355–361.
42. Stiskal M, Demsar F, Muhler A, et al. Contrast-enhanced MR imaging of two superparamagnetic RES-contrast agents: functional assessment of experimental radiation-induced liver injury. J Magn Reson Imaging 1999;10:52–60.
43. Bulte JW, Zhang S, van Gelderen P, et al. Neurotransplantation of magnetically labeled oligodendrocyte progenitors: magnetic resonance tracking of cell migration and myelination. Proc Natl Acad Sci USA 1999,96:15,256–15,261.
44. Shapiro EM, Skrtic S, Sharer K, Hill JM, Dunbar CE, Koretsky AP. MRI detection of single particles for cellular imaging. Proc Natl Acad Sci USA 2004;101:10,901–10,906.
45. Brooks PC, Stromblad S, Klemke R, Visscher D, Sarkar FH, Cheresh DA. Anti-integrin alpha v beta 3 blocks human breast cancer growth and angiogenesis in human skin. J Clin Invest 1995;96:1815–1822.
46. Winter PM, Caruthers SD, Kassner A, et al. Molecular imaging of angiogenesis in nascent Vx-2 rabbit tumors using a novel alpha(nu)beta3-targeted nanoparticle and 1.5 tesla magnetic resonance imaging. Cancer Res 2003;63:5838–5843.
47. Zhang Z, Kassner A, Lee J, et al. Multispectral analysis of physiologic MR imaging for tissue-specific clustering: application to gliomas postradiation therapy. In: Proceedings of 42nd Annual Meeting. Seattle, WA: American Society for Neuroradiology, 2004;p266.

9 Nuclear Imaging of Gliomas

Alexander M. Spence, David A. Mankoff,
Mark Muzi, and Kristin Swanson

Summary

This chapter reviews nuclear imaging of gliomas, both high- and low-grade, with emphasis on results from positron emission tomography (PET) with [F-18]-2-fluoro-2-deoxyglucose (FDG) for assessing energy metabolism. There are many additional advances beyond FDG-PET that are very exciting and potentially applicable in the management of gliomas. Biosynthesis in tumors occurs along several important broad fronts for DNA, proteins, and membrane lipids. Molecular imaging of these pathways is coming to the foreground. Hypoxia, a significant resistance mechanism that compromises the efficacy of radiotherapy and chemotherapy, can now be regionally quantified in vivo with PET. In the near future it is likely that the presence of mutant receptors, apoptosis, and angiogenesis will also be measurable with PET and new tracers.

Key Words: Brain tumor; glioma; PET; FDG; fluoromisonidazole; amino acids; thymidine; FLT; proliferation; acetate.

INTRODUCTION

Positron emission tomography (PET) provides the opportunity to image multiple dynamic biological processes in situ in brain tumors. [F-18]-2-fluoro-2-deoxyglucose (FDG) has been the most widely used tracer for nuclear imaging of gliomas, but this field is rapidly advancing and other processes aside from energy metabolism are being increasingly investigated. Imaging pathophysiology in vivo requires an understanding of the biology of tumors and their host organs at a molecular level. Knowledge gained from the test tube, tissue culture dish, or the microchip can be applied by nuclear imaging to whole tumors, host organs, and even multiple organ systems both simultaneously and quantitatively. PET is assuming an increasingly important role in the design of cancer treatments as well as monitoring the results earlier and more reliably.

The current standard noninvasive imaging procedures, X-ray computed tomography (CT) and magnetic resonance imaging (MRI), provide excellent anatomical precision and sensitivity. Unfortunately, their specificity in distinguishing neoplastic disease from vascular or inflammatory processes can be problematic in individual cases. Treatment effects including surgical trauma, corticosteroid-induced reduction of edema and contrast enhancement, and radionecrosis cannot always reliably be distinguished from tumor recurrence or response to therapy. As gliomas grow and infiltrate the normal cellular milieu, tumor cell density relative to the normal elements increases. T2 and fluid attenuated inversion recovery (FLAIR) mag-

From: *Current Clinical Oncology: High-Grade Gliomas: Diagnosis and Treatment*
Edited by: G. H. Barnett © Humana Press Inc., Totowa, NJ

Table 1
Metabolic Processes and Most Commonly Used Tracers To Study Them

Function	Tracers
Energy metabolism	[F-18]-2-fluoro-2-deoxyglucose (FDG)
	1-[C-11]glucose
	[O-15]O_2, [O-15]H_2O, [O-15]CO
Amino acid transport and incorporation	L-methyl-[C-11]methionine (MET)
	L-[C-11]tyrosine
	L-[F-18]fluorotyrosine
	L-[C-11]leucine
DNA synthesis	2-[C-11]thymidine
	methyl-[C-11]thymidine
	[F-18]-3'deoxy-3'-fluorothymidine (FLT)
Membrane/lipid biosynthesis	1-[C-11]acetate
	[C-11]choline
	[F-18]fluorocholine
Hypoxia	[F-18]fluoromisonidazole (FMISO)

netic resonance imaging (MRI) very ably define the margins of this advancing wave of pathology, but within a given abnormal volume the ratio of tumor to normal elements is not well defined. Magnetic resonance spectroscopy can profile some of the main chemical constituents of tumor and normal tissue but has limitations as does PET in that the volume of resolution is large relative to that provided by conventional MRI. As our understanding of pathology becomes increasingly molecular, especially in the brain where tissue sampling in vivo carries significant risks, it is imperative that we develop methods for measuring molecular pathologic processes as they progress over time. PET adds this capability to our clinical and research armamentarium. MRI and CT cannot estimate growth rate in a single setting whereas PET can provide quantitative measures of this with tracers of DNA, protein or membrane biosynthesis.

There are several uses for PET. For some of these our current experience is reasonably mature whereas for others more research is necessary *(1)*.

1. Detection.
2. Delineating tumors from non-neoplastic processes.
3. Grading and prognosis.
4. Localizing the optimum site for biopsy.
5. Distinguishing radionecrosis from recurrence.
6. Assessing response to therapy.
7. Predicting malignant degeneration in low-grade glioma (LGG).
8. Distinguishing high grade glioma (HGG) from LGG in MRI T1 gadolinium (Gd) nonenhancing tumors.
9. Designing therapy.

The main functions and tracers studied thus far with PET in gliomas are shown in Table 1.

ENERGY METABOLISM: [F-18]FLUORODEOXYGLUCOSE (FDG)

Glucose metabolism begins with transport from the serum to cells and continues through the process of phosphorylation catalyzed by hexokinase (*HK*), one of the most important enzymes controlling the rate of glucose utilization (Fig. 1). The product, glucose-6-phosphate (G6P)

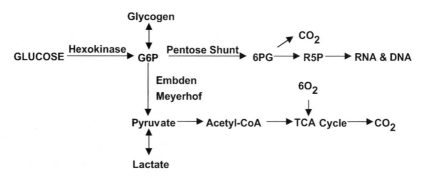

Fig. 1. The chief pathways followed by glucose intracellularly. Production of lactate in gliomas is increased, whereas in normal brain oxidation of glucose via the tricarboxylic acid cycle predominates. G6P, glucose-6-phosphate; 6PG, 6-phosphogluconic acid; R5P, ribose-5-phosphate; RNA, ribose nucleic acid; DNA, deoxyribose nucleic acid; Acetyl-CoA, acetyl coenzyme A; TCA, tricarboxylic acid cycle.

is the starting compound for glycogen synthesis, for the Embden–Meyerhof pathway (EMP) leading to lactate (glycolysis) or to pyruvate and entry to the tricarboxylic acid (TCA) cycle, and for the pentose shunt. Although malignant brain tumor tissue may show a respiratory quotient as low as 0.70, indicating some use of nonglucose substrates such as fatty acids or amino acids for energy, glucose is the chief source of energy *(2)*.

PET imaging with FDG is based on the fact that FDG, similar to glucose, is transported across the blood–brain barrier (BBB) and cell membranes and is phosphorylated by hexokinase to FDG-6-phosphate (FDG6P), which accumulates in tissues at a rate proportional to the rate of glucose utilization. FDG6P is not metabolized further along the glucose metabolic pathways, but is slowly dephosphorylated in the brain. FDG and glucose differ in their rates of transport and phosphorylation and respective volumes of distribution in brain or tumor tissue. This has been investigated and reported in detail but will not be reviewed here where emphasis will be on FDG *(3)*.

Grading and Prognosis

Di Chiro and coworkers pioneered the application of FDG-PET to gliomas *(4–6)*. HGG contained regions of high FDG uptake and lower grade gliomas lacked these regions (Fig. 2). In patients with grade III or IV astrocytic gliomas, FDG uptake correlated with survival *(7)*. Patients with ratios of tumor to contralateral normal brain glucose utilization greater than 1.4:1 had a median survival of 5 mo whereas patients with ratios of less than 1.4:1 showed median survival of 19 mo. The optimal cutoff levels for distinguishing LGG from HGG have been reported as 0.6 for the tumor-to-cortex (T/C) ratio and 1.5 for tumor-to-white matter (T/WM) ratio *(8)*. The sensitivity and specificity were 94 and 77%, respectively. The results of most other investigators of gliomas with FDG-PET agree *(9)*.

LGG present several diagnostic and management problems. Lesions that appear on MRI or CT scans to be low grade by virtue of lacking contrast enhancement or being calcified may remain apparently dormant for years or may progress to malignant behavior at unpredictable times in the future. Opinions vary widely about when to operate, irradiate, or treat with chemotherapy. These treatments, especially surgery and radiotherapy, carry significant risks of permanent neurological impairment. At presentation, when the MRI or CT scan shows no

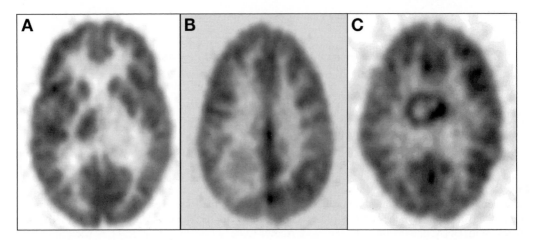

Fig. 2. (A) LGG of the left thalamus with FDG uptake ≤ normal white matter. **(B)** Intermediate-grade lesion of the right posterior white matter; FDG uptake is > normal white matter but < normal cortex. **(C)** HGG of the corpus callosum with FDG uptake > normal cortex.

enhancement to raise suspicion of anaplastic disease, the clinician does not want simply to observe and follow a malignant tumor delaying treatment that could control progression or even provide a response. On the other hand, causing neurological deficits by needlessly overtreating low-grade tumors is to be avoided if possible. Although MRI and CT cannot distinguish nonenhancing grade III or IV lesions from grade II, this may be possible with physiological imaging. Patients that have biopsy-proven LGG and FDG uptake in the tumor that is greater than white matter are at higher risk for progression and death than patients whose tumors show no areas of uptake greater than white matter *(10)*.

Localizing the Optimum Site for Biopsy

Many authors have presented convincing data and arguments that support the practice of selecting biopsy sites where the uptake of FDG is maximum to provide sampling of the most malignant areas of tumors (Fig. 3) *(11–13)*.

Dexamethasone Effect and Surgical Trauma

Steroid therapy does not appear to influence FDG uptake in recurrent anaplastic astrocytomas (AA) *(14)*. This was shown in five patients studied with FDG-PET before and after radiotherapy. In five nontumor-bearing patients following temporal lobectomy for epilepsy, no effect on FDG uptake from the surgical trauma was seen.

Radionecrosis vs Recurrence

From several recent series the sensitivity of FDG-PET for distinguishing recurrence of glioma from radionecrosis is typically 81 to 86%, although some results are higher, up to 100% *(15–19)*. Specificity is problematic in that estimates range from 22 to 92% *(16,17,19)*. The results of Ricci et al. are instructive. There were 31 patients suspected of harboring a recurrence in which the pathology was positive in 22 and negative in 9. With the cutoff of FDG uptake greater than normal white matter, the sensitivity was 86% and the specificity only 22% (positive predictive value, 73%; negative predictive value, 40%). With the cutoff greater than

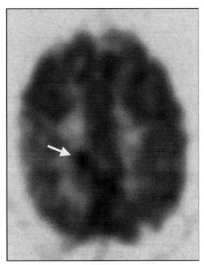

FDG

Fig. 3. Forty-six-year-old woman with a right parietal WHO grade II oligodendroglioma. The first biopsy attempt was too far posterior and was not diagnostic of tumor. The second biopsy (*white arrow*) directed by the FDG-PET proved the glioma diagnosis. Reprinted with permission from ref. *130*.

cortex the sensitivity was 73% and specificity 56% (positive predictive value, 80%; negative predictive value, 45%). Patients with irradiated malignant gliomas whose FDG-PET scans are hypometabolic consistent with radionecrosis may show in biopsy or resection specimens viable-appearing tumor cells that are incapable of proliferation. Also, a high percentage of post-treatment gliomas may be necrotic, as viewed by the pathologist or PET imaging specialist, but the tumor may still harbor viable cells that later lead to recurrence.

Assessing Response to Therapy

An important question with implications for clinical practice is whether changes in glucose metabolism are a reliable predictor of the response of malignant gliomas to therapeutic interventions. Successful radiotherapy (RT) of a tumor would be expected to kill tumor cells and cause a reduction of metabolism measured with FDG. That is, tumors that responded to treatment would show reduced metabolism and conversely, tumors that did not respond would show unchanged or increased metabolism. This hypothesis has been tested in patients scanned quantitatively with FDG within 2 wk pre- (Pre-RT) and/or 1 to 3 wk post-RT *(20,21)*. The results unexpectedly showed that an increase in metabolism, measured with FDG, from the beginning to end of RT correlated with longer survival whereas a decrease in metabolism was associated with shorter survival (Fig. 4).

Similar results, but involving chemotherapy, were reported for patients with recurrent glioblastoma studied with quantitative FDG-PET before and after a single cycle of 1,3-bis-(2-chloroethyl)-1-nitrosourea (BCNU) *(22)*. Following stereotactic radiosurgery (24–32 Gy) in a series of 19 tumors (mostly metastatic), Maruyama et al. reported that all but one of the tumors showed an increased uptake of FDG compared with Pre-RT levels *(23)*. This correlated with a decrease in the size of the tumors seen at later follow-up with CT or MRI.

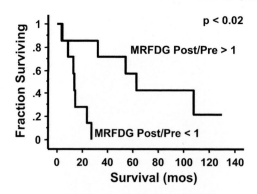

Fig. 4. These Kaplan Meier plots show survival results for 14 patients scanned with FDG both before and after RT. The patients were ranked from greatest to least value of the ratio of post-RT MRFDG over the pre-RT MRFDG and then split in two groups, higher 50% vs lower 50%. Survival was compared between the two groups. Two patients still alive were censored. The graphs show that an increase in metabolic rate from before to after RT correlates with longer survival.

How therapy could lead to increased metabolism and relatively better outcome is suggested from chemotherapy and radiotherapy experiments on tumor cultures and animal tumors (24–28). Increased transport has been considered one explanation. Infiltration of dead and dying tumor regions with metabolically active inflammatory elements has been reported following radiotherapy in rats bearing hepatomas implanted in the thigh (29,30). This could occur in responding gliomas and appear in the volume seen by PET as increased metabolism. Another speculative explanation is energy consumption for apoptosis (31,32). Lastly, an additional potential explanation is that therapy destroys tumor cells leading to an uncrowding effect that allows more active metabolism in surviving normal elements (i.e., within a volume of tissue the ratio and density of normal cells to tumor cells improves), leading to increased regional metabolism.

Another way to measure response to therapy is to assess metabolism at a single time following the intervention and hypothesize that longer survival correlates with lower metabolism. In 26 glioma cases from the study cited above, MRFDG measured shortly after RT did not correlate with survival (Fig. 5) (20). Although no prior studies have systematically and quantitatively examined the immediate post-RT time to correlate metabolic rate with outcome, examination of FDG uptake of malignant gliomas specifically at the time of clinical and/or radiographic recurrence has proven to be a significant predictor of survival (33).

In sum, multiple investigations have shown that high MRFDG preceeding treatment signifies more aggressive disease and shorter survival. Greater volume of FDG uptake likewise is associated with shorter survival (34). Comparisons of pre-treatment to post-treatment measurements for radio- or chemotherapy for primary or metastatic brain tumors have shown that increases in MRFDG correlate with longer, not shorter, survival. Lastly, immediate post-RT quantitative PET with FDG does not correlate with length of survival, whereas FDG uptake at the time of clinical and MRI determined recurrence does correlate with shorter survival.

Thus, for prognosis and grading before initial treatment or at recurrence, FDG-PET is clinically useful (33,35,36). For assessing response by pre- to post-treatment comparisons, there appears to be limited clinical usefulness. FDG-PET is not clinically useful for assessing

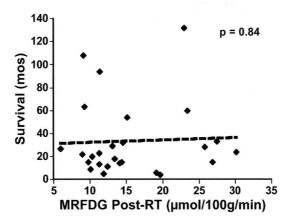

Fig. 5. This regression graph shows the data from studies performed on patients within 2–3 wk after RT ($n = 26$). There was no correlation between the post-RT MRFDG and survival.

response to radio- or chemotherapy immediately after the treatment is completed which is the time when it would be most helpful to clinicians to know whether a treatment has succeeded or not.

Therapy Planning

Conventional conformal RT for malignant gliomas consists of 1.8 to 2.0 Gy fractions that total around 60 Gy. Despite these doses, nearly inevitably there are in-field recurrences, progression and death. Doses as high as 70 to 90 Gy have been studied with the goal of providing better results than 60 Gy (37–40). There was no improvement in survival or local control, and recurrences developed in the volumes that received the high doses (38). Metabolic imaging with FDG-PET has been used to define the optimal volume in malignant gliomas for high-dose boost RT (34,41). Patients received 59.4 Gy in 33 fractions followed by an additional 20 Gy in 10 fractions directed at the FDG-PET defined volume of hypermetabolism plus a 0.5-cm margin. The median survival for 40 patients enrolled in this trial preliminarily is about 70 wk. Thus far, the study has shown no more radiation toxicity than would be expected from standard dosing. This pilot study shows that experimental radiotherapy protocols based on PET images are feasible and could in the future be designed to target regions of hypoxia, proliferation, protein synthesis or membrane biosynthesis.

OXYGEN METABOLISM AND BLOOD FLOW: [O-15]O$_2$, [O-15]H$_2$O, [O-15]CO

Oxygen metabolic rate (MRO$_2$), cerebral blood flow (CBF), oxygen extraction fraction (OEF), and cerebral blood volume (CBV) in malignant gliomas have all been examined by several groups (2,42–46). Among these studies there is consistency in showing that oxygen utilization is low relative to normal cortex despite an adequate supply of oxygen, at least macroscopically (i.e., there are adequate blood flow and blood oxygen levels to meet the metabolic demands of the tumors). Wise et al. in particular noted that both MRO$_2$ and OEF tend to be lower in malignant gliomas suggesting the tissue is not macroscopically ischemic (46).

Table 2
CBF, MRO₂ and OEF From Glioma and Contralateral Cortex (44)

Function (units)	Tumor	Contralateral cortex
CBF (mL/100 mL/min)	32 ± 9	32 ± 5
MRO$_2$ (mL/100 mL/min)	1.2 ± 0.6	2.8 ± 0.5
OEF	0.21 ± 0.07	0.47 ± 0.05

Table 2 shows data from seven patients with intermediate- or high-grade gliomas that illustrate the parameters relevant to oxygen metabolism (44). Note that blood flow in the tumors is the same as in uninvolved brain whereas MRO$_2$ and OEF are roughly half.

The utilization of oxygen relative to that of glucose, namely the metabolic ratio, is reduced in malignant gliomas (44,45). In normal brain the metabolic ratio is 5.2 moles of oxygen per mole of glucose whereas in gliomas it is 1.9 (44,47). A lower than normal metabolic ratio indicates that the tissue is breaking down glucose to lactate (glycolysis) and that nonoxidative metabolism of glucose is occurring. In the face of adequate blood flow and reduced oxygen extraction in tumors, the reduced metabolic ratio indicates that glycolysis is occurring under aerobic rather than anaerobic conditions (2).

Measurements of oxygen metabolism with PET in gliomas have not been as clinically useful as glucose measurements simply because the dominant energy source, glucose, undergoes glycolysis to lactate rather than oxidative breakdown. Measurements of glucose metabolism with FDG, therefore, have been more revealing of tumor tissue energetics than oxygen measurements.

HYPOXIA: [F-18]FLUOROMISONIDAZOLE (FMISO)

Although oxygen metabolism in gliomas differs from that in normal brain, the lack of oxygen, known as hypoxia, appears to be an important factor in determining glioma aggressiveness and response to therapy. It has been documented in several types of cancers that low-oxygen tension levels are associated with persistent tumor following RT and with the subsequent development of local recurrences (48–50). In gliomas, spontaneous necrosis suggests the presence of hypoxic regions that are radioresistant. Rampling et al. proved, by measurements with polarographic electrodes, that glioblastomas contain hypoxic regions (51). The percent pO$_2$ values <2.5 mmHg were between 10 and 69% with a median of 40%. In patients with AA the percent pO$_2$ values <2.5 mmHg were betweem 9 and 42 with a median of 20%.

The significance of hypoxia in the response of gliomas to radiotherapy has not been clarified completely. Treatment approaches based on eradication of hypoxic cell populations with radiotherapy have been either unsuccessful as reported for hypoxic cell radiosensitizers (52–54) or have been too toxic as reported following fast neutron therapy (55).

In the mid 1980s it was discovered that some radiosensitizing drugs (e.g., misonidazole) are selectively bound to molecules in viable hypoxic cells in vitro and in vivo (56,57). This has led to the development of [F-18]fluoromisonidazole (FMISO) as a hypoxia imaging agent with PET (58). The partition coefficient is essentially unity so the tracer is not retained in non-hypoxic tissues such as brain.

Reports of FMISO-PET imaging of gliomas are emerging (59–61). Liu et al. reported that FMISO was taken up in 14 of 18 brain tumors. Scott's group studied 13 newly diagnosed

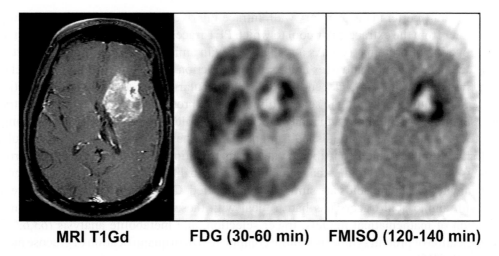

MRI T1Gd   FDG (30-60 min)   FMISO (120-140 min)

Fig. 6. Twenty-eight-year-old woman with a recurrent left frontotemporal malignant pleomorphic xanthoastrocytoma. MRI T1Gd (*left*), FDG (*middle*) and FMISO (*right*) images are co-registered. The patterns of FDG and FMISO uptake are distinctly different in both tumor and uninvolved brain. The region of irregular central necrosis is nearly the same in the FDG and FMISO images. Reprinted with permission from ref. *130.*

patients prior to surgery with both FMISO- and FDG-PET *(60)*. There was a correlation between FMISO uptake and tumor grade, and all high-grade lesions showed uptake that was frequently heterogeneous. There was some, but not complete, overlap between regions of FMISO uptake and FDG uptake. An example shown in Fig. 6 demonstrates heterogenous uptake that does not show conformity to the FDG region of uptake in these co-registered images.

Swanson et al. studied four glioma patients with FMISO-PET before, during, and after radiotherapy. There was an average decrease in MRI detectable tumor volumes (–28%) with a concurrent average increase in FMISO-positive hypoxic volumes (+10%) suggesting that the two imaging modalities provide distinctly different information in the assessment of radio-therapy response *(62)*.

These studies in aggregate show significant promise for FMISO-PET in gliomas but need to be extended to a larger patient population and examined at additional time points throughout the clinical course. Identifying the regional distribution of hypoxia may improve planning of resections and allow targeting higher doses of radiotherapy more precisely to the hypoxic areas.

AMINO ACID TRANSPORT AND INCORPORATION: [C-11]METHIONINE (C-11-MET), [F-18]FLUOROTYROSINE (F-18-TYR), [F-18]FLUOROETHYL-L-TYROSINE (F-18-FET), [C-11]TYROSINE (C-11-TYR)

The goal of PET imaging with labeled amino acids is to assess the protein synthetic process in growing tumors *(63)*. Most of the amino acids used for PET are transported by the L system. This has been documented by competition studies with other amino acids that use the same transporter *(64)*. Where the BBB is impaired, the exchange of amino acids can partially bypass the transporter in the capillary wall. Intracellularly, amino acids for protein synthesis come either from the extracellular pool to which PET tracers contribute or from the intracellular recycling of proteins (65). As a result, PET with amino acids measures transport plus amino acid incorporation and does not assess that fraction of protein synthesis that includes endogenous recycling (66). Depending on the particular amino acid, there are additional biochemical pathways leading in several directions for production of hormones, neurotransmitters, purines, pyrimidines and many other biomolecules. Incorporation in these nonprotein products cannot be distinguished from protein synthesis with PET. This is particularly true for methionine, which contributes via transmethylation reactions to several nonprotein products, as well as for tyrosine that is incorporated into dihydroxyphenylalanine. Degradation pathways for amino acids are similarly complicated. Consequently, the development of PET with amino acid tracers has had to deal with these complexities in the design and validation of mathematical models, tracer selection, and metabolite analysis (63,67–70). Quantification of protein synthesis is more complicated than quantification of glucose metabolism with FDG.

Transport contributes significantly to the uptake of amino acids in gliomas (69). In 15 patients studied with dynamic PET with L-2-[F-18]fluorotyrosine (F-18-TYR), there was a greater uptake in tumors than contralateral brain, but this resulted from a doubling of the transport rate, not the rate of incorporation into intracellular constituents. This increased transport did not correlate with Ga-68-ethylene-diamine tetraaacetic acid (EDTA) accumulation so that it was not due to breakdown of the BBB.

Whereas the goal of measuring protein synthesis rates with labeled amino acids has been complicated by the dominance of transport and the alternate biochemical directions that amino acids may follow, there are many observations in a large number of studies that have elevated the status of methionine and tyrosine in the PET arena. Amino acid uptake in normal brain is low relative to FDG uptake so that the tumor to normal tissue contrast is better with amino acid imaging than with FDG. It is especially interesting that the uptake of methionine in lesions lacking breakdown of the BBB suggests that there is upregulation of the transport process across the capillary wall (Fig. 7). This by itself is an interesting pathophysiological marker of the growth and metabolism of neoplasia. Particularly in the case of methionine, the distribution through several biosynthetic processes, including phospholipid synthesis, provides a broad measure of tumor growth. PCNA staining of histology specimens to assess proliferation correlated with methionine uptake in one study (71). In contrast, the relationship between C-11-TYR-PET measurements of protein synthesis and expression of Ki-67 antigen to assess proliferation and nucleolar organizer regions (NORs) to assess protein synthesis in paraffin sections has been reported (72). Protein synthesis rates ranged from 0.44 to 1.99 nmol/mL/min, Ki-67 ranged from 0.9 to 33.5 and AgNOR area ranged from 0.13 to 0.85 mm^2/cm^2. In this small group of patients there were no correlations among these measurements.

Detection

In a report of 50 cases, PET with [C-11]methionine (MET-PET) showed accumulation in 31 of 32 HGG (97% sensitivity) and 11 of 18 LGG (61%) (73); sensitivity as high as 98% has been published (74). Correlation between biopsy specimens and C-11-TYR-PET showed that PET detected the presence of tumor in 20 of 22 primary or recurrent lesions for a sensitivity of 91% (75). Compared with C-11-MET, O-(2-[F-18]fluoroethyl)-L-tyrosine (F-18-FET) PET findings in brain tumors are similar (76).

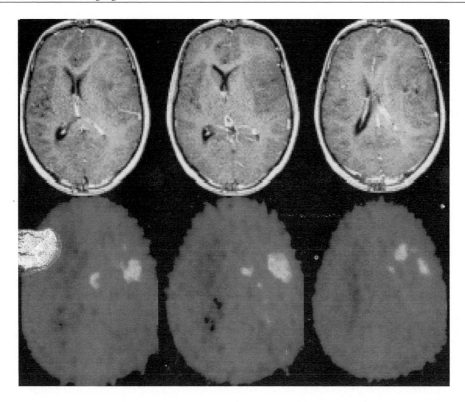

Fig. 7. A 15-yr-old boy presented with a large left frontoinsular tumor, without gadolinium uptake on MRI (*upper 3 images*). The diagnosis obtained from biopsy was that of an anaplastic oligodendroglioma. The C-11-MET pattern (*lower 3 images*) is that of an extremely hypermetabolic and heterogeneous lesion. The patient died 6 mo after the PET study, despite radiotherapy and chemotherapy. Adapted with permission from ref. *131*.

Grading and Prognosis

In an early study of 22 patients with gliomas, C-11-MET uptake was measured by a ratio of tumor to contralateral healthy brain and correlated with pathology grade *(77)*. For grade II gliomas ($n = 5$) the ratio was 1.0, grade III ($n = 5$) 1.7 and grade IV ($n = 12$) 2.3. Despite the small numbers, the differences between II and III, and II and IV were significant, but not between III and IV. Another report showed that tumor-to-mean cortical uptake (T/MCU) less than 2.1 was associated with survival greater than 5 yr whereas greater than 2.1 was associated with survival of 8 mo *(78)*. Other small studies of varied histological types of gliomas have shown the rate of uptake of C-11-MET in HGG to be significantly higher than in LGG but evaluation of malignancy in individual cases by MET-PET alone has been difficult *(71,73)*. Interestingly, C-11-MET uptake has been found to be greater in grade III oligodendroglioma than grade III astrocytoma, although the prognosis is generally better for oligodendroglioma than for astrocytic tumors *(74)*. In grade II lesions C-11-MET uptake was greater in untreated oligodendroglioma ($n = 6$) than astrocytoma ($n = 31$) or oligoastrocytoma ($n = 14$) *(79)*. One has to know both the histology and PET result for more complete grading and prognostication. For example, World Health Organization (WHO) grade II gliomas with a ratio of tumor/ normal brain greater than 2.2 were associated with poor outcome; for WHO grade III gliomas with a ratio greater than 2.8 there was a poor outcome *(74)*.

How well MET-PET or FDG-PET predict malignant degeneration in LGG was examined in a study confined to a group of patients who had WHO II fibrillary astrocytoma *(80)*. Thirteen patients received radiotherapy and seventeen did not. The T/C ratios for MET-PET and FDG-PET were no different between the groups at 94 mo, an interval during which malignant progression would have been expected. Malignant progression occurred at the same rate in both patient groups (3 in each group) at a mean postoperative interval of 46 mo. This suggests that malignant progression is not suppressed or enhanced by adjuvant RT in this patient group. Malignant recurrences showed higher T/C ratios than recurrences that were not malignant.

DNA BIOSYNTHESIS: 2-[C-11]THYMIDINE (TDR), [F-18]3'DEOXY-3'-FLUOROTHYMIDINE (FLT)

The most direct measure of tumor proliferation is the rate of DNA synthesis *(81–83)*. Of the four nucleosides used in DNA synthesis, only thymidine (TdR) is used in DNA and not RNA; therefore most tracer approaches for measuring proliferation have used a labeled form of TdR or an analog *(81,83–85)*.

The application of cellular proliferation imaging to brain tumors is supported by several investigations that examined the *S*-phase fraction (SPF) in series of astrocytic gliomas and established that there is a significant correlation between labeling index (LI) and histological grade *(86–89)*. Glioblastoma SPF averages about 8%, AA 4%, and low grade between 1 and 2%, with normal brain at or close to 0% *(88,89)*. Consequently, tracers of DNA synthesis potentially provide high contrast between tumor and normal brain in proportion to the grade and proliferation rate. Following RT the LIs in gliomas fall by roughly 50% such that cellular proliferation imaging may reliably measure response to treatment early after the intervention *(88,90)*.

The metabolic pathways traced by TdR and [F-18]-3'deoxy-3'-fluorothymidine (FLT), the chief analog of TdR used in PET, are illustrated in Fig. 8. Circulating TdR, extrinsic to the cell, is taken up and incorporated into DNA via the exogenous or salvage pathway. TdR enters cells by facilitated, nonenergy dependent transporters as well as active, Na+-dependent carriers *(91,92)*. Whereas TdR delivery from the blood to the cell is rapid in most somatic tissues, limited transport of TdR across the BBB makes transport a potentially rate limiting step in brain tumor imaging *(93,94)*.

Once inside the cell, TdR is phosphorylated three times to TdR tri-phosphate (TTP) before being incorporated into DNA *(81)*. The initial rate limiting step is phosphorylation by thymidine kinase-1 *(TK1)*, a cytosolic enzyme, to thymidine monophosphate (TMP). This supplements the production of TMP via the *de novo* pathway from deoxyuridine monophosphate catalyzed by thymidylate synthase. The ultimate rate-limiting step is the incorporation of TTP into DNA by DNA polymerase *(81,95)*. *TK1* is upregulated several-fold as cells pass from G1 to the *S*-phase of the cell cycle *(96)* so that retention of exogenous TdR tracers in the pathway to DNA synthesis largely reflects the activity of *TK1*. In the cell the salvage pathway competes with *de novo* synthesis from intracellular deoxyuridine, and therefore the rate of TdR uptake is affected by the relative utilization of the salvage and *de novo* pathways *(81,95)*. Tumors wherein the *de novo* pathway dominates DNA synthesis may be poorly imaged with PET tracers that are limited to following the salvage pathway *(97)*.

Thymidine labeling with C-11 in either the methyl or 2-position produced the earliest PET tracers for imaging cellular proliferation *(98–101)*. The use of these tracers is complicated by

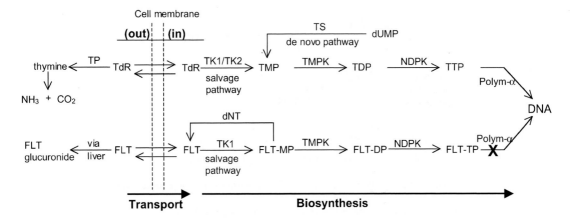

dNT: deoxynucleotidase
dUMP: deoxyuridine monophosphate
NDPK: nucleoside diphosphate kinase
Polym-α: DNA polymerase-α
TK1: thymidine kinase 1
TMPK: thymidylate kinase
TP: thymidine phosphorylase
TS: thymidylate synthase

Fig. 8. The metabolic pathways followed intracellularly by thymidine leading to incorporation in DNA and by FLT through phosphorylation steps in the exogenous (salvage) pathway. PET images measure tracer uptake via the exogenous pathway.

rapid metabolism, yielding $[C-11]-CO_2$ from 2-$[C-11]$-TdR and other labeled metabolites from methyl-$[C-11]$TdR *(102)*. The large pools of thymidine phosphorylase *(TP)* present in blood, liver, and spleen rapidly degrade TdR in vivo. This limits the incorporation of TdR into DNA and produces a large pool of labeled blood metabolites.

Images can be produced semi-quantitatively by injecting these tracers intravenously and collecting the emission data in the field of view of the PET scanner for up to 60 min *(103–105)*. The signal in the PET images includes not only the radioactivity of TdR bound in the DNA synthetic pathway but also the labeled unmetabolized TdR in the tumor plus that in the blood as well as circulating labeled metabolites, especially $[C-11]-CO_2$, some of which reenter the brain and tumor. The image as such is a composite of the bound TdR in the DNA synthetic pathway plus labeled precursor TdR and metabolic byproducts that contaminate the image. Importantly, this approach also does not distinguish the proportion of labeled unmetabolized TdR in the tissue that accumulates as a result of transport via a disrupted BBB vs the proportion that actually enters and binds in the DNA synthesis pathway.

Despite these confounding issues, a limited number of patient studies collected in this manner have been reported. Early on, Vander Borght et al. imaged 13 glioma-bearing patients with 2-$[C-11]$-TdR *(105)*. There were 10 high-grade and 3 low-grade, as well as 8 untreated and 5 recurrent tumors. They were imaged for 60 min but metabolites were not measured. The tumor-to-cortex uptake ratio was 1.27 ± 0.23 (standard deviation [SD]). However, no correlation was found between TdR uptake and tumor grade.

We have since developed and validated $[C-11]$-TdR labeled in the ring-2 position building on the work of Vander Borght *(103,105)*. The dominant metabolic product carrying the label

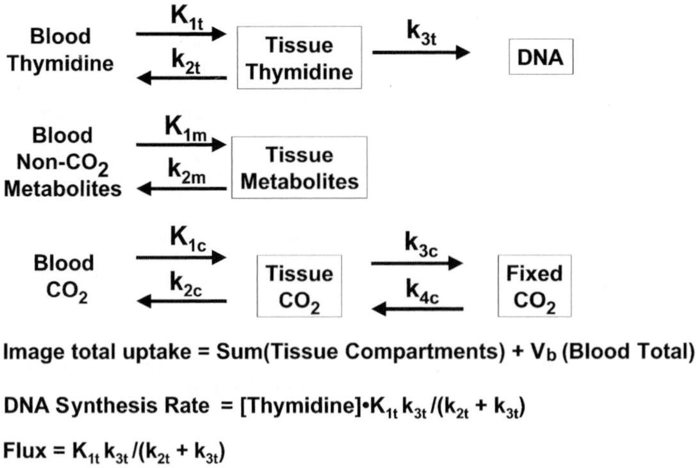

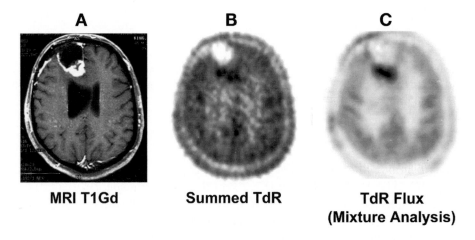

Fig. 9. Compartmental model for kinetics of [C-11]-CO_2 and 2-[C-11]-thymidine.

A   **B**   **C**

MRI T1Gd   **Summed TdR**   **TdR Flux (Mixture Analysis)**

Fig. 10. 2-[C-11]TdR images of a patient with a recurrent right frontal glioma. The MRI T1Gd(**A**) shows distinct contrast. The summed TdR image (**B**) shows uptake in the tumor but also shows the effect of metabolite uptake degrading the image. The TdR Flux (mixture analysis) image (**C**) shows the focus most clearly in the posterior aspect of the resection cavity. Reprinted with permission from ref. *103*.

is [C-11]-CO_2. This requires [C-11]-CO_2 injections and imaging prior to the injections of 2-[C-11]-TdR *(103)*. Blood metabolite analysis and kinetic modeling of dynamic plasma concentrations as well as imaging data are necessary to separate the contributions of [C-11]-TdR and [C-11]-CO_2 in the images. Analysis of the plasma and tissue kinetics of the [C-11]-CO_2 and 2-[C-11]-TdR data combined with compartmental modeling yields parameters from which a flux constant for exchange of TdR into DNA can be calculated as follows (Fig. 9):

$$\text{thymidine flux constant} = K_{\text{TdR}} = K_{1t} \cdot k_{3t}/(k_{2t} + k_{3t})$$

In this formulation, K_{TdR} represents retention of [C-11]-TdR into the DNA synthetic pathway and K_{1t} represents transport of [C-11]-TdR from blood to the intracellular space that may in largely result from disruption of the BBB.

MRI   **CO₂**   **TdR**

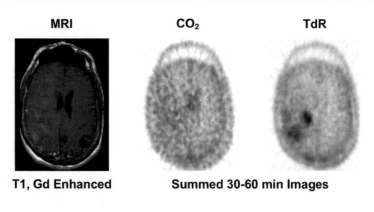

T1, Gd Enhanced   Summed 30-60 min Images

Time-Activity Curves

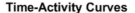

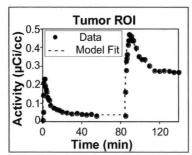
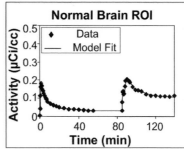

Fig. 11. MRI T1Gd, summed [C-11]-CO₂ and [C-11]-TdR images from a recurrent anaplastic mixed glioma with corresponding tissue time-activity curves below representing the tissue dynamic PET data in the tumor region of interest (ROI) and whole brain ROI. [C-11]-CO₂ was injected at $t = 0$ min and [C-11]-TdR was injected at $t = 85$ min. The initial peaks are from the [C-11]-CO₂ injection and the second peaks are due to the injection of [C-11]-TdR. These data were analyzed with the model shown in Fig. 9. Reprinted with permission from ref. *108*.

Examination of the summed image collected from 20 to 60 min after injection of 2-[C-11]-TdR (Fig. 10B) shows high background in the normal cortex, most likely on the basis of [C-11]-CO₂ that has accumulated from TdR metabolism elsewhere in the body. The image in Fig. 10C demonstrates the application of the kinetic model and mixture analysis to the dynamic TdR images and is an image of TdR flux, which indicates the rate of TdR incorporation into DNA with the model correction for labeled metabolites *(106,107)*. Comparison between the TdR summed and TdR flux images from mixture analysis (Fig. 10B vs 10C) shows the suppression of normal brain background and significant enhancement of tumor contrast in the calculated image, resulting in much better definition of the tumor.

More recently, detailed kinetic analysis of 2-[C-11]-TdR PET images in a group of 20 patients with a broad range of brain tumors was reported *(94,108)*. Validation of the modeling approach was achieved in that PET studies with sequential injections of [C-11]-CO₂ followed by 2-[C-11]-TdR provided dynamic images that allowed mathematical modeling (Fig. 9) to estimate K_{TdR} (retention) and K_{1t} (transport) with standard errors between 10 and 15%, respectively *(94)*. An example of the images and type of dynamic data are shown in Fig. 11. This patient had a recurrent right parietal anaplastic mixed glioma. For tumor, K_{TdR} (retention) and

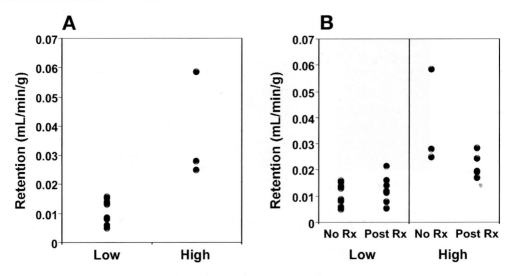

Fig. 12. Thymidine retention against tumor grade for untreated tumors (**A**) and tumor grade and treatment status (**B**). Reprinted with permission from ref. *108.*

K_{1t} (transport) were 0.059 and 0.081 mL/min/g respectively and for whole brain 0.016 and 0.011 mL/min/g respectively.

In the whole population of patients there was an association between transport (K_{1t}) and contrast-enhancement on MRI T1Gd in the expected direction of increased TdR transport into the tumors with contrast enhancement as an indication of BBB damage ($p < 0.001$). There was overlap between the estimated retention (K_{TdR}) for contrast enhancing and nonenhancing lesions which suggested that the flux constant was indeed measuring retention, not simply reflecting transport. TdR retention in untreated tumors (low grade, $n = 9$; high grade, $n = 3$) was significantly greater in the high-grade vs low-grade tumors despite low-population numbers ($p < 0.02$) (Fig. 12A). Previously treated patients with high-grade tumors tended to show lower TdR retention than those not yet treated, the lack of significance likely a result of the small number of cases (untreated, $n = 3$; treated, $n = 4$) ($p > 0.2$) (Fig. 12B). Also, there was no significant difference between patients with low-grade tumors that had received or had not received treatment ($p > 0.7$) (Fig. 12B).

One patient was scanned four times over the course of tumor progression and treatment. The time course of changes in K_{TdR} and K_{1t} are shown in Fig. 13. The tumor was a mixed grade II glioma at the time of the first scan when the model estimated a low level of retention. At the time of the second scan, MRI suggested that the tumor had transformed into a high-grade lesion, and the TdR retention (K_{TdR}) was also much higher. Partial resection confirmed a mixed grade III glioma. After treatment with both radiotherapy and chemotherapy (third scan), the model estimated a lower retention level, corresponding with residual contrast enhancement on MRI and a clinical course suggesting treated, but viable, tumor. One year later the patient was clinically well but had increased contrast enhancement on MRI, leading to the clinical question of active tumor vs radionecrosis. The kinetic analysis showed a decreased retention and increased transport rates, suggesting radionecrosis. The patient did well for 1 yr without additional treatment or evidence of tumor progression.

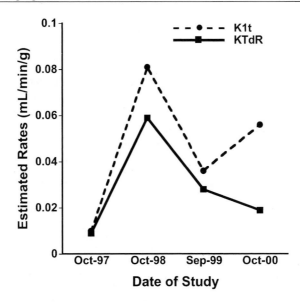

Fig. 13. Estimated flux constants and transport rates for a single patient scanned 4 times over the course of tumor progression and treatment: Oct-97, grade II mixed glioma diagnosed by biopsy; Oct-98, transformed to grade III followed by surgery, chemotherapy and radiotherapy; Sep-99, after therapy when retention and transport both were reduced; and Oct-00, increased contrast enhancement on MRI raising question of active tumor versus radionecrosis, but the kinetic analysis showed a decreased retention and increased transport rates consistent with a radionecrotic effect. Reprinted with permission from ref. *108*.

[F-18]FLUORO-L-THYMIDINE (FLT)

An alternate approach to imaging brain tumor cellular proliferation is to label TdR analogs with F-18 that are resistant to degradation by TP. This eliminates the background of labeled metabolites and provides a longer lived and more convenient tracer *(109)*. The leading compound for this is [F-18]-fluoro-L-thymidine (FLT) *(110,111)*. FLT is a selective substrate for *TK1* which is used for nuclear DNA replication, but only goes as far as the triphosphate along the DNA synthesis pathway shown in Fig. 8. FLT undergoes relatively little degradation after injection aside from production of the glucuronide in the liver. TP in the blood does not break it down. However, as with TdR the uptake of FLT is restricted by the BBB.

Several studies of tumors exposed in vitro to FLT have validated that its uptake correlates positively with *TK1* activity in cycling cells *(97,112)*. A study of the short-term metabolic fate of FLT in the DNA salvage pathway in exponentially growing A549 tumor cells has provided additional validation of the usefulness of FLT for imaging cellular proliferation *(113)*. *TK1* activity produced FLT-monophosphate (FLT-MP), which dominated the labeled nucleotide pool. Subsequent phosphorylations led to FLT-triphosphate (FLT-TP) that comprised about 30% of the metabolic pool after 1 h. A putative deoxynucleotidase (dNT), which degrades FLT-MP to FLT, provided the primary mechanism for tracer efflux from cells. In contrast, FLT-TP was resistant to degradation and highly retained.

The mathematical model describing the uptake of FLT is much simpler than that for TdR (Fig. 9) because the only metabolite in the plasma that needs to be measured is the glucuronide

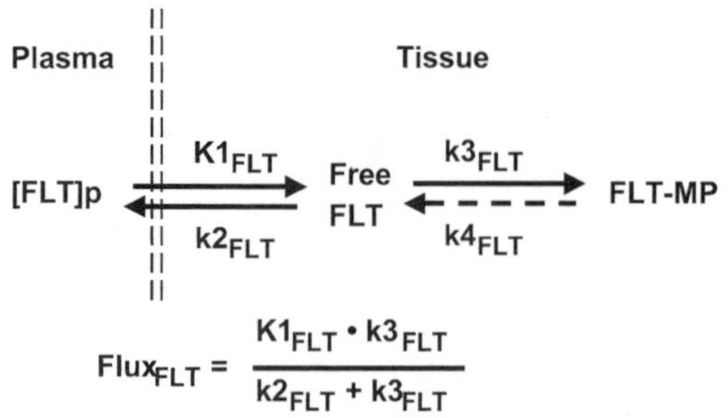

$$\text{Flux}_{FLT} = \frac{K1_{FLT} \cdot k3_{FLT}}{k2_{FLT} + k3_{FLT}}$$

Fig. 14. Two-compartment, 4 rate constant model for kinetics of FLT.

Table 3
FLT Modeling Results on the Patient shown in Fig. 15

	PreRT	PostRT
Parameter	*Right frontal tumor*	*Right frontal tumor*
ROI volume of ↑ uptake (cc)	19.0	33.8
Tumor volume encompassed by ↑ uptake (cc)	48.4	73.9
Flux (mL/min/g)	0.027	0.015
K1 (mL/min/g)	0.066	0.059

(Fig. 14). Similar to TdR, retention of FLT is reflected in the flux constant, K_{FLT}, and transport in K_{1FLT}:

$$\text{Flux constant} = K_{FLT} = K_{1FLT} \cdot k_{3FLT}/(k_{2FLT} + k_{3FLT})$$

Few brain tumor cases have been studied with FLT-PET. Sloan and coworkers reported 29 patients with gliomas at presentation or recurrence *(114–116)*. Tracer uptake was quantified as standard uptake value (SUV) which equals the tissue concentration of tracer normalized to the injected dose of tracer and body weight (i.e., SUV = tissue concentration of tracer/injected tracer dose/body weight). The value of the pixel in the image with the highest SUV is the SUVmax. From their results SUVmax of FLT correlated with tumor grade and MIB-1 immunolabeling for proliferation. SUVmax in normal brain was 0.32; LLG between 0.49 and 0.79; intermediate grade between 0.85- and 1.46; and HGG between 2.04 and 3.90. Uptake in areas of radionecrosis was low with SUVmax < 1.0. FLT uptake was seen exclusively in areas that showed contrast enhancement in MRI images *(116)*. These investigators also reported that brain tumor tissue biopsied shortly after FLT injection contained the labeled species largely in the form of phosphorylated FLT *(114)*.

Our preliminary work is illustrated in Table 3 and Figs. 15 and 16. In Table 3 and Fig. 15 the data and images are shown for a 67-yr-old man who had a bicentric gliosarcoma of the right frontal and temporal lobes. The right temporal lesion was resected and the frontal lesion was left untouched. FLT images were obtained both 2.5 wk before and 2.5 wk after 63 Gy of fractionated external beam RT. The K_{FLT} before RT for the frontal lesion was 0.030 mL/min/g and the tumor volume encompassed by increased FLT uptake was 48.4 cc. The images taken

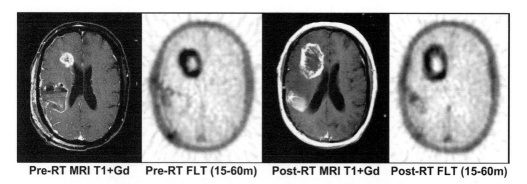

Pre-RT MRI T1+Gd   Pre-RT FLT (15-60m)   Post-RT MRI T1+Gd   Post-RT FLT (15-60m)

Fig. 15. Sixty-five-year-old man with a bicentric gliosarcoma in the right temporal lobe (resected) and the right frontal lobe (unresected). Labels under the images identify their sources and times.

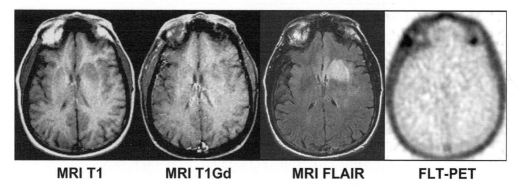

MRI T1   MRI T1Gd   MRI FLAIR   FLT-PET

Fig. 16. Sixty-one-year-old man who had a bifrontal AA. The MRI T1 and T1Gd show there was no contrast enhancement (i.e., no detectable breakdown of the BBB). The FLAIR image shows abnormality in the deep medial left frontal lobe. Other slices showed similar findings in the right frontal lobe. The FLT image shows no detectable uptake even though the microscopic examination of the tumor showed a MIB-1 labeling level of 10%.

after RT show that the volume had decidedly increased assessed by MRI T1Gd and the FLT volumes (73.9 cc), consistent with tumor progression by conventional standards *(117)*. However, the K_{FLT} was roughly halved after RT (0.017 mL/min/g) suggesting that growth rate had been reduced by the RT but not by enough to stabilize or shrink the tumor volume. The FLT-PET images clearly show an additional dimension to assessing response to therapy achievable by this approach. With additional therapy the patient survived a total of 10 mo from diagnosis.

Another illustrative case is shown in Fig. 16. This 61-yr-old man had a bifrontal AA that completely lacked contrast enhancement on MRI T1Gd at the time of clinical presentation; biopsy preceeded the FLT-PET by 20 d. The MIB-1 labeling level was 10%. The point here is that this malignant glioma had a high MIB-1 level but no breakdown of the BBB and little, if any, uptake of FLT. The tumor and brain K_{1FLT} levels were 0.006 and 0.011 mL/min/g, respectively, whereas the K_{FLT} flux constants were 0.003 mL/min/g. These numbers suggest very low transport into tumor and brain. Obviously, the essentially equal flux constants suggest but likely do not indicate that tumor and brain had the same proliferation rates since the tumor MIB-1 was 10%.

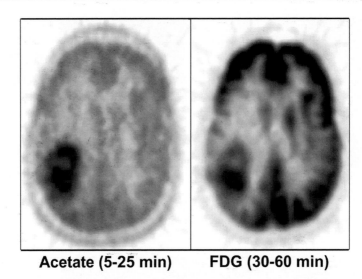

Acetate (5-25 min)   FDG (30-60 min)

Fig. 17. Thirty-nine-year-old women with a recurrent AA of the right frontoparietal region. The tumor to normal brain uptake is much better for the 1-[C-11]acetate than for the FDG. The tumor 1-[C-11]acetate SUV is 2.6 and the brain 1.0. SUV is (tissue concentration of tracer)/(injected tracer dose/body weight). Reprinted with permission from ref. *130*.

MEMBRANE BIOSYNTHESIS: [C-11]ACETATE, [C-11]CHOLINE, OR [F-18]FLUOROCHOLINE

The rationale for imaging membrane and lipid biosynthesis is that tumor growth requires both of these processes in parallel with DNA and protein synthesis. Studies of growth in additional dimensions may reveal clinically important biological insights. The tracers appropriate for this include 1-[C-11]acetate, [C-11]choline, or [F-18]fluorocholine. These will likely show retention in tumor tissue but not by gray matter, an important advantage over FDG (Fig. 17). For 1-[C-11]acetate, in particular, in nontumor regions of brain, C-11 will egress quickly as CO_2 via the tricarboxylic acid cycle.

1-[C-11]Acetate may be selectively taken up by glioma cells, because exogenous acetate is preferentially metabolized by astrocytes in the central nervous system and the uptake in astrocytes is by a carrier similar to the monocarboxylic acid transporter *(118)*. Transport across the BBB should be less problematic with 1-[C-11]acetate than with FLT, [C-11]TdR or amino acid tracers because the brain uptake index of acetate is higher than for these other compounds *(93,119)*. Further supporting the application of PET with 1-[C-11]acetate are the data of Yoshimoto and coworkers who measured uptake of 1-[C-14]acetate in vitro in four tumor cell lines and fibroblasts and showed a positive correlation between C-14 accumulation and growth estimated with [H-3]methyl TdR *(120)*.

Several studies in humans support the potential for 1-[C-11]acetate-PET in gliomas. Liu and others reported 14 gliomas (4 low grade, 10 high grade) imaged with 1-[C-11]acetate in 13 of which acetate uptake was higher than in gray matter *(121)*. In a second study, there was "intense" uptake of 1-[C-11]acetate in 18 of 25 brain tumors *(59)*. Although these studies in aggregate show significant promise for 1-[C-11]acetate in gliomas, they obviously need to be extended to a larger patient population and conducted with more rigorous quantitative methods at important decision-making points in the patient's clinical course.

[C-11]choline or [F-18]fluorocholine are alternative tracers that are being evaluated for lipid/membrane biosynthesis; early results in brain tumors have been encouraging *(122–125)*. However, Yoshimoto et al. have shown in uptake studies in cultured human tumors and fibroblasts that acetate distributes mainly in the lipid fraction whereas choline is converted to water-soluble metabolites *(126)*. Choline uptake could reflect choline transporter and/or choline kinase activity rather than lipid/membrane biosynthesis *(126)*.

CONCLUSIONS AND FUTURE DIRECTIONS

PET provides the opportunity to image multiple dynamic biological processes *in situ* in brain tumors. Energy metabolism and amino acid transport and incorporation are important components of the pathophysiology of gliomas about which molecular imaging is providing regional biological information that is useful in clinical practice. Imaging hypoxia is straight-forward and proliferation imaging with FLT shows significant promise. Neither has been exploited thoroughly enough to allow judgment of their potential benefit to the practice of neuro-oncology. Whereas cell division is the most distinguishing function of growth in tumors, probing membrane biosynthesis with PET and 1-[C-11]acetate or a choline tracer may yield information as helpful as protein or DNA synthesis. Because astrocytic gliomas frequently carry epidermal growth factor receptor mutations at a frequency that is related to grade, a PET tracer specific for this mutated receptor could be useful for grading and prognosis *(127)*. Methods for imaging angiogenesis are being developed as F-18-labeling of a cyclic RGD-containing glycopeptide, cyclo(-Arg- Gly-Asp-D-Phe-Lys(sugar amino acid)-), with 4-*nitro*phenyl 2-[F-18]fluoropropionate has been reported *(128)*. [F-18]-labeled annexin V is being tested as a new PET agent for quantitating tumor cell death and predicting response to therapy. Annexin V binds to surface membranes that have exposed phosphatidyl serine residues resulting from programmed cell destruction. Recently, a Tc-99m-labeled derivative has been shown to accumulate in late stage lung cancer and lymphoma in response to chemo-therapy *(129)*. As molecular pathways leading to and sustaining neoplasia become better understood, so will our capacity improve to measure them in vivo and intervene to the patient's advantage.

ACKNOWLEDGMENT

This work was supported by Grant No. CA42045 from the National Institutes of Health.

REFERENCES

1. Jager PL, Vaalburg W, Pruim J, de Vries EG, Langen KJ, Piers DA. Radiolabeled amino acids: basic aspects and clinical applications in oncology. J Nucl Med 2001;42:432–445.
2. Allen N. Respiration and oxidative metabolism of brain tumors. In: Kirsch WM, Paoletti EG, Paoletti P, eds. The Experimental Biology of Brain Tumors, Springfield: Charles C Thomas, 1972; 243–274.
3. Spence AM, Muzi M, Graham MM, et al. Glucose metabolism in human malignant gliomas measured quantitatively with PET, 1-[C-11]glucose and FDG: analysis of the FDG lumped constant. J Nucl Med 1998; 39:440–448.
4. Di Chiro G, Oldfield E, Bairamian D, et al. In vivo glucose utilization of tumors of the brain stem and spinal cord. In: Greitz T, Ingvar DH, Widen L, eds. The Metabolism of the Human Brain Studied with Positron Emission Tomography, New York: Raven Press, 1985;351–361.
5. Di Chiro G. Positron emission tomography using [18F] fluorodeoxyglucose in brain tumors: A powerful diagnostic and prognostic tool. Invest Radiol 1987;22:360–371.
6. Di Chiro G, DeLaPaz RL, Brooks RA, et al. Glucose utilization of cerebral gliomas measured by [18F] fluorodeoxyglucose and positron emission tomography. Neurology 1982;32:1323–1329.

7. Patronas NJ, Di Chiro G, Kufta C, et al. Prediction of survival in glioma patients by means of positron emission tomography. J Neurosurg 1985;62:816–822.

8. Delbeke D, Meyerowitz C, Lapidus RL, et al. Optimal cutoff levels of F-18 fluorodeoxyglucose uptake in the differentiation of low-grade from high-grade brain tumors with PET. Radiology 1995;195:47–52.

9. Padma MV, Said S, Jacobs M, et al. Prediction of pathology and survival by FDG PET in gliomas. J Neurooncol 2003;64:227–237.

10. De Witte O, Levivier M, Violon P, et al. Prognostic value of positron emission tomography with [18F]fluoro-2-deoxy-D-glucose in the low-grade glioma. Neurosurgery 1996;39:470–476.

11. Hanson MW, Glantz MJ, Hoffman JM, et al. FDG-PET in the selection of brain lesions for biopsy. J Comput Assist Tomogr 1991;15:796–801.

12. Herholz K, Pietrzyk U, Voges J, et al. Correlation of glucose consumption and tumor cell density in astrocytomas. A stereotactic PET study. J Neurosurg 1993;79:853–858.

13. Goldman S, Levivier M, Pirotte B, et al. Regional glucose metabolism and histopathology of gliomas. A study based on positron emission tomography-guided stereotactic biopsy. Cancer 1996;78:1098–1106.

14. Glantz MJ, Hoffman JM, Coleman RE, et al. Identification of early recurrence of primary central nervous system tumors by [18F]fluorodeoxyglucose positron emission tomography. Ann Neurol 1991;29:347–355.

15. Asensio C, Perez-Castejon MJ, Maldonado A, et al. The role of PET-FDG in questionable diagnosis of relapse in the presence of radionecrosis of brain tumors. Rev Neurol 1998;27:447–452.

16. Langleben DD, Segall GM. PET in differentiation of recurrent brain tumor from radiation injury. J Nucl Med 2000;41:1861–1867.

17. Maldonado A, Santos M, Rodriguez S, Ossola G, Liano H, Delgado JM. The role of PET-FDG in resolving diagnostic doubt: recurrence vs. radionecrosis in brain tumors (abs 124). Mol Imag Biol 2002;4:S32.

18. Patronas NJ, Di Chiro G, Brooks RA, et al. Work in progress: [18F] fluorodeoxyglucose and positron emission tomography in the evaluation of radiation necrosis of the brain. Radiology 1982;144:885–889.

19. Ricci PE, Karis JP, Heiserman JE, Fram EK, Bice AN, Drayer BP. Differentiating recurrent tumor from radiation necrosis: time for re-evaluation of positron emission tomography? AJNR Am J Neuroradiol 1998;19:407–413.

20. Spence AM, Muzi M, Graham MM, et al. FDG and glucose uptake in malignant gliomas before and after radiotherapy: correlation with outcome. Advances in Brief. Clinical Cancer Res 2002;8:971–979.

21. Hoekstra CJ, Paglianiti I, Hoekstra OS, et al. Monitoring response to therapy in cancer using [18F]-2-fluoro-2-deoxy-D-glucose and positron emission tomography: an overview of different analytical methods. Eur J Nucl Med 2000;27:731–743.

22. De Witte O, Hildebrand J, Luxen A, Goldman S. Acute effect of carmustine on glucose metabolism in brain and glioblastoma. Cancer 1994;74:2836–2842.

23. Maruyama I, Sadato N, Waki A, et al. Hyperacute changes in glucose metabolism of brain tumors after stereotactic radiosurgery: a PET study. J Nucl Med 1999;40:1085–1090.

24. Haberkorn U, Bellemann ME, Altmann A, et al. PET 2-fluoro-2-deoxyglucose uptake in rat prostate adenocarcinoma during chemotherapy with gemcitabine. J Nucl Med 1997;38:1215–1221.

25. Haberkorn U, Morr I, Oberdorfer F, et al. Fluorodeoxyglucose uptake in vitro: aspects of method and effects of treatment with gemcitabine. J Nucl Med 1994;35:1842–1850.

26. Haberkorn U, Oberdorfer F, Klenner T, et al. Metabolic and transcriptional changes in osteosarcoma cells treated with chemotherapeutic drugs. Nucl Med Biol 1994;21:835–845.

27. Haberkorn U, Reinhardt M, Strauss LG, et al. Metabolic design of combination therapy: use of enhanced fluorodeoxyglucose uptake caused by chemotherapy. J Nucl Med 1992;33:1981–1987.

28. Smith TA, Maisey NR, Titley JC, Jackson LE, Leach MO, Ronen SM. Treatment of SW620 cells with Tomudex and oxaliplatin induces changes in 2-deoxy-D-glucose incorporation associated with modifications in glucose transport. J Nucl Med 2000;41:1753–1759.

29. Kubota R, Yamada S, Kubota K, Ishiwata K, Tamahashi N, Ido T. Intratumoral distribution of fluorine-18-fluorodeoxyglucose in vivo: high accumulation in macrophages and granulation tissues studied by microautoradiography. J Nucl Med 1992;33:1972–1980.

30. Reinhardt MJ, Kubota K, Yamada S, Iwata R, Yaegashi H. Assessment of cancer recurrence in residual tumors after fractionated radiotherapy: a comparison of fluorodeoxyglucose, L-methionine and thymidine. J Nucl Med 1997;38:280–287.

31. Furuta M, Hasegawa M, Hayakawa K, et al. Rapid rise in FDG uptake in an irradiated human tumour xenograft. Eur J Nucl Med 1997;24:435–438.

32. Hasegawa M, Mitsuhashi N, Yamakawa M, et al. p53 protein expression and radiation-induced apoptosis in human tumors transplanted to nude mice. Radiat Med 1997;15:171–176.

33. Barker FG, Chang SM, Valk PE, Pounds TR, Prados MD. 18-Fluorodeoxyglucose uptake and survival of patients with suspected recurrent malignant glioma. Cancer 1997;79:115–126.

34. Tralins KS, Douglas JG, Stelzer KJ, et al. Volumetric analysis of fluorodeoxyglucose positron emission tomography in glioblastoma multiforme: prognostic information and possible role in definition of target volumes in radiation dose escalation. J Nucl Med 2002;43:1667–1673.

35. Alavi JB, Alavi A, Chawluk J, et al. Positron emission tomography in patients with glioma: A predictor of prognosis. Cancer 1988;62:1074–1078.

36. De Witte O, Lefranc F, Levivier M, Salmon I, Brotchi J, Goldman S. FDG-PET as a prognostic factor in high-grade astrocytoma. J Neurooncol 2000;49:157–163.

37. Chang CH, Horton J, Schoenfeld D, et al. Comparison of postoperative radiotherapy and combined postoperative radiotherapy and chemotherapy in the multidisciplinary management of malignant gliomas. A joint Radiation Therapy Oncology Group and Eastern Cooperative Oncology Group study. Cancer 1983;52: 997–1007.

38. Lee SW, Fraass BA, Marsh LH, et al. Patterns of failure following high-dose 3-D conformal radiotherapy for high-grade astrocytomas: a quantitative dosimetric study. Int J Radiat Oncol Biol Phys 1999;43:79–88.

39. Nelson DF, Diener-West M, Horton J, Chang CH, Schoenfeld D, Nelson JS. Combined modality approach to treatment of malignant gliomas—re-evaluation of RTOG 7401/ECOG 1374 with long-term follow-up: a joint study of the Radiation Therapy Oncology Group and the Eastern Cooperative Oncology Group. NCI Monogr 1988;6:279–284.

40. Salazar OM, Rubin P, Feldstein ML, Pizzutiello R. High dose radiation therapy in the treatment of malignant gliomas: final report. Int J Radiat Oncol Biol Phys 1979;5:1733–1740.

41. Tralins K, Stelzer KJ, Mankoff DA, et al. FDG-PET guided radiation dose escalation in the treatment of glioblastoma multiforme. In: Ninety-second Annual Meeting of the American Association for Cancer Research, New Orleans, LA, 2001.

42. Ito M, Lammertsma AA, Wise RJ, et al. Measurement of regional cerebral blood flow and oxygen utilisation in patients with cerebral tumours using 15O and positron emission tomography: analytical techniques and preliminary results. Neuroradiology 1982;23:63–74.

43. Lammertsma AA, Frackowiak RS. Positron emission tomography. Crit Rev Biomed Eng 1985;13:125–169.

44. Rhodes CG, Wise RJ, Gibbs JM, et al. In vivo disturbance of the oxidative metabolism of glucose in human cerebral gliomas. Ann Neurol 1983;14:614–626.

45. Tyler JL, Diksic M, Villemure JG, et al. Metabolic and hemodynamic evaluation of gliomas using positron emission tomography. J Nucl Med 1987;28:1123–1133.

46. Wise RJS, Thomas DGT, Lammertsma AA, Rhodes CG. PET scanning of human brain tumors. Prog Exp Tumor Res 1984;27:154–169.

47. Baron JC, Rougemont D, Soussaline F, et al. Local interrelationships of cerebral oxygen consumption and glucose utilization in normal subjects and in ischemic stroke patients: a positron tomography study. J Cereb Blood Flow Metab 1984;4:140–149.

48. Badib AO, Webster JH. Changes in tumor oxygen tension during radiation therapy. Acta Radiol Ther Phys Biol 1969;8:247–257.

49. Brizel DM, Dodge RK, Clough RW, Dewhirst MW. Oxygenation of head and neck cancer: changes during radiotherapy and impact on treatment outcome. Radiother Oncol 1999;53:113–117.

50. Nordsmark M, Overgaard M, Overgaard J. Pretreatment oxygenation predicts radiation response in advanced squamous cell carcinoma of the head and neck. Radiother Oncol 1996;41:31–39.

51. Rampling R, Cruickshank G, Lewis AD, Fitzsimmons SA, Workman P. Direct measurement of pO$_2$ distribution and bioreductive enzymes in human malignant brain tumors. Int J Radiat Oncol Biol Phys 1994;29: 427–431.

52. Davis LW. Malignant glioma—a nemesis which requires clinical and basic investigation in radiation oncology. Int J Radiat Oncol Biol Phys 1989;16:1355–1365.

53. Green SB, Byar DP, Strike TA, et al. Randomized comparisons of BCNU, streptozotocin, radiosensitizer, and fractionation of radiotherapy in the post-operative treatment of malignant glioma. Proc ASCO 1984; 3:260.

54. Nelson DF, Schoenfeld D, Weinstein AS, et al. A randomized comparison of misonidazole sensitized radiotherapy plus BCNU and radiotherapy plus BCNU for treatment of malignant glioma after surgery; preliminary results of an RTOG study. Int J Radiat Oncol Biol Phys 1983;9:1143–1151.

55. Griffin TW, Davis R, Laramore G, et al. Fast neutron radiation therapy for glioblastoma multiforme. Results of an RTOG study. Am J Clin Oncol 1983;6:661–667.

56. Chapman JD, Engelhardt EL, Stobbe CC, Schneider RF, Hanks GE. Measuring hypoxia and predicting tumor radioresistance with nuclear medicine assays. Radiother Oncol 1998;46:229–237.

57. Mathias CJ, Welch MJ, Kilbourn MR, et al. Radiolabeled hypoxic cell sensitizers: tracers for assessment of ischemia. Life Sci 1987;41:199–206.

58. Koh WJ, Bergman KS, Rasey JS, et al. Evaluation of oxygenation status during fractionated radiotherapy in human nonsmall cell lung cancers using [F-18]fluoromisonidazole positron emission tomography. Int J Radiat Oncol Biol Phys 1995;33:391–398.

59. Liu RS, Chu LS, Chu YK, Yen SH, Liao SQ, Yeh SH. Does β-oxidation occur in malignant neoplasm? A concurrent [C-11]acetate and [F-18]MISO study (abstract). J Nucl Med 1999;40 (suppl):239P.

60. Scott AM, Ramdave S, Hannah A, et al. Correlation of hypoxic cell fraction with glucose metabolic rate in gliomas with 18F-fluoromisonidazole (FMISO) and 18F-fluorodeoxyglucose (FDG) positron emission tomography (PET). J Nucl Med 2001;42:Abstract 250, 267P.

61. Valk PE, Mathis CA, Prados MD, Gilbert JC, Budinger TF. Hypoxia in human gliomas: demonstration by PET with fluorine-18-fluoromisonidazole. J Nucl Med 1992;33:2133–2137.

62. Swanson KR, Muzi M, Spence AM, Rajendran JG, Grierson JR, Krohn KA. PET imaging of glioma patients with FMISO and MRI provides distinct information in the assessment of radiation therapy (abstract). J Nucl Med 2004;45:266P.

63. Vaalburg W, Coenen HH, Crouzel C, et al. Amino acids for the measurement of protein synthesis in vivo by PET. Int J Rad Appl Instrum B 1992;19:227–237.

64. Bergstrom M, Ericson K, Hagenfeldt L, et al. PET study of methionine accumulation in glioma and normal brain tissue: competition with branched chain amino acids. J Comput Assist Tomogr 1987;11:208–213.

65. Smith CB, Deibler GE, Eng N, Schmidt K, Sokoloff L. Measurement of local cerebral protein synthesis in vivo: influence of recycling of amino acids derived from protein degradation. Proc Natl Acad Sci USA 1988; 85:9341–9345.

66. Widmann R, Kocher M, Ernestus RI, Hossmann KA. Biochemical and autoradiographical determination of protein synthesis in experimental brain tumors of rats. J Neurochem 1992;59:18–25.

67. Hawkins RA, Huang SC, Barrio JR, et al. Estimation of local cerebral protein synthesis rates with L-[1-11C]leucine and PET: methods, model, and results in animals and humans. J Cereb Blood Flow Metab 1989; 9:446–460.

68. Ishiwata K, Kubota K, Murakami M, et al. Re-evaluation of amino acid PET studies: can the protein synthesis rates in brain and tumor tissues be measured in vivo? J Nucl Med 1993;34:1936-1943.

69. Wienhard K, Herholz K, Coenen HH, et al. Increased amino acid transport into brain tumors measured by PET of L-(2-18F)fluorotyrosine [see comments]. J Nucl Med 1991;32:1338–1346.

70. Willemsen AT, van Waarde A, Paans AM, et al. In vivo protein synthesis rate determination in primary or recurrent brain tumors using L-[1-11C]-tyrosine and PET. J Nucl Med 1995;36:411–419.

71. Sato N, Suzuki M, Kuwata N, et al. Evaluation of the malignancy of glioma using 11C-methionine positron emission tomography and proliferating cell nuclear antigen staining. Neurosurg Rev 1999;22:210–214.

72. de Wolde H, Pruim J, Mastik MF, Koudstaal J, Molenaar WM. Proliferative activity in human brain tumors: comparison of histopathology and L-[1-(11)C]tyrosine PET. J Nucl Med 1997;38:1369–1374.

73. Ogawa T, Shishido F, Kanno I, et al. Cerebral glioma: evaluation with methionine PET. Radiology 1993; 186:45–53.

74. De Witte O, Goldberg I, Wikler D, et al. Positron emission tomography with injection of methionine as a prognostic factor in glioma. J Neurosurg 2001;95:746–750.

75. Pruim J, Willemsen AT, Molenaar WM, et al. Brain tumors: L-[1-C-11]tyrosine PET for visualization and quantification of protein synthesis rate. Radiology 1995;197:221–226.

76. Weber WA, Wester HJ, Grosu AL, et al. O-(2-[18F]fluoroethyl)-L-tyrosine and L-[methyl-11C]methionine uptake in brain tumours: initial results of a comparative study. Eur J Nucl Med 2000;27:542–549.

77. Derlon JM, Bourdet C, Bustany P, et al. [11C]L-methionine uptake in gliomas. Neurosurgery 1989;25:720–728.

78. Kaschten B, Stevenaert A, Sadzot B, et al. Preoperative evaluation of 54 gliomas by PET with fluorine-18-fluorodeoxyglucose and/or carbon-11-methionine. J Nucl Med 1998;39:778–785.

79. Herholz K, Holzer T, Bauer B, et al. 11C-methionine PET for differential diagnosis of low-grade gliomas. Neurology 1998;50:1316–1322.

80. Roelcke U, von Ammon K, Hausmann O, et al. Operated low grade astrocytomas: a long term PET study on the effect of radiotherapy. J Neurol Neurosurg Psychiatry 1999;66:644–647.

81. Cleaver JE. Thymidine metabolism and cell kinetics. Frontiers Biol 1967;6:43–100.

82. Livingston RB, Ambus U, George SL, Freireich EJ, Hart JS. In vitro determination of thymidine-[H-3] labeling index in human solid tumors. Cancer Res 1974;34:1376–1380.

83. Tannock IF, Hill RP (ed.) The Basic Science of Oncology, New York: McGraw-Hill, 1992.

84. Krohn KA, Mankoff DA, Eary JF. Imaging cellular proliferation as a measure of response to therapy. J Clin Pharmacol 2001;Suppl:96S–103S.

85. Mankoff DA, Dehdashti F, Shields AF. Characterizing tumors using metabolic imaging: PET imaging of cellular proliferation and steroid receptors. Neoplasia 2000;2:71–88.
86. Coons SW, Johnson PC, Pearl DK. Prognostic significance of flow cytometry deoxyribonucleic acid analysis of human astrocytomas. Neurosurgery 1994;35:119–125.
87. Lamborn KR, Prados MD, Kaplan SB, Davis RL. Final report on the University of California-San Francisco experience with bromodeoxyuridine labeling index as a prognostic factor for the survival of glioma patients. Cancer 1999;85:925–935.
88. Matsutani M. Cell Kinetics. In: Berger MS, Wilson CB, eds. The Gliomas, Philadelphia: WB Saunders Co, 1999;204–209.
89. Shibuya M, Ito S, Davis RL, Wilson CB, Hoshino T. A new method for analyzing the cell kinetics of human brain tumors by double labeling with bromodeoxyuridine *in situ* and with iododeoxyuridine in vitro. Cancer 1993;71:3109–3113.
90. Fujimaki T, Matsutani M, Takakura K. Analysis of BUdR (bromodeoxyuridine) labeling indices of cerebral glioblastomas after radiation therapy. J JPN Soc Ther Radiol Oncol 1990;2:263–273.
91. Damaraju VL, Damaraju S, Young JD, et al. Nucleoside anticancer drugs: the role of nucleoside transporters in resistance to cancer chemotherapy. Oncogene 2003;22:7524–7536.
92. Young JD, Cheeseman CI, Mackey JR, Cass CE, Baldwin SA. Gastrointestinal Transport, Molecular Physiology. In: Fambrough D, Benos D, Barrett K, Domowitz M, eds. Current Topics in Membranes, Vol. 50 San Diego, CA: Academic Press, 2000;329–378.
93. Cornford EM, Oldendorf WH. Independent blood–brain barrier transport systems for nucleic acid precursors. Biochim Biophys Acta 1975;394:211–219.
94. Wells JM, Mankoff DA, Muzi M, et al. Kinetic analysis of 2-[11C]thymidine PET imaging studies of malignant brain tumors: compartmental model investigation and mathematical analysis. Mol Imaging 2002;1:151–159.
95. Mankoff DA, Shields AF, Graham MM, Link JM, Eary JF, Krohn KA. Kinetic analysis of 2-[carbon-11] thymidine PET imaging studies: compartmental model and mathematical analysis. J Nucl Med 1998;39:1043–1055.
96. Sherley JL, Kelly TJ. Regulation of human thymidine kinase during the cell cycle. J Biol Chem 1988;263:8350–8358.
97. Schwartz JL, Tamura Y, Jordan R, Grierson JR, Krohn KA. Monitoring tumor cell proliferation by targeting DNA synthetic processes with thymidine and thymidine analogs. J Nucl Med 2003;44:2027–2032.
98. Christman D, Crawford EJ, Friedkin M, Wolf AP. Detection of DNA synthesis in intact organisms with positron-emitting (methyl-11C)thymidine. Proc Natl Acad Sci USA 1972;69:988–992.
99. Link JM, Grierson J, Krohn K. Alternatives in the synthesis of 2-[C-11]-thymidine. J Label Comp Radiopharm 1995;37:610–612.
100. Sundoro-Wu BM, Schmall B, Conti PS, Dahl JR, Drumm P, Jacobsen JK. Selective alkylation of pyrimidyldianions: synthesis and purification of 11C labeled thymidine for tumor visualization using positron emission tomography. Int J Appl Radiat Isot 1984;35:705–708.
101. Vander Borght T, Labar D, Pauwels S, Lambotte L. Production of [2-11C]thymidine for quantification of cellular proliferation with PET. Int J Rad Appl Instrum [A] 1991;42:103–104.
102. Shields AF, Lim K, Grierson J, Link J, Krohn KA. Utilization of labeled thymidine in DNA synthesis: studies for PET. J Nucl Med 1990;31:337–342.
103. Eary JF, Mankoff DA, Spence AM, et al. 2-[C-11]thymidine imaging of malignant brain tumors. Cancer Res 1999;59:615–621.
104. De Reuck J, Santens P, Goethals P, et al. [Methyl-11C]thymidine positron emission tomography in tumoral and non-tumoral cerebral lesions. Acta Neurol Belg 1999;99:118–125.
105. Vander Borght T, Pauwels S, Lambotte L, et al. Brain tumor imaging with PET and 2-[carbon-11]thymidine. J Nucl Med 1994;35:974–982.
106. O'Sullivan F. Metabolic images from dynamic positron emission tomography studies. Stat Methods Med Res 1994;3:87–101.
107. O'Sullivan F, Muzi M, Graham MM, Spence AM. Parametric imaging by mixture analysis in 3-D: Validation for dual-tracer glucose studies. In: Myers R, Cunningham V, Bailey D, Jones T, eds. Quantitation of Brain Function Using PET, Academic Press, Inc, 1996;297–300.
108. Wells JM, Mankoff DA, Eary JF, et al. Kinetic analysis of 2-[11C]thymidine PET imaging studies of malignant brain tumors: preliminary patient results. Mol Imaging 2002;1:145–150.
109. Shields AF, Grierson JR, Kozawa SM, Zheng M. Development of labeled thymidine analogs for imaging tumor proliferation. Nucl Med Biol 1996;23:17–22.
110. Grierson JR, Shields AF. Radiosynthesis of 3'-deoxy-3'-[(18)F]fluorothymidine: [(18)F]FLT for imaging of cellular proliferation in vivo. Nucl Med Biol 2000;27:143–156.

111. Shields AF, Grierson JR, Dohmen BM, et al. Imaging proliferation in vivo with [F-18]FLT and positron emission tomography. Nat Med 1998;4:1334–1336.

112. Rasey JS, Grierson JR, Wiens LW, Kolb PD, Schwartz JL. Validation of FLT uptake as a measure of thymidine kinase-1 activity in A549 carcinoma cells. J Nucl Med 2002;43:1210–1217.

113. Grierson JR, Schwartz JL, Muzi M, Jordan R, Krohn KA. Metabolism of 3'-deoxy-3'-[F-18]fluorothymidine (FLT) in proliferating A549 cells: validations for positron emission tomography (PET). Nucl Med Biol 2004:31:829–837.

114. Bendaly EA, Sloan AE, Dohmen BM, et al. Use of 18F-FLT-PET to assess the metabolic activity of primary and metastatic brain tumors (abstract). J Nucl Med 2002;43:111P.

115. Sloan AE, Bendaly EA, Dohman BM, et al. Use of 18F-FLT-PET to assess the metabolic activity of primary, recurrent and metastatic brain tumors (abs). Neuro-Oncology 2002;4:363.

116. Sloan AE, Shields AF, Kupsky W, et al. Superiority of [F-18]FLT-PET compared to FDG PET in assessing proliferative activity and tumor physiology in primary and recurrent intracranial gliomas. Neuro-Oncology 2001;3:345, Abstract 313.

117. Macdonald DR, Cascino TL, Schold SCJ, Cairncross JG. Response criteria for phase II studies of supratentorial malignant glioma. J Clin Oncol 1990;8:1277–1280.

118. Waniewski RA, Martin DL. Preferential utilization of acetate by astrocytes is attributable to transport. J Neurosci 1998;18:5225–5233.

119. Oldendorf WH. Clearance of radiolabeled substances by brain after arterial injection using a diffusible internal standard. In: Marks N, Rodnight R, eds. Research Methods in Neurochemistry, vol. 5. New York: Plenum Publishing Corporation, 1981:91–112.

120. Yoshimoto M, Waki A, Yonekura Y, et al. Characterization of acetate metabolism in tumor cells in relation to cell proliferation: acetate metabolism in tumor cells. Nucl Med Biol 2001;28:117–122.

121. Liu RS, Chang CP, Chu LS, et al. [C-11]acetate positron emission tomography in the detection of brain tumors: comparison with [F-18]fluorodeoxyglucose (abstract). J Nucl Med 1997;38 (suppl):240P.

122. DeGrado TR, Baldwin SW, Wang S, et al. Synthesis and evaluation of (18)F-labeled choline analogs as oncologic PET tracers. J Nucl Med 2001;42:1805–1814.

123. Hara T, Kondo T, Kosaka N. Use of 18F-choline and 11C-choline as contrast agents in positron emission tomography imaging-guided stereotactic biopsy sampling of gliomas. J Neurosurg 2003;99:474–479.

124. Ohtani T, Kurihara H, Ishiuchi S, et al. Brain tumour imaging with carbon-11 choline: comparison with FDG PET and gadolinium-enhanced MR imaging. Eur J Nucl Med 2001;28:1664–1670.

125. Shinoura N, Nishijima M, Hara T, et al. Brain tumors: detection with C-11 choline PET. Radiology 1997;202:497–503.

126. Yoshimoto M, Waki A, Yonekura Y, Fujibayashi Y. Acetate and choline as cell growth markers provide different perspectives of lipid synthesis. J Nucl Med 2001;42:275P.

127. Fredriksson A, Johnstrom P, Thorell JO, et al. In vivo evaluation of the biodistribution of 11C-labeled PD153035 in rats without and with neuroblastoma implants. Life Sci 1999;65:165–174.

128. Haubner R, Wester HJ, Weber WA, et al. Noninvasive imaging of alpha(v)beta3 integrin expression using 18F- labeled RGD-containing glycopeptide and positron emission tomography. Cancer Res 2001;61: 1781–1785.

129. Belhocine T, Steinmetz N, Hustinx R, et al. Increased uptake of the apoptosis-imaging agent 99mTc recombinant human annexin V in human tumors after one course of chemotherapy as a predictor of tumor response and patient prognosis. Clin Cancer Res 2002;8:2766–2774.

130. Spence AM, Mankoff DA, Muzi M. Positron emission tomography imaging of brain tumors. In: Meltzer CC, Drayer BP, eds. Neuroimaging Clinics North America, 13 (4), WB Saunders Co: Philadelphia. 2003:717–739.

131. Derlon JM, Chapon F, Noel MH, et al. Non-invasive grading of oligodendrogliomas: correlation between in vivo metabolic pattern and histopathology. Eur J Nucl Med 2000;27:778–787.

10 Magnetoencephalography

Michael P. Steinmetz, Jürgen Lüders, and Edward C. Benzel

Summary

Magnetoencephalography (MEG) combined with high-resolution magnetic resonance imaging (MRI) provides valuable insight into the dichotomy of structure and function. Information may be obtained quickly and noninvasively. Decisions may then be made prior to surgery regarding safety of surgical resection and/or determining the optimal surgical corridor. MEG and magnetic source imaging (MSI) may allow for maximum tumor resection and limit postoperative morbidity. In the future, MEG may be combined with other functional studies, such as fMRI, to provide a more complete picture of the brain's function relative to its anatomy.

Key Words: Magnetic source imaging; functional neurosurgery; image guided surgery; fMRI.

INTRODUCTION

Magnetoencephalography (MEG) is a noninvasive modality that is useful for the evaluation of brain function (1–5). By combining the anatomic information of high-resolution magnetic resonance imaging (MRI) to the functional data of MEG, a high-resolution, case-by-case map of brain function with respect to anatomy may be obtained. This is referred to as magnetic source imaging (MSI). MSI is useful in neurosurgical practice when preoperative planning is dependent upon the accurate determination of the location of functional or regions of eloquence (6). These eloquent regions are often distorted by pathology; therefore, it is critical to locate these areas in determining patient management (i.e., conservative treatment vs surgery) and to maximize resection without encroachment on eloquent regions. MSI also is valuable for the identification of epileptic foci and can provide insight into brain physiology and plasticity.

Just as electric current flow within a wire produces a surrounding magnetic field, current flow in neurons also produces a corresponding magnetic field (4). These fields may be detected and recorded and serve as the basis of MEG. Mathematical algorithms can then provide inferences on the three-dimensional (3D) spatial location of activated brain regions and the temporal sequence of activation of these regions.

Other functional imaging modalities, such as functional MRI (fMRI), single-photon emission computed tomography (SPECT), and positron emission tomography (PET) add great insight into brain function, but are limited in their temporal and spatial resolution and in their reliance on brain metabolism and hemodynamics. MEG allows real-time (on the order of milliseconds) processing, whereas fMRI and PET are limited by hemodynamic changes,

From: *Current Clinical Oncology: High-Grade Gliomas: Diagnosis and Treatment*
Edited by: G. H. Barnett © Humana Press Inc., Totowa, NJ

which may take seconds *(7)*. As such, MEG provides a direct measure of brain electrophysiology, while fMRI, SPECT, and PET measure changes that are only secondarily linked to actual physiology. Furthermore, the exact nature of this coupling is not completely understood *(8)*. The limitations of fMRI and PET may be especially true in the presence of high-grade gliomas (HGG) because of alterations in vasculature.

MEG METHODOLOGY

The extracranial magnetic field measured by MEG reflects postsynaptic intracellular current flow within the apical dendrites of pyramidal cells oriented parallel to the skull surface *(7)*. The resultant magnetic signal is typically very small. It is estimated that at least 30,000 neurons need to be simultaneously activated for the detection of extracranial fields *(9)*. Advanced technology is required to allow detection of this signal and ignore the significant background magnetic "noise."

The biomagnetometer is the device used to measure the neuromagnetic signal. It is usually configured as an axial gradiometer, typically consisting of two interconnected induction coils wound in opposition and separated by a few centimeters. The coils are in a superconducting state. This configuration allows the measurement of the spatial gradient of the magnetic field rather than the magnitude of the field *per se (4)*. It essentially renders the magnetometer insensitive to far field noise (e.g., power lines, and very sensitive to generated "nearby signals"). Another aid in decreasing background noise is the placement of the biomagnetometer in a magnetically shielded room. This room is typically made of a magnetically permeable material. Magnetic signal generated outside the room do not pass into the room, rather they flow through the walls of the chamber, around and away from the biomagnetometer.

The output device for the biomagnetometer is a SQUID (superconducting quantum interference device). The SQUID acts as a high-gain, low-noise, current-to-voltage converter that provides the output for the sensor system *(1,7)*. The voltage output of the SQUID can be made proportional to the magnetic field sensed *(10)*, and thus magnify the recorded signal. Figure 1 demonstrates a summary of the basic principals of MEG.

In order to localize in the magnetic signals that are changing in space and time, multiple sensors are needed. Sensor coils in a spherical cap are used to surround the head and thereby enable the sampling of a large volume.

Inferring the intracranial generators of measured extracranial magnetic signals is a "computationally illposed inverse problem; that is, not having a unique solution in absence of additional constraints" *(10)*. Modeling strategies have been developed to assist with this problem. The simplest model is the single equivalent current dipole description. The neuronal current distribution is modeled at each instant in time as a single current element enclosed within a sphere of uniform conducting tissue *(10)*. By assuming spherical symmetry, the differing electrical conductivity of the brain and skull may be ignored. This is problematic for source localization with electroencephalogram (EEG) where differing conductivities alter the recorded signal. The magnitude of the modeled magnetic field at the sensor position is compared with the observed signals, and a least-squares optimization procedure is performed *(10)*. This yields a focal source characterized by location, magnitude, and dipole orientation. This source may then be combined with high resolution MRI and provide anatomic localization of the functional anatomic area (MSI). The aforementioned modeling strategy is generally effective for the localization of certain brain activities such as movement of the digits of the hand, but it does not describe complex task paradigms or events occurring after the stimulus. Also, it does not provide temporal information. Multiple signal classification (MUSIC) algorithm

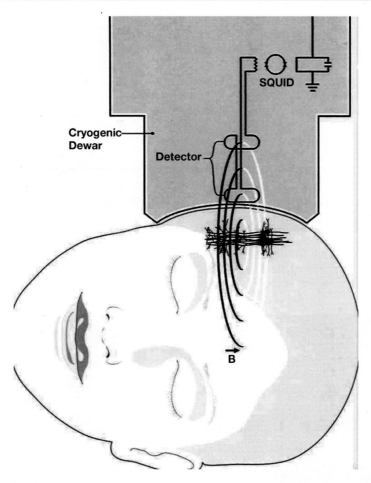

Fig. 1. Basic principles of MEG. Electrical activity in neurons generates a magnetic field, which may be read by the detector system. SQUID allows the signal to be magnified *(3)*.

(11,12) and magnetic field tomography (MFT) *(13,14)* incorporate this intrinsic information into improved source descriptions *(10)*.

The protocol for recording sensory evoked field (SEF) and motor evoked field (MEF) differs somewhat, depending on the imaging center performing the study. SEFs may be measured by delivering painless somatosensory stimulation using a compressed air-driven diaphragm attached to the fingertips, lips, and toes. In general, this provides a somatotopic representation of the sensory humunculs (Fig. 2). Alternatively, the median and/or the tibial nerve(s) may be electrically stimulated. Stimulation is applied for a set duration at psuedoradom interstimulus intervals. Epochs are recorded, including prestimulus time points to obtain baseline activity. The MEG epochs are averaged and filtered to improve signal-to-noise ratio. The single equivalent dipole (SED) model is used to identify the presumed neuronal source (see above). The SED that provides the strongest signal and best satisfies the model within the poststimulus range from 30 to 70 msec is chosen to represent the neuronal source *(15)*.

MEFs may be performed by brisk flexion movements of the index finger contralateral to the lesion every 3 to 5 s (Fig. 3). The MEF epochs beginning 2 s before and 1 s after movement onset are averaged after visual inspection and artifact rejection using the rectified surface

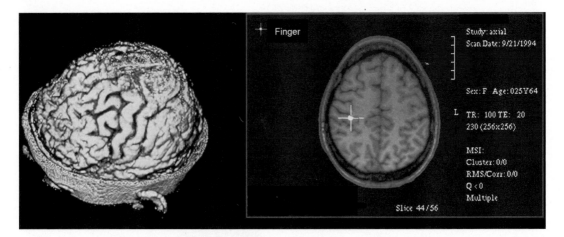

Fig. 2. Stimulation of the finger allows measurement of sensory evoked fields in the contralateral primary sensory cortex. Coregistration with high-resolution MRI (magnetic source imaging) permits identification of the postcentral gyrus, which may be traced on the 3D rendered image.

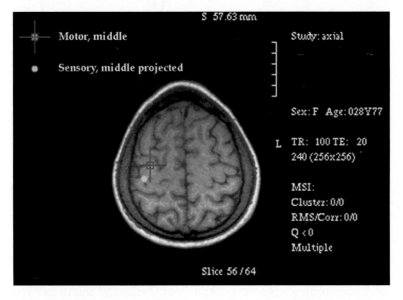

Fig. 3. MEFs may be measured by flexion and extension of the contralateral finger(s). Following coregistration with MRI the precentral sulcus may be identified. This may be combined with SEFs and the central region completely defined.

electromyogram (EMG) *(16)*. MEG dipoles are localized for the first pronounced peak in the MEF waveform. To accept a source localization (MEF and SEF), data-model correlations with greater than 98%, and a minimum of 95%, statistical confidence volume are required *(15)*.

Regardless of the data acquisition technique, the MEG derived source is co-registered with high-resolution MRIs. Anatomic landmarks and/or scalp fiducial markers along with electrical markers are used for this co-registration process. Estimates of error with the registration process are on the order of 4 mm. Thus, whereas MSI offers a temporal resolution of less than 1 ms, the practical spatial resolving power of sources ranges from 4 to 10 mm *(10)*.

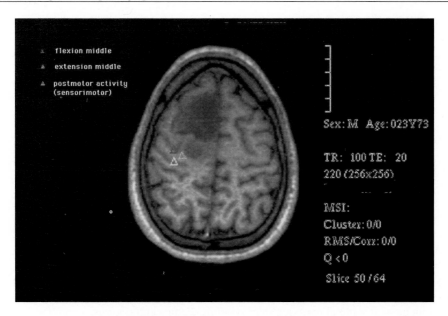

Fig. 4. MSI of a patient with a right frontal tumor. Prior to the MEG, the surgeon felt the tumor was involving the primary motor cortex and therefore surgical resection was too risky. MEG clearly demonstrated that the tumor only abuted the precentral gyrus making gross total resection possible.

CLINICAL APPLICATIONS

Pre-Surgical Mapping

MSI is ideal for the preoperative, noninvasive identification of eloquent brain regions. (Figs. 2 and 3) This information may aid in maximizing surgical resection while minimizing the case of any potential postoperative functional deficits. Furthermore, the knowledge gleaned may significantly aid in the clinical decision-making process (Fig. 4). The surgeon may discover that a tumor involves the functional cortex, such as sensorimotor and/or language areas , thus making resection too dangerous (Fig. 5). Biopsy and radiation may then be undertaken, if appropriate, rather than surgical resection or an "awake" technique utilized for intraoperative mapping. Alberstone et al. reported MSI in 26 patients with intracranial mass lesions *(6)*. In two of these patients surgery was not offered because of lesion location within functional cortex.

Brain tumors have been shown to potentially contain functional activity *(6,17)*. Knowledge of this activity preoperatively most certainly alters a surgical plan, solely based on anatomy. Preoperative MEG studies have demonstrated functional cortex located within radiographically defined tumors. Schiffbauer et al. found functional activity in 17% of grade III tumors and in 8% of grade IV tumors *(17)*. With this information preoperatively, a tailored surgical resection may be planned to spare the functional tissue.

Traditionally, anatomic studies such as MRI or intraoperative surgical navigation are used to tailor resection based on an "assumption" regarding the location of eloquent cortex. It has been demonstrated that it may be difficult to accurately localize eloquent regions on MRI. Furthermore, the pathology may further distort the anatomy (as well as physiology) and this may make it even more difficult to identify eloquent cortex by visualization alone. Sobel et al. *(18)* compared MSI with the visual inspection of anatomic MRIs for identifying the central

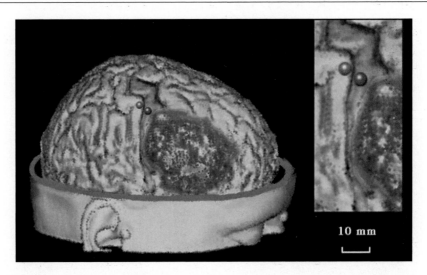

Fig. 5. 3D MSI model in a patient with a large right frontal lobe tumor. The tumor appears to be invading the primary motor cortex making complete resection impossible without compromising motor function. The patient underwent subtotal resection thus avoiding the precentral gyrus.

sulcus. The study demonstrated that the visual interpretation of MRIs may be inaccurate regarding the localization of the central sulcus; visual interpretation with MSI was accurate. This observation was especially true in a case where there was distortion resulting from the tumor. MEG, on the other hand, was readily able to identify functional regions, even in the face of anatomic distortion due to tumor (Fig. 6). In three patients reported by Alberstone et al., MSI correctly identified displacement of functional cortex *(6)*. In two cases, the somatosensory cortex was displaced posteriorly, whereas in one the auditory cortex was shifted posterior.

MEG/MSI may also be used to preoperatively determine the safest surgical corridor for tumors involving the central region. For example, a frontal approach rather than a posterior one may be chosen to avoid functional cortex. Alberstone et al. illustrated a case in which surgery was performed using a cone, despite contradictory information gained from a preoperative MSI study *(6)*. The patient developed a postoperative neurologic deficit that may have been avoided if the MEG information would have been utilized in planning the surgical approach.

Accuracy of MEG/MSI

Gallen et al. assessed MSI for the identification of the central sulcus, surgical risk, and to help determine the best operative approach *(19)*. All MSI identified points were found to be in agreement with intraoperative mapping. The standard deviation (SD) was determined to be around 6 mm. In localizing structures such as the pre or post-central sulcus, this uncertainty is acceptable.

Schiffbauer et al., quantitively compared MSI and electrophysiological cortical mapping (ECM) *(15)*. They found the distance between two corresponding points determined using MSI and ECM was 12.5 mm for somatosensory–somatosensory and 19mm for somatosensory–motor comparisons. The 6.5-mm increase in size separation was demonstrated in the antero-posterior direction. The authors concluded that preoperative MSI and intraoperative ECM show a favorable degree of quantitative correlation.

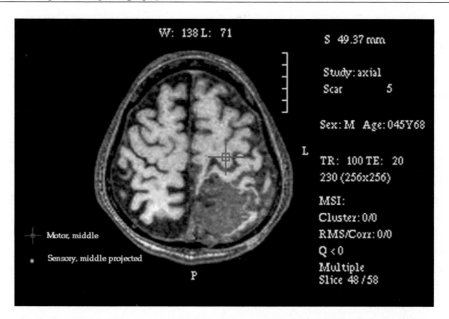

W: 138 L: 71

S 49.37 mm

Study: axial
Scar   5

Sex: M Age: 045Y68

TR: 100 TE: 20
230 (256x256)

MSI:
Cluster: 0/0
RMS/Corr: 0/0
Q < 0
Multiple
Slice 48 / 58

L

Motor, middle
Sensory, middle projected

P

Fig. 6. A large left parietal tumor has resulted in anterior displacement of the sensorimotor cortex. MEG correctly localized the primary motor and sensory cortices despite the displacement.

As discussed earlier, MEG is excellent at identifying the central sulcus, even when displaced by tumor. MSI correctly located functional regions in 3 of 26 patients when displaced by tumor *(6)*. Furthermore, it is highly reliable in identifying the postcentral gyrus. Using intraoperative cortical stimulation and/or cortical somatosensory evoked potentials, sources of somatosensory evoked fields correctly identified the postcentral gyrus is all patients as reported by Makela et al. *(20)*. It correctly identified the postcentral gyrus in 97% of cases in the report by Kober et al. *(16)*.

MEG is also able to reliably identify the precentral gyrus, although not as accurately as the postcentral gyrus. In the report by Kober et al., the central sulcus could only be correctly identified in 79% of cases by utilizing MEF *(16)*. This may result from the complex nature of the motor evoked field or difficulties with task performance. In patients presenting with a motor deficit, the MEG of motor responses may not be technically feasible in as many as 21% of cases *(16)*. In most situations, location of the central sulcus using sensory evoked fields should be sufficient. Although, identifying the precentral gyrus is useful in cases in which the central sulcus is not clearly visible due to tumor *(16)*.

Recently, MSI and MEG research have been extended to noninvasive identification of speech laterality and localization of speech centers. Sequential source-modeling of the late latency evoked field permits language laterality to be estimated and is largely consistent with Wada testing *(21)*. There has also been concordance noted with source localization of the late field activity and intraoperative mapping of language areas *(22)*. Future work will likely expand language localization and perhaps curtail or even avoid the need for intraoperative mapping.

The aforementioned studies have shown that it is often possible to localize functional areas in order to optimize a safe surgical resection in areas of eloquence. Intraoperative mapping with electrical stimulation is the gold standard; however, this adds time, cost, and potentially morbidity. MSI is noninvasive and has been shown to be comparable to electrical stimulation *(23)*. Furthermore, it may also be used as an adjunct to intraoperative cortical stimulation. By utilizing the preoperative MSI data on motor, sensory, and/or speech data, the size of craniotomy, and time required to perform intraoperative cortical stimulation may be significantly lessened.

Intraoperative Neuronavigation

The data obtained from MEG may be incorporated into a 3D neuronavigation system and used to aid in safe tumor removal *(24,25)*. Intraoperative decisions may be made regarding extent of tumor resection and in chosing the optimal surgical corridor. Firsching et al. reported their experience using MEG navigation in 30 patients with space occupying lesions around the central region *(24)*. Sensory evoked fields were identified in all patients preoperatively and superimposed on MRIs in their navigation workstation. Somatosensory evoked potentials were also used intraoperatively to locate the somatosensory cortex (phase-reversal technique). MEG agreed with phase reversal in all patients and permitted gross-total lesion resection in 28 patients and partial resection in 2 patients with gliomas. Following surgery, motor deficit improved in seven patients, was unchanged in five, and demonstrated a transient worsening in five. One patient had a worsened motor examination that failed to completely recover. The authors concluded that MEG-based neuronavigation is practical and safe for approaching tumors located or near the central region.

LIMITATIONS

The main limitation is the amount of confidence placed in the resolving power of MSI (i.e., resolution related error). The hardware contribution to this error is decreasing because of the development of detector arrays with greater than 100 channels and improved detector coils. The software or modeling contribution, however, may be large. Many sources may be simultaneously active, as opposed to a single source, and single-current dipole modeling at times may not be adequate. MUSIC and the MFT algorithms have been developed to address this type of situation and will likely decrease modeling error.

Further limitations exist when MEG/MSI is combined with neuronavigation. The navigation system's registration error must be included in the overall error of functional navigation. Moreover, the well-documented "brain-shift" phenomenon that occurs during craniotomy and limits modern neuronavigation systems must also be factored into the overall spatial resolutions of the study.

CONCLUSIONS

Magnetoencephalography combined with high-resolution MRI provides valuable insight into the dichotomy of structure and function. The information gleaned is valuable in that it is noninvasive, and is obtained relatively quickly. Preoperative decisions may be made based on functional information. For example, a surgical resection may be deemed too risky if the lesion involves eloquent areas such as the primary motor cortex or speech areas. Decisions may also be made regarding the safest surgical corridor for resection. Incorporating MEG data into neuronavigation allows the surgeon to use functional data for intraoperative decision making. Taken together, MEG/MSI may then allow maximum tumor resection and limit postoperative morbidity. In the future, MEG may be combined with other functional studies, such as fMRI, to provide a more complete picture of the brain's function relative to its anatomy.

ACKNOWLEDGMENT

The authors thank Dr. Ali Rezai for supplying the clinical images used in this chapter.

REFERENCES

1. Benzel EC, Lewine JD, Bucholz RD et al. Magnetic source imaging: a review of the Magnes system of biomagnetic technologies incorporated. Neurosurgery 1993;33:252–259.
2. Hamalainen M, Hari R, llmoniemi RE, et al. Magnetoencephalography: theory, instrumentation, and applications to noninvasive studies of the working brain. Rev Mod Physics 1993;65:413–498.
3. Lewine JD. Neuromagnetic techniques for the noninvasive analysis of brain function. In: Freeman SE, Fukushima E, Green ER, eds. Noninvasive Techniques in Biology and Medicine. San Francisco: San Francisco Press, 1990;33–74.
4. Lewine JD, Benzel EC, Baldwin NG, Orrison WW. Magnetoencephalography. In: Wilkins R, Rengachary S, eds. Neurosurgery, 2nd Ed. New York: McGraw-Hill, 1996;253–258.
5. Sato S. Magnetoencephalography. Adv Neurol 1990;54:1–284.
6. Alberstone CD, Skirboll SL, Benzel EC, et al. Magnetic source imaging and brain surgery: presurgical and intraoperative planning in 26 patients. J Neurosurg 2000;92:79–90.
7. Lewine JD, Orrison WW. Magnetic source imaging: basic principles and applications in neuroradiology. Acad Radiol 1995;2:436–440.
8. Kaufman L, Williamson SJ. Magnetic location of cortical activity. Ann NY Acad Sci 1982;388:197–213.
9. Williamson SJ, Kaufman L. Evolution of neuromagnetic topographic mapping. Brain Topogr 1990;3: 113–127.
10. Roberts TPL, Poeppel D, Rowley HA. Magnetoencephalography and magnetic source imaging. Neuropsychiatry Neuropsychol Behav Neurol 1998;11:49–64.
11. Mosher JC, Lewis PS, Leahy RM. Multiple dipole modeling and localization from spatio-temporal MEG data. IEEE Trans Biomed Eng 1992;39:541–557.
12. Sekihara K, Poeppel D, Marantz A, et al. Noise covariance incorporated MEG-MUSIC algorithm: A method for multiple-dipole estimation tolerant of the influence of background brain activity. IEEE Trans Biomed Eng 1997;44:839–847.
13. Ioannides AA. Brain function as revealed by current density analysis of magnetoencephalograpy signals. Physiol Meas 1993;14(suppl 4A):A75–A80.
14. Ioannides AA, Singh KD, Hasson R, et al. Comparison of single current dipole and magnetic field tomography analyses of the cortical response to auditory stimuli. Brain Topogr 1993;6:27–34.
15. Schiffbauer H, Berger MS, Ferrari P, Freudenstein D, Rowley HA, Roberts TPL. Preoperative magnetic source imaging for brain tumor surgery: a quantitative comparison with intraoperative sensory and motor mapping. J Neurosurg 2002;97:1333–1342.
16. Kober H, Nimsky C, Moller M, Hastreiter P, Fahlbusch R, Ganslandt O. Correlation of sensorimotor activation with functional magnetic resonsance imaging and magnetoencepahlography in presurgical functional imaging: a spatial analysis. Neuroimage 2001;14:1214–1228.
17. Schiffbauer H, Ferrari P, Rowley HA, Berger MS, Roberts TPL. Functional activity within brain tumors: a magnetic source imaging study. Neurosurgery 2001;49:1313–1322.
18. Sobel DF, Gallen CC, Schwartz BJ, et al. Locating the central sulcus: comparison of MR anatomic and magnetoencephalography. Am J Neuroradiol 1993;14:915–925.
19. Gallen CC, Sobel DF, Waltz T, et al. Noninvasive presurgical neuromagnetic mapping of somatosensory cortex. Neurosurgery 1993;33:260–268.
20. Makela JP, Kirveskari E, Seppa M, et al. Three-dimensional integration of brain anatomy and function to facilitate intraoperative navigation around the sensorimotor strip. Hum Br Map 2001;12:180–192.
21. Szymanski MD, Rowley HA, Roberts TPL. A hemispherically asymmetrical MEG response to vowels. Neuroreport 1999;10:2481–2486.
22. Roberts TPL, Ferrari P, Perry D, et al. Presurgical mapping with magnetic source imaging: comparisons with intraoperative findings. Brain Tumor Pathol 2000;17:57–64.
23. Gallen C, Schwartz BJ, Bucholz RD, et al. Presurgical localization of functional cortex using magnetic source imaging. J Neurosurg 1995;82:988–994.
24. Firsching R, Bondar I, Heinze HJ, et al. Practibility of magnetoencephalography-guided neuronavigation. Neurosurg Rev 2002;25:73–78.
25. Jannin P, Morandi X, Fleig OJ, Le Rumeur E, Toulouse P, Gibaud B, Scarabin JM. Integration of sulcal and functional information for multimodal neuronavigation. J Neurosurg 2002;96:713–723.

IV Management

11 General Considerations

Glen H. J. Stevens

Summary

The discipline of neuro-oncology has developed to allow the integration of complex care required for brain tumor patients. Patients with brain tumors suffer emotional and physical disabilities and often die of their disease over a short period of time. During that time they are faced with multiple treatment decisions often involving many disciplines. Patients may suffer from seizures, blood clots, and the effects of chronic steroid use. Further, they also take multiple medications that are likely to interact and lead to additional concerns. This chapter will deal with many of these common problems and provide practical solutions for a physician looking after brain tumor patients. Issues regarding antiepileptic drug use, driving restrictions, steroids use, fatigue, blood clots, and alternative therapy will be reviewed in detail so that the care of the brain tumor patient can be improved.

Key Words: Glioma; brain tumor; steroids; seizures; fatigue; blood clots; osteoporosis; alternative therapy.

BRAIN TUMORS AND SEIZURES

It has long been known that an association between brain tumors and seizure activity exists. As far back as 1882, Hughlings Jackson *(1)* noted seizures and epilepsy in patients with primary brain tumors. Penfield et al. *(2)*, in 1940 found seizure rates as high as 37% in glioblastoma multiforme (GBM) patients. It was also shown many years ago that tumor location could influence seizure activity. Tumors found in the primary motor and somatosensory cortex, are strongly associated with seizures but that may partly be the result of ease of diagnosis compared with seizures originating elsewhere. Other high-risk areas include the rest of the frontal lobe, temporal lobe, and perirolandic region *(3)*. It should be noted that seizures are a common presenting symptom in many low-grade tumors and that seizure frequency for the primary gliomas is inversely related to their malignancy (i.e., low-grade tumors are more likely to present with seizures) *(4)*. Seizure activity is thought to be neuronal in nature and hence, gliomas must somehow exert effects on neurons to cause seizure activity. Some tumors, such as dysembryoplastic neuroectodermal tumors and gangliogliomas, have neuronal elements within them and may cause seizures directly. Seizure mechanisms of action include alterations in synaptic connections, ion concentrations, neurotransmitters, or neuromodulators that increase excitability *(5)*. As will be discussed later, drugs that prevent second or third seizures may not prevent the first seizure. Using the Central Brain Tumor Registry of the United States (CBTRUS) *(6)*, which pooled brain tumor data between 1997 and 2001, it was estimated that 41,130 new cases of primary benign and malignant brain tumors would be diagnosed in 2004 *(6)*. There are also at least 170,000 brain metastases diagnosed per yr *(7)*.

From: *Current Clinical Oncology: High-Grade Gliomas: Diagnosis and Treatment*
Edited by: G. H. Barnett © Humana Press Inc., Totowa, NJ

It has been estimated that from 20 to 40% (62,000) of all brain tumor patients will have experienced at least one seizure prior to diagnosis and in those patients the need for anticonvulsant medication is rarely in question *(8)*.

Seizure Prophylaxis

Of patients who have not yet had a seizure, it is presumed that they are at risk and 20 to 45% (45,000) of those patients will eventually have a seizure *(8)*. Should we be treating those 145,000 patients prophylactically? In a study evaluating antiepileptic drug (AED) use in Rhode Island, 113 physicians from various disciplines (neurologists, oncologists, radiation oncologist, and neurosurgeons) were questioned about their practice. In newly diagnosed brain tumor patients, 55% of physician's routinely prescribed prophylactic AEDs. Most neurosurgeons did (81%) and most radiation oncologists did not (67%) *(9)*. To further address this issue, in 1999 the American Academy of Neurology pooled all the available data on AED use and brain tumors. The Quality Standards Subcommittee produced the following *(10)*:

AMERICAN ACADEMY OF NEUROLOGY POSITION STATEMENT

The subcommittee evaluated 12 studies that examined the ability of prophylactic AED use to prevent first seizure in newly diagnosed brain tumor patients. Four studies provided what was felt to be Class 1 type evidence and these trials then underwent a meta-analysis. The following recommendations were made:

"1. In patients with newly diagnosed brain tumors, anticonvulsant medications are not effective in preventing first seizures. Because of their lack of efficacy and their potential side effects, prophylactic anticonvulsants should not be used routinely in patients with newly diagnosed brain tumors (standard)."

"2. In patients with brain tumors who have not had a seizure, tapering and discontinuing anticonvulsants after the first postoperative week is appropriate, particularly in those patients who are medically stable and who are experiencing anticonvulsant-related side effects (guideline)."

In the meta-analysis, the issue of brain tumors, AED use, and driving was not adequately addressed and hence no specific recommendations were made. At this point each state determines driving restrictions for patients who have had seizures and will be reviewed in the next section.

Driving and Epilepsy

In the early 20th century when driver's licenses became common in the United States (US), people with epilepsy were excluded. In 1949, Wisconsin was the first state in the US permitting people with epilepsy to drive and specified a seizure free interval (SFI) of 2 yr. By 1987 Wisconsin had reduced the SFI to 3 mo *(11)*. The Marshfield Clinic completed a retrospective study comparing the accident rate of people with epilepsy and diabetes, to age matched controls in the same zip codes. The standardized accident rate for the diabetes group was 1.32; for the epilepsy group 1.33; and for the epilepsy group <25 yr old 1.79 *(12)*.

For brain tumor patients, seizures are only one of several factors that could define their ability to drive. Inability to drive can have a significant impact on a patient's quality of life and also their ability to maintain employment. "When can I drive?" is one of the most commonly asked questions in the brain tumor outpatient clinic. The answer to this question is not easily attained and is dependent on the state in which the patient resides. A consensus conference of the American Academy of Neurology, American Epilepsy Society, and the Epilepsy

Table 1
Favorable and Unfavorable Modifiers For Accessing Seizure Risk

Favorable Modifiers

- Seizures during medically directed medication change.
- Simple partial seizures that do not interfere with consciousness and/or motor control.
- Seizures with consistent and prolonged auras .
- Sleep deprived seizures.
- Established pattern of pure nocturnal seizures.
- Seizures related to acute illnesses that are not likely to recur.

Unfavorable modifiers

- Noncompliance with medication or lack of credibility.
- Increased number of seizures within 1 yr.
- Structural brain lesion such as a tumor.
- Alcohol or drug abuse within past 3 mo.
- Prior crashes caused by seizures in the last 5 yr.
- No correctable brain functional or metabolic condition.
- Frequent seizures after a seizure-free interval.

Foundation of America took place from May 31 to June 2, 1991 in Washington, D.C. Also included in this meeting were experts from the Department of Motor Vehicles (DMV), members of state Medical Advisory Boards (MAB), and people with epilepsy *(13)*. It was felt that the licensing decision should be made by the state DMV, not the treating physician, and that straightforward cases could be made independently by first level DMV staff. The treating physician should provide appropriate factual data and the opportunity to offer an opinion of licensure should they desire. The process should allow individual consideration and have an appeal process. A SFI of 3 mo was recommended starting from the date of the last seizure and should have associated favorable and unfavorable modifiers that could alter the interval (Table 1; not an inclusive list).

There was also unanimous agreement that patients should self-report and that physicians not be required to report to the DMV. It was also felt that there should be physician immunity for reporting and not reporting. A medical advisory board should exist in each state, the patient should be able to have voluntary license surrendering, and an appeal board should exist.

If we look at what the practice is 10 yr after the consensus meeting, it would appear that not much consensus had taken place. In a review by Krauss et al. *(14)* the seizure-free window for driving was not specified in ten states, including Ohio. A 3-mo interval was noted in 11 states, 6-mo in 18 states, 12-mo in 10 states and Washington, DC. Florida was the most rigid state with a 24-mo SFI policy.

In 1994 the SFI in Arizona was reduced from 12 to 3 mo. Motor vehicle crash reports from 3 yr before and after the change were reviewed. Overall, the crash rate secondary to seizures was small at <0.04% of all crashes. Seizures did account for 30% of all medically related crashes. There was no increase in seizure related crash rates *(15)*. Interestingly, only between 27 and 54% of patients with epilepsy report their seizures to the DMV. It is the physician's responsibility to raise the issue of driving with patients *(16)*. Patients driving behavior was evaluated in a prospective multicenter study (6 centers in the East and 1 in the Midwest) comprised of 367 patients ≥20 yr old undergoing presurgical evaluation for refractory epilepsy *(17)*. Sixty-five percent of patients reported having had a driver's license at some time during their seizure history and 37% had a current driver's license. Thirty-one percent had driven within the year and 27% had an accident resulting from a seizure. The probability of a male in his 20s driving within the year with a valid driver's license was 90%, whereas the probability of a patient in his/her 50s who had never had a valid driver's license was 2%.

Krauss et al. *(16)* completed a retrospective case control study of crash rates for seizure patients at Johns Hopkins University and the University of Maryland epilepsy clinic. The study was for the 12-mo preceding the study onset for crashes from mid-1996 to mid-1997 for controls. Clinical data was collected from chart reviews and phone interviews. They found that patients that were greater than 1-yr seizure free reduced the odds of an accident by 93%. For individuals seizure free ≥6 mo the odds were reduced by 85%. A 3-mo seizure-free period did not result in a significant reduction in automobile accidents.

For brain tumor patients, it is difficult to know how the existing data really relates to them as a group. At this point physicians should follow the rules of their state. It is important to always document discussions in the patient's medical record regarding driving and it is recommended that this be done with the first contact after a seizure.

Choice of Antiepileptic Drug

The two National Cancer Institute supported consortiums (New Approaches to Brain Tumor Therapy (NABTT) and North American Brain Tumor Consortium (NABTC)), are involved with evaluating new chemotherapeutic drugs in phase I and phase II clinical trials. Many AEDs may either induce or inhibit liver enzymes, thereby affecting other drugs (such as chemotherapy) metabolized in the liver. It is important then to determine the pharmacokinetics of chemotherapeutics so that appropriate doses can be used to assess clinical efficacy. Therefore, avoiding AEDs that are metabolized in the liver seems reasonable when possible. Table 2 shows a list of the current AEDs and their interaction with hepatic enzymes.

Within the past 10 yr, nine new AEDs have been introduced into the US market place increasing the choices for patients by approx 200% *(22)*. Although this increase causes confusion based on an apparent wealth of riches it also allows the physician to tailor treatment for specific groups of patients. Treatment decisions may be more important in the brain tumor population where individuals are often on multiple medications. One of the major differences between the "newer" and "older" AEDs is the potential for fewer drug interactions resulting from loss of hepatic enzyme induction as listed in Table 2. It should also be kept in mind that many of these drug–drug interactions are reciprocal.

HEPATIC P-450 SYSTEM

Drug metabolism is perhaps the most important mechanism by which drugs are eliminated in the body. Certain newer AEDs, such as Levetiracetam, are excreted essentially unchanged in the urine, but for most of the older AEDs, steroids, and chemotherapeutics, liver metabolism is critical. The cytochrome P-450 system or CYP is the main pathway of degradation for many substances *(23)*. Because many drugs are degraded by shared components of the CYP system, interactions are bound to happen. At least 12 CYP gene families have been identified with CYP 1, 2, and 3 involved in most drug metabolism. CYP are large heme-containing proteins that have substrate binding properties. They are located throughout the body but those most important for drug metabolism are located in the endoplasmic recticulum (ER) of the cyto-

Table 2

Group A—Anticonvulsants that induce hepatic metabolic enzymes	
Generic name	Trade name
Phenytoin	Dilantin
Carbamazepine	Tegretol
Phenobarbital	Phenobarbital
Primidone	Mysoline
Oxcarbazepine	Trileptal

Group B— Anticonvulsants that cause modest or no induction of hepatic metabolic enzymes	
Generic name	Trade name
Gabapentin	Neurontin
Lamotrigine	Lamictal
Valproic acid	Depakote, Depakene
Felbamate	Felbatol
Levetiracetam	Keppra
Tiagibine	Gabatril
Topiramate	Topamax
Zonisamide	Zonegram
Pregabalin	Lyrica

plasm of cells found in the gastrointestinal tract and liver. The isoforms CYP1A2, CYP2CP, CYP2C19, CYP2D6 and CYP3A4 are the most important for metabolism. Furthermore, it has been shown that up to 50% of all drugs are metabolized by the CYP3A4 system alone *(24)*. This is the most important system for most AED and chemotherapeutic drug metabolism. Interestingly, dexamethasone also induces CYP3A4. If patients were given both phenytoin (PHT) and dexamethasone (both inducers of the hepatic CYP system), the result would be lower serum levels of PHT for a given dose. Because PHT has nonlinear kinetics it would not be unusual for individuals on PHT and dexamethasone to become PHT toxic if the steroids are weaned and to become sub-therapeutic if the steroids are increased. We will look at camptotecin analogs as an example of AED-chemotherapy interaction. Irinotecan is metabolized by CYP3A4. In a recent trial looking at the pharmacokinetics of Irinotecan in adults with recurrent malignant glioma, it was noted that the maximal tolerated dose (MTD) was 3.5× greater for patients concurrently receiving a hepatic enzyme inducing AED *(25)*. The MTD for the hepatic enzyme induced group was 411 mg/m^2/wk and 117mg/m^2/wk for the group not on enzyme inducing AED. Similar results were seen in a trial by Fetell et al. *(26)* who found the MTD for paclitaxel given to glioblastoma patients to be 140 mg/m^2 in the nonhepatic enzyme inducing group, and 200 mg/m^2 in hepatic enzyme inducing group. On the other side of this is valproic acid (VPA), which is an enzyme inhibiting AED. Studies have shown toxic levels of chemotherapeutics resulting in increased bone marrow toxicity with individuals on VPA and cisplatin, etoposide, and nitrosoureas *(27)*.

ANTIEPILEPTIC DRUGS AND OSTEOPOROSIS

An unusual noted side effect of AEDs has been their potential effects on mineral density. A study by Kubata et al. *(28)*, performed bone density measurements (hip and spine) on 15 epileptic patients between the ages of 20 and 29 yr over a 7-yr period. The patients were most commonly on phenytoin or barbiturates. They reported a significant decrease in bone density over the 7-yr period. AED effects on bone density may be related to impaired vitamin D metabolism secondary to induced hepatic cytochrome P450 activity. As was discussed in the previous section on drug interactions, a similar situation occurs and results in decreased vitamin D through increased catabolism. It is also thought that 25 hydroxy-vitD is also affected resulting in decreased calcium absorption, secondary hyperparathyroidism, increased bone turnover, and a high rate of bone loss (29). In patients with high-grade malignant tumors, AED induced osteoporosis may be of less concern because of their limited life expectancy. However, with low-grade gliomas (LGG) this may become an issue of greater concern. In a recent study (30), women older than 65 yr taking AEDs had a 1.8-fold greater average rate of bone loss in the calcaneous than women not on AEDs and 1.7-fold greater average rate of loss at the hip over the 5.7 yr of the study. Whether brain tumor patients should be instructed to take supplements of vitamin D and calcium at this point is unknown. This patient population is also commonly on steroids which can hasten osteoporosis; therefore, this factor should also be taken into consideration when deciding whether to prophylax, for osteoporosis. Unless contraindicated, we will often recommend using supplements of calcium (1000–1500 mg/d) and vitamin D (400 IU/d).

Antiepileptic Drug Recommendations

If a patient does need to be on an AED, which medication should you chose? Because these patients are often on multiple medications and minimizing potential drug-to-drug interactions, as we have discussed, would be advantagous, there may be some benefit to using drugs which do not undergo hepatic metabolism (Table 2, class B). Wagner et al. (18) evaluated 26 brain tumor patients treated with Levetiracetam (LEV) which has little known effect on liver enzymes and has no protein binding (19). Eighteen patients with high-grade glioma (HGG) and 8 patients with LGG took part in the study. In 20 patients with persisting seizures, LEV produced a >50% reduction in seizure activity in 13 patients (67%). Of those 13 patients, 7 went on to be treated with monotherapy alone. Thirty-five percent of patients had mild side effects including dizziness, fatigue, and somnolence. One patient developed psychosis 4 wk into treatment and the drug was stopped. They concluded that the LEV may be a useful drug for brain tumor patients and that investigations into its use as monotherapy seemed reasonable. In a recent review of the pharmacokinetics of LEV in healthy volunteers, it was noted that 66% of LEV was excreted unchanged in the kidney, 24% was metabolized by hydrolysis of the acetamide group by a non-P450 dependent enzyme and that less than 2.5% was metabolized by the CYP enzymes (20). White et al. (21) recently reported on behavior problems that can be seen with patients taking levetiracetam. In their study of 553 patients, 38 of the patients (6.9%) discontinued LEV because of behavioral problems. Risk factors associated with LEV discontinuation included faster titration, history of psychiatric disorder, and diagnosis of symptomatic epilepsy. Our practice in general is to start (or convert) brain tumor patients that need AEDs to levetiracetam 500 mg bid for 1 wk then 1000 mg bid for 1 wk and finally 1500 mg bid. The choice of AED for any given patient should be individualized. Although more AEDs mean more options, well controlled clinical trials need to be completed to define which medications will best meet the means of brain tumor patients.

STEROIDS

Steroid use, its benefits and side effects, have been controversial since the 1960s when French first reported using them regularly in brain tumor patients (31,32). In the 1950s, while studying craniopharyngiomas, Ingraham noted a reduction in cerebral edema in patients using corticosteroids *(33)*. Dexamethasone (DMS) is a potent anti-inflammatory with a relative lack of mineralocorticoid activity. The DMS dose that the French empirically chose was 16 mg/d as this was the dose felt to give maximum clinical response. Renaudin et al. *(34)* escalated DMS dose to 96 mg/d and found some favorable responses and felt there were minimal complications encountered. There are no randomized controlled trials examining steroid use in malignant glioma patients. Despite this fact, it is common practice now to use DMS to decrease cerebral edema in glioma patients. The mechanism of action, however, remains controversial. Onishi *(35)* found that glucocorticoids exert their antiedema properties by acting directly on capillary endothelial cells, possibly through the inhibition of phophilipase A2 activity. Bodesch *(36)* studied operative tissue and found that both the water and electrolyte content of edematous tissue was reduced with dexamethasone. A positron emission tomography (PET) study by Jarden *(37)* looked at the time course of steroid action and found changes in brain tumor capillaries at 5 to 6 and 24 h, which may be responsible for some of the antiedema properties.

General concerns have been raised about the timing of steroid dose and how that might affect the interpretation of imaging. Buxton et al. *(38)* reported on a patient who initially had radiographic resolution of his tumor on contrasted computed tomography (CT) while on DMS 6 mg/d and was eventually diagnosed as a GBM by biopsy. These changes in enhancement related to steroid use are currently referred to as the "MacDonald Criteria" *(39)*. MacDonald and co-workers have reported on how steroid dose may affect interpretation of CT or magnetic resonance imaging (MRI) in malignant glioma patients. In an MRI study, ten symptomatic glioma patients were started on decadron 16 mg/d and underwent MRIs weekly. Interestingly, nine out of ten patients had a measurable reduction in the size of the gadolinium enhancing lesion or T2 signal. MRIs were reported as improved by the neuroradiologist in 7 out of 10 cases and cross-sectional tumor volume was decreased by at least 25% in 10 patients. Their recommendation was that patients who require increased steroid use for tumor progression that are going on a clinical trial should have a new MRI after a stable steroid dose of 2 wk duration which should serve as the baseline MRI. Failure to do this might increase the likelihood of false positive responses attributed by the investigational agent *(40)*. Similar findings were also found using CT scans, where 2 wk was the time period at which maximal steroid effect was seen *(41)*. Secondary to the above findings, the question of possible steroid antitumor effect on gliomas was raised. A study by Mackie et al. *(42)* using glioma cells suggested a cytostatic effect only without evidence for a cytotoxicity.

Another issue regarding steroids is their possible interaction with chemotherapeutic drugs and AEDs. Because decadron is a CYP3A4 inducer it can potentially affect other drugs that also undergo hepatic metabolism. If steroids act to decrease brain edema by affecting the blood–tumor and blood–brain barrier, then steroids might also affect the delivery of chemotherapeutic drugs to the central nervous system (CNS). Weller et al. *(43)* have gone so far as to recommend that, if possible, steroids be withdrawn from glioma patients so as to maximize the therapeutic effect of chemotherapy agents. It is common for patients on DMS to often require very high doses of phenytoin. Lachner *(44)* presented the case of a patient requiring >10 mg/kg/d of phenytoin to maintain therapeutic concentrations while on dexamethasone. Once the steroid was discontinued the phenytoin plasma level tripled. For these reasons, close monitoring of AED levels should be undertaken when drug interactions are known.

Steroid side effects have been well defined over time and usually worsen with higher dose and longer duration of use. Side effects include: weight gain, electrolyte disturbances, hyperglycemia, gastrointestinal irritation, osteoporosis, opportunistic infections (primarily *Can-*

dida but also *Pneumocistis carini* especially for those also on chemotherapy), thinning of skin, increased bruising, peripheral edema, vascular bone necrosis, insomnia, irritability, acne, cushingoid state, hypertension, and proximal myopathy *(45)*. Many of these effects are reversible with steroid reduction but they can cause serious quality of life issues. Because DMS has a long half-life, we generally recommend morning loading when possible to lessen some of the night-time side effects such as insomnia (i.e., for bid dosing we would recommend taking medication at breakfast and lunch instead of 8 AM and 8 PM). For steroid weaning we generally decrease DMS by 2 mg every 4 d as tolerated. It is important to emphasize to patients that steroid dosing is a mix of an art and science and that good doctor patient communication will allow the best care.

VENOUS THROMBOEMBOLISM

Venous thromboembolism (VTE) has long been known as a complication of cancer. Venous thromboembolisms are usually divided into deep venous thrombosis (DVT) and pulmonary embolism (PE). When DVTs affect the proximal veins of the lower extremities they are usually treated as a PE. We discuss VTE with all brain tumor patients at the initial consultation. Mechanism of action for VTE includes, venous stasis (immobility), intimal injury, and alterations in coagulation. In brain tumor patients, Sawaya et al. *(46)* has shown alterations in the fibrinolytic system and an underlying coagulopathy as causes of VTE. Other associations include age, prior DVT, smoking, oral contraceptives, and obesity. During surgery, brain tumor patients often have induced dehydration and hyperosmolality that increase the VTE risk. Malignant brain tumor patients have also been shown to display an increased risk of VTE with reports of upward of 28% of patients having symptomatic events *(47)*. At our institution we have a high index of suspicion for DVT and will order a duplex ultrasound on any suspected patient and on all postoperative patients on day three. The classic signs of DVT include calf pain, swelling, and erythema with a positive Homans sign (although all or none may be present). Approximately 25% of symptomatic patients that are investigated have a DVT *(48)*. A recent retrospective review at Johns Hopkins of 130 adult patients with gliomas found that 28% of patients developed VTE at a median of 4.8 mo after diagnosis *(49)*. Interestingly these patients were evaluated for VTE based on ABO blood group. The hazard ratios for thrombosis were 2.7 and 9.4 for patients with blood groups A ($p = 0.045$) and AB ($p < 0.0001$), respectively. A larger clinical trial is currently being conducted within the NABTT consortium validating these results. Data such as this might help define a subset of patients that should be treated prophylactically with anticoagulation. Management of VTE events includes prevention, pneumatic compression stockings, early mobilization, anticoagulation (coumadin, heparin, low-molecular-weight heparin), and an inferior vena cava (IVC) filter for patients that cannot be anticoagulated. In a recent trial from Goldhaber et al. *(50)*, they randomized 150 patients to enoxaparin 40 mg/d vs heparin 5000 U bid who were undergoing craniotomy for a brain tumor. All patients also received graduated compression stockings and intermittent pneumatic compression. The main outcome measure was DVT detected by venous ultrasound prior to hospital discharge. They reported no symptomatic DVTs or PE in any of the 150 patients. The overall rate of asymptomatic VTE was 9.3%, which was not different between the 2 groups. Ten of the 14 patients with DVT had deep calf involvement. They did not report any bleeding complications. For patients that develop a VTE and have an intracranial tumor there remain concerns about anticoagulation. Certain types of tumors are more prone to intracranial hemorrhage including renal cell carcinoma, melanoma, thyroid cancer, germ cell tumors, and choriocarcinomas *(51)*. Schiff and DeAngelis *(52)* reported on 3 of 42 metastatic patients with serious bleeding complications who were anticoagulated for VTE. In further review it was found that one patient received supratherapeutic doses of heparin and another patient who was on coumadin had a prothrombin time (PT) 4.8 times control. Several studies have examined anticoagulation in glioma patients. Ruff and Posner *(53)* reviewed 103 HGG patients on coumadin over 14 wk for VTE. There were two reported hemorrhages and one death. In 1990 Altschuler et al. *(54)* found no intracranial hemorrhagic events in 23 brain tumor patients over a 6-mo period. In that study, the PT was maintained at 1.25× control whereas in the Ruff study the PT was 2.5× control. Lastly, controversy exists about the use and efficacy of IVC filters. In a series of 42 brain tumor patients with IVC filters, Levin et al. *(47)* found that 26% had either filter or IVC thrombosis, 21% had a recurrent DVT, 9% developed a postphlebetic syndrome, and 12% had a recurrent pulmonary embolism.

Anticoagulation for brain tumor patients, especially those that have recently undergone craniotomy, makes all involved uneasy. Prevention, if possible, is the best strategy and for hospitalized patients we recommend compression stockings and early mobilization. For patients that require anticoagulation we recommend not giving a heparin bolus and for those that cannot be anticoagulated an IVC filter is an option.

FATIGUE

The neurologic disorder in which fatigue has been best evaluated is multiple sclerosis in which at least 78% of these patients suffer from fatigue and is often the most disabling symptom of this disease *(55)*. Similarly, in a study of over 1300 cancer patients, 58% of patients described problems with fatigue, yet less than 52% of those ever reported symptoms to their caregivers, and only 14% had received some type of treatment *(56)*. Perhaps the greatest obstacle to recognizing fatigue is in terms of definition as various health care professionals define fatigue differently based on their area of expertise. The most common complaint heard in our outpatient brain tumor clinic on a daily basis from patients, regardless of stage of treatment, is that they feel fatigue. This may be further defined as tiredness, exhaustion, muscle weakness, lethargy, or depression. Because fatigue can mean different things to physicians and patients it is imperative that the physician obtain a comprehensive history to better define what the patient is describing.

Treatment—General Considerations

- *Exercise:* this helps stimulate the appetite, maintain muscle mass.
- *Nutrition:* avoid refined sugars, which can alter blood glucose levels, that can cause fatigue as levels "spike" and then drop. Make sure hydration is adequate.
- *Limit caffeine and tobacco:* both of these act as CNS stimulants and can interfere with sleep.
- *Limit alcohol intake:* it is a CNS depressant, can affect other drugs metabolized in the liver and possibly affect seizure threshold.

No drugs have been approved by the Food and Drug Administration (FDA) for treatment of fatigue in brain tumor patients, however various medications have been used clinically over the years. Currently two clinical trials in brain tumor patients are looking at treating fatigue related problems (*http://www.clinicaltrials.gov*). The first trial is a "*Phase III Randomized trial of D-Methylphenidate To Improve Quality of Life in Patients Receiving Radiotherapy for Primary or Metastatic Brain Tumor.*" This is a placebo controlled trial. The second trial is a "*Pilot Randomized Study of Modafanil for Treatment of Fatigue and Neurobehavioral Dysfunction in Patients with Primary Brain Tumors.*" Meyer et al. *(57)* evaluated 30 primary brain tumor patients who received either 10, 20, or 30 mg of methylphenidate bid. All patients underwent neuropsychological assessment. They reported significant improvements in cognitive function at the 10 mg bid dose. Functional motor improvement was also noted. No increased seizure activity was noted and these gains were noted despite progression on MRI in at least half of the cases. An abstract was presented at the Society for Neuro-oncology (SNO) meeting in Toronto in November 2004 evaluating the effect of Donepezil in previously irradiated brain tumor patients *(58)*. Patients were given donepezil at 5 mg/d for 6 wk and then 10 mg/d for 18 wk. They reported an improvement in the health-related quality of life and mood as measured by Functional Assessment of Cancer Therapy for Brain (FACT-BR) and Profile of Mood States (POMS). Patients also reported a significant reduction in fatigue. Further clinical trials are required looking for ways to improve patient quality of life and in particular fatigue.

ALTERNATIVE/COMPLIMENTARY TREATMENT

Alternative medicine has been defined as the use of various treatment modalities that are not usually used in traditional medicine, taught in medical schools, or covered by insurance companies. Terminology, however, is changing and these treatments are being incorporated more and more into traditional therapies and hence the term complimentary medicine is now used more frequently (Complimentary-Alternative Medicine [CAM]). In 1991, the National Institutes of Health (NIH) established the office for Alternative Medicine to address the growing use of these treatments. It has been estimated that two-thirds of the American population has used some form of CAM *(59)*. Of importance, 70% of those patients using CAM did not disclose this use to their physician *(60)*. In 1998 the Alternative Medicine office changed its name to the National Center for Complimentary and Alternative Medicine (NCCAM). Alternative therapies include things such as imagery, biofeedback, acupuncture, reiki, dietary supplements, herbal products, and traditional Chinese medicine. The NCCAM web site is: *http://www.nccam.nih.gov* and can be used for more detailed information beyond the scope of this review.

The Glioma Outcome project or "GO" was a physician directed project with the goal of improving the care of brain tumor patients. A total of 788 HGG patients were enrolled. The project collected data on the use of alternative therapies by glioma patients. An abstract of this data was presented at the Society for Neurooncology meeting in 2000 *(61)*, which evaluated data from the first 520 patients. Patients were asked about alternative therapy use within 3 wk of glioma surgery and at 3-mo intervals after that. Forty-nine percent of patients used at least one alternative therapy during their treatment. The most frequently used treatments included meditation and prayer (28%), high-dose vitamins (23%), and herbs (18%). Interestingly, alternative therapy use at some point (49%) was greater than the use of chemotherapy (25%), or those who enrolled in clinical trials (21%). An earlier study by Verhoef et al. *(62)* out of Canada also found that alternative therapy in glioma patients is common (24%). In that trial, conducted in Southern Alberta, 167 patients were evaluated using a prospectively administered questionnaire. Verhoef et al. felt alternative medicine use resulted from the patients' need to perceive that they have some autonomy in the management and treatment for their tumor. Clearly, these are evolving fields that require closer evaluation. Because it is obvious that patients are looking to other sources of treatment, we as a community need to evaluate these "therapies" in clinical trials. It is also imperative that when asking patients and caregivers about medications that it includes over-the-counter and herbal medications. As an example, grapefruit juice has been shown to be a CYP-450 inhibitor and St. John's Wort a CYP-450 inducer. This information can be found at *http://medicine.iupui.edu/flockhart/*.

CONCLUSIONS

The overall treatment of brain tumor patients remains a challenge. Although mortality remains a primary concern, morbidity and quality of life are issues that neuro-oncologists are in a unique position to address on a daily basis. Issues related to AED use, chemotherapies, steroids, and combinations lead to drug interactions that can affect patient response to treatment. Fatigue remains a primary problem of almost all brain tumor patients with new drugs currently being investigated in clinical trials. VTE events occur in a high frequency in cancer patients and a high index of suspicion is warranted. Patients continue to use alternative therapies and it is important to address this use with them. A collaborative team approach with attention to detail should help improve not only mortality but certainly morbidity and quality of life for brain tumor patients.

REFERENCES

1. Jackson JH. Localized convulsions from tumor of the brain. Brain 1882;5:364–374.
2. Penfield W, Erickson TC, Tarlov J. Relation of intracranial tumors and symptomatic epilepsy. Arch Neurol Psychiatry 1940;44:300–315.
3. Penfield W, Jasper H. Epilepsy and the functional anatomy on the human brain. Boston, MA, Little Brown and Company. 1954;288–291.
4. Wen PY, Marks PW. Medical management of patients with brain tumors. Curr Opinions Oncol 2002;14: 299–307.
5. Scaller B, Ruegg SJ. Brain tumors and seizures: pathophysiology and its implications for treatment revisited. Epilepsia 2003;44:1223–1232.
6. Primary brain tumors in the United States. Central Brain Tumor Registry of the United States. Chicago: Statistical Report 1997–2001.
7. Landis SH, Murray T, Bolden S, Wingo PA. Cancer statistics, Cancer J Clin 1999;49:8–31.
8. Posner JB. Neurologic complications of cancer. Philadelphia: FA Davis, 1995.
9. Glantz MJ, Cole BF, Friedberg MH, et al. A randomized, blinded, placebo controlled trial of divalproex sodium prophylaxis in adults with newly diagnosed brain tumors. Neurology 1996;46:985–991.
10. Glantz MJ, Cole BF, Forsyth PA, et al. Practice parameter: anticonvulsant prophylaxis in patients with newly diagnosed brain tumors: report of the quality standards subcommittee of the American Academy of Neurology. 2000;54:1886–1893.
11. Hansotia P. Epilepsy and driving regulations in Wisconsin. Epilepsia 1994;35:685–687.
12. Hansotia P, Broste SK. The effect of epilepsy or diabetes mellitus on the risk of automobile accidents. N Engl J Med 1991;324:22–26.
13. American Academy of Neurology, American Epilepsy Society, and the Epilepsy Foundation. Consensus statements, sample statutory provisions, and model regulations regarding driver licensing and epilepsy. Epilepsia 1994;35:696–705.
14. Krauss GL, Ampaw L, Krumholz A. Individual state driving restrictions for people with epilepsy in the US. Neurology 2001;57:1780–1785.
15. Drazkowski JF, Fischer RS, Sirven JI, et al. Seizure related vehicle crashes in Arizona before and after reducing the driving restriction from 12 to 3 months. Mayo Clin Proc 2003;78:819–825.
16. Krauss GL, Krumholz A, Carter RC, Li G, Kaplan P. Risk factors for seizure-related motor vehicles crashes in patients with epilepsy. Neurology 1999;52:1324–1329.
17. Berg AT, Vickery BG, Sperling MR, et al. Driving in adults with refractory localization-related epilepsy. Neurology 2000;54:625–630.
18. Wagner GL, Wilms EB, Van Donselaar CA, Vecht CH J,. Levetiracitam: preliminary experience in patients with primary brain tumors. Seizure 2003;12:585–586.
19. Patsalos PN. Pharmakokinetic profile of levetiracetam: toward ideal characteristics. Pharmacol Ther 2000;85:77–85.
20. Benedetti MS, Whomsley R, Nicholes JM, Young C, and Battes E.Pharmacokinetics and metabolism of 14C-levetiracetam, a new antiepileptic agent in healthy volunteers. Eur J Clinic Pharmacol. 2003;59(8–9): 621–630.
21. White JR, Walczak TS, Leppik IE, et al. Discontinuation of levetiracetam because of behavioral side effects: a case-contol study. Neurology 2003; 61:1218–1221.

22. Cole AJ. Initial individualized selection of long-term anticonvulsant drugs by neurologists. Neurology suppl 2004;63(10): S1–S2.

23. Wrighton SA, Stevens JC. The human hepatic cytochromes P450 involved in drug metabolism Crit Rev Toxicol 1992;22:1–21.

24. Nelson DR, Koymans L, Kamataki T, et al. P450 super family: update on new sequences, gene mapping, accession numbers and nomenclature. Pharmacogenetics 1996;6:1–42.

25. Gilbert MR, Supko JG, Batchelor T, et al. Phase I clinical trial and pharmacokinetics study of irinotecan in adults with recurrent malignant glioma. Clin Cancer Res 2003;9:2940–2949.

26. Fetell MR, Grossman SA, Fischer JD, et al. Preirradiation paclitaxel in glioblastoma multiforme: eficacy, pharmacology, and drug interactions. J Clin Oncol 1997;15:3121–3128.

27. Bourg V, Lebrun C, Chichmahian RM, et al. Nitrosourea-cisplatinum based chemotherapy associated with valproate: increase of haematologic toxicity. Ann Oncol 2001;12:217–219

28. Kubota F, Kifune A, Shibata N, et al. Bone mineral density of epileptic patients on long-term antiepileptic drug therapy: a quantitative digital radiography study. Epilepsy Res 1999;33:93–97.

29. Hahn TJ, Birge SJ, Scara CR, Avioli. Phenobarbital induced alterations in vit D metabolism. J Clin Invest 1972;51:741–748.

30. Ensrund WE, Walczak TS, Blackwell T, et al. Antiepileptic drug use increases rates of bone loss in older women: a prospective study. Neurology 2004;62:2051–2057.

31. French LA, Galicich JH. The use of steroids for control of cerebral edema. Clin Neurosurg 1964;10: 212–223

32. French LA. The use of steroids in the treatment of cerebral edema. Bull NY Acad Med 1966;42:301–311

33. Ingraham FD, Matson DD, McLaurin RL. Cortisone and ACTH as Cortisone and ACTH as an adjuvant to the surgery of craniopharyngioma N Engl J Med 1952;246:568–571, 1952.

34. Renaudin J, Fewer D, Wilson CB, Boldrey EB, Calogero J, Enot KJ. Dose dependency of decadron in patients with partially excised brain tumors. J Neurosurg 1973;39: 302–305.

35. Onishi T, Sher PB, Posner JB, Shapiro WR. Capillary permeability factor secreted by malignant brain tumor. J Neurosurg 1990;72:245–251.

36. Bodsch W, Rommel T, Ophjoff BG, Menzel J. Factors responsible for the retention of fluid in human tumor edema and the effects of dexamethasone. J. Neurosurg 1987;67: 250–257.

37. Jarden JO, Dhawan V, Moeller JR, Strother SC, Rottenberg DA, The time course of steroid action on blood-to-brain and blood-to-tumor transport of 82Rb. A Positron Emission Tomography Study. Ann Neurol 1989; 25:239–245.

38. Buxton N, Phillips N, Robertson I. The case of the disappearing glioma. J Neurol Neurosurg Psych 1997; 63:520–521.

39. Macdonald DR, Cascino LT, Schold SC, Cairncross JG. Response criteria for phase II studies of supratentorial malignant glioma. J Clin Oncol 1990;8:1277–1280.

40. Watling CJ, Donald HL, Macdonald DR, Cairncross JG. Corticosteroid-induced magnetic resonance imaging changes in patients with recurrent malignant glioma. J Clin Oncol 1994;12:1886–1889.

41. Cairncross JG, Macdonald DR, Pexman JHW, et al. Steroid-induced CT changes in patients with recurrent malignant glioma. Neurology 1988;38:724–726.

42. Mackie AE, Freshney RL, Akturk F, Menzel J. Factors responsible for the retention of fluid in human glioma cells: relationships to cytostasis. Br J Cancer 1988;58 (Suppl. IX):101–107.

43. Weller M, Schmidt C, Roth W, Dichgans J. Chemotherapy of human malignant glioma: prevention of efficacy by dexamethasone? Neurology 1997;48:1704–1709.

44. Lachner TE. Interaction of dexamethasone with phenytoin. Pharmacotherapy 1991;11:344–347.

45. Wen PY. Diagnosis and management of brain tumors. In: Black PM, Loeffler JS, eds. Cancer of the Nervous System. Cambridge, MA:Blackwell Scientific;1997:106–127.

46. Sawaya R, Glas-Greenwalt P. Postoperative venous thromboembolism and brain tumors. Part II: Hemostsis profile. J Neurooncol 1992;14:127–134.

47. Brandes AA, Scelzi E, Salmistraro G, et al. Incidence of risk of thromboembolism during treatment of high grade gliomas: a prospective study Eur J Cancer 1997;33:1592–1596.

48. Cogo A, Lensing A, Prandoni P, Hirsh J. Distribution of thrombosis in patients with symptomatic deep vein thrombosis: implications for simplifying the diagnosis process with compression ultrasound. Arch Intern Med 1993;153:2777–2780.

49. Streiff MB, J Segal, SA Grossman, TS Kinckler, EG Weir. ABO blood group is a potent risk factor for venous thromboembolism in patients with malignant gliomas. Cancer 2004;100:1717–1723.

50. Goldhaber SZ, Dunn K, Gerhard-Herman M, Park JK, Black PM. Low rate of venous thromboembolism after craniotomy for brain tumor using multimodality prophylaxis. Chest 2002;122:1933—1937.

51. Levin JM, Schiff D, Loeffler JS, Fine HA, Black PM, Wen PY. Complications of therapy for venous thromboembolic disease in patients with brain tumors.Neurology 1993;43:1111–1114.

52. Schiff D, DeAngelis LM. Therapy of venous thrombolembolism in patients with brain metastases. Cancer 1994;73:493–498.

53. Ruff RL, Posner JB. The incidence and treatment of peripheral venous thrombosis in patients with glioma. Ann Neurol 1983;13:334–336.

54. Altschuler E, Moosa H, Selker RG, Vertosick FT, Jr. The risk and efficacy of anticoagulant therapy in the treatment of thromboembolic complications in patients with primary malignant brain tumors. Neurosurgery 1990;27:74–77.

55. Freal JE, Kraft GH, Coryell JK. Symptomatic fatigue in multiple sclerosis. Arch Phys Med Rehabil 1984;65:135–138.

56. Stone P, Richards M, RA'Hern R, Hardy J. A study to investigate the prevalence, severity and correlates of fatigue among patients with cancer on comparison with a control group of volunteers without cancer. Ann Oncol 2000;11:561–567.

57. Meyer CA, Weitzner MA, Valentine AD, Levin VA. Methylphenidate therapy improves cognition, mood, and function of brain tumor patients. J Clinical Oncology 1998;16:2522–2527.

58. Shaw EG, Rosdhal R, D'Aostino RB, Lovato J Jr, Naughton M, Rapp S. A phase II study of Donepezil in irradiated brain tumor patients: effect on health related quality of life and mood. Neuro-oncology 2004;6:358 (abstract)

59. Kessler RC, Bavis RB, Foster DF, et al. Long-term trends in the use of complimentary and alternative medical therapies in the United States. Ann Intern Med 2001;135:262–268.

60. Eisenbery DM, Davis RB, Ettner SL, et al. Trends in alternative medicine use in the United States, 1990–1997: results of a follow-up national survey. JAMA 1998;280:1569–1575.

61. Hariharan S, Landolfi J, More J, et al. Alteraternative therapy use by malignant glioma patients: data from the glioma outcomes project. Neuro-oncology 2000;2:A92 p. 268.

62. Verhoef MJ, Hagan N, Pelletier G, Forsyth P. Alternative therapy use in neurologic diseases: use in brain tumor patients. Neurology 1999;52;617–622.

12 Surgical Techniques

Gene H. Barnett

Summary

The development of surgical navigation systems (SNS) has revolutionized the surgical management of high-grade glioma. The most common procedures using this technology are biopsy and craniotomy. Biopsy is often the procedure of choice when a histological diagnosis is desired, or when open resection is too risky or unnecessary. Stereotactic biopsy has low morbidity, high rates of diagnosis (albeit with a small risk of undergrading HGG), and may provide tissue for both histologic and molecular diagnoses. SNS may also be used to placed catheters for cyst drainage, brachytherapy, and convection enhanced delivery—a relatively new technique for infusing therapeutic agents through the brain. Extent of resection is becoming increasingly recognized as important to outcome in HGG. Navigation may be used to locate or tailor the bone flap, locate the tumor, or assist with assessment of resection completeness. It is important for the surgeon to consider the impact of gross brain movement due to loss of cerebrospinal fluid (so-called brain shift) as well as local tissue distortions when navigating using preoperatively acquired imaging. With proper care, use of SNS can limit morbidity and enhance resection for some patients with HGG.

Key Words: Surgery; brain biopsy; stereotaxic techniques; craniotomy; ommaya reservoir; intraoperative MRI; stereotactic radiosurgery.

INTRODUCTION

The principal surgical procedures for malignant gliomas are biopsy and craniotomy for debulking and cytoreduction *(1–5)*. Biopsy has evolved from open or free-hand procedures solely for histologic diagnosis to precise, image-guided techniques using frame or frameless stereotaxy for both histologic and molecular diagnosis *(2,6–12)*. Traditional associated procedures include tumor cyst aspiration *(13)*, placement of catheters for attachment to subcutaneous reservoirs or diversion systems (shunts) *(13,14)*, placement of radioactive "seeds" for brachytherapy *(15,16)*, and injection of chemotherapeutic agents. Placement of catheters for convection-enhanced delivery of a new generation of antitumoral agents is emerging as an important new procedure for the treatment of malignant gliomas *(17–22)*.

The era where the "only good craniotomy is a big craniotomy" for brain tumor has been supplanted by one where minimal access craniotomies guided by surgical navigation systems are the standard for elective resection of high-grade gliomas *(5,23–32)* and may be augmented by intraoperative imaging such as magnetic resonance imaging (MRI) *(33–47)*. The importance of aggressive, safe resection of these tumors is now supported by class I evidence *(48, 49)* and new methods of optimizing extent of resection of enhancing tumor are on the horizon.

In this chapter the basic principals of these common surgical procedures are reviewed and emerging applications explored.

From: *Current Clinical Oncology: High-Grade Gliomas: Diagnosis and Treatment*
Edited by: G. H. Barnett © Humana Press Inc., Totowa, NJ

STEREOTACTIC BRAIN BIOPSY
General Principals

Soon after the development of computerized imaging techniques such as computerized tomography (CT) and magnetic resonance imaging (MRI), surgeons began to devise methods of extracting the inherent 3-dimensional (3D) information within these image data and use them to direct surgical procedures using frame-stereotactic techniques *(1,5,50–53)*. Fore-most among these procedures was brain biopsy for the purpose of histologic diagnosis. Advances in technologies allowed for the development of stereotaxy systems without frames *(23,25,26,54–57)*. Today, most image-guided stereotactic brain biopsies are performed using guidance from surgical navigation systems (SNSs) or so-called "frameless stereotaxy" *(8–10,58–62)*. Regardless of whether frames are used or not, the general principals of biopsy target and trajectory selection are constant, as are many nuances of the surgical procedure.

Patients selected for stereotactic brain biopsy are typically those where a histologic diagnosis is desired, the outcome of that diagnosis will potentially change management, and open surgical tumor resection is either not necessary or desirable—on the basis of location, co-morbidities, or possibility that the lesion is better treated nonsurgically (e.g., primary central nervous system lymphoma [PCNSL]. Today, additional molecular information may also be a motivator for biopsy, such as determining the status of chromosomes 1p and 19q in anaplastic oligodendroglioma where their loss is predictive of chemosensitivity and overall better prognosis with treatment *(63)*.

Once the decision for biopsy has been made, then a target needs to be selected. Most high-grade gliomas (HGG) enhance, at least peripherally, and some authors advocate targeting the peripheral rim of enhancement in ring-enhancing tumors. Others prefer to target the center, even if necrotic, and then advance or withdraw the biopsy device based on intraoperative frozen section to obtain diagnostic tissue. In this manner, the ability to eventually obtain diagnostic tissue is virtually assured (unless prevented by early bleeding) *(64)* and the chance for missing the edge of the tumor (owing to the small but real errors in sterotactic application accuracy) is obviated. In nonenhancing tumors or otherwise homogenously appearing lesions, additional neuroimaging studies such as positron emission tomography using radiolabeled flurodeoxyglucose (FDG-PET), magnetic resonance spectroscopy (MRS), or magnetic resonance perfusion or CT blood volume may provide more rational targets than identifiable on conventional CT and MRI *(7,65–72)* Angiography is not routinely used.

The general principles of trajectory planning include (in order of importance) avoiding vascular structures, avoiding eloquent brain, and minimizing the length of the surgical trajectory. A corollary to the first principle is to avoid traversing multiple pial or ependymal planes as MRI-occult, relatively immobile vessels often reside on these surfaces.

Our preferred technique and results for performing stereotactic brain biopsy using SNS has been reported elsewhere and a brief review is presented here *(2)*. Markers ("fiducials") are affixed to the scalp with adhesive or cyanoacrylate. We often will also mark the outline of the fiducial with indelible ink as a reference should the fiducial fall off prior to surgery. When an ultra-high accuracy biopsy is necessary (such as for some brainstem and posterior fossa procedures), then skull implanted fiducials are placed, typically the day of surgery, resulting in accuracy that equals or exceeds that of conventional frames *(73–77)*. The appropriate image studies are obtained. This is usually a T1-weighted volume acquisition after administration of intravenous gadolinium contrast. A target and trajectory are selected (Fig. 1).

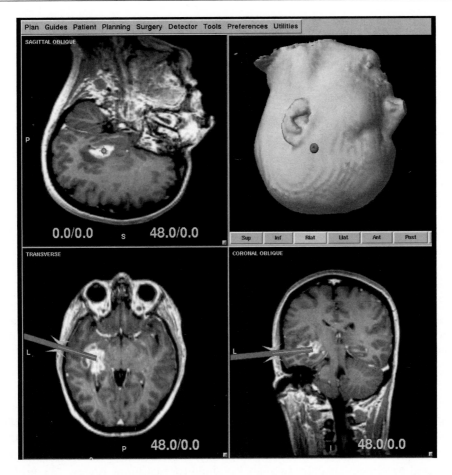

Fig. 1. Plan for biopsy of a high-grade gliomas as presented on a contemporary surgical navigation system.

Although many surgeons perform these procedures with the patient under a local anesthetic with sedation, the author prefers a general anesthetic so as to avoid potential self-extraction from a frame or fixation device either from agitation or seizure, and to avoid emergency intubation in the event of significant hemorrhage. Contemporary neuroanesthetic techniques are sufficiently advanced to the point that we have not seen complications related to the use of general anesthetic in this setting. For frameless biopsies, the head is secured in a three-point fixation device and a dynamic reference frame (DRF) attached to allow the SNS to track head movements during the procedure (Fig. 2).

The fiducials and images are co-registered using the methodology of the specific stereotactic system and the surgical trajectory mapped onto the patient's scalp. Hair in the immediate region is clipped (78), the scalp cleansed with and iodine-containing solution, and the area draped. Often an "eye drape" is used to define the surgical field. Although some surgeons perform bur holes, it is the belief of the author that twist drill holes are sufficient in the vast majority of cases. An approximate 1-cm incision is made, centered on the surgical trajectory. The twist drill is guided by an apparatus which has been adjusted using the target and trajectory features of the navigation system (79) and the inner table perforated. The dura is then punc-

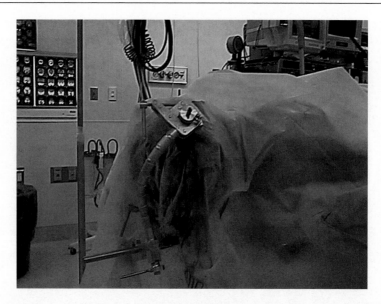

Fig. 2. General setup for stereotactic procedures on HGG using surgical navigation. The head is secured in a three-point fixation device to which a dynamic reference frame is attached (not shown) that allows compensation for head movement. An extra-large instrument holder secured to a stereotactic guide block can be used to accurately direct a biopsy instrument to the target in a high-grade gliomas.

tured using electrocautery. A preset depth for the biopsy instrument can be determined from information provided by the SNS, or the biopsy device may be attached to encoders that allow it to be tracked in real time using the SNS. The (side cutting) instrument is advanced to the target site and specimens (usually two) are obtained for histologic review. We prefer frozen section analysis although many centers use cytologic smear techniques *(80)*. If the tissue is nondiagnostic, adjustments are made to the depth of the biopsy instrument, usually at 1-cm increments). If nondiagnostic because of necrosis, the author usually starts to withdraw the instrument, however if nondiagnostic because of gliosis, the author may be more likely to advance if it is suspected that the device is shallow becuase of brain sagging resulting from gravity and loss of cerebrospinal fluid (CSF). The surgeon should carefully inspect the surgical trajectory to discern the likelihood of being too deep, shallow, or a true "miss" to some side.

If venous bleeding is encountered it can usually be managed by a combination of head elevation, irrigation of the outer lumen of the biopsy instrument using a narrow gage spinal needle, and periodic mechanical clearing of the lumen with a stylet *(81)*. These procedures are continued until fluid in the canula remains clear and pulsates with the cardiac cycle. These procedures rely on the opening of the biopsy instrument's outer cannula being left at the original site of biopsy and not rotated or withdrawn. Arterial bleeding may require additional efforts such as pharmacologic lowering of blood pressure and direct injection of small volumes of thrombin *(81)*. These methods only work if the source of the bleeding is local. If bleeding results from remote avulsion of the vessel, the outcome is often catastrophic or may require emergency craniotomy. Once controlled, intraoperative bleeding does not necessarily mean that further biopsies cannot be considered (but usually not at the same site)—the surgeon should balance anticipated risk vs need for diagnosis. Immediate postoperative imaging should be considered in patients with significant bleeding during the procedure and/or new deficit.

When satisfactory tissue has been obtained and hemostasis secured, the biopsy instrument is withdrawn, the scalp closed with vertical interrupted mattress sutures, the hair washed with shampoo, and a small dressing stapled in place. The head is removed from the fixation device and the patient awakened. A CT scan without contrast is obtained about 2 h later. If the CT shows no evidence of bleeding (or blood less than 1 cm in maximum dimension), the patient is neurologically unchanged from their preoperative status, and there was not intraoperative bleeding, the patient is sent to a regular nursing floor. In some cases, discharge home the day of the procedure may be reasonable *(60,82)*, although outpatient stereotactic brain biopsy is not currently reimbursed by the Centers for Medicare and Medicaid Services.

Contemporary series of stereotactic brain biopsies are diagnostic in 90 to 100 percent of cases with serious morbidity or mortality less than 10 and 1% percent, respectively *(1,2,5,7,9,10,60,61,64,81–83)*. Intracranial infections such as abscesses or meningitis are rare. Sampling error (i.e., underestimating the maximum grade of the lesion) may occur in 10 to 20% of cases *(67,71)* but may be mitigated by use of some of the enhanced targeting techniques cited above *(59,66,69,70)*.

Stereotactic brain biopsy has evolved into a relatively safe, accurate means to establish the histologic and molecular diagnosis of high-grade gliomas. Methodologies using nonlinear stereotaxis *(84)* or robotics *(85)* may further enhance the efficacy and safety of brain biopsy and related procedures.

Related Procedures

Cyst Drainage and Subcutaneous Reservoir

HGG are not infrequently associated with cyst formation. The rates of production and consistency (thin vs viscous) of the fluid are quite variable. The stereotactic techniques of biopsy cited above can be directly applied to drain a cyst as a one time procedure (with or without instillation of a chemical or radioactive agent—rarely used for HGG). Typically, these cysts are recurrent and placement of a catheter coupled to a subcutaneous reservoir may allow for episodic drainage of the cyst without resorting to additional operative procedures *(13,14)*. Such devices work well for cysts where the fluid accumulates relatively slowly or is too viscous for continuous drainage (as with a shunt). Similarly, catheters may be implanted into cerebral ventricles, or other diversion procedures performed such as third ventriculostomy, when normal CSF outflow has been obstructed by tumors thereby resulting in a "trapped" ventricle *(86,87)*. It is important to remember that the portion of the catheter that is to allow for drainage should be targeted for the center of the cyst and that the depth should be referenced to some rigid cranial or extracranial reference. If referenced to the visible surface of the brain after the brain has begun to sag (shift) from gravity and loss of CSF, the ultimate location of the catheter may prove to be too deep. Also, the catheter should be secured well at the surface of the skull so that it is not pushed deeper when the scalp is closed. After successful drainage, new cysts may form or the device may become infected or blocked requiring revision of the system. Nonetheless, stereotactic placement of intratumoral catheters for continuous or episodic percutaneous drainage are important surgical tools in the management of some HGG.

Brachytherapy

The notion that a strategic boost of radiation dose to the enhancing tumor or resection bed (where most recurrences occur) was the basis for brachytherapy as a treatment for newly diagnosed or recurrent malignant gliomas. Despite much enthusiasm in the early 1990s that the temporary implantation of high-activity radioactive seeds in such situations may lead to

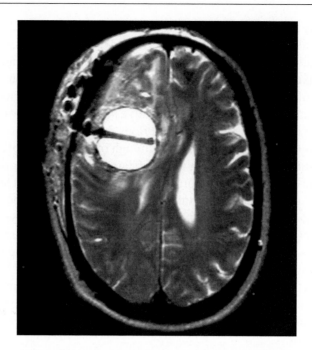

Fig. 3. An implanted balloon for liquid brachytherapy of HGG as shown on a T2-weighted MRI. Although initial results appear promising, this was also true for other forms of brachytherapy and stereotactic radiosurgery and was subsequently disproved when subjected to randomized trials.

improved outcome in patients with HGG *(88–90)*, subsequent randomized trials have failed to find a survival advantage from this type of brachytherapy *(91,92)*. In fact, dose escalation by this or any other means beyond contemporary radiotherapy (e.g., stereotactic radiosurgery) has not been shown to be of benefit when subjected to randomized trials *(93,94)*. The extended survival of patients with grade III or IV gliomas found in most series appears to have resulted largely from selection bias. As such, brachytherapy with temporary sources is rarely used today for HGG because of its high toxicity, apparent ineffectiveness, and the existence of other means to deliver regional radiation boosts less invasively. Stereotactic techniques have also been used for implantation of permanent radioactive seeds and new devices use liquid brachytherapy temporarily placed in balloons within tumor resection beds (Fig. 3) *(95)* and although the results again appear promising, their efficacy has not been established by class I evidence.

Convection Enhanced Delivery (CED)

Several new "targeted" therapies of malignant gliomas require unusual means of delivery so as to avoid systemic complications and optimize delivery not only to solid tumor, but to the brain around tumor harboring infiltrating tumor cells. Delivery of an agent as a single bolus results in limited penetration and exponential falloff of dose as its distribution is through the process of diffusion. Continuous, slow infusion of a stable substance, capable of distribution through the extracellular matrix of the brain, at rates that do not produce cavitation and cyst formation allows for high concentrations to be delivered centimeters away from the point of infusion *(17–22,96)*. This process, typically known as convection enhanced delivery,

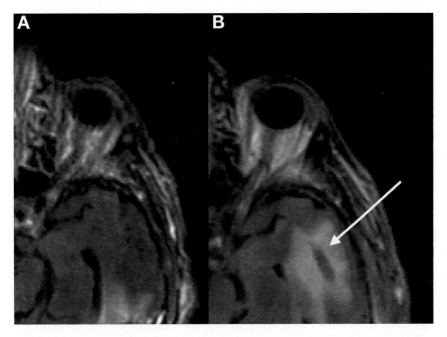

Fig. 4. (A) FLAIR image of temporal lobe prior to catheter placement for convection enhanced delivery (CED) of immunotoxin. **(B)** FLAIR image of same patient after 4 d of CED—note wide distribution of fluid as shown by region of high signal. Arrow points to catheter.

is becoming increasingly important and may become a common means of treating HGG in the near future. Although the technique remains relatively new, several observations regarding this approach appear valid. The catheter itself should be small with a single outlet at its tip. This point of delivery should be within the white matter and not tumor. The length of catheter from the tip to any pial surface should be sufficiently long to preclude backflow of the infused agent into the subarachnoid space with associated loss of diffusion and possible local surface toxicities (Fig. 4).

Prediction of distribution of the infusion remains difficult as is optimal selection of catheter placement. Computerized approaches of predicting flow and, therefore, ideal catheter placement are underway and may make CED more reliable and effective as a means to deliver local therapies of high-grade gliomas.

MINIMAL ACCESS CRANIOTOMY

General Principals

Traditionally, large craniotomies were necessary when operating on HGG because these were largely exploratory procedures, guided only by the inferences of the neurologic examination, angiography and ventriculography *(30,32)*. Surface features such as the presence of arterialized veins or other alterations in appearance such as color or texture could indicate the location of a subcortical tumor, often supplemented by palpation. Hemostatic and anesthetic techniques were also less advanced and a large craniotomy was thought to facilitate access to potential sources of bleeding and managing intraoperative brain swelling.

The development of computerized imaging such as CT and the application of frame then frameless stereotactic guidance has led to an era where the size of craniotomies have become minimal—often just a few centimeters in diameter when accessing a deep tumor, and just large enough to encompass one that comes to the surface of the brain *(5,23,27,28,58)*. A thorough discussion on the topic and approaches of craniotomy for malignant gliomas is beyond the scope of this chapter, however general principles are presented.

EXTENT OF RESECTION

It is accepted that surgical resection of a HGG is often beneficial when a percutaneous stereotactic biopsy is too risky, or when the patient is symptomatic from mass effect or medically refractory seizures. However, the concept that removing the majority of a HGG improves prognosis has been controversial for decades because of the lack of class I evidence *(48)* despite a wealth of, at times conflicting, reports on the topic *(97–100)*. Although the preponderance of literature, particularly in recent years, support the observation that near complete resection of a HGG improves survival, virtually all are plagued by the possibility that an insidious selection bias has skewed the results. That is, those patients that will inherently live longer will be those that have disease where near-total resections are feasible either on anatomic grounds (e.g., unifocal, accessible, and unilateral) or where a more aggressive approach would be favored (e.g., younger age, better performance status, good general health—"good surgical candidate"). It has only been recently that there is class I evidence to support this long held belief that aggressive, safe surgical resection is an important favorable prognostic factor, even in the elderly *(49)*.

Given that aggressive, safe resection of enhancing high-grade tumor is desirable (and presumably the bulk of the rare, nonenhancing HGG), it is natural to use guidance adjunct to enhance the extent of tumor that can be safely be removed. Today most surgeons use surgical navigation for these purposes.

NAVIGATION-ASSISTED MINIMAL ACCESS CRANIOTOMY
Preoperative Planning

MRI remains the cornerstone of preoperative decision making and planning in surgery for HGG. The location of the tumor is generally clear (although subtleties of anatomy can be distorted beyond recognition) and the function of surrounding brain tissues inferred *(101)*. Lesions that cross the midline or have substantial ependymal or leptomeningeal involvement are often treated less aggressively or denied surgery at all. Further information on cortical function can be obtained by functional MRI. However, the spatial resolution of fMRI is limited to about 1 cm and likely relates to changes in venous blood oxygenation downstream from the actual site of neural activation. Previous surgery or radiotherapy may lead to inaccurate localization or lateralization of function. Nonetheless, fMRI is often a valuable tool in the overall planning of a case and determining the need for and nature of intraoperative neurophysiology and awake techniques *(37)*.

Conventional navigation imaging (usually high-resolution volume MRI with contrast) provides substantial anatomic data on surface and ventricular anatomy (Fig. 5), but little information on white matter tracts. Diffusion tensor imaging is a specialized MRI method of extracting directional water diffusion information that correlates with the directionality of white matter tracts *(102,103)*. These data are often color coded to denote tracts that are left–right, front–back, or up–down (and vice versa) in their orientation. The method can be taken a step further to track these neural bundles by placing a "seed" along a tract, then allowing the

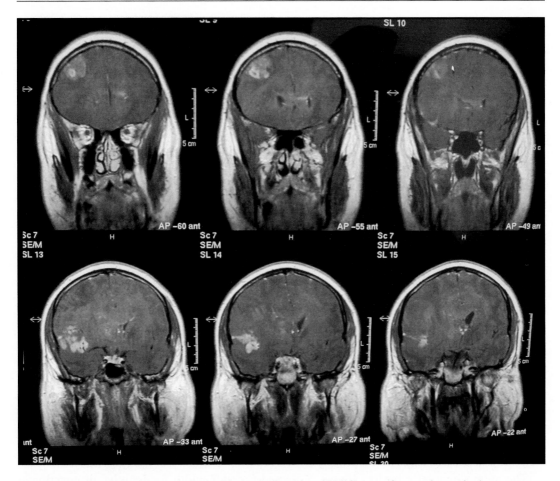

Fig. 5. Volume MRI with contrast showing relationship of HGG to surface and ventricular anatomy.

computer to trace a "fiber" along that bundle. So-called "fiber tracking" may allow for better visualization of the distortion, displacement or replacement of key pathways by HGG and allow for better planning and decisions regarding intraoperative white matter stimulation *(104)* awake craniotomy or other monitoring techniques (Fig. 6).

Taking structure and function into account, a surgical plan is devised—usually placing a target within the lesion and defining a safe entry corridor if the lesion is subcortical. Most of these procedures are done with the patient under a general anesthetic. The head is secured in a fixation device to the operating table and the dynamic reference frame secured to the fixation device. (For awake procedures the fixation device is still used as a mounting point for the DRF, but it is not secured to the table, but allowed to "float" on a pillow.) The scalp fiducials are touched with the SNS pointing device (usually a hand-held wand) and co-registered with their locations on the image data sets. The wand is used to map the surgical trajectory onto the patient's scalp and define the boundaries of the craniotomy. The craniotomy need be large enough to encompass the surface component of the tumor and can be as small as 3 or 4 cm in diameter when the lesion is deep. Oblique or wand oriented displays are generally better used for this purpose than the standard triplanar (axial, coronal, sagittal) display.

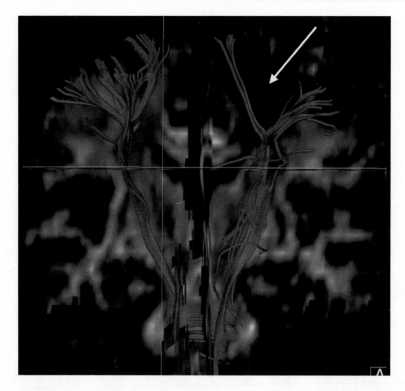

Fig. 6. Diffusion tensor imaging derived "fiber tracking" showing the corticospinal tract "split" and displaced by intervening tumor in motor strip (*arrow*).

The author generally prefers linear, *S*-shaped (greater width for length), or curvilinear incisions depending on location and cosmetic considerations (Fig. 7). It is our impression that they heal better and that they also allow for greater flexibility at time of reoperation where the tumor may no longer be within the confines of a horseshoe or other "flap." Hair is typically clipped in a narrow strip *(78)* along the incision and, the wound cleansed and draped. Muscle is divided or reflected as indicated and the navigation device used to map out the extent of the craniotomy. One or more burr holes are fashioned and a craniotome used to create a free bone flap. For parasagittal tumors such as HGG in the superior frontal or parietal gyri, navigation is used to identify the true location of the superior sagittal sinus and the bone flap created lateral to the sinus. The bone flap need be large enough to allow direct access to the tumor that comes to the underlying brain surface and can be more limited in size (2–3 cm) when the tumor is entirely subcortical. For frontal or temporal lobectomies the bone flap is centered at the posterior superior aspect of the lobectomy. Navigation is used to confirm the superficial tumor boundaries—generally these respect sulci, at least in part. It is probably safer to perform subpial dissections in these areas rather than dissect the sulcus and risk

Fig. 7. *(opposite page)* Typical sequence of steps in a minimal access craniotomy. **(A)** Fiducials are placed in stereotypical manner. **(B)** Hair is clipped along prospecitive linear incision. **(C)** Retractors are placed.

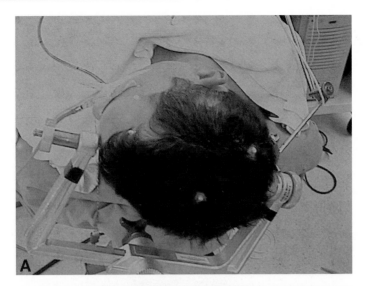

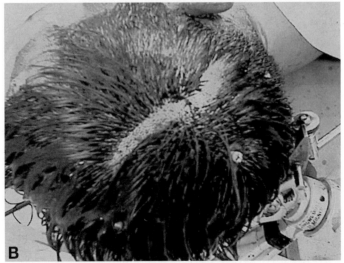

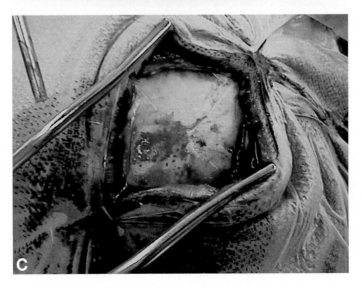

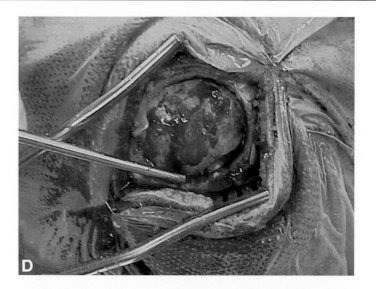

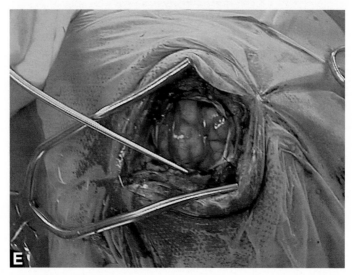

Fig. 7. *(continued)* Typical sequence of steps in a minimal access craniotomy. **(D)** A small craniotomy is fashioned and dural tacking sutures placed. **(E)** The dura is opened in a cruciate fashion.

vascular injury, however this is not always possible if the tumor has infiltrated the pia. Using navigation, the superficial boundary is usually entirely defined and then dissection carried deeper. Often there is a clear textural or visual difference between the solid, enhancing tumor and the surrounding "brain around tumor" (BAT), although this may be subtle and this region may be more or less firm than the BAT. The region of enhancement usually has neovascularization that is apparent under magnification. If the tumor has gross necrosis it is important to remove not only it, but also the enhancing tissue around it. Often it is necessary to amputate the superficially defined tumor in order to work at depth. When a gross total or maximal resection has been achieved, it is worthwhile to sweep the tumor cavity with the navigation

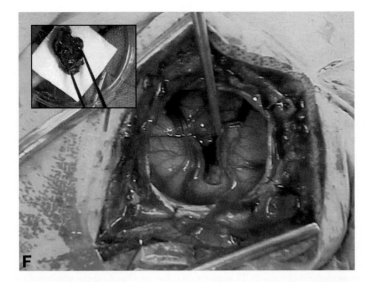

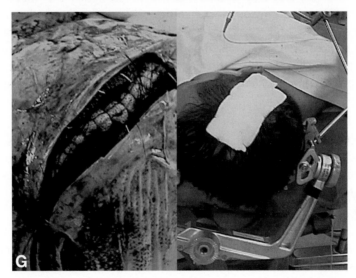

Fig. 7. *(continued)* Typical sequence of steps in a minimal access craniotomy. **(F)** The tumor is resected in an *en bloc* fashion *(inset)*. Cerebrotomy is directed between large surface veins. **(G)** Closure *(left)* and dressing *(right)*.

wand to look for regions that may have escaped resection, particularly projections of tumor beyond the more spherical core. It is important to bear in mind that resection will cause the tumor cavity not only to shift in location as the brain sinks (so-called "brain shift") but also to contract such that the navigation system will suggest that there is more tumor beyond that that truly remains in most cases. The author has found that filling the cavity with large cotton balls will re-expand the cavity to roughly its preoperative dimensions and allow for more useful information from navigation at this point. Of course, intraoperative imaging (i.e., CT, ultrasound, and MRI) can also be used as a reality check at this time *(33–35,38,44)*. Methods to mathematically predict brain shift remain investigational *(105,106)*. Also, prior to resection and significant shift, catheters or other small markers may be placed stereotactically around the periphery of the tumor, thereby providing landmarks that are, more or less, independent of shift *(68)*. Recent trials of a fluorescent agent to visually indicate the location and extent of residual HGG have proved promising as a means to maximize resection *(107)*.

Intracavitary treatment can be considered before closure. This includes biodegradable wafers laden with a chemotherapeutic agent, intraoperative radiotherapy, placement of a container for postoperative liquid brachytherapy, or catheters for CED as discussed above. Although a water-tight closure is often desirable, dural approximation followed by layers of fibrin glue and cellulose gel, compressed by a securely affixed bone flap provide good protection against postoperative CSF leakage. The scalp is closed with a running vertical mattress suture providing a combination of an excellent cosmetic result and an additional barrier to fluid leakage. The scalp and hair are washed with shampoo, rinsed, and a sterile dressing stapled in place. The overall technique is modified as necessary depending on the specifics of the case and surgical findings.

Postoperatively, and barring complications, the patient is observed overnight in the recovery room or intermediate care unit. The next day he or she is then mobilized, a new baseline MRI obtained, and Doppler ultrasounds of the lower limb veins obtained to test for deep vein thrombosis. Previous assessments have shown that most patients are discharged within a few days of surgery. If there are new deficits, imaging should be obtained to try to determine if this is likely temporary or permanent, and the appropriate support services (e.g., physical, occupational, or speech therapy) consulted and rehabilitation assessments obtained.

CONCLUSIONS

Surgery for HGG is useful in the diagnosis and treatment of these disorders. When feasible, aggressive resection of the enhancing component appears to improve outcome over biopsy alone. Advanced applications such as convection enhanced delivery of selective agents are promising new techniques in the treatment of these disorders.

ACKNOWLEDGMENTS

The author wishes to thank Ms. Christine Moore and Ms. Martha Tobin for their assistance with the preparation of this manuscript.

REFERENCES

1. Apuzzo ML, Chandrasoma PT, Cohen D, Zee CS, Zelman V. Computed imaging stereotaxy: experience and perspective related to 500 procedures applied to brain masses. Neurosurgery 1987;20(6):930–937.
2. Barnett GH, Miller DW, Weisenberger J. Brain biopsy using frameless stereotaxy with scalp applied fiducials: Experience in 218 cases. J Neurosurg 1999;91:569–576.
3. Barnett GH. Minimal Access Craniotomy. In: Barnett GH, Roberts DW, Maciunas RJ, eds. Image-Guided Neurosurgery: Clinical Applications of Surgical Navigation. St. Louis, MO: Quality Medical Publishing Inc. 1998;63–71.
4. Barnett GH. Stereotactic techniques in the management of brain tumors. Contemp Neurosurg 1997;19(10): 1–9.
5. Gomez H, Barnett GH, Estes ML, Palmer J, Magdinec M. Stereotactic and computer-assisted neurosurgery at the Cleveland Clinic. Review of 501 consecutive cases. Cleve Clin J Med 1993;60:399–410.
6. Barnett GH, Miller DW. Brain biopsy and related procedures. In: Barnett GH, Roberts DW, Maciunas RJ, eds. Image-Guided Neurosurgery: Clinical Applications of Surgical Navigation. St. Louis, Misouri; Quality Medical Publishing Inc. 1998;181–191.
7. Bernays RL, Kollias SS, Khan N, Brandner S, Meier S, Yonekawa Y. Histological yield, complications, and technological considerations in 114 consecutive frameless stereotactic biopsy procedures aided by open intraoperative magnetic resonance imaging. J Neurosurg 2002;97(2):354–362.

8. Dorward NL, Paleologos TS, Alberti O, Thomas DG. The advantages of frameless stereotactic biopsy over frame-based biopsy. Br J Neurosurg 2002;16(2):110–118.

9. Gralla J, Nimsky C, Buchfelder M, Fahlbusch R, Ganslandt O. Frameless stereotactic brain biopsy procedures using the Stealth Station: indications, accuracy and results. Zentralbl Neurochir 2003;64:166–170.

10. Grunert P, Espinosa J, Busert C, et al. Stereotactic biopsies guided by an optical navigation system: technique and clinical experience. Minim Invasive Neurosurg. 2002;45(1):11–15.

11. Kelly PJ, Earnest F 4th, Kall BA, Goerss SJ, Scheithauer B. Surgical options for patients with deep-seated brain tumors: computer-assisted stereotactic biopsy. Mayo Clin Proc 1985;60(4):223–229.

12. Paleologos TS, Dorward NL, Wadley JP, Thomas DG. Clinical validation of true frameless stereotactic biopsy: analysis of the first 125 consecutive cases. Neurosurgery 2001;49(4):830–835.

13. Al-Anazi A, Bernstein M. Modified stereotactic insertion of the Ommaya reservoir. Technical note. J Neurosurg. 2000;92(6):1050–1052

14. Rogers LR, Barnett G. Percutaneous aspiration of brain tumor cysts via the Ommaya reservoir system. Neurology 1991;41:279–282.

15. Sneed PK, Gutin PH, Larson DA et al. Patterns of recurrence of glioblastoma multiforme after external irradiation followed by implant boost. Int J Radiat Oncol Biol Phys 1994;29:719–727.

16. Suh JH, Barnett GH. Brachytherapy for brain tumor. Hematol Oncol Clin North Am 1999;13(3):635–650, viii–ix.

17. Croteau D, Walbridge S, Morrison PF, et al. Real-time in vivo imaging of the convective distribution of a low molecular-weight tracer. J Neurosurg 2005;102:90–97.

18. Mamot C, Nguyen JB, Pourdehnad, et al. Extensive distribution of liposomes in rodent brains and brain tumors following convection-enhanced delivery. J Neuro-Oncology 2004;68:1–9.

19. Nguyen TT, Pannu YS, Sung C, et al. Convective distribution of macromolecules in the primate brain demonstrated using computed tomography and magnetic resonance imaging. J Neurosurg 2003;98:584–590.

20. Saito R, Bringas JR, McKnight TR, et al. Distribution of liposomes into brain and rat brain tumor models by convection-enhanced delivery monitored with magnetic resonance imaging. Cencer Res 2004;64:2572–2579.

21. Saito R, Bringas JR, Panner A, et al. Convection-enhanced delivery of tumor necrosis factor-related apoptosis-inducing ligand with systemic administration of temozolomide prolongs survival in an intracranial glioblastoma xenograft model. Cancer Res 2004;64:6858–6862.

22. Voges J, Reszka R, Gossmann A, et al. Image-guided convection-enhanced delivery and gene therapy for glioblastoma. Ann Neurol 2003;54:479–487.

23. Barnett GH, Kormos DW, Steiner CP, Weisenberger J. Use of a frameless, armless stereotactic wand for brain tumor localization with two-dimensional and three-dimensional neuroimaging. Neurosurgery 1993;33:674–678.

24. Barnett GH. Surgical navigation for brain tumors. In: Winn HR ed. Youman's Neurological Surgery, 5th Ed. Philadelphia: WB Saunders 2004.

25. Doshi PK, Lemmieux L, Fish DR, Shorvon SD, Harkness WH, Thomas DG. Frameless stereotaxy and interactive neurosurgery with the ISG viewing wand. Acta Neuroschir Suppl Iwien 1995;64:49–53.

26. Golfinos JG, Fitzpatrick BC, Smith LR, Spetzler RF. Clinical use of a frameless stereotactic arm: results in 325 cases. J Neurosurg 1995;83:197–205.

27. Guthrie BL, Adler JR Jr. Computer-assisted preoperative planning, interactive surgery, and frameless stereotaxy. Clin neurosurg 1992;38:112–131.

28. Kelly PJ, Kall BA, Goerss S Earnest F 4th. Computer-assisted stereotaxic laser resection of intra-axial brain neoplasms. J Neurosurg 1986;64:427–439.

29. Kelly PJ. Volumetric stereotactic surgical resection of intra-axial brain mass lesions. Mayo Clin Proc 1988; 63:1186–1198.

30. McDermott MW. Intracranial Gliomas. In: Barnett GH, Roberts DW, Maciunas RJ, eds. Image-Guided Neurosurgery: Clinical Applications of Surgical Navigation. St. Louis, MO: Quality Medical Publishing Inc. 1998;77–86.

31. Murphy MA, Barnett GH, Kormos DW, Weisenberger J. Astrocytoma resection using an interactive frameless stereotactic wand. An early experience. J Clinical Neuroscience 1994;1:33–37.

32. Walters CL, Schmidek HH. Surgical management of intracranial gliomas. In: Schmidek HH, Sweet WH, eds. Operative neurosurgical techniques: Indications, methods and results. Philadelphia: WB Saunders 1988;431–450.

33. Bernstein M, Al-Anazi AR, Kucharczyk W, Manninen P, Bronskill M, Henkelman M. Brain tumor surgery with the Toronto open magnetic resonance imaging system: preliminary results for 36 patients and analysis of advantages, disadvantages, and future prospects. Neurosurgery 2000;46(4):900–907.

34. Bohinski RJ, Kokkino AK, Warnick RE, et al. Glioma resection in a shared-resource magnetic resonance operating room after optimal image-guided frameless stereotactic resection. Neurosurgery 2001;48:731–742.

35. Gering DT, Nabavi A, Kikinis R, et al. An integrated visualization system for surgical planning and guidance using image fusion and an open MR. J Magn Reson Imaging 2001;13:967–975.

36. Hall WA, Kowalik K, Liu H, Truwit CL, Kucharczyk J. Costs and benefits of intraoperative MR-guided brain tumor resection. Acta Neurochir 2002;85:137–142.

37. Hall WA, Liu H, Maxwell RE, Truwit CL. Influence of 1.5-Tesla intraoperative MR imaging on surgical decision making. Acta Neurochir Suppl. 2003;85:29–37.

38. Kanner AA, Vogelbaum MA, Mayberg MR, Weisenberger JP, Barnett GH. Intracranial navigation by using low-field intraoperative magnetic resonance imaging: preliminary experience. J Neurosurg 2002;97(5):1115–1124.

39. Lindseth F, Kaspersen JH, Ommedal S, et al. Multimodal image fusion in ultrasound-based neuronavigation: improving overview and interpretation by integrating preoperative MRI with intraoperative 3D ultrasound. Comput Aided Surg 2003;8:49–69.

40. Nabavi A, Black PM, Gering DT, et al. Serial intraoperative magnetic resonance imaging of brain shift. Neurosurgery 2001;48:787–797.

41. Nimsky C, Ganslandt O, Cerny S, Hastreiter P, Greiner G, Fahlbusch R. Quantification of, visualization of, and compensation for brain shift using intraoperative magnetic resonance imaging. Neurosurgery 2000;47:1070–1079.

42. Nimsky C, Ganslandt O, Hastreiter P, Fahlbusch R. Intraoperative compensation for brain shift. Surg Neurol 2001;56:357–365.

43. Siomin V, Barnett G. Intraoperative imaging in glioblastoma resection. Cancer J 2003;9:91–98.

44. Trobaugh JW, Richard WD, Smith KR, Bucholz RD. Frameless stereotactic ultrasonography: Method and applications. Comput Med Imaging Graph 1994;18:235–246.

45. Tummala RP, Chu RM, Liu H, Truwit CL, Hall WA. Optimizing brain tumor resection. High-field interventional MR imaging. Neuroimaging Clin N Am 2001;11:673–683.

46. Unsgaard G, Gronningsaeter A, Ommedal S, Nagelhaus Hernes TA. Brain operations guided by real-time two-dimensional ultrasound: new possibilities as a result of improved image quality. Neurosurgery 2002;51:402–411.

47. Unsgaard G, Ommedal S, Muller T, Gronningsaeter A, Nagelhaus Hernes TA. Neuronavigation by intraoperative three-dimensional ultrasound: initial experience during brain tumor resection. Neurosurgery 2002;50:804–812.

48. Evidence-Based Medicine Working Group. Evidence-based medicine. A new approach to teaching the practice of medicine. JAMA 1992;68(17):2420–2425.

49. Vuorinen V, Hinkka S, Farkkila M, Jaaskelainen J, Debulking or biopsy of malignant glioma in elderly people–randomised study. Acta Neurochir (Wien) 2003;145(1):5–10.

50. Brown RA. A computerized tomography-computer graphics approach to stereotaxic localization. J Neurosurg 1979;50(6):715–720.

51. Couldwell WT, Apuzzo ML. Initial experience related to the use of the Cosman-Roberts-Wells stereotactic instrument. Technical note. J Neurosurg 1990;72(1):145–148.

52. Heilbrun MP, Roberts TS, Apuzzo ML, Wells TH Jr, Sabshin JK. Preliminary experience with Brown-Roberts-Wells (BRW) computerized tomography stereotaxic guidance system. J Neurosurg 1983;59(2):217–222.

53. Lunsford LD, Martinez AJ. Stereotactic exploration of the brain in the era of computed tomography. Surg Neurol. 1984;22(3):222–230.

54. Maciunas RJ, Galloway RL Jr, Fitzpatrick JM, et al. A universal system for interactive image-directed neurosurgery. Stereotact Funct Neurosurg 1992;58:108–113.

55. Roberts DW, Strohbehn JW, Friets EM, Kettenberger J, Hartov A. The stereotactic operating microscope: accuracy refinement and clinical experience. Acta Neurochir Suppl (Wien) 1989;46:112–114.

56. Roberts DW, Hartov A, Kennedy FE, Miga MI, Paulsen KD. Intraoperative brain shift and deformation: a quantitative analysis of cortical displacement in 28 cases. Neurosurgery 1998;43(4):749–758

57. Smith KR, Frank KJ, Bucholz RD. The NeuroStation—a highly accurate, minimally invasive solution to frameless stereotactic neurosurgery. Comput Med Imaging Graph 1994;18:247–256.

58. Adler JR. Surgical guidance now and in the future: the next generation of instrumentation. Clin Neurosurg 2002;49:105–114.

59. Hall WA, Martin A, Liu H, Truwit CL. Improving diagnostic yield in brain biopsy: coupling spectroscopic targeting with real-time needle placement. J Magn Reson Imaging 2001;13(1):12–15.

60. Kaakaji W, Barnett GH, Bernhard D, Warbel A, Valaitis K, Stamp S. Clinical and economic consequences of early discharge of patients following supratentorial stereotactic brain biopsy. J Neurosurg 2001;94(6):892–898.

61. Kulkarni A, Bernstein M. Stereotactic biopsy. In: Bernstein M, Berger M. eds. Neurooncology: the essentials.. New York:Thieme Medical Publishers Inc. 2000;122–129.

62. Moriarty TM, Quinones-Hinojosa A, Larson PS, et al. Frameless stereotactic neurosurgery using intraoperative magnetic resonance imaging: stereotactic brain biopsy. Neurosurgery 2000;47(5):1138–1145; discussion 1145–1146.

63. Cairncross JG, Ueki K, Zlatescu MC, et al. Specific genetic predictors of chemotherapeutic response and survival in patients with anaplastic oligodendrogliomas. J Natl Cancer Inst 1998;90(19):1473–1479.

64. Field M, Witham TF, Flickinger JC, Kondziolka D, Lunsford LD. Comprehensive assessment of hemorrhage risks and outcomes after stereotactic brain biopsy. J Neurosurg 2001;94(4):545–551.

65. Barnett GH. The role of image-guided technology in the surgical planning and resection of gliomas. J Neuro-Oncol 1999;42(3):247–258.

66. Burtscher IM, Skagerberg G, Geijer B, Englund E, Stahlberg F, Holtas S. Proton MR spectroscopy and preoperative diagnostic accuracy: an evaluation of intracranial mass lesions characterized by stereotactic biopsy findings. AJNR Am J Neuroradiol 2004;21(1):84–93.

67. Friedman WA, Sceats DJ Jr, Nestok BR, Ballinger WE Jr. The incidence of unexpected pathological findings in an image-guided biopsy series: a review of 100 consecutive cases. Neurosurgery 1989;25(2):180–184.

68. Hassenbusch SJ, Anderson JS, Pillay PK. Brain tumor resection aided with markers placed using stereotaxis guided by magnetic resonance imaging and computed tomography. Neurosurgery 1991;28(6):801–805.

69. Martin AJ, Liu H, Hall WA, Truwit CL. Preliminary assessment of turbo spectroscopic imaging for targeting in brain biopsy. AJNR Am J Neuroradiol 2001;22(5):959–968.

70. Pirotte B, Goldman S, Brucher JM, et al. PET in stereotactic conditions increases the diagnostic yield of brain biopsy. Stereotact Funct Neurosurg 1994;63(1-4):144–149.

71. Roessler K, Czech T, Dietrich W, et al. Frameless stereotactic-directed tissue sampling during surgery of suspected low-grade gliomas to avoid histological undergrading. Minim Invasive Neurosurg 1998;41(4):183–186.

72. Soo TM, Bernstein M, Provias J, Tasker R, Lozano A, Guha A. Failed stereotactic biopsy in a series of 518 cases. Stereotact Funct Neurosurg 1995;64(4):183–196.

73. Galloway RL, Maciunas RJ, Latimer JW. The accuracies of four stereotactic frame systems: an independent assessment. Biomed Instrum Tech 1991;25:457–460.

74. Maciunas RJ, Galloway RL, Latimer JW, Galloway RL Jr. The application accuracy of stereotactic frames. Neurosurgery 1994;35(4):682–694.

75. Maurer CR Jr, Fitzpatrick JM, Wang MY, Galloway RL Jr, Maciunas RJ, Allen GS. Registration of head volume images using implantable fiducial markers. IEEE Trans Med Imaging 1997;16(4):447–462.

76. Wang MY, Maurer CR Jr, Fitzpatrick JM, Maciunas RJ. An automatic technique for finding and localizing externally attached markers in CT and MR volume images of the head. IEEE Trans Biomed Eng 1996;43(6):627–637.

77. West JB, Fitzpatrick JM, Toms SA, Maurer CR, Maciunas RJ. Fiducial Point Placement and the Accuracy of Point-based, Rigid Body Registration. Neurosurgery 2001;48(4):810–816; discussion 816–817.

78. Winston KR. Hair and neurosurgery. Neurosurgery 1992;31:320–329.

79. Barnett GH, Steiner CP, and Weisenberger J. Target and trajectory guidance for interactive surgical navigation systems. Stereotact Funct Neurosurg 1996;66:91–95.

80. Brainard JA, Prayson RA, Barnett GH. Frozen section evaluation of stereotactic brain biopsies: diagnostic yield at the stereotactic target position in 188 cases. Arch Pathol Lab Med 1997;121(5):481–484.

81. Chimowitz MI, Barnett GH, Palmer J. Treatment of intractable arterial hemorrhage during stereotactic brain biopsy with thrombin. Report of three patients. J Neurosurg 1991;74(2):301–303.

82. Bhardwaj RD, Bernstein M. Prospective feasibility study of outpatient stereotactic brain lesion biopsy. Neurosurgery. 2002;51(2):358–361.

83. Devaux BC, O'Fallon JR, Kelly PJ. Resection, biopsy and survival in malignant glial neoplasms. A retrospective study of clinical parameters, therapy and outcome. J Neurosurg 1993;78:767–775.

84. Grady MS, Howard MA, Dacey RG, et al. Experimental study of the magnetic stereotaxis system for catheter manipulation within the brain. J Neurosurg 2000;93(2):282–288.

85. Nathoo N, Cavusoglu MC, Vogelbaum MA, Barnett GH. In Touch with Robotics: Neurosurgery for the Third Millennium. Neuosurgery 2005;56(3):421–433.

86. Luciano MG, Rhoten RLP, Barnett GH. Hydrocephalus. In: Barnett GH, Roberts DW, Maciunas RJ, eds. Image-Guided Neurosurgery: Clinical Applications of Surgical Navigation. St. Louis, Misouri;Quality Medical Publishing Inc. 1998;149–162.

87. Rhoten RL, Luciano MG, Barnett GH. Computer-assisted endoscopy for neurosurgical procedures: technical note. Neurosurgery 1997;40(3):632–637.

88. Bernstein M, Laperriere N, Glen J, Leung P, Thomason C, Landon AE Brachytherapy for recurrent malignant astrocytoma. Int J Radiat Oncol Biol Phys 1994;30(5):1213–1217.

89. Larson DA, Gutin PH, Leibel SA, Phillips TL, Sneed PK, Wara WM. Stereotaxic irradiation of brain tumors. Cancer 1990;65(3 Suppl):792–799.

90. Prados MD, Gutin PH, Phillips TL, et al. Interstitial brachytherapy for newly diagnosed patients with malignant gliomas: the UCSF experience. Int J Radiat Oncol Biol Phys 1992;24(4):593–597.

91. Laperriere NJ, Leung PM, McKenzie S, et al. Randomized study of brachytherapy in the initial management of patients with malignant astrocytoma. Int J Radiat Oncol Biol Phys 1998;41(5):1005–1011.

92. Selker RG, Shapiro WR, Burger Pet al. The Brain Tumor Cooperative Group NIH Trial 87-01: a randomized comparison of surgery, external radiotherapy, and carmustine versus surgery, interstitial radiotherapy boost, external radiation therapy, and carmustine. Neurosurgery 2002;51(2):343–355.

93. Barnett GH and Suh JH. Stereotactic radiosurgery for gliomas. In: Pollock BE ed. Contemporary Stereotactic Radiosurgery: Technique and Evaluation., Armonk, NY:Futura Publishing Company; 2002:265–279.

94. Souhami L, Seiferheld W, Brachman D, et al. Randomized comparison of stereotactic radiosurgery followed by conventional radiotherapy with carmustine to conventional radiotherapy with carmustine for patients with glioblastoma multiforme: report of radiation therapy oncology group 93–05 protocol. Int J Radiation Oncology Biol Phys 2004;60:853–860.

95. Tatter SB, Shaw EG, Rosenblum ML, Karvelis KC, et al. An inflatable balloon catheter and liquid 125I radiation source (GliaSite Radiation Therapy System) for treatment of recurrent malignant glioma: multicenter safety and feasibility trial. J Neurosurg 2003;99(2):297–303.

96. Broaddus WC, Gillies GT, Kucharczyk J. Minimally invasive procedures. Advances in image-guided delivery of drug and cell therapies into the central nervous system. Neuroimaging Clin N Am 2001;11:727–735.

97. Laws ER, Parney IF, Huang W, et al. Survival following surgery and prognostic factors for recently diagnosed malignant glioma: data from the Glioma Outcomes Project. J Neurosurg 2003;99(3):467–473.

98. Lunsford LD, Niranjan A. The rationale for rational surgery for fibrillary astrocytomas. Clin Neurosurg 2001; 48:20–36.

99. Rostomily RC, Spence AM, Duong D, et al. Multimodality management of recurrent adult malignant gliomas: results of a phase II multiagent chemotherapy study and analysis of cytoreductive surgery. Neurosurgery 1994;35:378–388.

100. Simpson JR, Horton J, Scott C, et al. Influence of extent of surgical resection on survival in patients with glioblastoma multiforme: results of three consecutive Radiation Therapy Oncology Group (RTOG) clinical trials. Int J Radiat Oncol Biol Phys 1993;26:239–244.

101. Barnett GH. Definition of Functional Anatomy. In: Barnett GH, Roberts DW, Maciunas RJ, eds. Image-Guided Neurosurgery: Clinical Applications of Surgical Navigation. St. Louis, MO; Quality Medical Publishing Inc. 1998;205–214.

102. Berman JI, Berger MS, Mukherjee P, Henry RG. Diffusion-tensor imaging-guided tracking of fibers of the pyramidal tract combined with intraoperative cortical stimulation mapping in patients with gliomas. J Neurosurg 2004;101(1):66–72.

103. Coenen VA, Krings T, Axer H, et al. Intraoperative three-dimensional visualization of the pyramidal tract in a neuronavigation system (PTV) reliably predicts true position of principal motor pathways. Surg Neurol 2003;60:381–390.

104. Keles GE, Lundin DA, Lamborn KR, Chang EF, Ojemann G, Berger MS. Intraoperative subcortical stimulation mapping for hemispherical perirolandic gliomas located within or adjacent to the descending motor pathways: evaluation of morbidity and assessment of functional outcome in 294 patients. J Neurosurg 2004; 100(3):369–375.

105. Hartkens T, Hill DL, Castellano-Smith ADet al. Measurement and analysis of brain deformation during neurosurgery. IEEE Trans Med Imaging 2003;22:82–92.

106. Hastreiter P, Engel K, Soza G, et al. Remote computing environment compensating for brain shift. Comp Aided Surg 2003;8:169–179.

107. Stummer W, Reulen H-J. Prospektiv-randomisierte Studie zur fluoreszenzgestützten Resektion maligner Gliome mit 5-Aminolävulinsäure. MANUALHirntumoren und primäre Tumoren des Rückenmarks. Tumorzentrum München und W. Zuckschwerdt Verlag München. 2004;203–206.

13 Radiation Therapy

Hiral K. Shah and Minesh P. Mehta

Summary

The role of radiation therapy in the management of high-grade gliomas was established by a series of prospective randomized trials. Subsequently, numerous attempts to improve outcomes with dose escalation, radiation sensitizers, neutrons, and brachytherapy have been unsuccessful. The lack of success with these approaches may be a consequence of poor target volume definition, tumor repopulation, or innate radioresistance. Until recently, the role of chemotherapy in the management of glioblastoma multiforme was unclear, but a large phase III randomized trial conclusively demonstrated a survival advantage of temozolomide delivered concurrently with radiation and in the adjuvant setting. The role of chemotherapy in the management of anaplastic astrocytoma and anaplastic oliodendroglioma remains to be defined. Current focus is on the identification of molecular pathways unique to high-grade gliomas that may serve as targets for future therapeutic agents.

Key Words: Glioblastoma multiforme; anaplastic astrocytoma; anaplastic oligodendroglioma; radiation therapy.

INTRODUCTION

The role of postoperative radiation therapy (RT) for high-grade gliomas (HGG) has been established through prospective randomized trials. The survival benefit is clear, but modest. Institutional dose escalation experience for World Health Organization (WHO) grade IV glioblastoma multiforme has been promising, but larger randomized trials have not demonstrated a benefit beyond 60 Gy. This may be a consequence of inadequate imaging resulting in poor target definition, relative radioresistance, accelerated tumor repopulation, patient selection differences between phase II and III trials, or the innate biases inherent in uncontrolled phase II trials. Most clinical trials of adjuvant chemotherapy for GBM have not yielded statistically significant clinical benefit, although some advantage is deduced from meta-analysis of these trials. A recent phase III trial has demonstrated that the addition of temozolomide (TMZ) to radiotherapy produces a survival advantage. However, this benefit is still modest and in order to rapidly evaluate novel agents and conserve clinical resources, the Radiation Therapy Oncology Group (RTOG) has devised the recursive partitioning analysis (RPA) classification model to which results of smaller, but appropriately powered phase II trials are compared, with the expectation that this "screening" process might yield promising agents which would subsequently be evaluated in larger phase III trials.

Patients diagnosed with WHO grade III anaplastic astrocytoma (AA) have a significantly better prognosis than GBM; however, dose intensification with particle therapy, brachytherapy, radiosensitizers, or chemotherapy has not shown a conclusive clinical benefit, and in fact,

From: *Current Clinical Oncology: High-Grade Gliomas: Diagnosis and Treatment*
Edited by: G. H. Barnett © Humana Press Inc., Totowa, NJ

there is even a suggestion that these intensification approaches might paradoxically have resulted in a reduction in survival. Randomized clinical trials have failed to show categorical benefit from chemotherapy, although a recent meta-analysis suggests a small benefit. Currently there is significant interest in incorporating TMZ for these tumors, and randomized clinical trials are ongoing.

WHO grade III anaplastic oligodendroglioma (AO), both pure and mixed (but with a predominant oligodendroglial component) represent a very unique tumor with specific chromosomal abnormalities which predict for improved outcomes with the use of chemotherapy or radiotherapy. The RTOG recently reported on a large, randomized trial in which adjuvant procarbazine, carmustine and vincristine (PCV) was not shown to be of benefit in terms of overall survival, although progression-free survival was somewhat improved, especially for AO patients with loss of at least one copy of 1p and 19q. There are preliminary data establishing the activity of TMZ for this disease and hence there is significant interest in further defining the value of this agent for AO.

GLIOBLASTOMA MULTIFORME

The role of postoperative radiation therapy for patients with GBM was established by a landmark randomized trial that compared best supportive care to carmustine (BCNU) and/or external beam radiation to a dose of 50 to 60 Gy (1). Postoperative RT was associated with a median survival time (MST) of 35 wk compared with 14 wk for best supportive care. The combination of BCNU and RT did not improve median survival but did increase survival at 18 mo. These results were validated by studies reported by Kristiansen et al. (2) and Andersen et al. (3), both reporting significant improvement in survival with the addition of posterative-operative RT. Laperriere et al. analyzed six published randomized trials of postoperative RT compared with best supportive care for patients with GBM and demonstrated a relative risk of survival of 0.81 with the addition of postoperative RT (4). The results of these randomized trials are summarized in Table 1.

Dose Response Relationship

The Brain Tumor Study Group (BTSG) also reported a radiotherapy dose vs response relationship, with patients receiving 60 Gy having a MST of 42.0 wk compared with a MST of 28.0 wk for patients receiving 50 Gy and a MST of 13.5 wk for patients receiving $\leq$ 45 Gy (5). These data are summarized in Table 2. These results were corroborated by a United Kingdom Medical Research Council (UKMRC) trial which randomized patients to 45 Gy in 20 fractions and 60 Gy in 30 fractions and demonstrated that patients in the higher dose arm had a significantly longer MST (12 –9 mo; $p = 0.007$) (6). Phillips et al. performed a randomized trial comparing 35 Gy in 10 fractions ($n = 32$) to 60 Gy in 30 ($n = 36$) fractions for patients with GBM and AA and demonstrated a MST of 8.7 mo (7.4–10.7 mo) with the former regimen and 10.3 mo (7.8–14.0 mo) with the latter regimen. These results were not statistically significant ($p = 0.37$), likely a result of the small number of patients in each arm (7).

These early trials frequently involved treatment of the entire brain. The advent of computed tomography (CT) and magnetic resonance imaging (MRI) facilitated improved tumor localization and advances in treatment planning allowed delivery of conformal radiotherapy to precisely defined volumes. Additionally, the work of Kelly et al. (8) and Hochberg et al. (9) demonstrated that microscopic extension is predominantly confined to a few centimeters around the enhancing tumor and the primary site of treatment failure is recurrence at the

Table 1
Randomized Trials of Postoperative Radiotherapy

Ref.	n	Randomization scheme	Results
(1)	222*	Postoperative BCNU, RT, BCNU +RT, or best supportive care	Patients receiving RT had significantly longer MST (35 wk) than patients receiving BCNU alone (MST 18.5 wk) or best supportive care (MST 14.0 wk) (p = significant)
(2)	118	Postoperative RT, RT + bleomycin, or supportive care	MST with RT alone 10.2 mo compared with 5.2 mo with supportive care (p = significant)
(3)	108	Postoperative RT compared to best supportive care	Postoperative RT significantly improves survival compared to best supportive care ($p < 0.05$)
(37)	33	Postoperative RT and BCNU compared to BCNU alone	MST with BCNU alone 30 wk compared with 44.5 wk for RT + BCNU (p = ns)
(38)	171	Postoperative PCV ± RT	MST with PCV alone 42 wk compared with 62 wk for PCV+ RT (p = .028)
(39)	358*	Postoperative Semustine, RT, Semustine +RT, BCNU +RT	Patients receiving RT had significantly longer MST(36–51 wk) than patients receiving Semustine alone (MST 24 wk) (p = significant)

*Valid study group.

Table 2
Radiotherapy Dose Vs Response Relationship for GBM

Dose (Gy)	MS (wk)	25% Surv	p
0	18	N/A	N/A
<45	14	N/A	Ns
50	28	52	<0.001
55	36	57	<0.001
60	42	68	<0.001

Abbr: MS, median survival; 25% Surv, 25th percentile survival.

original tumor site in 90% of patients. These findings support the role of partial field irradiation. This was prospectively evaluated by Shapiro et al. in the Brain Tumor Cooperative Group Trial (BTCG) 8001 which randomized patients to three different chemotherapy regimens (10). In the early years of the trial all patients were treated with whole brain radiation to 60.2 Gy but later patients were randomized to whole brain radiotherapy or whole brain irradiation to 43 Gy with a boost of 17.2 Gy to the preirradiation contrast enhancing volume with a 2-cm margin. They reported no significant difference in survival between the different radiation volumes.

Dose Escalation

In most biological systems, radiation exhibits stochastic properties. In cell–culture systems, when survival curves as a function of dose are generated, a dose-dependant response,

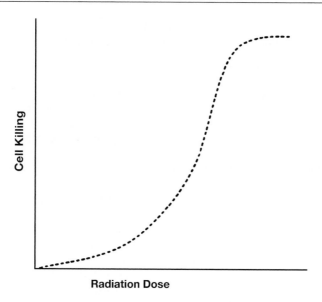

Fig. 1. Radiation therapy dose response relationship.

with an initial "shoulder" and subsequent slope is clearly identified. These cell-survival curves are best described by a linear–quadratic function. In the human context, very clear dose-dependent phenomena such as hair loss, cataract formation, skin reactions, and xerostomia can be quantified. These clinical dose-response curves are characterized by a sigmoidal shape, with low doses initially producing a relatively flat response curve, but demonstrating an upward response-inflection after a certain threshold dose, beyond which the response slope is large for a minimal change in dose; at much higher doses, there is a flattening of the curve, resulting in lower incremental gain. One example of such a dose-response relationship is illustrated in Fig. 1. For malignant brain tumors such as GBM, most therapeutic trials have explored the 0 to 60 Gy dose range, a few hyperfractionation trials have explored doses up to 80 Gy and brachytherapy trials have reached 100 to 120 Gy. Although the dose-response phenomenon across this large range has not been prospectively evaluated, a review of the composite data from various clinical trials and institutional experiences (Fig. 2) suggest the possibility of a shallow dose-response effect.

Based on these composite data, one may hypothesize that further improvement in clinical results may be possible with dose escalation beyond the conventional 60 Gy. However, in a recent phase I trial from the University of Michigan, no clear survival benefit was identified for GBM patients receiving doses approaching 90 Gy *(11)*. The failure to demonstrate any survival advantage with dose escalation in large randomized and some institutional trials is possibly a result of one or more of the following barriers: (1) inadequate imaging resulting in a geographic miss, (2) innate tumor radioresistance, and (3) accelerated tumor repopulation.

GEOGRAPHIC MISS

Current radiotherapy planning incorporates MRI data to determine treatment volumes. Initially, a large field encompassing the T2-signal abnormality including surrounding edema with a 2- to 3-cm margin is treated to 45 Gy with a subsequent boost to the T1-contrast

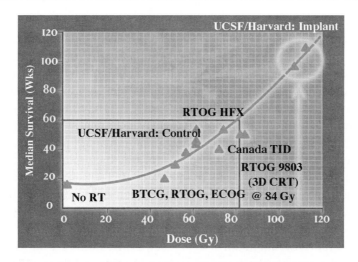

Fig. 2. Composite data of clinical outcomes with dose escalation.

enhancing region with a 1- to 2-cm margin for a total dose of 59.4 Gy. The accurate definition of these fields, especially the boost field, is critical. Otherwise, a geographic miss will result. The likelihood of a geographic miss with whole brain radiation may seem implausible, but many of these trials boosted regions with a high likelihood of microscopic disease. If there is viable tumor outside of the boost region then the treatment is destined to fail.

Magnetic resonance spectroscopy (MRS) is a noninvasive imaging tool that can distinguish between tumor bearing regions, normal tissues, and necrosis based on the metabolic profile of the tissue. The three main cerebral metabolites are choline-containing compounds (Cho), the total creatine pool, and *N*-acetylaspartate (NAA). An increase in Cho containing compounds relative to NAA correlates closely with tumor infiltration; a corresponding increase in creatine predicts for a malignant neoplastic process such as GBM. Researchers at the University of California San Francisco (UCSF) compared radiotherapy planning based on standard MRI to MRS for 34 patients with HGG *(12)*. In their study, they found that metabolically active tumor extended outside the T2 region in 88% of patients. Additionally, defining the boost volume as the T1-contrast enhancing region with a 2-cm margin missed metabolically active tumor by as much as 2.8 cm.

To demonstrate the importance of MRS in predicting clinical outcomes, Graves et al. performed MRS and standard MRI on patients with recurrent GBM who met criteria for gamma-knife radiosurgery *(13)*. Patients were planned using MRI data. Based on the results of the preradiosurgery MRS, patients were scored as 0 to 1 (pretreatment MRS confined to the radiosurgery target) and 2 to 3 (pretreatment MRS was beyond the radiosurgery target by <5 or >5 cm, respectively). Patients in category 2 to 3 had a significantly shorter time to progression and lower 1-yr survival time. These data clearly suggest that conventional MRI is likely inadequate at identifying the true extent of tumor that needs to be boosted; as long as this remains poorly defined, radiotherapy is doomed to fail, irrespective of dose.

The use of positron emission tomography (PET) with radiolabeled 2-[18F]fluoro-2-deoxy-D-glucose (FDG) has been used clinically to determine sites of metastatic disease based on the principle that tumor cells will incorporate more glucose within the cell and metabolize it more rapidly than normal cells. Its utility in gliomas is limited secondary to increased background cortical activity that makes it difficult to delineate tumor volumes. Jacobs et al, examined combining MRI, FDG-PET, PET with radiolabeled *methyl*-[¹¹C]-L-methionine (MET) or radiolabeled 3'-deoxy-3'-[18F]fluoro-L-thymidine (FLT) and demonstrated that the latter twoO modalities were very sensitive noninvasive modalities for imaging gliomas *(14)*. Investigators at the University of California Los Angeles (UCLA) have utilized F-18 dopa imaging for gliomas with promising preliminary data; these advances may afford imaging technologies with superior ability to distinguish the true extent of malignant glioma *(15)*. Conventionally, PET data have not served as an adequate source for treatment planning because of limited anatomic detail; however, with the advent of integrated PET-CT devices, both functional and corresponding anatomic data are readily available, which can further be fused to MR image sets, thereby providing unprecedented sophistication in the level of detail available for treatment planning.

Thus, the incorporation of functional imaging such as MRS and PET into three-dimensional (3D) radiotherapy planning has the potential to improve target volume delineation, reduce the likelihood of a geographic miss, and may facilitate demonstration of a clinical benefit to dose escalation.

INNATE RADIORESISTANCE

To demonstrate improved clinical outcomes from dose escalation, issues regarding the radioresistance of the tumor must be addressed.

Hypoxic Cell Modifiers. From a radiobiological perspective, it is well documented that hypoxic cells are more radioresistant, by a factor of 2.5 to 3, compared with oxic cells *(16)*. Hypoxia is commonly encountered in malignant glioma, and is believed to result in dysregulation in the expression of hypoxia-induced factor 1α (HIF1 α), which regulates transcription of vascular endothelial growth factor (VEGF), a major proangiogenic protein. Thus, the fact that hypervascularity, high levels of VEGF expression and hypoxia are all intimately linked in GBM is therefore no surprise. Twelve randomized studies of hypoxic cell sensitizers, misonidazole, metronidazole, or nimorazole have been conducted. These agents produced significant radiosensitization in vitro; however, all of the clinical trials, with the exception of one small study, have not detected a significant advantage for hypoxic cell sensitizers. Overgaard et al. performed a meta-analysis of these combined trials and did not detect a significant survival advantage for hypoxic cell sensitizers in malignant glioma *(17)*.

RSR 13 is a synthetic allosteric modifier of hemoglobin that reduces its oxygen binding affinity resulting in greater unloading of oxygen in tissue. The New Approaches to Brain Tumor Therapy consortium (NABTT) conducted a phase II trial utilizing daily RSR 13 prior to RT for GBM patients *(18)*. This regimen was well-tolerated and resulted in a median survival time of 12.3 mo which compared favorably to results from 3 other trial conducted between 1993 to 1999 utilizing Paclitaxel, 9-AC, and CI-980. These data, however, were not superior to historic controls from the NABTT database.

Halogenated Pyrimidines. There has been significant interest in the use of halogenated pyrimidines, bromodeoxyuridine (BudR) and iododeoxyuridine (IudR) as radiosensitizers. The incorporation of these compounds into DNA of rapidly dividing cells "weakens" the DNA structure and makes it mores susceptible to ionizing radiation. Gliomas represent an ideal target for the study of such radiosensitizers because highly proliferating tumor cells are surrounded by nonproliferating normal brain tissue that shows little to no DNA incorporation of the halogenated pyrimidines. Radiosensitizers are only effective in cells that take up the agent. If even 10% of tumor cells do not incorporate the agent, it will be difficult to demonstrate any advantage. To maximize the proportion of tumor cells incorporating halogenated pyrimidines, a phase I study was conducted utilizing a continuous infusion of IudR for 28 d with hyperfractionated accelerated radiotherapy *(19)*. Even with improvement in the pharmacokinetics of IudR with continuous infusion, survival data could not be interpreted as clinically advantageous.

Prados et al. reviewed 2 RTOG trials and the Northern California Oncology Group (NCOG) trial that included over 1700 patients to determine the impact of BudR on patients with GBM and AA *(20)*. Univariate analysis favored the use of BudR for GBM patients and proportional hazard regression model indicated a benefit for GBM patients receiving BudR (*RR* = 0.83).

Motexafin-Gadolinium (MGd). MGd is a unique MRI detectable radiosensitizer that depletes ascorbate and co-factor NADPH, which metabolically stresses tumor cells through adenosine triphosphate (ATP) depletion and predisposes cells to undergo apoptosis. Recent data suggest that MGd inhibits ribonucleotide reductase, a key enzyme that is upregulated in most neoplasms to support the enhanced requirement for DNA synthesis. MGd inhibits potentially lethal damage repair and sublethal damage repair. In preclinical trials it has been shown to enhance radiation responses and demonstrates selective uptake and accumulation in tumors. Ford et al. reported the results of a phase I trial of 33 GBM patients who received RT concurrently with MGd *(21)*. Kaplan-Meier estimate of MST of 17.6 mo for patients treated with MGd compared with MST of 12.9 mo for 33 matched patients in the RTOG database. In a recent composite analysis of 56 GBM patients from the preceding phase I trial, together with a smaller phase II trial of MGd, the median survival was 14.7 mo. The 45 patients who received 6 0mg/kg of MGd had a 6- and 12-mo survival of 93% and 75% respectively (personal communication; see Phan, MD, Pharmacyclics Inc; submitted to SNO 2004).

Radiosensitizing Chemotherapy. The use of low-dose concurrent chemotherapy as a radiosensitizer has improved outcomes in patients with head and neck cancer and cervical cancer. Stupp et al. tested this hypothesis in GBM patients with TMZ. TMZ is an oral alkylating agent that penetrates the blood–brain barrier (BBB) with a plasma to cerebrospinal fluid (CSF) ratio of 30 to 40%. Based on promising phase II trials, Stupp et al. conducted a large (*n* = 573) phase III randomized trial of radiotherapy with or without concurrent TMZ and demonstrated a 3 mo improvement in both median and overall survival (MST: 12–15 mo; *p* < 0.0001) for patients receiving concurrent TMZ and RT *(22)*. Currently the RTOG is conducting phase II trials of TMZ in combination with other chemotherapeutic and molecularly targeted agents in patients with GBM, including CPT-11, the farnesyl transferase inhibitors Sarasar. R115777, and MGd.

Epidermal Growth Factor Receptor (EGFR) Inhibitors. The epidermal growth factor receptor (EGFR) belongs to a family of at least four *trans*-membrane cell-surface receptors. Structurally, these complex proteins have an extracellular domain with specific binding affinity for particular ligands such as epidermal growth factor (EGF), a growth factor that after binding induces dimerization and phosphorylation of EGFR through an enzyme, receptor tyrosine kinase (RTK), located on the intracellular domain of EGFR. This activated complex is involved in signaling through several cytoplasmic pathways that are activated by a series of phosphorylation reactions, catalyzed by other kinases, and results in the transduction of signal from the cell surface to the nucleus. Within the nucleus, the arrival of such a signal results in transcriptional activation of specific genes, and hence synthesis/expression of regulatory proteins which affect a host of cellular phenotypic responses such as cell–cycle regulation, apoptosis, growth-arrest, growth-acceleration, neoangiogenesis, and differentiation.

EGFR is overexpressed in about 40% of patients with GBM *(23)*. Barker et al. examined the UCSF database of GBM patients and identified 174 tumor specimens to determine a correlation between EFGR status and response to radiation. A three-tier system was used to score EGFR status: 0 indicated no staining, 1 indicated light or focal staining, and 2 indicated strong staining. Radiation response was based on comparison between pre-RT and post-RT contrast enhanced CT or MRI. In their analysis, there was strong correlation ($p = 0.046$) between EGFR score of 0 and odds of better radiation response compared with EGFR scores of 2. Not all studies, however, support this observation. In an analysis of tissue microarray prepared from 155 GBM patients enrolled on RTOG trials, specimens were stained using a mouse monoclonal antibody (MAb) specific for the extracellular binding domain of EGFR to detect total EGFR (including wild-type-both phosphorylated and unphosphorylated isoforms with some cross-reactivity with EGFRvIII, a mutant variant commonly seen in GBM). The intensity of total EGFR expression was measured by computerized quantitative image analysis and correlated with clinical outcome. No association between EGFR expression and survival was identified on a multivariate analysis *(24)*. These results were corroborated by Buckner et al. who analyzed EGFR overexpression in malignant glioma patients enrolled on the North Central Cancer Treatment Group (NCCTG) trial and did not find a correlation between EGFR overexpression and survival in patients with GBM *(25)*.

Preclinical experiments demonstrate that blockade of the EGFR pathway, either using antibodies such as C225 specific to EGFR, or inhibitors of RTK such as ZD-1839, or other interventions of this cascade (i.e., blocking a key enzymatic step, farnesylation, through farnesyl transferase inhibitors), results in altered cellular behavior, particularly, a shift from a growth-advantaged to a disadvantaged status *(26)*. In the face of an external potentially lethal stimulus such as radiation, inhibition of the EGFR pathway enhances apoptosis, reduces proliferative capacity, diminishes angiogenesis, and ultimately provides a method for enhanced tumor kill, or radiopotentiation. Additional preclinical data indicate a synergistic effect of EGFR blockade and radiation. The RTOG has recently completed a trial using ZD-1839 with radiotherapy for GBM *(27)*.

ACCELERATED TUMOR REPOPULATION

Accelerated tumor repopulation is a well-recognized phenomenon that occurs in rapidly proliferating tumors during a conventional multifraction radiotherapy regimen. This acceleration in proliferation during the radiotherapy regimen increases the likelihood that viable tumor clonogens maybe present at the completion of treatment. Traditionally, dose escalation experiments have involved increasing the number of fractions; however, it is possible that the addition of fractions at the end of radiotherapy may not compensate for the acceleration in tumor repopulation. Accelerated fractionation (AF) attempts to minimize tumor acceleration by shortening the overall duration of radiotherapy by increasing the number of daily fractions, or effectively delivering more dose per day. A similar phenomenon occurs in several other malignancies, including head and neck cancer and lung cancer where randomized trials with AF have demonstrated improvements in local control and survival.

Accelerated Fractionation and Radiosurgery. RTOG Trial 83-02 was a dose escalation trial with either hyperfractionated radiotherapy (HF RT) (1.2 Gy bid to 64.8, 72, 76.8, or 81.6 Gy) or accelerated hyperfractionation (AHF) (1.6 Gy bid to 48 or 54.4 Gy) *(28)*. Though the dose delivery in the AHF arm was feasible and associated with tolerable toxicity, the mean survival time (MST) of these patients was 10.2 mo compared with 11.6 mo for HF RT. The lack of benefit with AHF maybe a result of the low biologically equivalent doses utilized in the AHF arm. The RTOG recently closed a phase II trial examining weekly fractionated stereotactic radiotherapy (FSRT) boost (5 or 7 Gy) during a course of conventional 6-wk radiotherapy to overcome tumor repopulation. This trial used significantly higher total doses and its results are keenly awaited.

Potentially, single fraction radiosurgery boost could be viewed as a form of AHF, although the total doses achievable through this approach are limited because of the use of a single radiosurgery fraction. In a recently completed RTOG phase III trial, the addition of a stereotactic radiosurgery boost to external beam radiotherapy and BCNU did not improve survival *(29)*.

Brachytherapy. Brachytherapy involves insertion of permanent or temporary radioactive sources within tumor harboring tissues. One of the advantages of brachytherapy is the rapid reduction in dose that allows higher doses to be delivered to high-risk areas while minimizing radiation exposure to surrounding normal tissues. It has been used as a method for dose escalation with promising institutional reports. There have been two randomized trials of external beam radiotherapy with or without interstitial ^{125}I brachytherapy, but neither have demonstrated a survival benefit for interstitial brachytherapy *(30,31)*. With conventional brachytherapy, there is typically a several week delay between the completion of external beam radiotherapy and initiation of brachytherapy. During this delay there is ample time for tumors to repopulate. The Gliasite device is a catheter inserted intraoperatively into the tumor bed which allows inflation of various sized balloons into which a radioisotope is subsequently instilled to deliver a high dose of radiation to the surgical margin and a modest peritumoral bed, of approx 1- to 2-cm depth. Unlike standard brachytherapy, there is limited radiation dose to the center resulting in a lower incidence of reoperation for necrosis. The radiation dose is delivered over a period of 3 to 5 d to overcome accelerated repopulation. The target area (tumor bed + 1–2 cm) receives at least 100% of the prescribed dose, typically 40 to 60 Gy. Currently no adequate clinical trials in newly diagnosed GBM patients with this device have been conducted. This device maybe most valuable in GBM patients undergoing a total or near-total resection or as a method of palliation in patients with recurrent disease in whom a significant resection can be achieved.

RPA Classification System

From these various trials, it becomes evident that patients with GBM represent a heterogeneous group; however, an adequate staging system has never been developed. The Radiation Therapy Oncology Group (RTOG) has analyzed an extensive database of prospectively treated patients (primarily with surgery, radiotherapy and alkylating chemotherapy), and using a statistical method known as recursive partitioning analysis (RPA), have developed six prognostic groups, referred to as RTOG RPA classes I–VI for classifying patients with high grade gliomas *(32)*. Patients can be segmented into classes using eight variables: age, histology, Karnofsky Performance Score (KPS), mental status, neurological function, symptom duration, extent of resection, and radiotherapy dose. This is illustrated in Fig. 3 with corresponding clinical outcomes summarized in Table 3. GBM patients are represented in classes III–VI, and their median survival ranges from 4.6 to 17.9 mo.

The RPA classification permits evaluation of new therapeutic approaches in combination with radiotherapy using a series of small phase II trials, in which patients are categorized by RPA class and outcomes are compared with the historic database. Promising agents can be further studied in phase III trial. This approach allows maximum resource utilization and allows early identification of potentially promising agents in management of patients with GBM.

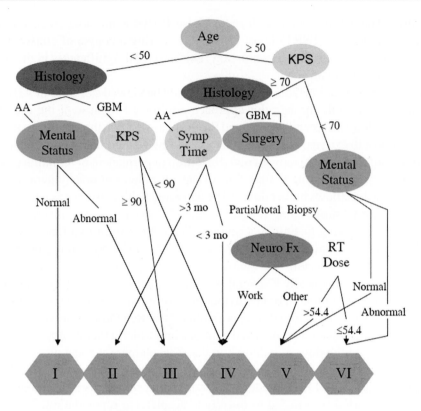

Fig. 3. RPA classification of HGG.

Table 3
Survival Based on RPA Classification

RPA class	n	MST (mp)	% 2-yr survival
I	139	58.6	76
II	34	37.4	68
III	175	17.9	35
IV	457	11.1	15
V	395	8.9	6
VI	263	4.6	4

ANAPLASTIC ASTROCYTOMA

Traditionally, patients with anaplastic astrocytoma (AA) have been included in trials with GBM patients. It became clear very early that patients with AA (MST 36 mo) had a significantly better survival than patients with GBM (MST <12 mo). Newer trials therefore evaluate AA patients separately from GBM patients. Attempts to improve survival have included the use of chemotherapy, radiosensitizers, and neutron therapy. Laramore et al. analyzed the RTOG experience treating AA with conventional radiotherapy, chemoradiotherapy and the addition of neutrons, demonstrating median survival values of 3, 2.3 and 1.7 yr *(33)*. Thus, paradoxically it appears that intensifying treatment leads to worse outcome.

RTOG trial 94–04 examined the role of the radiosensitizer bromodeoxyuridine (BudR) in addition to radiotherapy and PCV chemotherapy for patients with AA, excluding GBM. This phase III trial demonstrated no survival advantage with BudR .

Currently the RTOG is conducting a randomized trial for patients with AA to determine whether BCNU or TMZ is the optimal chemotherapy regimen during and after radiotherapy.

ANAPLASTIC OLIGODENDROGLIOMA

These rare tumors represent a unique clinical situation from the perspective of radiotherapy. They typically carry a more favorable prognosis than their astrocytic counterparts with a MST of 60 mo. The better survival observed for oligodendroglioma is also reflected in its improved responsiveness to both radiotherapy and chemotherapy. Recent molecular analysis suggests that subsets of these tumors are characterized by chromosomal losses of 1p and/or 19q. Patients with AO that have these chromosomal deletions exhibit exquisite sensitivity to radiation and chemotherapy *(34)*. The RTOG conducted a randomized phase III trial to determine the value of preradiation PCV chemotherapy. This trial also confirmed loss of 1p and 19q as significant prognostic factors, but did not demonstrate a specific survival benefit to the use of PCV *(35)*.

TMZ has been used for patients with recurrent AO. Chinot et al. treated 48 patients who experienced a recurrence after receiving PCV with TMZ and reported a 44% radiographic response rate, with 15 patients experiencing a complete response *(36)*. Based on the lower toxicity of TMZ, a pilot RTOG trial addressing the role of postoperative, pre-RT TMZ for newly diagnosed AO has recently been completed.

RADIOTHERAPY TECHNIQUES

Radiation therapy can be delivered using either external beam techniques of varying degrees of sophistication, or through highly localized isotope placement, known as brachytherapy. There are several different options, each with specific advantages and disadvantages. Brachytherapy approaches are most effective at delivering highly localized radiation and avoiding irradiation of normal tissue, but they are limited because of their invasive nature. External beam radiotherapy approaches have evolved and recently become very sophisticated (e.g., FSRT, IMRT) allowing the ability to conformally shape the radiation beam to minimize normal tissue exposure. This has been achieved by improvement in tumor targeting, using sophisticated treatment planning programs capable of permitting image-fusion of multiple different datasets (i.e., CT, MRI, MRS, and PET) as well as significant improvement in immobilization and localization processes, allowing a reduction in the size of the error margin that is typically built into radiotherapy treatment plans. For patients with HGG, the initial treatment field includes the MRI defined T2-signal abnormality, including edema, with a 2- to 3-cm margin that is treated to 45 Gy in 1.8 Gy per fraction. The boost field is defined by the T1-contrast enhancing region on the MRI with a 1- to 2-cm margin and is treated to an additional 14.4 Gy in 1.8 Gy per fraction for a total dose of 59.4 Gy.

SIDE EFFECTS OF RADIOTHERAPY

Acute Reactions

Acute reactions are those that occur during and immediately following completion of a course of external beam radiation therapy. Using current technologies, these reactions are usually rare and clinically readily manageable. These include skin reactions, typically dry desquamation and some degree of erythema, which are managed with local ointments. Temporary alopecia within the radiation field is a common sequela. Fatigue may be observed with radiation therapy, but is often a function of several other variables such as age, performance status, underlying medical status, and extent of brain being irradiated.

Subacute Reactions

Subacute reactions may occur several weeks or months after completion of radiation therapy. When large volumes of the brain are treated, especially in younger patients, lethargy and somnolence may be observed in approx 3 mo. In children, this is specifically described as an acute somnolence syndrome. Rarely, some patients may develop localized demyelination resulting in nausea, vomiting, ataxia, dysphasia, and cerebellar ataxia. This is usually self-limiting. If the lacrimal gland(s) are included in the radiation portal, dry-eye may result; similarly, a keratoconjunctivitis may develop if the cornea is not protected.

Late Complications

Late complications of radiotherapy occur from several months to several years after completion of therapy. The exact incidence of these complications is unclear because a substantial proportion of patients are either short-term survivors or have a component of both tumor progression and delayed radiation morbidity. Radiation necrosis in the absence of tumor progression is not commonly encountered when total doses are kept under 60 Gy. However, necrosis in concert with viable tumor is commonly seen, especially in patients with malignant glioma. With sequential CT imaging, a mineralizing angiopathy can be identified, characterized by loss of white matter, enlarged ventricles and microcalcifications. This occurs as a consequence of radiation injury to small vessels, and clinically may result in impairment of intellectual function, especially memory and mathematical ability. In severe cases, this may result in significant dementia, ataxia, and confusion. Significant white matter atrophy may be an accompaniment on imaging studies. The clinical sequela of these changes frequently manifest as neurocognitive impairment. Several factors have now been identified as contributory to overall neurocognitive decline in these patients, including the tumor itself, surgery, radiation, and chemotherapy. In addition, host factors such as underlying diseases, especially those disease characterized by microvascular changes (e.g., diabetes, hypertension, smoking, stroke, and cardiovascular insufficiency) also contribute to this. Specific radiotherapy parameters that influence the risk profile for neurocognitive decline include fraction size, total dose, and volume irradiated. Therefore, current radiotherapy paradigms, in general, avoid large fraction irradiation, with radiosurgery representing an exception to this rule. More importantly, 3D and conformal techniques are evolving and hold promise for reducing the volume of normal brain irradiated. These approaches are of significance, since no effective therapy exists for the patient suffering neurocognitive decline after radiotherapy.

REFERENCES

1. Walker MD, Alexander E, Jr, Hunt WE, et al. Evaluation of BCNU and/or radiotherapy in the treatment of anaplastic gliomas. A cooperative clinical trial. J Neurosurg 1978;49(3):333–343.
2. Kristiansen K, Hagen S, Kollevold T, et al. Combined modality therapy of operated astrocytomas grade III and IV. Confirmation of the value of postoperative irradiation and lack of potentiation of bleomycin on survival time: a prospective multicenter trial of the Scandinavian Glioblastoma Study Group. Cancer 1981;47(4):649–652.
3. Andersen AP. Postoperative irradiation of glioblastomas. Results in a randomized series. Acta Radiol Oncol Radiat Phys Biol 1978;17(6):475–484.

4. Laperriere N, Zuraw L, Cairncross G, Cancer Care Ontario Practice Guidelines Initiative Neuro-Oncology Disease Site G. Radiotherapy for newly diagnosed malignant glioma in adults: a systematic review. Radiother Oncol 2002;64(3):259–273.

5. Walker MD, Strike TA, Sheline GE. An analysis of dose-effect relationship in the radiotherapy of malignant gliomas. Int J Radiat Oncol Biol Phys 1979;5(10):1725–1731.

6. Bleehen NM, Stenning SP. A Medical Research Council trial of two radiotherapy doses in the treatment of grades 3 and 4 astrocytoma. The Medical Research Council Brain Tumour Working Party. Br J Cancer 1991; 64(4):769–774.

7. Phillips C, Guiney M, Smith J, Hughes P, Narayan K, Quong G. A randomized trial comparing 35Gy in ten fractions with 60Gy in 30 fractions of cerebral irradiation for glioblastoma multiforme and older patients with anaplastic astrocytoma. Radiother Oncol 2003;68(1):23–26.

8. Kelly PJ, Daumas-Duport C, Kispert DB, Kall BA, Scheithauer BW, Illig JJ. Imaging-based stereotaxic serial biopsies in untreated intracranial glial neoplasms. J Neurosurg 1987;66(6):865–874.

9. Hochberg FH, Pruitt A. Assumptions in the radiotherapy of glioblastoma. Neurology 1980;30(9):907–911.

10. Shapiro WR, Green SB, Burger PC, et al. Randomized trial of three chemotherapy regimens and two radio-therapy regimens and two radiotherapy regimens in postoperative treatment of malignant glioma. Brain Tumor Cooperative Group Trial 8001. J Neurosurg 1989;71(1):1–9.

11. Chan JL, Lee SW, Fraass BA, et al. Survival and failure patterns of high-grade gliomas after three-dimensional conformal radiotherapy. J Clin Oncol 2002;20(6):1635–1642.

12. Pirzkall A, McKnight TR, Graves EE, et al. MR-spectroscopy guided target delineation for high-grade glio-mas. Int J Radiat Oncol Biol Phys 2001;50(4):915–928.

13. Graves EE, Nelson SJ, Vigneron DB, et al. A preliminary study of the prognostic value of proton magnetic resonance spectroscopic imaging in gamma knife radiosurgery of recurrent malignant gliomas. Neurosurgery 2000;46(2):319–326; discussion 26–28.

14. Jacobs AH, Winkler A, Dittmar C, et al. Molecular and functional imaging technology for the development of efficient treatment strategies for gliomas. Technol Cancer Res Treat 2002;1(3):187–204.

15. Chen W CT, Kamdar N. Imaging gliomas with FDOPA and FLT, compared with FDG. In: Society of Nuclear Medicine 2004.

16. Hall E. Radiobiology for the Radiobiologist, 5th Ed. Philadelphia:Lippincott, Williams & Wilkins; 2000.

17. Overgaard J. Clinical evaluation of nitroimidazoles as modifiers of hypoxia in solid tumors. Oncol Res 1994; 6(10–11):509–518.

18. Kleinberg L, Grossman SA, Carson K, et al. Survival of patients with newly diagnosed glioblastoma multiforme treated with RSR13 and radiotherapy: results of a phase II new approaches to brain tumor therapy CNS consortium safety and efficacy study. J Clin Oncol 2002;20(14):3149–3155.

19. Schulz CA MM, Badie B, et al. Continuous 28 day iododeoxyuridine infusion and hyperfractionated accel-erated radiotherapy for malignant glioma: A phase I clinical study. Int J Radiat Oncol Biol Phys 2004;59(4): 1007–1115.

20. Prados MD, Scott CB, Rotman M, et al. Influence of bromodeoxyuridine radiosensitization on malignant glioma patient survival: a retrospective comparison of survival data from the Northern California Oncology Group (NCOG) and Radiation Therapy Oncology Group trials (RTOG) for glioblastoma multiforme and anaplastic astrocytoma. Int J Radiat Oncol Biol Phys 1998;40(3):653–659.

21. Ford J SW, Mehta MP, et al. Comparison of survival of patients in the phase I study of Motexafin Gadolinium (MGd) with radiation therapy (RT) for glioblastoma multiforme (GBM), with a matched cohort of patients from the RTOG RPA glioma data base. In: American Society of Clinical Oncology; 2003.

22. Stupp R MP, Mason WP, van den Bent MJ, et al. Radiotherapy plus concomittant and adjuvant temozolomide for glioblastoma. N Engl J Med 2005;352:987–996.

23. Barker FG 2nd, Simmons ML, Chang SM, et al. EGFR overexpression and radiation response in glioblastoma multiforme. Int J Radiat Oncol Biol Phys 2001;51(2):410–418.

24. Seiferheld W, Chakravarti A, Ang KK, et al. Overexpression of the epidermal growth factor receptor (EGFR), as determined by EGFR immunostaining on tissue microarrays, fails to demonstrate prognostic value for patients with glioblastoma multiforme: a report from RTOG 7401, 7918, 8302, 8409, 9006, 9305, 9602, and 9806. IInt J Radiat Oncol Biol Phys 2002;54(2 Supp 1):96.

25. Buckner JC AK, Ballman K, et al. Immunohistochemical detection of EGFRvIII and prognostic significance in patients with malignant glioma enrolled in NCCTG clinical trials. In: American Society of Clinical Oncol-ogy; 2004.

26. Huang SM, Harari PM. Modulation of radiation response after epidermal growth factor receptor blockade in squamous cell carcinomas: inhibition of damage repair, cell cycle kinetics, and tumor angiogenesis. Clin Cancer Res 2000;6(6):2166–2174.

27. Chakravarti A, Dicker A, Mehta M. The contribution of epidermal growth factor receptor (EGFR) signaling pathway to radioresistance in human gliomas: a review of preclinical and correlative clinical data. Int J Radiat Oncol Biol Phys 2004;58(3):927–931.
28. Werner-Wasik M, Scott CB, Nelson DF, et al. Final report of a phase I/II trial of hyperfractionated and accelerated hyperfractionated radiation therapy with carmustine for adults with supratentorial malignant gliomas. Radiation Therapy Oncology Group Study 83–02. Cancer 1996;77(8):1535–1543.
29. Souhami L SW, Brachman D, et al. Randomized comparison of radiosurgery followed by conventional radiotherapy with carmustine to conventional radiotherapy with carmustine for patients with Glioblastoma multiforme: Report of Radiation Therapy Oncology Group 93-05 protocol. Int J Radiat Oncol Phys 2004; 60(3):853–860.
30. Laperriere NJ, Leung PM, McKenzie S, et al. Randomized study of brachytherapy in the initial management of patients with malignant astrocytoma. Int J Radiat Oncol Biol Phys 1998;41(5):1005–1011.
31. Selker RG, Shapiro WR, Burger P, et al. The Brain Tumor Cooperative Group NIH Trial 87-01: a randomized comparison of surgery, external radiotherapy, and carmustine versus surgery, interstitial radiotherapy boost, external radiation therapy, and carmustine. Neurosurgery 2002;51(2):343–355; discussion 55--57.
32. Curran WJ, Jr., Scott CB, Horton J, et al. Recursive partitioning analysis of prognostic factors in three Radiation Therapy Oncology Group malignant glioma trials.[see comment]. J Natl Cancer Inst 1993;85(9):704–710.
33. Laramore GE, Martz KL, Nelson JS, Griffin TW, Chang CH, Horton J. Radiation Therapy Oncology Group (RTOG) survival data on anaplastic astrocytomas of the brain: does a more aggressive form of treatment adversely impact survivalInt J Radiat Oncol Biol Phys 1989;17(6):1351–1356.
34. Cairncross JG, Ueki K, Zlatescu MC, et al. Specific genetic predictors of chemotherapeutic response and survival in patients with anaplastic oligodendrogliomas. J Natl Cancer Inst 1998;90(19):1473–1479.
35. Cairncross J SW, Shaw E, et al. An intergroup randomized controlled clinical trial (RCT) of chemotherapy plus radiation (RT) versus RT alone for pure and mixed anaplastic oligodendrogliomas: Initial report of RTOG 94-02. In: American Society of Clinical Oncology 2004.
36. Chinot OL, Honore S, Dufour H, et al. Safety and efficacy of temozolomide in patients with recurrent anaplastic oligodendrogliomas after standard radiotherapy and chemotherapy. J Clin Oncol 2001;19(9):2449–2455.
37. Shapiro WR, Young DF. Treatment of malignant glioma. A controlled study of chemotherapy and irradiation. Arch Neurol 1976;33(7):494–450.
38. Sandberg-Wollheim M, Malmstrom P, Stromblad LG, et al. A randomized study of chemotherapy with procarbazine, vincristine, and lomustine with and without radiation therapy for astrocytoma grades 3 and/or 4. Cancer 1991;68(1):22–29.
39. Walker MD, Green SB, Byar DP, et al. Randomized comparisons of radiotherapy and nitrosoureas for the treatment of malignant glioma after surgery. N Engl J Med 1980;303(23):1323–1329.

14 Brachytherapy

Marcus L. Ware, P. K. Sneed,
and Michael W. McDermott

Summary

Surgical resection alone is insufficient in the treatment of malignant gliomas because of the extensive infiltration of tumor cells into surrounding normal brain. Even with adjuvant external beam radiation therapy (EBRT), median survival times are poor. Local recurrence eventually results in death for these patients. Thus, radiation therapy that targets the focal area of the initial tumor occurrence may be useful. Clinical evidence suggests that successful radiation treatment of malignant gliomas is dose dependent. However, treatment with doses of EBRT greater than 60 Gy is not beneficial to patients. In most cases, treatment of the bed of surgical resection with radiosurgery is impractical because of the large volume of the tumor resected as well as the risk of radiation necrosis. Brachytherapy is an appealing modality in such cases because it permits the delivery of localized radiation therapy to the area at greatest risk for recurrence.

Key Words: Brachytherapy; isotopes; recurrent HGG.

INTRODUCTION

The discovery of radioactivity by Henri Becquerel in1896 ushered in a scientific era that gave rise to many discoveries. Radioactivity was first applied therapeutically for cancer in 1902, when radiation was used to treat a cancer involving the palate and pharynx *(1)*. Interstitial brachytherapy—in which a sealed radioactive source, or "seed," is placed in or near a tumor to deliver high doses of radiation to tumor cells while minimizing exposure of surrounding normal tissue—was first used to treat a tumor of the central nervous system (CNS) in 1912, when Hirsch used the technique to treat a pituitary tumor *(2)*. The first glioma treated with a radioactive source implanted directly into the tumor cavity was treated by Frazier in 1914 *(3)*.

Between the early 1950s and the late 1980s, new radioisotopes were developed that brought about a renewed and concerted interest in interstitial brachytherapy for the treatment of brain tumors. The focus of this intense clinical activity was primary and recurrent malignant gliomas. Major efforts in the development of phase I and II trials at the University of California, San Francisco (UCSF) involved the use of stereotactically implanted, temporary high-activity iodine-125 (I-125) sources either alone or in combination with interstitial hyperthermia *(4–9)*. The early phase II studies suggested a survival benefit for patients with newly diagnosed tumors and reasonable control of tumor for patients with a recurrence. However, further analysis suggested that the differences seen reflected an unintended bias based on the selection

From: *Current Clinical Oncology: High-Grade Gliomas: Diagnosis and Treatment*
Edited by: G. H. Barnett © Humana Press Inc., Totowa, NJ

of the patients in the studies *(10)*. It was not until the phase III trials of interstitial brachytherapy performed by Laperriere et al. *(11)* in Toronto and by the Brain Tumor Cooperative Group *(12)* that the technique was evaluated in a prospective randomized fashion and compared against standard treatment. Neither of the trials showed any survival benefit, and those results led to a dramatic decline in the practice of brachytherapy for primary and recurrent malignant gliomas. Since then, a number of studies have evaluated the use of brachytherapy for malignant gliomas at initial presentation and at recurrence. This chapter reviews the radiobiology of treatment with brachytherapy, as well as studies that evaluate the efficacy of this treatment modality.

RATIONALE FOR BRACHYTHERAPY TREATMENT

Surgical resection alone is insufficient in the treatment of malignant gliomas because of the extensive infiltration of tumor cells into surrounding normal brain. Even with adjuvant external beam radiation therapy (EBRT), median survival times are poor, ranging from 9 to 12 mo for glioblastoma multiforme (GBM) *(13,14)*. Most patients treated for malignant glioma have locally persistent disease despite an apparent gross-total resection, with 80% of recurrent tumors arising within 2 cm of the primary site *(15,16)*. Local recurrence eventually results in death for these patients. Thus, radiation therapy that targets the focal area of the initial tumor occurrence may be useful.

Clinical evidence suggests that successful radiation treatment of malignant gliomas is dose dependent *(8)*. However, treatment with doses of EBRT greater than 60 Gy is not beneficial to patients *(13)*. In most cases, treatment of the bed of surgical resection with radiosurgery is impractical because of the large volume of the tumor resected as well as the risk of radiation necrosis. Brachytherapy is an appealing modality in such cases because it permits the delivery of localized radiation therapy to the area at greatest risk for recurrence.

From any point source, the radiation dose delivered to tissue decreases rapidly with increasing distance from the source. While the fall-off in the dose rate does not correspond exactly to the inverse square law, the dose to the tumor site is very conformal and the dose to surrounding normal brain is significantly less than dosages delivered using EBRT. The ultimate goal of any irradiation technique is a high degree of conformity of the dose and limited irradiation of normal tissue. With either the temporary or permanent brachytherapy implants, the dose distribution depends on the number of sources implanted within the site, the spatial relationship of the sources to one another, the energy of the emitted photon, and the attenuation or absorbance by the surrounding tissues. Dose rates from interstitial brachytherapy commonly range from 0.4 to 0.6 Gy/h, as compared with approx 1.8 to 2 Gy/min with high-energy linear accelerator systems. For any specified total dose delivered, the lower the dose rate, the smaller is the biologic effect of the given dose *(17–24)*. Thus, one would expect brachytherapy to be safer and more effective than teletherapy, based on proximity of the radiation source to the target of interest as well as the relatively low rate of radiation-dose delivery.

RADIOBIOLOGY OF BRACHYTHERAPY

Biologic Properties of Commony Used Isotopes

The isotopes most often used for interstitial brachytherapy are I-125 and iridium-192 (Ir-192). For intracavitary brachytherapy, phosphorus-32 (P-32) and yttrium-90 (Y-90) are the agents most commonly used. The half-life of these isotopes, the energy emitted, and the half-value in tissues for these isotopes are shown in Table 1.

Table 1
Isotopes Used in Interstitial/Intracavitary Brachytherapy

| Isotope | T1/2 | Interstitial brachytherapy (26) | |
		Energy of emitted γ-rays (mean)	Half-value layer in tissue (mm)
Iodine-125	60.2 days	28 KeV	20 mm
Iridium-192	74.2 days	380 KeV	70 mm

| Isotope | T1/2 | Intracavitary brachytherapy | |
		Energy of emitted γ-rays (mean)	Half-value layer in tissue (mm)
Phosphorus-32	14.2 days	0.69 MeV	0.8 mm
Yttrium-90	2.7 days	0.93 MeV	1.1 mm

The half-value in tissues refers to the distance within tissue over which the dose is reduced by one half because of the absorbance of energy by the tissue. The total dose delivered by using brachytherapy depends on the isotopes used, the number of sources, the total radiation activity, and the duration of the implant. For interstitial brachytherapy, I-125 is a lower-energy isotope that emits γ-rays in the range of 27 to 35 keV, as compared with Ir-192 with higher energy emitted at 300 to 610 keV. Lower-energy photons are attenuated to a greater degree by surrounding tissue, thus reducing the radiation dosage to the normal tissue surrounding the tumor site and affording better radiation safety for patients and their family, nurses, and surgeons. Whereas temporary high-activity and permanent low-activity I-125 sources are implanted directly by the surgeon using radiation safety precautions, most Ir-192 systems require some sort of remote after-loading device. The tissue penetration of radiation from the isotopes is also reflected in the half-value level in tissue, which is more than three times as great for Ir-192 as it is for I-125. The low-energy photons of I-125 do have prominent photoelectric absorption that depends on the atomic number of the interposed tissue (25). Therefore, when there are elements in surrounding tissue that have a high atomic number, such as bone, the absorption of photons from I-125 will be much greater than absorption of photons from Ir-192. Thus, in many cases, after craniotomy and permanent implantation of I-125 sources, the radiation measured at 1 meter from the patient may be almost undetectable or it may be easily shielded by a very thin layer of lead lining a hat (26).

With low-energy isotopes used for intracavitary treatments such as P-32 and Y-90, most of the radiation dose is deposited in the first few millimeters of the cyst wall or tumor, and little radiation reaches normal tissues (27–29). In contrast with the case with permanent or temporary high I-125 brachytherapy implants, it is not possible to confirm the source distribution by postoperative imaging in order to calculate the dose distribution. One assumes that, within the volume of the cyst, the isotope is distributed equally, and on that basis the dosage calculations are made preoperatively. For the intracavitary treatment of craniopharyngiomas, which have a long epithelial cell-cycle time, effective doses of 200 to 250 Gy are delivered over five half-lives of the isotope, which is approx 71 d for P-32. Because the half-value layer of beta particles from P-32 is only 0.8 mm in tissue, treatment of mixed, solid, and cystic tumors with this technique is not recommended. Surgeons who have aspirated cysts several days after the injection of P-32 have found that the radioactivity in the recovered material is lower than anticipated, suggesting that there may be a "plating" phenomenon of some isotope up against the cyst wall. This "plating" of some of the isotope up against the cyst wall which may not allow for uniform distribution of the isotope within the cyst. The larger the cyst, the higher is the actual dose to the cyst wall because of this phenomenon.

Biology of DNA Repair in Tumor Cells and Normal Cells

One of the main advantages of brachytherapy is related to the radiation biology of continuous low-dose irradiation, which tends to substantially damage proliferating tumor cells while allowing normal tissue a chance for repair of sublethal damage *(19,21,22,24,30)*. Normal tissue is more efficient at repairing the sublethal damage, but as the dose rate increases there is less separation of this effect; the higher the dose rate, the lower is the total dose at which damage to normal tissue is observed. Cells commonly respond to DNA damage from ionizing radiation by activating cell-cycle checkpoints. These checkpoints permit cells to correct possible DNA damage before proceeding through the cell cycle. Ionizing radiation induces arrest in the G_1, S, and G_2 phases of the cell cycle *(31)*. In addition, cell survival data have shown that cells are most sensitive to radiation during mitosis and G2, are less sensitive in G1, and are least sensitive during the latter part of S phase *(32,33)*. Continuous irradiation with brachytherapy also fosters a buildup of damage by synchronizing tumor cells within the cell cycle, particularly the G2-M phase *(34)*. This synchronization of cells may account for some of the improved tumor cell kill achieved with brachytherapy.

It has long been known that hypoxic cancer cells are resistant to radiation therapy. Ionizing radiation damages DNA by first forming reactive oxygen species after interacting with water. The protective effects of hypoxia were initially believed to be a reflection of decreased oxygen as a source of radiation-induced radicals. However, recent studies have shown that hypoxia is the principal physiologic stimulus for hypoxia-inducible factor 1 (HIF-1) *(35)*. HIF-1 is a transcriptional regulator that leads to the expression of vascular endothelial growth factor (VEGF) and basic fibroblast growth factor (bFGF), which may act to prevent radiation-induced cell death *(36,37)*. Brachytherapy theoretically would be useful in treating transiently hypoxic cells by delivering radiation during the period of reoxygenation that occurs during the course of low-dose rate continuous brachytherapy *(38)*.

BRACHYTHERAPY FOR NEWLY DIAGNOSED HIGH-GRADE GLIOMAS

In the 1980s and 1990s, most of the information from brachytherapy trials for newly diagnosed malignant gliomas was based on phase II studies. Scharfen et al. *(7)* at UCSF reported median survival of 88 wk for patients with GBM, 142 wk for those with nonGBM, and 226 wk for those with low-grade glioma (LGG). Of the 307 patients in this study, 124 (40%) required reoperation after brachytherapy; and of the 124 patients who had reoperation, 6 (5%) had necrosis only, 36 (29%) had tumor only, and 82 (66%) had both tumor and necrosis. The median survival of reoperated patients did not differ significantly. The mortality rate for the series was 0.7% and the acute complication rate was 7.8%. Sneed et al. *(39)* analyzed the results of brachytherapy boost in 159 GBM patients treated at UCSF and found that, on multivariate analysis, age was the only significant independent predictor of outcome. For the 18- to 29.9-yr-old age group the 2-yr survival rate was 78%; and for the 50- to 59.9-yr-old group the 2-yr survival rate was 25%. The median survival rate for the youngest age group was not yet reached at the time of analysis and was 77 wk in the older age group. Again, these results were from a selected group of patients evaluated in prospective phase II studies.

UCSF investigators went on to conduct a phase III trial evaluating the use of brachytherapy alone as compared with the use of brachytherapy plus hyperthermia for patients with newly diagnosed GBM (9,40). Their rationale for using hyperthermia was that hyperthermia kills tumor cells exponentially as a function of temperature above 41°C, and that it inhibits the repair of sublethal damage (9,40). Hyperthermia is also effective against cells that tend to be resistant to radiation. The goal of this trial was to try to maintain fairly high temperatures of at least 42.5°C for 30 min immediately before and after brachytherapy, using interstitial microwave antennas to heat tumors and interstitial thermometry to record temperatures. Thirty-nine patients were randomized to the "brachytherapy alone" group and 40 to the "combined treatment" group. Whether by intent-to-treat analysis or by an analysis of only patients in each group who actually received brachytherapy, the time to tumor progression and the median survival time were significantly longer for the brachytherapy-plus-hyperthermia group. The median survival time in the hyperthermia group was 95 wk, and was 76 wk in the group undergoing brachytherapy alone. Multivariate analysis revealed that, after adjusting for significant prognostic factors such as age and Karnofsky Performance Scale (KPS) score, a longer survival time was significantly associated with the use of brachytherapy plus hyperthermia. This was the first prospective clinical trial to show a survival benefit with the addition of hyperthermia to irradiation at any body site.

Subsequent clinical studies evaluating brachytherapy for primary malignant gliomas included prospective randomized trials conducted by Laperriere et al. (11) in Toronto and by the Brain Tumor Cooperative Group (National Institutes of Health trial 87–01) (12). Laperriere et al. (11) reported the results of a trial conducted between 1986 and 1996 in which 140 patients were randomized either to receive I-125 brachytherapy implants after an open operation and EBRT or to undergo only an open operation plus EBRT. Two types of analyses were performed on the two patient groups: both intent-to-treat analysis and analysis of only those patients who actually received the implant. Of the 71 patients who were randomized to the brachytherapy group, only 63 actually received an implant. In the intent-to-treat analysis, there was no significant difference in median survival times between the surgery-plus-EBRT group (13.2 mo) and the brachytherapy group (13.8 mo; $p = 0.24$). For the 63 patients who actually received the implant, the median survival time was 15.7 mo; and multivariate analyses revealed a trend toward improved survival in that group, although it was not significant. Most of the brachytherapy implants were placed through use of one or two catheters, and the median prescription volume was 42.3 cc. Reoperation was required for 31% of the patients in the implant group and 33% of the patients in the surgery-plus-EBRT group. Complications directly attributable to the I-125 implant occurred in 24% of patients. There was no significant difference in the recurrence sites between the groups, recurrence occurring locally in 93% of the surgery-plus-EBRT group and in 82% of the implant group. Although there was no significant difference in the KPS scores at 6 and 12 mo after randomization, the patients receiving an implant had a significantly higher dexamethasone requirement at both time intervals. The investigators concluded their report by indicating that brachytherapy implants did not provide any significant improvement in survival in the management of patients with malignant glioma. A subsequent study from the same group evaluated the quality of life in patients who had participated in this trial (41). There was no difference between the two study groups in their KPS and quality-of-life scores during the first year of follow-up review, but there was a significant deterioration in the KPS scores during the first year as compared with the baseline

Table 2
Results of Brachytherapy Boost for Malignant Glioma

Investigators	Year	No. patients	Pathology	Median survival (mo)
Sneed et al. *(9)*	1998	33	GM	17.5 (no heat)
		35	GM	19.6 (heat)
Videtic et al. *(62)**	1999	53	GM	17.0
		22	AA	38.0
Laperriere et al. *(11)*	1998	69	GM	13.2 (no implant)
		71	GM	13.8 (implant)
Selker et al. *(12)*	2002	107	GM	13.4 (no implant)
		123	GM	14.7 (implant)

Notes: *Denotes a permanent low-activity implant.

scores. For both groups, during the first year of follow-up review there was a statistically significant deterioration in selected items on the quality-of-life assessment, including self-care, speech, concentration, cognitive functioning, and physical symptoms.

The Brain Tumor Cooperative Group (BTCG) trial was the second phase III trial reported that evaluated the use of brachytherapy in treating newly diagnosed malignant glioma (Table 2) *(12)*. It included 299 patients randomized into 2 study arms between December 1987 and April 1994. Each group was followed for an additional 3 yr. After 29 patients were excluded from analysis, the valid study group consisted of 270 patients. Of those, 137 patients received standard treatment consisting of surgical resection plus EBRT and BCNU chemotherapy, and 133 had I-125 brachytherapy after undergoing resection followed by EBRT and BCNU chemotherapy. The initial 64 patients who were randomized to either study arm received whole brain radiation therapy and a cone-down boost. After May 1989, the protocol was amended so that EBRT was delivered to the tumor border plus a 3-cm margin. All patients in both study groups received BCNU at 200 mg/m^2 every 8 wk; and all received their first dose of BCNU at 16 to 48 h before their first EBRT treatment. For all 270 patients in the valid study group, prognostic factors such as age and KPS score were equally matched. Both groups consisted predominantly of patients with GBM, but patients with anaplastic astrocytoma (AA), anaplastic oligodendroglioma (AO), and malignant mixed glioma were also included. Patients with GBM made up 80.5% of the standard therapy group and 89.8% of the brachytherapy group. There was no significant difference in survival times overall between the brachytherapy group (68.1 wk) and the standard therapy group (58.8 wk). Age and KPS score were significant predictors of outcome in both groups. In the subgroup of patients with GBM, the median survival time in the group receiving the brachytherapy implant was 64 wk, as compared with 58.1 wk in the standard therapy group ($p = 0.169$). As expected, the survival time for patients with non-GBM (145.3 wk) was significantly longer than for those with GBM (59.7 wk). Evaluation of differences in survival times between patients undergoing only a biopsy as compared with those undergoing gross-total resection showed that the extent of resection was not a significant predictor of outcome in either the standard therapy group or the brachytherapy group. Among the patients who had brachytherapy, median survival time was 63 wk for those who had only a biopsy, and was 68.1 wk for those who had gross-total resection. For patients in the standard treatment arm, median survival was 58.8 wk for those undergoing a biopsy and 58.7 wk for those undergoing resection. The investigators concluded that there was no survival advantage with the addition of I-125 brachytherapy for the management of patients with malignant glioma.

One criticism of the early brachytherapy clinical trials was that the favorable survival rates could be accounted for simply by the criteria for the selection of patients alone *(42)*. Florell et al. *(10)*, reviewing a series of patients with newly diagnosed GBM who were referred to a regional cancer center, found that only about 30% of the patients were eligible for brachytherapy based on imaging studies and KPS score alone. The patients eligible for brachytherapy tended to be younger and to have more extensive surgical resection prior to brachytherapy and have higher KPS prior to any treatment. The eligible patients survived longer than patients who were not eligible, even though both groups were treated in a standard fashion with open operation and EBRT. The investigators used these findings to support the notion that selection alone had a significant influence on the results regarding outcome after brachytherapy. In another report of a phase II study *(43)*, at least 25% of the patients selected for brachytherapy after the completion of EBRT had tumor recurrence during the course of EBRT. These patients were eliminated from the brachytherapy group because of the tumor recurrence. The elimination of patients with early recurrence of tumors after early recurrence could possibly improve survival in the brachytherapy group.

Taking the opposite position, Videtic et al. *(44)* reported data from a retrospective review of nonrandomized patients with malignant glioma undergoing brachytherapy who were analyzed with respect to volume of the implant and the Radiation Therapy Oncology Group (RTOG) recursive partitioning analysis (RPA) criteria *(45)*. Between 1991 and 1998, 75 patients were treated with surgery and brachytherapy followed by fractionated EBRT; 53 (71%) of the patients had GBM. The median survival time was 17 mo for patients with GBM, with survival of 40% at 2 yr. The greatest impact from brachytherapy was seen for the poorest prognostic classes (V/VI), with 25% improvement in median survival for the brachytherapy group compared with RTOG historical data (11.1 vs 8.9 mo) and even more improvement in survival at 2 yr (29 vs 6%). The investigators concluded that selection factors alone did not account for the improved survival in their patients. In their series, patients were implanted at the time of operation, before they underwent EBRT. Thus, in this group, brachytherapy appeared to have a positive effect.

BRACHYTHERAPY FOR RECURRENT HIGH-GRADE GLIOMAS

The first trials of brachytherapy for patients with malignant glioma were focused on patients with recurrent tumor *(7,8,46–56)*. The earliest trials used temporary high-activity interstitial brachytherapy, whereas the most recent reports have been on the use of permanent low-activity brachytherapy implants (Table 3). As of now, there has not been a phase III randomized trial of interstitial brachytherapy for patients with recurrent malignant glioma. In a series of retrospective reviews published between 1995 and 2000, median survival times for patients with recurrent GBM or recurrent malignant glioma ranged from 9.5 to 16 mo. Reported rates of reoperation after brachytherapy for recurrent tumor ranged from 27.8 to 54%. In a review of the entire brachytherapy experience at UCSF that was published in 1992, the reoperation rate ranged from 36 to 47% depending on the initial diagnosis *(7)*. Reoperation was associated with a significantly prolonged survival time. Shrieve et al. *(55)* presented an interesting analysis of survival and reoperation rates for patients with recurrent malignant glioma treated with either temporary high-activity brachytherapy implants or radiosurgery. The median survival times were comparable in the two groups: 11.5 mo for the brachytherapy group and 10.2 mo for the radiosurgery group. The risk of need for reoperation appeared to

Table 3
Results of Brachytherapy Implant for Recurrent Glioma

Investigators	Year	No. patients	Diagnosis	Median survival (mo)
Gaspar et al. (57)*	1999	59	MG	16.0
Patel et al. (58)*	2000	40	GM	10.8
Tatter et al. (61)	2003	21	MG	12.7
		15	GM	8.0
Larson et al. (23)*	2004	38	GM	12.0

Notes:*Denotes permanent low-activity implant.

be slightly higher in the brachytherapy group, at 64% as compared with 33% in the radiosurgery group at 12 mo. It should be noted however that the target volumes for treatment were three times greater in the brachytherapy group than in the radiosurgery group.

The use of permanent low-activity brachytherapy sources has received attention because it results in a lower incidence of symptomatic radiation necrosis requiring reoperation. Halligan et al. (50) in 1996 treated 18 patients with recurrent GBM with a permanent low-activity brachytherapy implant, achieving a median survival of 64 wk. None of their patients required reoperation for symptomatic radiation necrosis. Gaspar et al. (57), in 1999, reported 59 patients undergoing brachytherapy for recurrent GBM and recurrent malignant glioma. Only 3 (5%) patients required reoperation for symptomatic radiation necrosis. Median survival for the group with GBM was 0.9 yr and for the group with tumors other than GBM was 2.04 yr. In their study, factors predictive of a poor outcome were GBM histology, age greater than 60 yr, implant target volume greater than 17 cc, and tumor location within the corpus callosum or thalamus.

Patel et al. (58) reported results of therapy for 40 patients with recurrent GBM receiving permanent I-125 implants. No patient developed symptoms attributable to radiation necrosis, and none required reoperation. Time to tumor progression was 25 wk after implantation. The extent of tumor resection showed a trend toward improved survival after reoperation and brachytherapy at 51 wk for patients who had gross-total resection as opposed to 43 wk for those who had subtotal resection, although this difference was not significant ($p = 0.58$). In contrast, progression-free survival was significantly better in patients who had gross-total resection (31 wk) as opposed to subtotal resection (17 wk). Those patients younger than 60 yr of age at the time of brachytherapy did significantly better than those older than 60 yr. There was also a trend for those patients who had a high MIB-1 staining index to have shorter time to tumor progression and worse survival rate than those with a low staining index, although these differences again were not statistically significant.

Larson et al. (23) recently reported their experience in 38 patients with recurrent GBM who had permanent low-activity brachytherapy seeds implanted between June 1997 and May 1998 at UCSF. At a 5-mm depth, the dosage achieved locally at infinite decay time was 300 Gy and the median initial dose rate was 15 cGy/h. Of the 37 patients included in the analysis, the median survival after brachytherapy was 52 wk and the time to tumor progression clearly established with 36 patients was 16 wk. Of the 37 tumors, 34 had recurred and two were censored at the time of latest follow-up review or magnetic resonance imaging. Only age was a significant predictive factor in survival in multivariate analysis. The investigators compared the results from 35 patients with permanent implants and 54 patients with temporary implants who met the same criteria for inclusion in a survival comparison. In a multivariate Cox proportion hazards model, adjusting for age, KPS score, and log of the tumor implant volume, there was no significance difference in survival between the historical high-activity brachytherapy group and the reported permanent low-activity brachytherapy implant group. Kaplan–Meier curves showed similar survival patterns. Of the patients in the reported study, 63% underwent some form of salvage therapy. Four patients underwent reoperation for presumed recurrent tumor; pathologic evaluation revealed recurrent tumor in three of the patients, and gliosis without recurrent tumor in one patient. As all four patients were asymptomatic, none required craniotomy for symptomatic radiation necrosis. The investigators concluded that permanent I-125 brachytherapy for recurrent progressive GBM was well tolerated, and survival times were comparable to similar groups of patients treated with high-activity temporary brachytherapy implants.

Simon et al. *(59)* reported a study of 42 patients who were treated with Ir-192 implantation. A dose of 40 to 60 Gy was delivered to the periphery of the tumor over a period of 7 to 12 d using a 70% prescription isodose line. The dosage rates ranged from 0.4 to 0.5 Gy/h. Twenty-four patients required reoperation for radiation necrosis. The median survival was 50 wk, with a 1-yr survival rate of 48% and a 2-yr survival of 11%. In multivariate analysis, only tumor volume and KPS score were significant predictors of outcome.

RECENT DEVELOPMENTS IN BRACHYTHERAPY

Dempsey et al. *(60)* and Tatter et al. *(61)* have described a high activity brachytherapy delivery device that utilizes a liquid I-125 isotope. An inflatable silicon balloon reservoir attached to a catheter is placed into the resection cavity and filled postoperatively with the liquid I-125 radionuclide solution. The balloon assumes a relatively spherical shape and the surrounding tissue may conform to the shape of this balloon. Previously investigators have shown a homogenous dose within the target volume that was superior to seed implants; however, there was a slight increase in the volume of normal tissue receiving 50 to 75% the prescribed tissue dose *(60)*. Tatter et al. *(61)* reported a phase I study evaluating the safety and performance of this system in the treatment of 21 patients with recurrent malignant glioma. The primary end point of the trial was successful performance by the device. Fifteen patients with recurrent GBM, five with recurrent AA, and one with AO were treated. All the patients had undergone standard therapy with surgery and EBRT. Eleven patients had received chemotherapy and two had undergone radiosurgery. After resection of the recurrent glioma, the Silastic® balloon catheter (GliaSite®) was inserted into the resection cavity and inflated to determine the appropriate balloon volume for later inflation. Then a combination of Iotrex®, an aqueous I-125 radiation source, and saline was injected into the catheter to inflate the balloon to the predetermined size. The combination treatment is known as the GliaSite® RTS. The device delivered radiation to the surrounding tissue at 41 to 61 cGy/h, delivering mean doses of 40 to 60 Gy to a mean depth of 6 to 9 mm from the resection margin over the course of 70 to 140 h. The total activity of Iotrex® ranged from 73 to 459 mCi. The device functioned as intended in all cases, and 20 of the 21 patients received the prescribed dose. One patient received only 40% of the dose because of an error in mixing the Iotrex® with intravenous contrast medium. There were three adverse events related to the device: one pseudomeningocele, one infection, and one case of chemical meningitis. No patient developed symptomatic radiation necrosis. Although the median time for follow-up review was not reported, the total follow-up period was 21.8 wk. All patients died of recurrent tumor during the follow-up period. In

6 of the 14 patients treatment failure occurred within the brachytherapy volume. The median survival time after GliaSite® RTS therapy was 8 mo for patients with GBM and 17.9 mo for those with AA or AO. The investigators concluded that the delivery system was safe and efficiently delivered the prescribed dose of radiation. This group plans future studies of both newly diagnosed and recurrent brain tumors.

THE FUTURE OF BRACHYTHERAPY

Although interstitial brachytherapy is still used to treat brain tumors—including recurrent malignant glioma, newly diagnosed and recurrent brain metastases, recurrent benign and malignant meningiomas, and some skull-based tumors—a number of studies have shown that it is not of any great benefit to patients who have malignant glioma. For long-term survivors of brachytherapy, it appears that the trade-off may be neurologic deficit from radiation necrosis and the side effects of long-term steroid use.

Temporary high-dose brachytherapy for newly diagnosed GBM was not beneficial in two phase III trials, and in light of those results many groups have abandoned further investigation of brachytherapy for malignant glioma. Although a UCSF study showed that permanent low-activity I-125 brachytherapy and temporary high-activity brachytherapy have similar efficacy against recurrent progressive GBM (23), we no longer offer brachytherapy for patients with recurrent GBM because of the short time to tumor progression. More recently, a prospective phase I/II clinical trial at UCSF was designed to evaluate the toxicity of permanent I-125 brachytherapy implantation followed by hyperfractionated EBRT with a dose regimen of 100 cGy bid to a total dose of 60 Gy. The trial was terminated because of concern over significant radiation toxicity, although long-term follow-up evaluations are ongoing for some of the long-term survivors in this group. Currently, we have no active trials of brachytherapy for malignant glioma at UCSF, but rather are focusing our efforts in local treatment on convection-enhanced delivery strategies. Despite the many theoretical benefits of brachytherapy, it is unlikely, after 20 yr of effort, that new brachytherapy strategies will have a significant impact on the outcome from this disease.

REFERENCES

1. Dutreix J, Tubiana M, Pierquin B. The hazy dawn of brachytherapy. Radiother Oncol 1998;49:223–232.
2. Hirsch O. Die operative Behandlung von Hypophysistumoren nach endonasalen Methoden. Arch Laryngol Rhinol 1912;26:529–686.
3. Frazier C. The effects of radium emanations upon brain tumors. Surg Gynecol Obstet 1920;31:236–239.
4. Gutin PH, Prados MD, Phillips TL, et al. External irradiation followed by an interstitial high activity iodine-125 implant "boost" in the initial treatment of malignant gliomas: NCOG study 6G-82-2. Int J Radiat Oncol Biol Phys 1991;21:601–606.
5. McDermott MW, Sneed PK, Gutin PH. Interstitial brachytherapy for malignant brain tumors. Semin Surg Oncol 1998;14:79–87.
6. Prados MD, Gutin PH, Phillips TL, et al. Interstitial brachytherapy for newly diagnosed patients with malignant gliomas: the UCSF experience. Int J Radiat Oncol Biol Phys 1992;24:593–597.
7. Scharfen CO, Sneed PK, Wara WM, et al. High activity iodine-125 interstitial implant for gliomas. Int J Radiat Oncol Biol Phys 1992;24:583–591.
8. Sneed PK, Lamborn KR, Larson DA, et al. Demonstration of brachytherapy boost dose-response relationships in glioblastoma multiforme. Int J Radiat Oncol Biol Phys 1996;35:37–44.
9. Sneed PK, Stauffer PR, McDermott MW, et al. Survival benefit of hyperthermia in a prospective randomized trial of brachytherapy boost +/- hyperthermia for glioblastoma multiforme. Int J Radiat Oncol Biol Phys 1998;40:287–295.
10. Florell RC, Macdonald DR, Irish WD, et al. Selection bias, survival, and brachytherapy for glioma. J Neurosurg 1992;76:179–183.

11. Laperriere NJ, Leung PM, McKenzie S, et al. Randomized study of brachytherapy in the initial management of patients with malignant astrocytoma. Int J Radiat Oncol Biol Phys 1998;41:1005–1011.

12. Selker RG, Shapiro WR, Burger P, et al. The Brain Tumor Cooperative Group NIH Trial 87-01: a randomized comparison of surgery, external radiotherapy, and carmustine versus surgery, interstitial radiotherapy boost, external radiation therapy, and carmustine. Neurosurgery 2002;51:343–355; discussion 355–347.

13. Chang CH, Horton J, Schoenfeld D, et al. Comparison of postoperative radiotherapy and combined postoperative radiotherapy and chemotherapy in the multidisciplinary management of malignant gliomas. A joint Radiation Therapy Oncology Group and Eastern Cooperative Oncology Group study. Cancer 1983;52:997–1007.

14. Fine HA, Dear KB, Loeffler JS, et al. Meta-analysis of radiation therapy with and without adjuvant chemotherapy for malignant gliomas in adults. Cancer 1993;71:2585–2597.

15. Burger PC, Dubois PJ, Schold SC, Jr., et al. Computerized tomographic and pathologic studies of the untreated, quiescent, and recurrent glioblastoma multiforme. J Neurosurg 1983;58:159–169.

16. Burton EC, Prados MD. Malignant gliomas. Curr Treat Options Oncol 2000;1:459–468.

17. Armour EP, Wang ZH, Corry PM, et al. Sensitization of rat 9L gliosarcoma cells to low dose rate irradiation by long duration 41 degrees C hyperthermia. Cancer Res 51991;1:3088–3095.

18. Bernstein M, Gutin PH. Interstitial irradiation of brain tumors: a review. Neurosurgery 1981l9:741–750.

19. Fowler JF. Why shorter half-times of repair lead to greater damage in pulsed brachytherapy. Int J Radiat Oncol Biol Phys 1993;26:353–356.

20. Fu KK, Phillips TL, Kane LJ, et al. Tumor and normal tissue response to irradiation in vivo: variation with decreasing dose rates. Radiology 1975;114:709–716.

21. Hall EJ. The promise of low dose rate: has it been realized? Int J Radiat Oncol Biol Phys 1978;4:749–750.

22. Hall EJ. Radiation dose-rate: a factor of importance in radiobiology and radiotherapy. Br J Radiol 1972;45: 81–97.

23. Larson DA, Suplica JM, Chang SM, et al. Permanent iodine 125 brachytherapy in patients with progressive or recurrent glioblastoma multiforme. Neuro-oncol 2004;6:119–126.

24. Schultz CJ, Geard CR. Radioresponse of human astrocytic tumors across grade as a function of acute and chronic irradiation. Int J Radiat Oncol Biol Phys 1990;19:1397–1403.

25. Krishnaswamy V. Dose distribution around an 125I seed source in tissue. Radiology 1978;126:489–491.

26. McDermott MW, Gutin PH, Berger MS, et al. Interstitial and intracavitary irradiation of brain tumors. In: Winn HR, ed. Neurologcal Surgery, vol. 4. Philadelphia: Elsevier; 2003: 4095–4109.

27. Backlund EO. Colloidal radioisotopes as part of a multi-modality treatment of craniopharyngiomas. J Neurosurg Sci 1989;33:95–97.

28. Backlund EO, Axelsson B, Bergstrand CG, et al. Treatment of craniopharyngiomas—the stereotactic approach in a ten to twenty-three years' perspective. I. Surgical, radiological and ophthalmological aspects. Acta Neurochir (Wien) 1989;99:11–19.

29. Coffey RJ, Lunsford LD. The role of stereotactic techniques in the management of craniopharyngiomas. Neurosurg Clin N Am 1990;1:161–172.

30. Ling CC, Chui CS. Stereotactic treatment of brain tumors with radioactive implants or external photon beams: radiobiophysical aspects. Radiother Oncol 1993;26:11–18.

31. Pawlik TM, Keyomarsi K. Role of cell cycle in mediating sensitivity to radiotherapy. Int J Radiat Oncol Biol Phys 2004;59:928–942.

32. Sinclair WK, Morton RA. Variations in X-Ray Response During the Division Cycle of Partially Synchronized Chinese Hamster Cells in Culture. Nature 1963;199:1158–1160.

33. Sinclair WK, Morton RA. X-Ray and Ultraviolet Sensitivity of Synchronized Chinese Hamster Cells at Various Stages of the Cell Cycle. Biophys J 1965;97:1–25.

34. Knox SJ, Sutherland W, Goris ML. Correlation of tumor sensitivity to low-dose-rate irradiation with G2/M-phase block and other radiobiological parameters. Radiat Res 1993;135:24–31.

35. Semenza GL. HIF-1: mediator of physiological and pathophysiological responses to hypoxia. J Appl Physiol 2000;88:1474–1480.

36. Bussink J, Kaanders JH, van der Kogel AJ. Tumor hypoxia at the micro-regional level: clinical relevance and predictive value of exogenous and endogenous hypoxic cell markers. Radiother Oncol 2003;67:3–15.

37. Moeller BJ, Cao Y, Li CY, et al. Radiation activates HIF-1 to regulate vascular radiosensitivity in tumors: role of reoxygenation, free radicals, and stress granules. Cancer Cell 2004;5:429–441.

38. Ling CC, Spiro IJ, Mitchell J, et al. The variation of OER with dose rate. Int J Radiat Oncol Biol Phys 1985;11:1367–1373.

39. Sneed PK, Prados MD, McDermott MW, et al. Large effect of age on the survival of patients with glioblastoma treated with radiotherapy and brachytherapy boost. Neurosurgery 1995;36:898–903; discussion 903–894.

40. Sneed PK, Larson DA, Gutin PH. Brachytherapy and hyperthermia for malignant astrocytomas. Semin Oncol 1994;21:186–197.
41. Bampoe J, Laperriere N, Pintilie M, et al. Quality of life in patients with glioblastoma multiforme participating in a randomized study of brachytherapy as a boost treatment. J Neurosurg 2000;93:917–926.
42. Haines SJ. Moving targets and ghosts of the past: outcome measurement in brain tumour therapy. J Clin Neurosci 2002;9:109–112.
43. Barker FG, 2nd, Prados MD, Chang SM, et al. Radiation response and survival time in patients with glioblastoma multiforme. J Neurosurg 1996;84:442–448.
44. Videtic GM, Gaspar LE, Zamorano L, et al. Implant volume as a prognostic variable in brachytherapy decision-making for malignant gliomas stratified by the RTOG recursive partitioning analysis. Int J Radiat Oncol Biol Phys 2001;51:963–968.
45. Curran WJ, Jr., Scott CB, Horton J, et al. Recursive partitioning analysis of prognostic factors in three Radiation Therapy Oncology Group malignant glioma trials. J Natl Cancer Inst 1993;85:704–710.
46. Bernstein M, Laperriere N, Glen J, et al. Brachytherapy for recurrent malignant astrocytoma. Int J Radiat Oncol Biol Phys 1994;30:1213–1217.
47. Chamberlain MC, Barba D, Kormanik P, et al. Concurrent cisplatin therapy and iodine 125 brachytherapy for recurrent malignant brain tumors. Arch Neurol 1995;52:162–167.
48. Coffey RJ, Friedman WA. Interstitial brachytherapy of malignant brain tumors using computed tomography-guided stereotaxis and available imaging software: technical report. Neurosurgery 1987;20:4–7.
49. Gutin PH, Phillips TL, Wara WM, et al. Brachytherapy of recurrent malignant brain tumors with removable high-activity iodine-125 sources. J Neurosurg 1984;60:61–68.
50. Halligan JB, Stelzer KJ, Rostomily RC, et al. Operation and permanent low activity 125I brachytheraphy for recurrent high-grade astrocytomas. Int J Radiat Oncol Biol Phys 1996;35:541–547.
51. Leibel SA, Gutin PH, Wara WM, et al. Survival and quality of life after interstitial implantation of removable high-activity iodine-125 sources for the treatment of patients with recurrent malignant gliomas. Int J Radiat Oncol Biol Phys 1989;17:1129–1139.
52. Loeffler JS, Alexander E, 3rd, Hochberg FH, et al. Clinical patterns of failure following stereotactic interstitial irradiation for malignant gliomas. Int J Radiat Oncol Biol Phys 1990;19:1455–1462.
53. Loeffler JS, Alexander E, 3rd, Wen PY, et al. Results of stereotactic brachytherapy used in the initial management of patients with glioblastoma. J Natl Cancer Inst 1990;82:1918–1921.
54. McDermott MW, Gutin PH, Larson DA, et al. Interstitial brachytherapy. Neurosurg Clin N Am 1990;1: 801–824.
55. Shrieve DC, Alexander E, 3rd, Wen PY, et al. Comparison of stereotactic radiosurgery and brachytherapy in the treatment of recurrent glioblastoma multiforme. Neurosurgery 1995;36:275–282; discussion 282–274.
56. Sneed PK, Gutin PH, Prados MD, et al. Brachytherapy of brain tumors. Stereotact Funct Neurosurg 1992; 9:157–165.
57. Gaspar LE, Zamorano LJ, Shamsa F, et al. Permanent 125iodine implants for recurrent malignant gliomas. Int J Radiat Oncol Biol Phys 43:977–982, 1999
58. Patel S, Breneman JC, Warnick RE, et al. Permanent iodine-125 interstitial implants for the treatment of recurrent glioblastoma multiforme. Neurosurgery 2000;46:1123–1128; discussion 1128–1130.
59. Simon JM, Cornu P, Boisserie G, et al. Brachytherapy of glioblastoma recurring in previously irradiated territory: predictive value of tumor volume. Int J Radiat Oncol Biol Phys 2002;53:67–74.
60. Dempsey JF, Williams JA, Stubbs JB, et al. Dosimetric properties of a novel brachytherapy balloon applicator for the treatment of malignant brain-tumor resection-cavity margins. Int J Radiat Oncol Biol Phys 1998;42: 421–429.
61. Tatter SB, Shaw EG, Rosenblum ML, et al. An inflatable balloon catheter and liquid 125I radiation source (GliaSite Radiation Therapy System) for treatment of recurrent malignant glioma: multicenter safety and feasibility trial. J Neurosurg 2003;99:297–303.
62. Videtic GM, Gaspar LE, Zamorano L, et al. Use of the RTOG recursive partitioning analysis to validate the benefit of iodine-125 implants in the primary treatment of malignant gliomas. Int J Radiat Oncol Biol Phys 1999;45:687–692.

15 Radiosurgery

John H. Suh and Gene H. Barnett

Summary

Radiation therapy is an important treatment option for patients with high-grade gliomas (HGG). Because the majority of patients fail locally, various strategies have been investigated to improve tumor control. Stereotactic radiosurgery (SRS) is one method of focally escalating radiation dose while minimizing dose to normal brain. Although some institutional results have shown improved survival for some patients, others have questioned this benefit because patient selection is known to influence survival. The results from the Radiation Therapy Oncology Group (RTOG 93–05) phase III study did not demonstrate a survival advantage for patients undergoing radiosurgery in addition to radiation therapy and chemotherapy. Current trials are evaluating the use of chemotherapy or radiation sensitizers to improve results. Based on the two negative randomized trials of brachytherapy and one negative randomized trial of radiosurgery for newly diagnosed glioblastoma multiforme, the use of radiosurgery is limited in these tumors.

Key Words: Stereotactic radiosurgery; glioblastoma multiforme; high-grade glioma.

INTRODUCTION

Studies from the Brain Tumor Cooperative Group (BTCG) established the benefit of radiation therapy in several phase III studies. BTCG 6901 was a four armed randomized trial that demonstrated the superiority of whole brain radiation therapy to supportive care *(1)*. BTCG 7201 was a four armed randomized trial that showed the superiority of whole brain radiation therapy over chemotherapy alone *(2)*. BTCG 8001 was a phase III trial that randomly assigned patients to one of three chemotherapy regimens followed by whole brain radiation therapy (WBRT) *(3)*. Patients enrolled between 1982 and 1983 were further randomized to WBRT or WBRT followed by a cone down boost. No survival advantage was seen with the use of WBRT. Based on these results, the initial course of radiation therapy usually consists of treatment of the region of edema defined on T2-weighted images followed by a cone down defined by the resection cavity or region of residual enhancement after surgery.

Although radiation therapy is an important component in managing high-grade gliomas (HGG), the outcomes with radiation therapy are poor. As a result, a number of trials have been conducted over the past two decades exploring the use of different chemotherapy agents and radiation sensitizers. Unfortunately, these trials have not changed the outlook for these patients. A number of different radiation therapy strategies have also been explored in hopes of improving the therapeutic ratio. One strategy that gained popularity in the 1990s was focal irradiation using brachytherapy or stereotactic radiosurgery.

From: *Current Clinical Oncology: High-Grade Gliomas: Diagnosis and Treatment*
Edited by: G. H. Barnett © Humana Press Inc., Totowa, NJ

This chapter reviews the rationale, radiobiology, clinical results, and future direction of stereotactic radiosurgery for high-grade glioma patients. The use of fractionated radiosurgery or stereotactic radiation therapy will not be discussed.

RATIONALE FOR STEREOTACTIC RADIOSURGERY

Because the majority of patients fail within the resection cavity or region of enhancing tumor, the concept of focally escalating radiation dose to these regions appears oncologically sound as more radiation dose may provide better tumor control and survival. Successive BTCG studies from 1966 to 1975, analyzed with respect to radiation dose, noted an improvement in survival with increasing dose: 28 wk for patients receiving 45.9 to 51.7 Gy, 36 wk for 52.9 to 58 Gy, and 42 wk for 58.5 to 62.0 Gy (4). A randomized trial from the United Kingdom Medical Research Council comparing 4500 cGy in 20 fractions to 6000 cGy in 30 fractions also showed survival benefit for the higher dose arm (12 vs 9 mo; $p = 0.007$) (5).

Two Radiation Therapy Oncology Group (RTOG) studies evaluating the use of 7000 cGy external beam radiation therapy and the use of hyperfractionated radiation therapy (6480 cGy to 8160 cGy) did not demonstrate improved survival (6,7). Because the use of higher doses of conventional radiation (6000–7000 cGy) has potential toxicities, such as radiation necrosis, with no apparent survival benefit, focal irradiation techniques such as brachytherapy were explored.

The initial results with brachytherapy showed promise (8–10). The placement of temporary or permanent radioactive sources, such as iodine-125, focally escalated radiation dose while providing a steep dose gradient from the edge of the tumor bed. Although the morbidity from the procedure was high, the improved survival appeared to justify the high rates of reoperation. Given these encouraging results from brachytherapy, some investigators felt radiosurgery techniques would be easier and safer to use in tumors of various size, shape and location.

Unlike brain metastases, HGG are not considered an ideal target for SRS because of their large size at presentation, irregular radiographic appearance, and infiltrative borders. These tumors are also hypoxic, acute responding, and intertwined with normal brain tissue (11–13). In addition, tumor cells are present beyond their enhancing borders with 80% of patients recurring within 2 cm of the primary tumor (14,15). Despite these unfavorable characteristics, the role of radiosurgery was investigated in hopes of improving the poor results of HGG patients.

RADIOBIOLOGY

When SRS was introduced, one major concern was the effect that a high single fraction of radiation would have against normal brain tissue. The traditional dogma in radiation oncology was to fractionate in order to minimize normal tissue damage; therefore, some were concerned that the therapeutic ratio would worsen with radiosurgery. Because HGG are composed of a mixture of solid tumor cells, combination of brain and tumor cells, and normal brain with isolated tumor cells at the periphery, a high dose of a SRS may have the intended effect on tumor cells, but a deleterious effect against normal tissue. Fortunately, the steep dose gradient that is achieved with multiple intersecting beams or arcs and close conformality of the isodose lines to the target allow for a beneficial therapeutic ratio because the radiobiologic effect is high.

To better understand the effects of radiation and normal tissue, Fowler proposed the biologically effective dose (BED) as a measure of effect to compare various fractionation schemes.

For radiosurgery, Larson modified this formula so that one could approximate BED by the following equation:

$$BED\ (n) = nd\ (1 + d/(\alpha/\beta))$$

where n is the number of fractions, d is the dose per fraction, nd is the total dose, and α and β represent the linear quadratic model for cell survival (16). Although this formula would support the concept of fractionation, the benefits were less than expected suggesting SRS was a reasonable choice for small tumors. Because HGG are considered early responding tissues surrounded by late-responding normal tissue, Larson predicted that an acceptable therapeutic ratio was obtained because the dose to tumor was much higher than normal tissues.

In an in vivo rat C6 glioma model, Kondziolka studied the histological responses after radiosurgery and different fractionated radiation therapy schedules (17). The response to SRS was generally greater than the biologically equivalent doses of fractionated radiation therapy. No difference was observed in tumor diameter or survival benefit for SRS or fractionated radiation treatments.

PRIMARY MANAGEMENT

Two randomized studies using brachytherapy have been completed for patients with newly diagnosed HGG. Laperriere reported the results of a phase III trial from Princess Margaret Hospital, which was a 2 arm trial comparing 5000 cGy/25 fractions external beam radiation therapy followed by brachytherapy boost (5000 cGy I-125 implant) to 6000 cGy/30 fractions of external beam radiation therapy (18). The median survival was not statistically different for either anaplastic gliomas or glioblastoma multiforme (GBM) patients. Selker reported the results of BTCG 8701, which was phase III trial of I-125 implant followed by external beam radiation therapy (6020 cGy/34 fractions) with 1,3-bis(2-chloroethyl)-1-nitrosurea (BCNU) vs external beam radiation therapy (6020 cGy/34 fractions) with BCNU (19). Like the Princess Margaret trial, no survival difference was noted.

One of the earliest papers reporting the use of radiosurgery as a boost for malignant gliomas was from Loeffler at the Joint Center for Radiation Therapy (20). The survival results for the 23 GBM and 14 anaplastic astrocytoma (AA) patients were impressive. As a result, other institutions investigated the use of SRS in conjunction with radiation therapy. The results from some institutions did not, however, corroborate the findings from the Joint Center for Radiation Therapy. Table 1 summarizes the various published institutional results (21–28). Of note, the best results are from institutions with the smallest median tumor volume, which demonstrates the importance of patient selection in determining outcome (29).

Given the conflicting results in the literature, the Joint Center for Radiation Therapy, University of Florida at Gainesville, and University of Wisconsin at Madison performed a multi-institutional review of their data (30). The median survival for the 115 GBM patients was an impressive 24 mo with 2-yr survival of 40%. Compared with the results of the RTOG recursive partitioning analysis (RPA), the median and 2-yr survivals were significantly improved, especially for the class III–VI patients. KPS was the only significant predictor of outcome on multivariate analysis.

Although single institution and multi-institutional results suggested a benefit to SRS boost, some investigators believed that the improved survival was a result of selection bias rather than true treatment effect, similar to the effect seen with brachytherapy (31). Curran and colleagues reviewed the RTOG database of malignant glioma patients enrolled in three consecutive trials (RTOG 74-01, 79-18, 83-02) (32). Of the 1743 patients enrolled on these

Table 1

Institutional Results of Stereotactic Radiosurgery for Newly Diagnosed HGG

	No. patients	Tumor type	Median tumor volume (cc)	Median dose (cGy)	Median survival (mo)
Shrieve (22)	78	GBM	9.4	1200	19.9
Kondziolka (28)	107 (65 primary)	45 GBM	6.5 (mean)	1550 (mean)	20
		20 AA	6.0 (mean)	1520 (mean)	56
Masciopinto (21)	31	GBM	16.4	1174	9.5
Nwokedi(23)	31	GBM	25	1710	25
Gannett(24)*	30	17 GBM	24 (all patients)	1000 (all patients)	13
		10 AA	28		
Shenouda (25)	14	GBM	<34	2000	10
Selch (26)	35 (18 primary)	12 GBM	20 (all patients)	3000 (all patients)	9
		6 AA			
Buatti (27)	11	6 GBM	14 (all patients)	1250 (all patients)	17
		5 AA			

Note:*Included anaplastic mixed oligoastrocytoma and two patients with a gliosarcoma.

studies, 1578 had sufficient information to analyze factors that influenced survival. This study analyzed 26 pretreatment characteristics and 6 treatment-related variables using recursive partitioning analysis (RPA). This analysis stratified patients into 6 distinct classes of malignant glioma patients with survivals ranging from 4.6 to 58.6 mo. Significant factors included age (most significant factor), mental status, histology, working status, extent of surgery, and Karnofsky performance status (KPS) (most significant factor for patients age 50 or older). Further analysis of RTOG 83-02, a randomized phase I/II study of hyperfractionated radiation therapy, into potentially SRS-eligible (11.9% of study patients) and ineligible patients demonstrated superior median survival times (14.4 vs 11.9 mo) and 18-mo survival rates (40 vs 27%) *(33)* for SRS eligible patients. Multivariate analysis revealed SRS eligibility to be strongly predictive of outcome.

Given the controversy surrounding the use of SRS in newly diagnosed GBM patients, the RTOG initiated a randomized phase III trial of SRS followed by radiation therapy (6000 cGy/ 30 fractions) with BCNU (80 mg/m^2 days 1–3 of radiation therapy, then every 8 wk for a total of 6 cycles) vs radiation therapy with BCNU *(34)*. Patients with supratentorial unifocal GBM who were 18 years of age or older with a KPS of > 60 and a postoperative tumor measuring less than 4 cm in maximum diameter were eligible for this study.

From February 1994 to September 2000, 203 patients with GBM were entered into this study. Pretreatment patient characteristics were well balanced between the arms. With a median follow-up of 44 mo, the median survival (14.1 mo for the non-SRS arm vs 13.7 mo for the SRS arm) and RTOG RPA class III or IV survival were not significantly different. In both arms, 90% of the failures presented as a component of local progression. Quality of life (Spitzer index) and cognitive function (mini-mental status) were not different in either arm.

RECURRENT DISEASE

At the same time investigators were exploring the use of SRS for newly diagnosed patients, some centers were also evaluating the role of SRS for recurrent HGG patients. Because many of these patients had limited treatment options, SRS appeared to be a potentially good option with results that were comparable or better than the available salvage therapies. Unlike the newly diagnosed patients, no randomized trial has been performed evaluating the use of SRS vs chemotherapy or other salvage modality. Table 2 lists the published institutional results *(35–40)*.

The largest published institutional series of recurrent HGG is from the Joint Center of Radiation Therapy. The study had 86 patients with recurrent GBM *(35)*. Median tumor volume was 10.1 cc (2.2 to 83 cc range). The median actuarial survival was 10.2 mo with 12- and 24-mo survival rates of 45 and 19%, respectively. The only factors that were predictive of outcome were younger age and smaller tumor volume. The actuarial risk for reoperation was 33% at 1-yr and 48% at 2-yr with the risk being proportional to volume.

Larson reported the multi-institutional experience of 189 glioma patients treated at eight gamma knife radiosurgery centers *(40)*. One hundred thirty-two patients had recurrent gliomas (World Health Organization [WHO] Grade I, 4 patients; WHO Grade II, 35 patients; WHO Grade III, 27 patients; and WHO Grade IV, 66 patients). Brachytherapy criteria were applied to these patients to determine if patients were eligible for brachytherapy. For the recurrent GBM patients, the median survival was 57 wk and 40 wk for the brachytherapy eligible and ineligible patients, respectively. For the recurrent AA patients, the median survival was not reached and 53 wk for the brachytherapy eligible and ineligible patients, respectively.

Table 2
Institutional Results of SRS for Recurrent HGG

	No. patients	Tumor type	Tumor volume (cc)	Median dose (cGy)	Median survival (mo)
Shrieve (35)	86*	GBM	10.1	1300	10.3
Cho (38)	46*	27 GBM 15 AA	10 (all pts)	1700 (all patients)	11 (all pts)
Kondziolka (27)	107 (42 recurrent)	19 GBM 23 AA	6.5 (mean) 6.0 (mean)	1550 (mean) 1520 (mean)	30 (all patients)
Sanghavi (36)	30	8 Gr III 22 Gr IV	7.2 (all patients)	1200 (all patients)	11 7
Park (39)	23	GBM	9.9	1500	10.3
Chamberlain (37)	20**	5 GBM 10 AA	17 (all patients)	1340 (all patients)	7 (all patients)

Notes: *Included patients with astrocytoma or anaplastic oligodendroglioma.
**Included patients with fibrillary astrocytoma and primitive neuroectodermal tumor.

TOXICITY OF STEREOTACTIC RADIOSURGERY

Acute complications from SRS are generally minimal and usually transient. These side effects may include infection or numbness at a pin site, headache, seizure, nausea, vomiting, fatigue, and exacerbation of existing neurologic symptoms. To prevent some of these side effects, many centers premedicate and discharge patients on corticosteroids. For those patients with a history of seizures, some centers also give antiseizure medications. The most common late toxicities include radiation necrosis, steroid dependency, and exacerbation of neurologic symptoms such as motor weakness, numbness, or gait difficulties. Given the difficulty in distinguishing between radiation necrosis and recurrent/persistent tumor, the reoperation rates have varied widely. In the RTOG 9305 study, the incidence of Grade III or higher toxicity was not significantly different in either arm *(34)*.

RTOG 9005 was a phase I/II dose escalation study that evaluated the maximum tolerated dose of SRS for patients with recurrent brain metastases and gliomas *(41)*. This was an important trial that demonstrated that cooperative group radiosurgery trials could be performed in and helped establish the SRS doses for newly diagnosed and recurrent malignant brain tumors. Based on the results of this study, the maximum tolerated doses were 2400 cGy for lesions <20 mm in diameter, 1800 cGy for lesions 21 to 30 mm, and 1500 cGy for lesions 31 to 40 mm. Of note, the maximum tolerated dose was not reached for lesions < 20 mm in diameter because of the investigators' reluctance to further escalate the dose. In multivariate analysis, maximum tumor diameter, tumor dose, and KPS were associated with significantly increased risk for Grade III–V neurotoxicity. The actuarial risk for radiation necrosis was 5, 8, 9, and 11% at 6, 12, 18, and 24 mo, respectively. Recurrent glioma patients were rarely able to taper off steroids. Table 3 lists the RTOG CNS toxicity criteria used for this study.

Because radiation necrosis is a potential complication of radiosurgery, accurate diagnosis of this entity is important. To help differentiate radiation necrosis from recurrent tumor, positron emission tomography (PET), single photon emission CT (SPECT), magnetic resonance spectroscopy (MRS), or biopsy may be needed to help with diagnosis *(42–46)*. The use of corticosteroids usually helps decrease the edema and mass effect associated with radiation necrosis. In addition, hyperbaric oxygen may improve neurological symptoms associated with radiation necrosis *(47)*. Intraoperative MRI is useful in facilitating removal of radiation necrosis *(48)*.

FUTURE DIRECTIONS

Some investigators are trying to improve outcomes by combining SRS with chemotherapy or radiation sensitizers. Others are exploring new imaging modalities to improve treatment planning. The James Cancer Center at Ohio State University is currently evaluating the use of Motexafin Gadolinium, a redox modulator, with SRS for newly diagnosed GBM as part of an NCI-sponsored phase I study (Grecula, personal communication). Landy and colleagues reported some encouraging results on the use of estramustine, an oral chemotherapeutic agent, for patients with newly diagnosed and recurrent malignant gliomas undergoing – gamma knife radiosurgery *(49)*. PET and MRS are being explored to help define tumor volumes and aid treatment planning *(43,50)*.

CONCLUSION

Similar to brachytherapy, stereotactic radiosurgery initially had many enthusiastic proponents for this type of dose escalation. Based on two negative randomized trials with brachytherapy and one negative trial with SRS, we do not believe that SRS should be part of the routine management of most patients with newly diagnosed HGG. In addition, the costs associated with SRS and lack of improved quality of life further the argument against SRS in this setting and as such we recommend enrollment of these patients on to clinical trials testing novel agents or radiation strategies. For recurrent HGG, scientific evidence remains sparse. SRS may be a viable option in some cases, but these patients should be offered clinical trials as well.

REFERENCES

1. Walker MD, Alexander E Jr, Hunt WE, et al. Evaluation of BCNU and/or radiotherapy in the treatment of anaplastic gliomas. A cooperative clinical trial. J Neurosurg 1978;49:333–343.
2. Walker MD, Green SB, Byar DP, et al. Randomized comparisons of radiotherapy and nitrosoureas for the treatment of malignant glioma after surgery. N Engl J Med 1980; 303:1323–1329.
3. Shapiro WR, Green SB, Burger PC, et al. Randomized trial of three chemotherapy regimens and two radiotherapy regimens in postoperative treatment of malignant glioma. J Neurosurg 1989; 71:1–9.
4. Walker MD, Strike TA, Sheline GE. An analysis of dose-effect relationship in the radiotherapy of malignant gliomas. Int J Radiat Oncol Biol Phys 1979; 5:1725–1731.
5. Bleehen NM, Stennin SP. A Medical Research Council trial of two radiotherapy doses in the treatment of grades 3 and 4 astrocytomas. Br J Cancer 1991;64:769–774.
6. Nelson DF, Diener-West M, Weinstein AS, et al. A randomized comparison of misonidazole sensitized radiotherapy plus BCNU and radiotherapy plus BCNU for treatment of malignant glioma after surgery: Final report of an RTOG study. Int J Radiat Oncol Biol Phys 1986;12:1793–1800.
7. Nelson DF, Curran WJ Jr, Scott C, et al. Hyperfractionated radiation therapy and bis-chloroethyl nitrosurea in the treatment of malignant glioma-possible advantage observed at 72.0 Gy in 1.2 Gy bid fractions: report of the RTOG protocol 8302. Int J Radiat Oncol Biol Phys 199325:193–207.
8. Gutin PH, Prados MD, Phillips TL, et al. External irradiation followed by an interstitial high activity iodine-125 implant "boost" in the initial treatment of malignant gliomas: NCOG study 6G-82-2. Int J Radiat Oncol Biol Phys 1991;21:601–606.
9. Prados MD, Gutin PH, Phillips TL, et al. Highly anaplastic astrocytoma: a review of 357 patients treated between 1977 and 1989. Int J Radiat Oncol Biol Phys 1992;23:3–8.
10. Gutin PH, Leibel SA, Wara WM, et al. Recurrent malignant gliomas: survival following interstitial brachytherapy with high-activity iodine-125 sources. J Neurosurg 1987;67:864–873.
11. Zietman AL, Suit HD, Tomkinson KN, et al. The response of two human tumor xenografts in fractionated irradiation. The derivation of alpha/beta ratios from growth delay, tumor control, and in vitro cell survival assays. Int J Radiat Oncol Biol Phys 1990;18:569–575.
12. Marin LA, Smith CE, Langston MY, et al. Response to glioblastoma cell lines to low dose rate irradiation. Int J Radiat Oncol Biol Phys 1991;21:397–402.
13. Raza SM, Lang FF, Aggarwal BB, et al. Necrosis and glioblastoma: a friend or a foe? A review and a hypothesis. Neurosurg 2002;51:2–12.
14. Hochberg FH, Pruitt A. Assumptions in the radiotherapy of glioblastoma. Neurol 1980;30:907–911.
15. Wallner KE, Galicich JH, Krol G, et al. Patterns of failure following treatment for glioblastoma multiforme and anaplastic astrocytoma. Int J Radiat Oncol Biol Phys 1989;16:1405–1409.
16. Larson DA, Flickinger JC, Loeffler JS. The radiobiology of radiosurgery. Int J Radiat Oncol Biol Phys 1993; 25:557–561.
17. Kondziolka D, Somaza S, Comey C, et al. Radiosurgery and fractionated radiation therapy: comparison of different techniques in an in vivo rat glioma model. J Neurosurg 1996;84:1033–1038.
18. Laperriere NJ, Leung PM, McKenzie S, et al. Randomized study of brachytherapy in the initial management of patients with malignant astrocytoma. Int J Radiat Oncol Biol Phys 1998;41:1005–1011.
19. Selker RG, Shapiro WR, Burger P, et al. The Brain Tumor Cooperative Group NIH trial 87-01: a randomized comparison of surgery, external beam radiotherapy, and carmustine versus surgery, interstitial radiotherapy boost, external radiation therapy, and carmustine. Neurosurg 2002;51:343–355.
20. Loeffler JS, Alexander E 3d, Shea WM, et al. Radiosurgery as part of the initial management of patients with malignant gliomas. J Clin Oncol 1992;10:1379–1385.
21. Masciopinto JE, Levin AB, Mehta MP, et al. Stereotactic radiosurgery for glioblastoma: a final report of 31 patients. J Neurosurg 1995;82:530–535.

22. Shrieve DC, Alexander E, Black PM, et al. Treatment of patients with primary glioblastoma multiforme with standard postoperative radiotherapy and radiosurgical boost: prognostic factors and long-term outcome. J Neurosurg 1999;90:72–77.

23. Nwokedi EC, DiBiase SJ, Jabbour S, et al. Gamma Knife stereotactic radiosurgery for patients with glioblastoma multiforme. Neurosurg 2002;50:41–46.

24. Gannett D, Stea B, Lulu B, et al. Stereotactic radiosurgery as an adjunct to surgery and external beam radiotherapy in the treatment of patients with malignant gliomas. Int J Radiat Oncol Biol Phys 1995;33:461–468.

25. Shenouda G, Souhami L, Podgorsak EB, et al. Radiosurgery and accelerated radiotherapy for patients with glioblastoma. Can J Neurol Sci 1997;24:110–115.

26. Selch MT, Ciacci JD, De Salles AA, et al. Radiosurgery for primary malignant brain tumors. In: AA De Salles, SJ Goetsch, eds. Stereotactic Surgery and Radiosurgery. Madison, WI:Medical Physics Pub. 1993; 335–352.

27. Buatti JM, Friedman WA, Bova FJ, et al. Linac radiosurgery for high-grade gliomas: the University of Florida experience. Int J Radiat Oncol Biol Phys 1995;32:205–210.

28. Kondziolka D, Flickinger JC, Bissonette DJ, et al. Survival benefit of stereotactic radiosurgery for patients with malignant glial neoplasms. Neurosurg 1997;41:776–783.

29. Loeffler JS, Shrieve DC, Alexander E III. Radiosurgery for glioblastoma multiforme: the importance of selection criteria. Int J Radiat Oncol Biol Phys 1994;30:731–733.

30. Sarkaria JN, Mehta MP, Loeffler JS, et al. Radiosurgery in the initial management of malignant gliomas: survival comparison with the RTOG recursive partitioning analysis. Radiation Therapy Oncology Group. Int J Radiat Oncol Biol Phys 1995;32:931–941.

31. Florell RC, Macdonald DR, Irish WD, et al. Selection bias, survival, and brachytherapy for glioma. J Neurosurg 1992;76:179–83.

32. Curran WJ, Scott CB, Horton J, et al. Recursive partitioning analysis of prognostic factors in three Radiation Therapy Oncology Group malignant glioma trials. J Natl Cancer Inst 1993;85:704–710.

33. Curran WJ Jr, Scott C, Weinstein AS, et al. Survival comparison of radiosurgery-eligible and ineligible malignant glioma patients treated with hyperfractionated radiation therapy and carmustine: a report of Radiation Therapy Oncology Group 83-02. J Clin Oncol 1993;11:857–862.

34. Souhami L, Seiferheld W, Brachman D, et al. Randomized comparison of stereotactic radiosurgery followed by conventional radiotherapy with carmustine to conventional radiotherapy with carmustine for patients with glioblastoma multiforme: report of Radiation Therapy Oncology Group 93-05 protocol. Int J Radiat Oncol Biol Phys 2004;60:853–860.

35. Shrieve DC, Alexander E, Wen PY, et al. Comparison of stereotactic radiosurgery and brachytherapy in the treatment of recurrent glioblastoma multiforme. Neurosurg 1995;36:275–282.

36. Sanghavi S, Skrupky R, Badie B, et al. Recurrent malignant gliomas treated with radiosurgery. J Radiosurg 1999;2:119–125.

37. Chamberlain MC, Barba D, Kormanik P, et al. Stereotactic radiosurgery for recurrent gliomas. Cancer 1994; 74:1342–1347.

38. Cho KH, Hall WA, Gerbi BJ, et al. Single dose versus fractionated stereotactic radiosurgery for recurrent high-grade gliomas. Int J Radiat Oncol Biol Phys 1999;45:1133–1141.

39. Park JL, Suh JH, Barnett GH, et al. Survival after stereotactic radiosurgery for recurrent glioblastoma multiforme. J Radiosurg 2000;3:169–175.

40. Larson DA, Gutin PH, McDermott M, et al. Gamma knife for glioma: selection factors and survival. Int J Radiat Oncol Biol Phys 1996;36:1045–1053.

41. Shaw E, Scott C, Souhami L, et al. Single dose radiosurgical treatment of recurrent previously irradiated primary brain tumors and brain metastases: Final report of RTOG 90-05. Int J Radiat Oncol Biol Phys 2000;47: 291–298.

42. Chao ST, Suh JH, Raja S, et al. The sensitivity and specificity of FDG-PET in distinguishing recurrent brain tumor from radionecrosis in patients treated with stereotactic radiosurgery. J Cancer 2001;96:191–197.

43. Graves EE, Nelson SJ, Vigneron DB, et al. A preliminary study of the prognostic value of proton magnetic resonance spectroscopic imaging in gamma knife radiosurgery of recurrent malignant gliomas. Neurosurg 2000;46:319–326.

44. Kline JL, Noto RB, Glantz M. Single-photon emission CT in the evaluation of recurrent brain tumor in patients treated with gamma knife radiosurgery or conventional radiation therapy. Am J Neuroradiol 1996;17:1681–1686.

45. Schlemmer HP, Bachert P, Herfarth KK, et al. Proton MR spectroscopic evaluation of suspicious brain lesions after stereotactic radiotherapy. Am J Neuroradiol 2001;22:1316–1324.

46. Schwartz RB, Hsu L, Kacher DF, et al. Intraoperative dynamic MRI: localization of sites of brain tumor recurrence after high-dose radiotherapy. J Magn Reson Imaging 1998;8:1085–1089.
47. Warnick RE, Gessell LB, Breneman JC, et al. Hyperbaric oxygen is an effective treatment for radiation necrosis of the brain. [Abstract] Neurosurg 2002;51:560.
48. McPherson CM, Warnick RE. Results of contemporary surgical management of radiation necrosis using frameless stereotaxis and intraoperative magnetic resonance imaging. J Neuro-oncol 2004;68: 41–47.
49. Landy H, Markoe A, Potter P, et al. Pilot study of estramustine added to radiosurgery and radiotherapy for treatment of high grade glioma. J Neuro-Oncol 2004;67:215–220.
50. Levivier M, Wikler D Jr, Massager N, et al. The integration of metabolic imaging in stereotactic procedures including radiosurgery: a review. J Neurosurg 2002;97 (Suppl): 542–550.

16 Chemotherapy

Manmeet Singh Ahluwalia and David M. Peereboom

Summary

The role of systemic chemotherapy in high-grade gliomas (HGG) continues to evolve. The use of chemotherapy for central nervous system (CNS) malignancies poses specific challenges related to drug delivery and interactions with anticonvulsants. Chemotherapy has become standard in the adjuvant therapy of HGG. For patients with chemotherapy-sensitive subgroups of pure and mixed anaplastic oligodendrogliomas, chemotherapy represents the preferred initial therapy. Chemotherapy is often used for patients with recurrent HGG. The efficacy of chemotherapy for patients with HGG is likely to improve substantially with the advent of new drugs with novel mechanisms of action, markers to select patients likely to benefit from chemotherapy, new methods to enhance drug delivery, and strategies to circumvent drug resistance.

Key Words: High-grade glioma; chemotherapy; pre-irradiation chemotherapy; glioblastoma, anaplastic oligodendroglioma; recurrent glioma; blood–brain barrier.

PRINCIPLES OF CHEMOTHERAPY FOR CENTRAL NERVOUS SYSTEM MALIGNANCIES

Treatment of high-grade gliomas (HGG) with systemic chemotherapy poses challenges unique to brain tumors. Foremost is the blood–brain barrier (BBB) which impairs delivery of adequate concentrations of most chemotherapeutic agents to the tumor. The BBB is maintained by interaction between astrocytes and endothelial cells that protect the brain from the foreign and undesirable molecules. This membrane lacks intercellular fenestrations, has high-electrical resistance and low-ionic permeability rendering it relatively impermeable to many water-soluble compounds *(1)*. Most cytotoxic drugs traverse the BBB by passive diffusion while some use specific endothelial cell transport mechanisms to gain access to the central nervous system (CNS). Gadolinium enhancement, however, most likely signifies disruption of the BBB that may allow access of chemotherapeutic agents although the degree of penetration is unknown. To cross the BBB, chemotherapy agents administered systemically must be less than approx 200 daltons in size, lipid soluble, not bound to plasma proteins, and minimally ionized. Most cytotoxic agents do not meet these criteria, and when administered systemically only a small proportion of the drug reaches the CNS. Several strategies have attempted to overcome the BBB. Intra-arterial (with or without BBB disruption) *(2)* and convection enhanced delivery (CED) *(3)* have been used to deliver agents (e.g., carboplatin, etoposide, paclitaxel) that do not cross BBB.

Most patients receive chemotherapy after radiotherapy. Whereas a transient increase in BBB permeability occurs early in the course of radiation therapy, long-term damage to the

From: *Current Clinical Oncology: High-Grade Gliomas: Diagnosis and Treatment*
Edited by: G. H. Barnett © Humana Press Inc., Totowa, NJ

Table 1
Metabolism of Anticonvulsant Drug Agents

Anticonvulsant drugs that induce hepatic metabolic enzymes

Generic name	Trade name
Phenytoin	Dilantin
Carbamazepine	Tegretol
Phenobarbital	Phenobarbital
Primidone	Mysoline
Oxcarbazepine	Trileptal

Anticonvulsant drugs with modest or no induction of hepatic metabolic enzymes

Generic name	Trade name
Gabapentin	Neurontin
Lamotrigine	Lamictal
Valproic Acid	Depakote, Depakene
Levetiracetam	Keppra
Tiagibine	Gabitril
Topiramate	Topimax
Zonisamide	Zonegran

microvasculature impairs drug delivery to the viable tumor *(4)*. In addition, radiation-induced hypoxia likely reduces the proportion of dividing cells thereby rendering the tumor less sensitive to chemotherapy *(4)*. The formation of necrotic and fibrotic tissue within the irradiated tumor further reduces the likelihood of tumor shrinkage and confounds the radiographic assessment of response to chemotherapy. Radionecrosis can mimic tumor progression many months after radiotherapy and can give the false impression of chemotherapy failure.

Certain aspects of chemotherapy pertain specifically to the treatment of brain tumors. For example, acute worsening of cerebral edema can complicate regimens that require significant hydration such as those that contain cisplatin *(5)*. Other regimens such as BCNU/cisplatin can cause abrupt reductions in serum anticonvulsant levels that can precipitate seizures *(6)*. Conversely, anticonvulsants can markedly affect the serum levels of chemotherapeutic agents *(7)*. Hepatic enzyme inducing anticonvulsant drugs (Table 1) decrease the serum concentrations of chemotherapeutic drugs that are metabolized through the P-450 cytochrome enzyme pathway (P-450) (Table 2) *(7,8)*. Other drugs commonly used in patients with HGG can also interact with these chemotherapeutic agents (Table 2).

ASSESSMENT OF RESPONSE

Measurement of tumor response to chemotherapy is important not only in clinical trials but also in clinical practice. Markers of radiographic responses are traditionally defined as follows:

- Partial response (PR): Less than 50% decrease in tumor size on imaging (computed tomography [CT]/magnetic resonance imaging [MRI]). (Tumor size is defined by the sum of the products of bi-dimensional measurements.)
- Minor response (MR): 25 to –50% decrease in tumor size on imaging.
- Stable disease (SD): Less than 25% change in tumor size after chemotherapy.
- Progressive disease: Tumor enlargement less than 25 % on chemotherapy.

Table 2
Metabolism of Selected Chemotherapeutic Agents

Chemotherapeutic agents metabolized by P-450
Irinotecan
Lomustine
Vincristine
Tamoxifen
Paclitaxel
Etoposide
Cis-retinoic acid
Chemotherapeutic agents not metabolized by P-450
Temozolomide
Procarbazine
Carmustine
Thalidomide

As applied to brain tumors, the modified McDonald criteria require that the patient be on stable or decreasing doses of steroids in order to meet the above measures of complete, partial response, and stable disease *(9)*. Given the difficulties in tumor assessment by imaging, these measures have limited utility in assessment of chemotherapy efficacy in brain tumors, especially after radiotherapy. Furthermore, many newer targeted agents can provide meaningful durations of progression-free survival in the absence of disease regression.

Survival parameters are much more useful in measurement of treatment efficacy in HGG. Progression-free survival (PFS) and overall survival have become the preferred measures of efficacy. Difficulties still arise in the determination of time of progression and this parameter can vary significantly with the interval between assessments (e.g., MRI obtained every 2 mo vs 3 mo). For tumors with a relatively short survival time such as glioblastoma multiforme (GBM), these variables can have significant effects on assessment of PFS. Therefore, 6-mo PFS (the proportion of patients free from progression at 6 mo) is probably the most useful measure of efficacy particularly in patients with recurrent gliomas. For newly diagnosed patients, median survival and 1- and 2-yr survivals are the most commonly used benchmarks.

PROGNOSTIC VARIABLES

An understanding of the prognostic variables is critical not only in the assessment and management of patients with HGG but also in the interpretation of clinical trial reports. The most important prognostic factors identified for adults with HGG are age (< 40, 40-60, >60 yr), tumor histology (anaplastic astrocytoma [AA] vs GBM vs. anaplastic oligodendroglioma [AO]), performance status (Karnofsky performance status, [KPS] 70 vs 60) and the extent of resection *(10–12)*. For a given histology, younger patients live significantly longer than older patients *(13)*.

A landmark analysis of prognostic factors by the Radiation Therapy Oncology Group (RTOG) used recursive partitioning to divide patients into six prognostic classes (Tables 3 and 4) *(12)*. These classes have markedly different prognoses depending primarily on histology, age, and KPS. Thus the results of clinical trials must be interpreted in light of these prognostic classes.

Table 3
Classes Divided on Basis of Age, Histology, and Performance Status *(12)*

HGG: RTOG recursive partition analysis

Class I:	Age <50, AA, normal mental status.
Class II:	Age ≥ 50, AA, ST > 3 mo.
Class III:	Age <50, AA, abnormal mental status.
Class IV:	Age <50, GBM, KPS 90–100.
Class IV:	Age <50, GBM, KPS <90.
Class IV:	Age ≥50, AA, KPS >70, ST <3 mo.
Class IV:	Age ≥50, GBM, KPS <90, ST < 3 mo, WNFx.
Class V:	Age ≥50, KPS ≥70, GBM, NWNFx.
Class V:	Age ≥50, KPS ≥70, GBM, RT dose >54.4 Gy.
Class V:	Age ≥50, KPS <70, normal mental status.
Class VI:	Age ≥50, KPS <70, abnormal mental status, RT dose <54.4 Gy.

Abbr: AA, anaplastic astrocytoma; GBM, glioblastoma multiforme; KPS, Karnofsky performance status; ST, symptom time; WNFx, working neurological function; NWNFx, nonworking neurological function; MS, mental status

Table 4
Prognosis Based on RPA Class *(12)*

Class	Median survival (mo)	2-yr survival
I	59	76
II	37	68
III	18	35
IV	11	15
V	9	6
VI	5	4

A given agent will appear more efficacious in a clinical trial with a predominance of class I or II patients compared to a study with mainly class V or VI patients.

CHEMOTHERAPEUTIC AGENTS

Single Agents

Multiple agents have been reported to have activity against HGG, mostly on the basis of small phase II trials. Table 5 lists agents most commonly used for these patients *(14–17,19–34)*. The only single agents that have been tested in phase III trials are BCNU, procarbazine, temozolomide, and streptozoticin *(14–19)*. Several randomized phase II trials have tested single agents but these studies are not designed or powered to make comparisons between agents *(20)*.

Drug Combinations

Multiple drug combinations have been tested in the treatment of HGG. The most common combination has been PCV (procarbazine, CCNU, vincristine). It is still used occasionally as a first line regimen in AO and AA but it has been largely replaced by temozolomide in this setting because pf the higher incidence of nonhematological toxicity and dose-limiting cumu-

Table 5
Selected Agents Active Against HGG

Agent	Primary mechanism of action	Toxicities particular to agent	Comments	Refs.
Nitrosoureas (BCNU, CCNU ACNU)	DNA alkylation	Myelosuppression, cumulative and often irreversible; pulmonary fibrosis	BCNU, CCNU most commonly used. BCNU also used in implantable wafers	(14,15,17,19,21)
Temozolomide	DNA methylation	Myelosuppression, noncumulative	The most commonly used agent in gliomas; relatively low toxicity profile	(16,22,23)
Procarbazine	DNA alkylation	Interaction with MAO inhibitors and tyramine-rich foods	Used mostly in PCV combination regimen	(20,24)
Irinotecan	Topoisomerase I inhibition	Diarrhea can be severe	Marked effect on serum levels by P450-active AEDs	(25–27)
Isotretinoin (cis retinoic acid)	Differentiating agent	Chelitis, teratogenic	Well tolerated, mainly cytostatic	(28,29)
Tamoxifen	PKC inhibition	Deep vein thrombosis	Used in high doses (160–240 mg/d)	(30–34)

Abbr: MAO, monoamine oxidase; AED, antiepileptic drug; PKC, protein kinase C.

271

Table 6
Drug Combinations

Procarbazine, CCNU/lomustine, vincristine (PCV)	*(35)*
Cyclophosphamide and vincristine	*(36)*
Cisplatin/Carboplatin and etoposide	*(37,38)*
Procarbazine, etoposide and vincristine	*(39)*
Procarbazine and high dose tamoxifen	*(33)*
Ifosfamide, carboplatin and etoposide (ICE)	*(40)*
Procarbazine/BCNU and temozolomide	*(41,42)*
Cisplatin and temozolomide	*(43)*
Mecholorethamine, vincristine and procarbazine	*(44)*
Irinotecan and bevacizumab	*(44a)*
Imatinib and hydroxyurea	*(44b)*

lative myelosuppression of PCV. Other drug regimens used are given in Table 6 *(33,35–44)*. None of these combinations, however, have produced a significant improvement in time to progression (TTP) or overall survival (OS).

Several new combination therapies have been reported for patients with recurrent or progressive HGG. Selected regimens appear in Table 6. These newer regimens have begun to incorporate targeted agents and will hopefully improve efficacy with minimal or no worsening of toxicity.

ADJUVANT CHEMOTHERAPY

Adjuvant chemotherapy refers to treatment applied at diagnosis as an adjunct to definitive surgery and/or radiotherapy. The goal of adjuvant chemotherapy is to increase cell kill, to improve survival, and ultimately to enhance the cure or response rate. The role of adjuvant chemotherapy has been controversial despite multiple prospective randomized clinical trials over the past 30 yr. Several trials demonstrated a modest survival benefit with the addition of chemotherapy *(14,45)*. Unfortunately, almost all of these trials included both GBM and anaplastic glioma so that conclusions about particular histologies with divergent behaviors could not be made. The most recent such trial by Stupp and colleagues, however, included only patients with GBM and established temozolomide as standard in the initial treatment for this histology *(16)*. This study of patients with newly diagnosed GBM compared radiotherapy alone to radiotherapy with temozolomide given during and after radiotherapy. The median overall survival was improved significantly in the temozolomide arm (14.6 vs 12.1 mo; $p <$ 0.001). Two-year survival was also improved (26 vs 11%). Thus, radiotherapy with temozolomide has become standard therapy for patients with newly diagnosed GBM. The next generation of clinical trials will build on this regimen in phase II and III trials. As the Stupp trial included temozolomide both during and after radiotherapy, it is unknown whether the benefit of radiation and temozolomide occurs as a result of concurrent low-dose therapy and/or subsequent full-dose therapy. It is known that radiotherapy does cause transient opening of the BBB which could improve drug delivery during concurrent therapy *(45a)*. Future randomized trials of initial therapy for HGG might compare standard concurrent and post-radiation temozolomide to either concurrent or post-radiation temozolomide alone in an effort to answer this question as well as to reduce the costs of adjuvant chemotherapy.

Table 7
Phase III Trials of Radiation Treatment With and Without Chemotherapy for Newly Diagnosed HGG

Regimens	Result	Accrual	Ref.
RT vs RT/BCNU	No change in median survival	222	(14)
RT vs MeCCNU vs RT/BCNU vs RT/MeCCNU	Trend toward 18-m survival advantage with RT /BCNU as compared with RT alone.	358	(15)
RT vs RT/PCV	No difference in survival	674	(47)
RT vs RT/TMZ Glioblastoma only	2.5-mo survival advantage in RT/TMZ arm	573	(16)

Most investigators have regarded PCV as standard adjuvant therapy for patients with AA on the basis of a 1990 report of the Northern California Oncology Group (NCOG) study *(35)*. This trial randomized patients with HGG to adjuvant PCV or BCNU. In the subset of 73 patients with AA, adjuvant therapy with PCV increased the median survival to157 wk as compared with 82 wk with BCNU. A subsequent analysis of these data, however, cast doubt on the superiority of PCV in this setting *(46)*. This report had pooled data of 4 RTOG trials over 15 yr involving over 400 patients. The authors concluded that PCV did not confer a survival benefit over BCNU in the adjuvant treatment of patients with AA. Given the substantially greater toxicity of PCV, this regimen has largely fallen out of favor as first line treatment of patients with AA but it is commonly used at recurrence after temozolomide. A current Intergroup trial compares BCNU or CCNU with temozolomide and may define standard initial therapy for this patient group.

A 1993 meta-analysis of eight randomized controlled trials (RCT) concluded that the addition of nitrosoureas to radiation increased 1-yr survival by 10 %and 2-yr survival by 8.6% in patients with HGG *(49)*. Patients less than 60 yr of age benefited more from chemotherapy as compared with the elderly. A more recent meta-analysis in 2002 evaluated over 3000 patients from 12 RCT (11 published, 1 unpublished) and provided clear evidence of a small survival benefit for patients treated with chemotherapy in addition to radiation therapy *(50)*. There was a 2-mo improvement in median survival and a 15%relative decrease in the risk of death.

PRE-IRRADIATION OR NEOADJUVANT CHEMOTHERAPY

Neoadjuvant chemotherapy refers to treatment given at diagnosis before other modalities such as radiation. It has several potential advantages. First, neoadjuvant chemotherapy allows early treatment of the infiltrating tumor cells that may be at or beyond the border of the radiation field. Second, neoadjuvant chemotherapy allows true assessment of the efficacy of the chemotherapy. Such information is important at the time of tumor progression in deciding whether treatment with the same regimen might be helpful. Finally, new agents are most effectively screened for activity in this setting *(51)*. If a given agent has no efficacy in newly diagnosed patients, it will not help patients with recurrent tumors, and further testing in these patients can be avoided. The risk of tumor progression during chemotherapy, however, is significant, particularly for patients with GBM. The neoadjuvant trial design for patients with HGG requires very close monitoring. Most such trials appropriately mandate repeat imaging every 4 wk during pre-irradiation chemotherapy.

Table 8
Phase III Trials of Various Chemotherapy Regimens Added
to Radiation Therapy in Patients with Newly Diagnosed HGG

Regimens	Result	Accrual	Ref.
BCNU BCNU/Methylprednisolone Methylprednisolone Procarbazine	BCNU improved median survival as compared to other agents	527	(17)
BCNU BCNU/Procarbazine BCNU/Hydroxyurea procarbazine/VM-26	Median survival equivalent in all arms.	510	(18)
BCNU vs streptozotocin (19)	No change in median survival; streptozotocin more toxic regimen	557	(19)
BCNU vs PCV (20)	Median survival equivalent for GBM. In AA, PCV superior	148	(35)
BCNU vs BCNU/Cisplatin (21)	No change in median survival BCNU cisplatin more toxic.	219	(48)

Studies of pre-irradiation chemotherapy have shown mixed results. A study by Grossman et al. reported a partial response (PR) rate of 42% in 52 patients with HGG treated with BCNU and cisplatin; 53% of the patients remained stable (5). A recent French study, however, reported PRs in only 19% of the patients (52). These discrepancies also underline the heterogeneous nature of HGG. Despite great interest in neoadjuvant chemotherapy in the last decade, this approach has not yet produced evidence of prolonged survival as compared with adjuvant chemotherapy in HGG. Whereas theoretically attractive, pre-irradiation chemotherapy for GBM and AA should not be administered outside of a clinical trial. As more effective agents are developed, however, neoadjuvant chemotherapy may develop a role in the management of HGG.

ANAPLASTIC OLIGODENDROGLIOMA

In contrast to GBM, AO are unusually chemosensitive tumors. Chemosensitivity in this tumor type is marked by chromosome 1p deletion in the tumor (53–54). In addition, AO may harbor loss of 19q; however, deletion of 19q without 1p deletion does not translate into chemosensitivity. Patients who have loss of both 1p and 19q have marked and often times durable responses to chemotherapy associated with prolonged survival with and without radiation. Those patients whose tumors have loss of 1p but either do not have 19q loss or have other genetic alterations (e.g., TP53 mutation, PTEN mutation, 10q loss, endothelial growth factor receptor [EGFR] amplification or CDKN2A loss) can respond to chemotherapy but with a shorter duration of response than those patients with loss of both 1p and 19q (54).

AO that lack 1p deletion are less chemosensitive. These tumors can be divided into 2 groups: those with TP53 mutation who respond to chemotherapy but recur quickly and those who lack TP53 mutation and act like GBM showing poor response to chemotherapy (54). The chemosensitivity of AO is attributed mainly to inability of these tumors to repair DNA damage induced by alkylating agents (55). Hence molecular diagnosis of 1p/19q loss provides a rational basis for clinical decisions. Patients with 1p deletions could be treated safely with chemotherapy alone with radiotherapy deferred until disease progression *(53)*. Chemotherapy is increasingly preferred over radiation therapy as initial treatment after surgical resection *(56,57)*. Those with intact 1p are frequently treated with concurrent chemotherapy and radiotherapy although in the context of a clinical trial chemotherapy is reasonable as initial treatment *(57a)*

For patients with AO, the combination of procarbazine, CCNU, and vincristine (PCV) has been the most widely used chemotherapy with responses in up to 75% *(58,59)*. The response rates are similar with or without prior radiation treatment *(60)*. Recently six patients with recurrent or progressive AO were treated with intensive PCV regimen followed by stem cell support, two showed CR while the other four had PR *(61)*. As many as 30% of the patients treated with PCV have significant myelosuppression and are unable to complete six cycles of chemotherapy. Therefore, temozolomide rather than PCV has become the most common first line agent for patients with AO. In a phase II trial, patients with AO treated with temozolomide as first line agent showed a response rate of 53% *(62)*. In a retrospective study 9 out of 10 (90%) patients who had 1p deletion responded to temozolomide as compared with 2 out of 6 (33%) who had intact 1p *(63)*.

In recurrent AO, PCV is an option if not previously used. In recurrent AO previously treated with PCV response rates of 44 to 50% have been achieved with temozolomide *(23,64)* making it a suitable second-line option. Four out of ten patients (40%) responded to etoposide and carboplatin, whereas 15% responded to paclitaxel *(65)*.

Because of their chemosensitivity and durable responses to treatment, AO serve as a useful setting for neoadjuvant trials with quality-of-life (QOL) measures. Several such trials are in progress *(66)*. Whereas standard therapy for this group of patients is controversial, treatment of patients with anaplastic gliomas is based increasingly on genetics rather than on histology. Patients with 1p deletions are often treated first with chemotherapy with radiation reserved for use at the time of progressive disease. Patients with 1p intact often receive radiation at diagnosis but this approach is also the subject of clinical trials *(66)*.

RECURRENT HIGH-GRADE GLIOMAS

For recurrent HGG no standard chemotherapy exists with the possible exception of PCV for chemotherapy sensitive AO. Whereas temozolomide is approved by the United States Food and Drug Administration (FDA) for recurrent AA, and in Europe for recurrent GBM, this agent is almost always used at diagnosis, largely obviating its role in the recurrent setting. Furthermore, approval of this agent was based on a single phase II data for each tumor type *(20,67)*. Repeat therapy with this agent is reasonable for the exceptional patient who experiences a prolonged response (e.g., 6-mo progression-free interval after completion of treatment) to initial therapy. An alternative strategy is the use of a different treatment schedule of the same drug; one example of this approach is the use of low-dose temozolomide (75 mg/m^2 daily $\leftrightarrow$ 42 d every 56 d) in the patient who has received standard dose temozolomide. Unlike the mechanisms of bolus dosing chemotherapy, such "metronomic" schedules of chemotherapy could produce second responses to the same agent by virtue of anti-angiogenic properties *(68)* and depletion of methylguanine-methyl transferase, an important DNA repair enzyme (see below section on "Modulation of Drug Resistance and Delivery").

If feasible, surgical resection, or experimental agents or delivery techniques such as convection-enhanced delivery are the preferred treatment modalities for most patients with recurrent gliomas. Chemotherapy, however, can be useful for certain patients. Those most likely to benefit are young patients with low tumor bulk and good performance status. Outside of

Table 9
Outcomes and Prognostic Factors in Recurrent Gliomas:
Response and Survival Rates *(69)*

Response	GBM *(n = 225)*	AA *(n = 150)*	Total *(n = 375)*
CR+PR %	6	14	9
6 month PFS %	15	31	21
1 yr PFS %	8	20	12
1 yr OS %	21	47	32
Median PFS(wk)	9	12	10
Median OS (wk)	25	47v	30

clinical trials, single-agent temozolomide or nitrosoureas like carmustine or lomustine are most commonly used although any of the agents listed in Table 5 represent viable options. Given the better safety profile temozolomide is often the preferred agent.

The goal of chemotherapy for recurrent HGG is to stabilize the tumor (i.e., to slow or stop its growth.) Because of the limited activity of systemic chemotherapy in this setting, QOL needs to be addressed in clinical trials. Therefore, one must have a detailed discussion with the patient and the patient's family regarding the goals, prognosis, and toxicities of the therapy before offering chemotherapy in this setting. One trial of temozolomide has demonstrated improvements with QOL in this patient population *(67)*.

As a result of the difficulties inherent in measurement of radiographic response in gliomas, PFS has emerged as an important response parameter in studies of recurrent HGG. An analysis of the MD Anderson database of multiple clinical trials has become a benchmark for historical control data *(69)*. The most commonly used parameters are 6-mo PFS, which for AA is approx 30% and for GBM approx 15%.

Future therapies for patients with recurrent HGG are the subject of multiple phase I or II clinical trials both by single institutions and by cooperative groups. Some of the classes of agents are listed in Table 10.

STRATEGIES TO IMPROVE CHEMOTHERAPEUTIC EFFICACY IN HIGH-GRADE GLIOMAS

Imroved Patient Selection

Three areas of advance have occurred that can improve selection of patients for chemotherapy. Analysis of 1p and 19q status in AO has been discussed above (see section on "Anaplastic Oligodendroglioma") and is commonly used to select patients who could be treated with chemotherapy as initial therapy. Two additional markers may improve the ability to select patients who might benefit for chemotherapy.

Methylguanine-methyl transferase (MGMT) is a ubiquitous cellular enzyme responsible in large part for resistance to the cytotoxic action of DNA alkylating agents (e.g., temozolomide, carmustine, lomustine, procarbazine) in HGG. Inactivation of MGMT impairs the ability of the cell to repair DNA damage. Methylation of the MGMT gene promoter in the cells of HGG inactivates the enzyme. Correlative studies performed on tumor samples in the randomized GBM trial of radiotherapy with or without temozolomide *(16)* determined that patients whose

Table 10
Selected New Classes of Agents in Clinical Trials for HGG

Class of agent	Examples
Differentiating agents	Retinoids, phenylacetate, phenylbutyrate
Histone deacetylase inhibitors	Depsipeptide
EGFR tyrosine kinase inhibitors	Erlotinib
Pan HER kinase inhibitors	GW572016
Iinhibitors of mammalian target of rapamycin (mTOR)	Temsirolimus (CCI779), RAD001
Inhibitors of *Ras* signaling (farnesyl transferase inhibitors)	Tipifarnib (R115777)
Inhibitors of Raf	Sorafenib (BAY 43-9006)
Integrin antagonists	Cilengitide (EMD 121974)
Endothelin receptor antagonist	Atrasentan
Mitotic kinesins	SB 715992
Proteasome Inhibitors	Bortezomib (PS-341)
Cycloxygenase2 inhibitors	Celecoxib
PARP inhibitors	ABT 472
VEGF inhibitors	Bevacizumab
Platelet derived growth factor inhibitors	Imatinib

tumors had methylation of the MGMT promoter survived longer than whose MGMT promoter was unmethylated *(69a)* In the future, methylation status may serve as a marker to select patients who are more likely to benefit from alkylating agents. For example, patients with methylated MGMT might benefit from additional strategies to inactivate MGMT such as scheduling alterations that could deplete the enzyme. The large Intergroup randomized GBM trial (RTOG 0525) stratifies patients according to MGMT promoter status to evaluate prospectively the utility of this marker as a selection tool.

Similar molecular determinants have been investigated in patients who received inhibitors of EGFR kinase *(69b)* Coexpression of the EGFR deletion mutant variant III (EGFRvIII) and the tumor-suppressor protein PTEN in recurrent HGG is associated with responsiveness to EGFR kinase inhibitors. Such markers could conceivably become part of patient selection criteria for use of these agents.

MODULATION OF DRUG RESISTANCE AND DELIVERY

Drug resistance and restricted delivery beyond the BBB remain major limitations in the chemotherapy treatment of HGG. Attempts to circumvent these barriers by increased local drug delivery include the use of chemotherapy-impregnated wafers, convection enhanced delivery (see Chapter 18), and intra-arterial chemotherapy. One technique not yet in clinical practice is the use of a fenestrated balloon catheter for the local infusion of chemotherapy. Modulation of DNA repair and administration of high-dose chemotherapy represent attempts at a systemic level to circumvent drug resistance and to improve dose intensity.

Carnustine wafers (3.8% BCNU impregnated wafers) are biodegradable polymers containing BCNU. These wafers can be implanted into the surgical resection cavity to deliver BCNU directly into the tumor. Randomized trials have shown a modest survival benefit both in recurrent and in newly diagnosed patients *(70–71)*. A recently formulated BCNU wafer contains 20% BCNU (as compared with the standard 3.8% wafer) and is in clinical trials.

High-dose chemotherapy with stem cell rescue attempts to circumvent dose-limiting myelosuppression by administration of high-dose chemotherapy followed by autologous stem cell rescue. Small trials using high-dose BCNU or high-dose thiotepa/carboplatin followed by autologous stem cell rescue have reported promising results *(72,73)*. Nonetheless, this approach has generally not been adopted for HGG because of the inherent chemotherapy resistance of these tumors. High-dose chemotherapy for newly diagnosed AO appears feasible with some long-term survivors *(74)*. With the development of more effective agents, high-dose chemotherapy may develop a niche in the therapy of patients with good performance status and chemotherapy sensitive tumors.

What about IA combo? Intra-arterial delivery of chemotherapy attempts to deliver high local concentrations of drug with smaller systemic doses thereby reducing the systemic side effects. The ideal agent for intra-arterial delivery is one that is lipophilic, small in size, and undergoes rapid systemic inactivation. Nitrosoureas fulfill these criteria and have been used in several trials *(75,76)*. Two series of selected patients with recurrent HGG showed encouraging results using IA carboplatin and intravenous cyclophosphamide with osmotic disrupton of the BBB *(76a,76b)*. Because of toxicity and technical difficulty, however, intra-arterial chemotherapy has not been used extensively in treatment of HGG. The lack of efficacy reflects the recurring problem with intrinsic drug resistance of most HGG.

Because MGMT mediates resistance to DNA alkylating agents, it is an ideal target for biochemical modulation of anti tumor drug resistance *(77)*. O^6-benzyl guanine (O^6BG) causes substantial depletion of MGMT in tumors in phase I trials *(78,78a)* This agent is currently in a phase III trial of patients with newly diagnosed GBM in which patients receive radiotherapy, BCNU with or without O^6BG. Of interest, the maximum tolerated dose of BCNU in the combination regimen is 20% of the MTD as a single agent (40 vs 200 mg/m^2 every 6 wk) raising the question as to whether this substantially lower dose will provide a therapeutic advantage.

Another strategy for depletion of MGMT is to alter the schedule of administration of temozolomide. Protracted low-dose administration (e.g., 14 or 21 d) or higher doses of alternating schedules can deplete plasma MGMT activity by approx 70% *(79)*. Whether such reductions in MGMT will translate into improved therapy is under study. To date, multiple small trials have examined alternate dosing schedules for temozolomide for HGG with results that are therefore difficult to interpret. A large Intergroup randomized trial for patients with newly glioblastoma (RTOG 0525) will compare standard dose temozolomide with extended dose temozolomide in an effort to deplete MGMT. The investigators will stratify patients according to the methylation status of the MGMT promoter. This stratification will allow the investigators to determine whether this marker of MGMT activity can predict efficacy and whether pharmacologic MGMT depletion can capitalize on inactivation of the enzyme.

SUMMARY

The role of cytotoxic chemotherapy for HGG continues to evolve. As the biology of HGG becomes better understood, more effective and less toxic strategies will be developed. In addition, new agents that effectively cross the BBB and overcome mechanisms of drug resistance will be incorporated into combinations with targeted molecules to enhance the multimodality management of HGG.

REFERENCES

1. Muldoon LL, Pagel MA, Kroll RA, Roman-Goldstein S, Jones RS, Neuwelt EA. A physiological barrier distal to the anatomic blood-brain barrier in a model of transvascular deliver. Am J Neuroradiol 1999;20:217–222.
2. Ashby LS, Shapiro WR. Intra-arterial cisplatin plus oral etoposide for the treatment of recurrent malignant glioma: a phase II study. J Neurooncol 2001;51:67–86.
3. Mardor Y, Roth Y, Lidar Z, et al. Monitoring response to convection-enhanced taxol delivery in brain tumor patients using diffusion-weighted magnetic resonance imaging. Cancer Res 2001;61:4971–4973.
4. Sheline GE, Wara WM, Smith V. Therapeutic irradiation and brain injury. Int J Radiat Oncol Biol Phys. 1980;6:1215–1228.
5. Grossman SA, Wharam M, Sheidler V, et al. Phase II study of continuous infusion carmustine and cisplatin followed by cranial irradiation in adults with newly diagnosed high-grade astrocytoma. J Clin Oncol. 1997;15:2596–2603.
6. Grossman SA, Sheidler VR, Gilbert MR. Decreased phenytoin levels in patients receiving chemotherapy. Am J Med. 1989;87:505–510.
7. Grossman SA, Hochberg F, Fisher J, et al. Increased 9-aminocamptothecin dose requirements in patients on anticonvulsants. NABTT CNS Consortium. The New Approaches to Brain Tumor Therapy. Cancer Chemother Pharmacol. 1998;42:118–126.
8. Fetell MR, Grossman SA, Fisher JD, et al. Preirradiation paclitaxel in glioblastoma multiforme: efficacy, pharmacology, and drug interactions. New Approaches to Brain Tumor Therapy Central Nervous System Consortium. J Clin Oncol. 1997;15:3121–3128.
9. McDonald DR, Cascino TL, Schold SC Jr, Cairncross JG. Response criteria for phase II studies of supratentoral malignant glioma. J Clin Oncol 1990;8:1277–1280.
10. Eagen RT, Scott M. Evaluation of prognostic factors in chemotherapy of recurrent brain tumors. J Clin Oncol. 1983;1:38–44.
11. Nelson DF, Nelson JS, Davis DR, Chang CH, Griffin TW, Pajak TF. Survival and prognosis of patients with astrocytoma with atypical or anaplastic features. J Neurooncol. 1985;3:99–103.
12. Curran WJ Jr, Scott CB, Horton J, et al. Recursive partitioning analysis of prognostic factors in three Radiation Therapy Oncology Group malignant glioma trials. J Natl Cancer Inst 1993;85:704–710.
13. Byar DP Green SB, Strike TA, et al. Prognostic factors for malignant gliomas. In Walker MD (ed). Oncology of the nervous system. Boston. Marinus Nijhoff, 1983:379–395.
14. Walker MD, Alexander E Jr, Hunt WE, et al. Evaluation of BCNU and/or radiotherapy in the treatment of anaplastic gliomas. A cooperative clinical trial. J Neurosurg 1978;49:333–343.
15. Walker MD, Green SB, Byar DP, et al. Randomized comparisons of radiotherapy and nitrosoureas for the treatment of malignant glioma after surgery. N Engl J Med 1980;303:1323–1329.
16. Stupp R, Mason WP, van den Bent MJ, et al. European Organisation for Research and Treatment of Cancer Brain Tumor and Radiotherapy Groups; National Cancer Institute of Canada Clinical Trials Group. Radiotherapy plus concomitant and adjuvant temozolomide for glioblastoma. N Engl J Med 2005;352:987–96.
17. Green SB, Byar DP, Walker MD, et al. Comparisons of carmustine, procarbazine, and high-dose methylprednisolone as additions to surgery and radiotherapy for the treatment of malignant glioma. Cancer Treat Rep 1983;67:121–132.
18. Shapiro WR, Green SB, Burger PC, et al. Randomized trial of three chemotherapy regimens and two radiotherapy regimens and two radiotherapy regimens in postoperative treatment of malignant glioma. Brain Tumor Cooperative Group Trial 8001. J Neurosurg 1989;71:1–9.
19. Deutsch M, Green SB, Strike TA, et al. Results of a randomized trial comparing BCNU plus radiotherapy, streptozotocin plus radiotherapy, BCNU plus hyperfractionated radiotherapy, and BCNU following misonidazole plus radiotherapy in the postoperative treatment of malignant glioma. Int J Radiat Oncol Biol Phys 1989;16:1389–1396.
20. Yung YK, Albright RE, Olson J, et al. A phase II study of temozolomide vs procarbazine in patients with glioblastoma at first relapse. Brit J Cancer 2000;83:588–593.
21. Westphal M, Hilt DC, Bortey E, et al. A phase 3 trial of local chemotherapy with biodegradable carmustine (BCNU) wafers (Gliadel wafers) in patients with primary malignant glioma. Neuro-oncol 2003;5:79–88.
22. Dhodapkar M, Rubin J, Reid JM, et al. Phase I trial of temozolomide (NSC 362856) in patients with advanced cancer. Clin Cancer Res 1997;3:1093–1100.
23. van den Bent MJ, Chinot O, Boogerd W, et al. Second-line chemotherapy with temozolomide in recurrent oligodendroglioma after PCV (procarbazine, lomustine and vincristine) chemotherapy: EORTC Brain Tumor Group phase II study 26972. Ann Oncol 2003;14:599–602.

24. Rodriguez LA, Prados M, Silver P, Levin VA. Reevaluation of procarbazine for the treatment of recurrent malignant central nervous system tumors. Cancer 1989;64:2420–2423.

25. Hare CB, Elion GB, Houghton PJ, et al. Therapeutic efficacy of the topoisomerase I inhibitor 7-ethyl-10-(4-[1-piperidino]-1-piperidino)-carbonyloxy-camptothecin against pediatric and adult central nervous system tumor xenografts. Cancer Chemother Pharmacol 1997;39(3):187–191.

26. Friedman HS, Petros WP, Friedman AH, et al. Irinotecan therapy in adults with recurrent or progressive malignant glioma. J Clin Oncol 1999;17:1516–1525.

27. Gruber ML, Buster WP. Temozolomide in combination with irinotecan for treatment of recurrent malignant glioma. Am J Clin Oncol 2004;27:33–38.

28. Meyskens FL Jr, Goodman GE, Alberts DS. 13-Cis-retinoic acid: pharmacology, toxicology, and clinical applications for the prevention and treatment of human cancer. Crit Rev Oncol Hematol 1985;3:75–101.

29. Wismeth C, Hau P, Fabel K, et al. Maintenance therapy with 13-cis retinoid acid in high-grade glioma at complete response after first-line multimodal therapy—a phase-II study. J Neurooncol 2004;68:79–86.

30. Couldwell WT, Antel JP, Yong VW. Protein kinase C activity correlates with the growth rate of malignant gliomas: Part II. Effects of glioma mitogens and modulators of protein kinase C. Neurosurgery 1992;31:717–724.

31. Couldwell WT, Hinton DR, Surnock AA, et al. Treatment of recurrent malignant gliomas with chronic oral high-dose tamoxifen. Clin Cancer Res 1996;2:619–622.

32. Zhang W, Yamada H, Sakai N, Niikawa S, Nozawa Y. Enhancement of radiosensitivity by tamoxifen in C6 glioma cells. Neurosurgery 1992;31:725–729; discussion 729–730.

33. Brandes AA, Ermani M, Turazzi S, et al. Procarbazine and high-dose tamoxifen as a second-line regimen in recurrent high-grade gliomas: a phase II study. J Clin Oncol 1999;17:645–650.

34. Chamberlain MC, Kormanik PA. Salvage chemotherapy with tamoxifen for recurrent anaplastic astrocytomas. Arch Neurol 1999;56:703–708.

35. Levin VA, Silver P, Hannigan J, et al. Superiority of post-radiotherapy adjuvant chemotherapy with CCNU, procarbazine, and vincristine (PCV) over BCNU for anaplastic gliomas: NCOG 6G61 final report. Int J Radiat Oncol Biol Phys 1990;18:321–324.

36. Longee DC, Friedman HS, Albright RE Jr, et al. Treatment of patients with recurrent gliomas with cyclophosphamide and vincristine. J Neurosurg 1990;72:583–588.

37. Buckner JC, Brown LD, Cascino TL, et al. Phase II evaluation of infusional etoposide and cisplatin in patients with recurrent astrocytoma. J Neurooncol 1990;9:249–254.

38. Watanabe K, Kanaya H, Fujiyama Y, Kim P. Combination chemotherapy using carboplatin (JM-8) and etoposide (JET therapy) for recurrent malignant gliomas: a phase II study. Acta Neurochir (Wien) 2002;144:1265–1270.

39. Hellman RM, Calogero JA, Kaplan BM. VP-16, vincristine and procarbazine with radiation therapy for treatment of malignant brain tumors. J Neurooncol 1990;8:163–166.

40. Sanson M, Ameri A, Monjour A, et al. Treatment of recurrent malignant supratentorial gliomas with ifosfamide, carboplatin and etoposide: a phase II study. Eur J Cancer 1996;32A:2229–2235.

41. Newlands ES, Foster T, Zaknoen S. Phase I study of temozolamide (TMZ) combined with procarbazine (PCB) in patients with gliomas. Br J Cancer 2003;89:248–251.

42. Chang SM, Prados MD, Yung WK, et al. Phase II study of neoadjuvant 1, 3-bis (2-chloroethyl)-1-nitrosourea and temozolomide for newly diagnosed anaplastic glioma: a North American Brain Tumor Consortium Trial. Cancer 2004;100:1712–1716.

43. Brandes AA, Basso U, Reni M, et al. Gruppo Italiano Cooperativo di Neuro-Oncologia. First-line chemotherapy with cisplatin plus fractionated temozolomide in recurrent glioblastoma multiforme: a phase II study of the Gruppo Italiano Cooperativo di Neuro-Oncologia. J Clin Oncol 2004;22:1598–1604.

44. Coyle T, Baptista J, Winfield J, et al. Mechlorethamine, vincristine, and procarbazine chemotherapy for recurrent high-grade glioma in adults: a phase II study. J Clin Oncol 1990;8:2014–2018.

44a. Stark-Vance V. Bevacizumab and CPT-11 in the treatment of relapsed malignant glioma. Neuro-Oncol 2005;7:369 (abstr 342).

44b. Dresemann G. Imatinib and hydroxyurea in pretreated progressive glioblastoma multiforme: a patient series. Ann Oncol. 2005;16:1702–1708.

45. Chang CH, Horton J, Schoenfeld D, et al. Comparison of postoperative radiotherapy and combined postoperative radiotherapy and chemotherapy in the multidisciplinary management of malignant gliomas. A joint Radiation Therapy Oncology Group and Eastern Cooperative Oncology Group study. Cancer 1983;52:997–1007.

45a. van Vulpen M, Kal HB, Taphoorn MJ, El-Sharouni SY. Changes in bloodbrain barrier permeability induced by radiotherapy: Implications for timing of chemotherapy? Oncol Rep 2002;9:683–688.

46. Prados MD, Scott C, Curran WJ Jr, Nelson DF, Leibel S, Kramer S. Procarbazine, lomustine, and vincristine (PCV) chemotherapy for anaplastic astrocytoma: A retrospective review of radiation therapy oncology group

protocols comparing survival with carmustine or PCV adjuvant chemotherapy. J Clin Oncol 1999;17:3389–3395.

47. Medical Research Council Brain Tumor Working Party. Randomized trial of procarbazine, lomustine, and vincristine in the adjuvant treatment of high-grade astrocytoma: a Medical Research Council trial. J Clin Oncol 2001;19:509–518.

48. Grossman SA, O'Neill A, Grunnet M, et al. Phase III study comparing three cycles of infusional carmustine and cisplatin followed by radiation therapy with radiation therapy and concurrent carmustine in patients with newly diagnosed supratentorial glioblastoma multiforme: Eastern Cooperative Oncology Group Trial 2394. J Clin Oncol 2003;21:1485–1491.

49. Fine HA, Dear KB, Loeffler JS, Black PM, Canellos GP. Meta-analysis of radiation therapy with and without adjuvant chemotherapy for malignant gliomas in adults. Cancer 1993;71:2585–2597.

50. Stewart LA. Chemotherapy in adult high-grade glioma: a systematic review and meta-analysis of individual patient data from 12 randomised trials. Lancet 2002;359:1011–1018.

51. Grossman SA, Fisher JD, Piantadosi S, Brem H. The New Approaches to Brain Tumor Therapy (NABTT) CNS Consortium: Organization, objectives and activities. Cancer Control 1998;5:107–114.

52. Mathieu NT, Genet D, Labrousse F, et al. Pre-irradiation chemotherapy for newly diagnosed high grade astrocytoma. Anticancer Res 2004;24:1249–1253.

53. Cairncross JG, Ueki K, Zlatescu M, et al. Specific genetic predictors of chemotherapeutic and survival in patients with anaplastic oligodendrogliomas. J Natl Cancer Inst 1998;90:1473–1479.

54. Ino Y, Betensky RA, Zlatescu MC, et al. Molecular subtypes of anaplastic oligodendroglioma: implications for patient management at diagnosis. Clin Cancer Res 2001;7:839–845.

55. Perry JR, Louis DN, Cairncross JG. Current treatment of oligodendrogliomas. Arch Neurol 1999;56:434–436.

56. Fortin D, Cairncross GJ, Hammond RR. Oligodendroglioma: an appraisal of recent data pertaining to diagnosis and treatment. Neurosurgery 1999;45:1279–1291; discussion 1291.

57. Paleologos NA. Oligodendroglioma. Curr Treat Options Neurol 2001;3:59–66.

57a. Peereboom DM, Kaur H, Wood L, et al. Phase II multicenter study of 7/7 dosing of temozolomide in patients with newly diagnosed pure and mixed anaplastic oligodendroglioma. Neuro-oncol 2005;7:401 (abstr 470).

58. Cairncross G, Macdonald D, Ludwin S, et al. Chemotherapy for anaplastic oligodendroglioma. National Cancer Institute of Canada Clinical Trials Group. J Clin Oncol 1994;12:2013–2021.

59. van den bent MJ. Chemotherapy of Oligodendroglial tumors: current developments. Forum 2000;10: 108–118.

60. Bouffet E, Jouvet A, Thiesse P, Sindou M. Chemotherapy for aggressive or anaplastic high grade oligodendrogliomas and oligoastrocytomas: better than a salvage treatment. Br J Neurosurg 1998;12:217–222.

61. Zander T, Nettekoven W, Kraus JA, et al. Intensified PCV-chemotherapy with optional stem cell support in recurrent malignant oligodendroglioma. J Neurol 2002;249:1055–1057.

62. van den Bent MJ, Taphoorn MJ, Brandes AA, et al. Phase II study of first-line chemotherapy with temozolomide in recurrent oligodendroglial tumors: the European Organization for Research and Treatment of Cancer Brain Tumor Group Study 26971. J Clin Oncol 2003;21:2525–2528.

63. Chahlavi A, Kanner A, Peereboom D, Staugaitis SM, Elson P, Barnett G. Impact of chromosome 1p status in response of oligodendroglioma to temozolomide: preliminary results. J Neurooncol 2003;61:267–73.

64. Chinot OL, Honore S, Dufour H, et al. Safety and efficacy of temozolomide in patients with recurrent anaplastic oligodendrogliomas after standard radiotherapy and chemotherapy. J Clin Oncol 2001;19:2449–2455.

65. Chamberlain MC, Kormanik PA. Salvage chemotherapy with paclitaxel for recurrent oligodendrogliomas. J Clin Oncol 1997;15:3427–3432.

66. Peereboom D, Kaur H, Wood L, et al. Phase II multicenter study of dose-intense (7days on/7days off) temozolomide in patients with newly diagnosed pure and mixed anaplastic oligodendroglioma. J Neuro-oncol 2003;5:353.

67. Yung WK, Prados MD, Yaya-Tur R, et al. Multicenter phase II trial of temozolomide in patients with anaplastic astrocytoma or anaplastic oligoastrocytoma at first relapse. Temodal Brain Tumor Group. J Clin Oncol 1999;17:2762–2771, erratum: J Clin Oncol 1999;17:3693.

68. Kerbel RS, Kamen BA. The anti-angiogenic basis of metronomic chemotherapy. Nature Reviews. Cancer 2004;4:423–436.

69. Wong ET, Hess KR, Gleason MJ, et al. Outcomes and prognostic factors in recurrent glioma patients enrolled onto phase II clinical trials. J Clin Oncol. 1999;17:2572–2578.

69a. Hegi ME, Diserens AC, Gorlia T, et al. MGMT gene silencing and benefit from temozolomide in glioblastoma. N Engl J Med. 2005;352:997–1003.

69b. Mellinghoff IK, Wang MY, Vivanco I, et al.. Molecular determinants of the response of glioblastomas to EGFR kinase inhibitors. N Engl J Med 2005;353:2012–2024.

70. Brem H, Piantadosi S, Burger PC, et al. Placebo-controlled trial of safety and efficacy of intraoperative controlled delivery by biodegradable polymers of chemotherapy for recurrent gliomas. The Polymer-brain Tumor Treatment Group. Lancet 1995;345:1008–1012.

71. Westphal M, Hilt DC, Bortey E, et al. Ram Z. A phase 3 trial of local chemotherapy with biodegradable carmustine (BCNU) wafers (Gliadel wafers) in patients with primary malignant glioma. Neuro-oncology 2003;5:79–88.

72. Johnson DB, Thompson JM, Corwin JA, et al. Prolongation of survival for high-grade malignant gliomas with adjuvant high-dose BCNU and autologous bone marrow transplantation. J Clin Oncol 1987;5:783–789.

73. Chen B, Ahmed T, Mannancheril A, Gruber M, Benzil DL. Safety and efficacy of high-dose chemotherapy with autologous stem cell transplantation for patients with malignant astrocytomas. Cancer 2004;100:2201–2207.

74. Abrey LE, Childs BH, Paleologos N, et al. High-dose chemotherapy with stem cell rescue as initial therapy for anaplastic oligodendroglioma. J Neuro-oncol 2003;5:127–134.

75. Newton HB, Slivka MA, Stevens CL, et al. Intra-arterial carboplatin and intravenous etoposide for the treatment of recurrent and progressive non-GBM gliomas. J Neuro-oncol 2002;56:79–86.

76. Chow KL, Gobin YP, Cloughesy T, et al. Prognostic factors in recurrent glioblastoma multiforme and anaplastic astrocytoma treated with selective intra-arterial chemotherapy. Am J Neurorad 2000;21:471–478.

76a. Doolittle ND, Miner ME, Hall WA, et al. Safety and efficacy of a multicenter study using intraarterial chemotherapy in conjuction with osmotic opening of the blood-brain barrier for the treatment of malignant brain tumors. Cancer 2000;88:637–647.

76b. Fortin D, Desjardins A, Benko A, et al. Enhanced chemotherapy delivery by intraarterial infusion and blood-brain barrier disruption in malignant brain tumors. Cancer 2005;103:2606–2615.

77. Pegg AE, Dolan ME, Moschel RC. Structure, function, and inhibition of O6-alkylguanine-DNA alkyltransferase. Prog Nucleic Acid Res Mol Biol 1995;51:167–223.

78. Spiro TP, Gerson SL, Liu L, et al. O^6-benzylguanine: a clinical trial establishing the biochemical modulatory dose in tumor tissue for alkyltransferase-directed DNA repair. Cancer Res 1999;59:2402–2510.

78a. Quinn JA, Desjardins A, Weingart J, et al. Phase I trial of temozolomide plus o6-benzylguanine for patients with recurrent or progressive malignant glioma. J Clin Oncol 2005;23:7178–7187.

79. Tolcher AW, Gerson SL, Denis L, et al. Marked inactivation of O^6-alkylguanine-DNA alkyltransferase activity with protracted temozolomide schedules. Br J Cancer 2003;88:1004–1011.

17 Nursing Considerations

Kathleen Lupica and Gail Ditz

Summary

The diagnosis of a malignant brain tumor is a stressful and traumatic event for patients and families. Management of patients with a malignant brain tumor requires a team effort where nursing plays a unique role. Neuro-oncology nurses are nurses who care for patients with primary and metastatic cancers of the central nervous system and patients with neurologic complications from their systemic cancer or treatments. These nurses face unique challenges when caring for patients with high-grade gliomas. Nurses provide care to these patients in many settings, from initial diagnosis to death, and in a wide variety of roles. Nurses are constantly attempting to recognize, prevent, and treat complications whether at the bedside, in the outpatient department, or by telephone triage and support. General nursing concerns for this patient population focus on the following: patient and family education, symptom management, and appropriate referrals. The focus of nursing care is to improve survival and maintain quality of life through recognition of symptoms and knowledgeable symptom control.

Key Words: Caregivers; quality-of-life; deep vein thrombosis; steroid management; symptom management; nursing roles; seizure management; patient education; fatigue; social support; emotional distress.

INTRODUCTION

Neuro-oncology nurses are nurses who deal with patients with primary and metastatic cancers of the central nervous system (CNS) and patients with neurologic complications from their systemic cancer or treatments. These nurses face unique challenges especially when caring for patients with high-grade gliomas (HGG). Despite recent treatment advances, life expectancy remains limited even with aggressive treatment. Focus is on improving survival and maintaining quality-of-life. Neuro-oncology nurses apply their knowledge to understand the relationship between anatomy and the patient's symptoms in order to anticipate symptoms and possible complications. They must also appreciate the significant impact of the diagnosis on patients and their families.

Multidisciplinary treatment approaches for these patients include conventional treatment such as surgery, radiation, and chemotherapy, as well as specialized treatments and clinical trials. These patients and their families have unique needs and challenge nurses to use their knowledge, skill, and compassion to the highest level *(1)*. Patients diagnosed with a malignant brain tumor face an array of concerns regarding treatment choices, follow-up care, and risk of recurrence. Malignant brain tumors can cause significant physical and cognitive impairment that greatly impacts the patient and family. The impact of the diagnosis of a brain tumor

From: *Current Clinical Oncology: High-Grade Gliomas: Diagnosis and Treatment*
Edited by: G. H. Barnett © Humana Press Inc., Totowa, NJ

on the patient and family is overwhelming and unique because of the direct effect on the brain and thus on the mind, personality, memory, the concept of self, and the ability to function independently. Patients can undergo dramatic changes over the course of their illness that impact not only the patient, but the family, staff, and other caregivers.

Management of patients with malignant brain tumors requires a team effort where nursing plays a unique role. Depending on the level of education of the individual nurse and local state laws, the role of the nurse can vary from a supervisory role—where all decisions must be made by the treating physician—to an independent practitioner. Advanced practice nurses, in many fields, may make independent decisions regarding patient management, medication management, and order therapies and diagnostic tests. Some of the more unique roles available to neuro-oncology nurses are discussed later in this chapter. General nursing concerns focus on patient and family education, symptom management, and appropriate referrals.

PATIENT AND FAMILY EDUCATION

Informed patients often cope better and informed families are better equipped to offer care and support (2). Patients and families should be urged to be active participants in their care. Patient and family education occurs throughout the continuum of the disease. Information must be provided in both verbal and written forms and continually repeated and reinforced. Important periods requiring education along the disease course are at initial presentation of symptoms, hospitalization, diagnosis, initiation of new treatments or procedures, recurrence, and at end-of-life.

Information needs change over time. Patients and families require factual information regarding their particular diagnosis, treatment options, managing their medications, handling common symptoms and side effects, and recognizing medical emergencies. The key is to empower patients and families to effectively manage their own care. Also important are specific details on the likely course(s) of their illness and the supportive resources available to them over the course of their disease. The key is to provide accurate information so that patient and families can make informed decisions. Desperate families who have not been given adequate information may make decisions based on misinformation in the media, on the Internet, and from well-intentioned friends and family members. Information provided should be easy to understand and accurate. Adequate education can decrease anxiety and sustain confidence. Ideally, patient education materials need to be written at a ninth grade level or below and include simple words, short sentences, be reasonable in length, and in large print, usually 12 point or higher. They should also include, whenever appropriate, instructional graphics (3).

The team should encourage questions. Patients should be advised to keep a diary or journal and to write down questions and prioritize their concerns. This can result in office visits that are less frantic and can reduce the number of phone calls. Patients should be urged to bring someone with them to all appointments. Information should be provided in a calm and comforting manner. The key is to maintain an open line of communication between the team, the patient, and the patient's family over the course of the illness and to ensure that the communication and information is comprehensive and consistent. Continual teaching and reinforcement of previous teaching as well as interpretation of outside information is key to an open line of communication between everyone. The focus is on answering questions, providing information, and constantly repeating information. It is imperative to involve the family and other caregivers at all times. Patients will do better with complex treatment if they are informed and understand the goal of treatment (4).

Medications and Chemotherapy

Patients and families should be educated regarding all medications and treatments prescribed. The drug's indications for use, expected outcomes, appropriate dosing schedules, potential side effects, and symptoms of toxicity should be reviewed. Patients and families who receive adequate education are more likely to be compliant regarding their medications and treatments. Potential interactions with foods and other drugs including alcohol and over-the-counter (OTC) medications, such as vitamins and supplements, should be included. Caregivers and patients should be educated on the importance of reporting all alternative health practices to their health care providers *(5)*. They should also be provided with legitimate sources for complementary and alternative treatments.

PREOPERATIVE ASSESSMENT AND EDUCATION OF THE NEUROSURGICAL PATIENT

Preoperative Education

Preoperative education for the patient with a high-grade CNS malignancy is a unique challenge to nurses. Management of this patient population involves multiple treatment modalities and requires ongoing vigilance of a multidisciplinary team to detect and treat newly diagnosed and recurrent tumors. Multiple studies have indicated that preoperative education significantly reduces pre- and postoperative anxiety. Certainly, with the addition of a potential malignant diagnosis, and the often rapid succession of events from diagnosis to surgery, patient and family education is a cornerstone in this population.

Preoperative education can broadly cover the entire surgical experience of the patient. Patients need to be educated on their individual surgical procedure, medication use and potential side effects, necessary neurodiagnostic testing (preoperative and over the continuum), and education regarding how to identify and prevent the more common postoperative complications such as deep vein thrombosis (DVT) and wound infection. A detailed history and a physical examination are the basis of every patient evaluation, and will aid in decision-making before surgical intervention. Many institutions use Critical Pathways to delineate the inpatient and outpatient care required during the perioperative period *(6)*. Outpatient visits are necessary to medically optimize patients prior to surgery and to provide crucial patient education by the nursing staff. The patient should be provided with both verbal and written information pertinent to their diagnosis, procedure, and plan of care.

It is important to have a complete medication list from the patient including not only prescription drugs but OTC medications, vitamins, "as needed" drugs, as well as herbal supplements and preparations. The medication list should be reviewed at every visit with the patient and changes made as necessary. Aspirin and aspirin containing preparations, anticoagulants, nonsteroidal anti-inflammatories (NSAIDs), and vitamins, minerals, and herbal medications should be stopped prior to surgery. The length of cessation varies from physician to physician and individual institutional policies. Anesthesiologists are conducting research to determine exactly how certain herbals interact with certain anesthetics. They are finding that certain herbal medicines may prolong the effects of anesthesia; other medications may increase the risks of bleeding or raise blood pressure *(7)*. Certain oral hypoglycemics also need to be discontinued at some point prior to surgery, depending on the individual drug, and can be identified during the review of medications. Patients and their families need to be educated on what medications to stop prior to surgery, as well as what medications are necessary to take the morning of their procedure, despite their nothing to eat or drink after midnight status.

A battery of tests is routinely ordered preoperatively and throughout the patient's course of treatment. In addition to routine preoperative laboratory studies, it is important to remember to monitor anticonvulsant levels and make necessary adjustments accordingly. Multiple neurodiagnostic tests may be ordered for the patient with a HGG. It is important the patient be educated on the rationale for these studies, which include:

- *Cerebral angiograpy:* Invasive method of visualizing cerebral vascular structures.
- *Cerebrospinal Fluid (CSF) flow scan:* Used to evaluate CSF flow abnormalities, particularly in patients with leptomeningeal disease or tumors within the ventricular system *(8).*
- *Computed Tomography (CT):* Helpful in evaluating soft tissue, edema, bony lesions, calcifications, or hemorrhage. If a contrast agent is used, it is usually iodine-based and patients who are allergic to iodine should inform their health care providers before undergoing a CT scan with contrast.
- *Electroencephalogram (EEG):* Used to document seizure activity, seizure focus and focal slowing of brain waves.
- *Functional MRI (fMRI):* Detects physiological changes during physical and cognitive activity; may be used for evaluation of language, sensory, and motor function.
- *Lumbar puncture/spinal tap:* Helpful in diagnosing of leptomeningeal involvement.
- *Magnetic resonance angiography (MRA):* Noninvasive method of visualizing vascular structures.
- *Magnetic resonance imaging (MRI):* Shows structure in three planes, with and without contrast (gadolinium). MRI is the examination of choice for primary brain tumors.
- *Magnetic resonance spectroscopy (MRS):* Measures the level of metabolites, ratio of choline to creatine to help differentiate necrosis or scarring from malignancy. The level of metabolites in tumors is different from that of normal brain tissue; the presence of lactate may suggest a higher grade tumor.
- *Magnetic resonance venogram (MRV):* Noninvasive method of visualizing venous structures and patency of cerebral sinuses.
- *Positron emission tomography scan F-18 fluorodeoxyglucose (FDG):* Measures tissue metabolism; currently the most effective method to differentiate treatment related necrosis or scarring (hypometabolic) vs tumor (hypermetabolic). Aggressive tumors generally have a higher rate of metabolism and therefore a higher uptake of FDG.
- *Stereotactic MRI and CT:* Studies done preoperatively for surgical localization purposes to provide computer-assisted, three-dimensional surgical guidance.
- *Thallium 201 single-photon emission computed tomography (SPECT):* May help differentiate tumor versus radiation necrosis.
- *WADA:* Cerebral angiography with addition of neurologist present testing for definitive language and memory dominance.

One of the nurse's main responsibilities during this diagnostic period is to provide information about the necessary tests, however, the emotional impact of the possibility of a brain tumor or its recurrence can cause extreme stress. The impact of the diagnosis is dependent on the extent the patient is able to understand the information and how it will affect their life. It is important to develop individualized teaching plans that are flexible and can adapt to the patient's broad range of physical and emotional needs.

Education about postoperative concerns should begin preoperatively. Numerous complications and problems can develop after a craniotomy. The nurse is responsible for monitoring the patient for the development of complications and implementing preventative measures when possible *(9).* Within the medical community, DVT is a well-recognized problem in persons with brain cancer *(10).* Postoperatively, routine lower extremity ultrasounds should be ordered to assess for DVT. Consideration should be given to preoperatively screen high-risk patients. Routine postoperative instruction includes diligent education regarding daily wound inspection and wound care. Special attention needs to be given to the patient and family regarding signs and symptoms of infection, or CSF leak, and instructions to call the office immediately if questions or concerns arise. Permanents, dyes, or hair bleaching should be avoided for at least 4 wk. Patients should be knowledgeable regarding postoperative swelling and preventative factors such as sleeping with the head elevated on pillows and keeping active and out of bed during the day. Heavy lifting (anything over twenty pounds) should be avoided for about 6 wk, gradually increasing, as tolerated thereafter. Teach the patient to avoid activity that requires bending at the waist and demonstrate proper body mechanics by bending at the knees. It should be mentioned to avoid any activity requiring them to hold their breath, such as the Valsalva maneuver. Encourage ambulation, with walking being the exercise of choice, and caution patients to use the railing when climbing stairs. Patients should not drive or return to work until their physician releases them. Educate the patient that headaches are to be expected, but if they persist or increase despite pain medication, they should notify their doctor's office. Prescription pain medication should only be taken as needed, usually in the first few days postoperatively, and OTC medication, such as acetaminophen (1000 mg), may be taken for minor pain. It is important to educate the patient that narcotic pain medication is constipating and the use of laxatives and stool softeners is safe to control constipation. Make sure the patient and their family has the physician's office and emergency phone numbers.

It is important to include not only the patient in the education process, but their family and support system as well, as cognitive deficits are common in this patient population. Encourage family members to accompany the patient to appointments to assist in information gathering and to provide the necessary emotional support. It is a unique challenge of the neurosurgical oncology nurse to prepare the patient for the surgical process. The dynamic nature of the disease as well as the patient's perspective and knowledge of their diagnosis provides many opportunities for education in this patient population.

Disease Specific

Patients need to understand their particular diagnosis, symptoms, anticipated course, and potential side effects and complications. Education should be provided regarding the tumor type and grade, location, and possible effects on brain function. Patients and families often need to be reassured that the presenting signs and symptoms of malignant brain tumors are often easy to misdiagnose initially and that there are no effective screening tools for early detection. This information may help relieve any guilt they may be experiencing by thinking that they missed something or were misled.

Reproductive counseling regarding sexual function and fertility is often overlooked given the patient's potentially terminal disease but all patients should be educated regarding sexual and reproductive issues. Many female patients may experience premature menopause, irregular menstrual cycles, and infertility. Infertility can be permanent, particularly in men and women over the age of 40. Patients need to be educated regarding their prognosis so that they can make informed decisions regarding future childbearing. Males may choose to bank sperm prior to undergoing treatment. Females may chose to undergo egg retrieval but this requires considerably more time and expense and therefore the need to initiate therapy as soon as possible may not provide enough time to retrieve viable eggs *(8)*. Patients should be counseled to use reliable contraception and that it is important to avoid pregnancy during chemotherapy and radiation. A waiting period following treatment is recommended for women patients who are considering pregnancy. Adjustments may need to be made in the patient's medication if a woman chooses to pursue pregnancy in order to eliminate drugs that may be teratogenic. Treatments and medications can also cause decreased libido and sexual dysfunction. Some patients may lose the desire for sexual relations as a result of fatigue, tumor location, treatment, medication, depression, or body image changes. Patients should be asked about this important aspect of their life so that adjustments can be made whenever possible to improve sexual function.

SYMPTOM MANAGEMENT

Primary malignant brain tumors are among the most difficult human malignancies to manage *(11)*. Although we are typically unable to cure the underlying disease, knowledgeable symptom control can significantly improve the patient's quality of life and promote survival. Recognition of symptoms and effective interventions to control symptoms requires a multidisciplinary approach *(12)*. Symptoms are often unique and individual, hence, difficult to predict and may be caused by the disease itself or as a result of treatments. Symptoms described by patients over the course of their disease are often vague, confusing, and difficult to diagnose. While symptom based research in primary brain tumor patients has been limited, studies on cancer patients show a correlation between the severity of fatigue and other symptoms such as pain, depression, sleep disturbance and anxiety. Symptoms can have a significant effect on functional status and quality of life *(13)*. Patients need to be educated when to call the doctor and what doctor to call. Symptoms may worsen during the course of treatment and can temporarily decrease a patient's level of functioning. The key is to recognize urgent symptoms requiring an office visit or emergency room visit versus those that may be treatable by telephone triage. Nurses are constantly attempting to recognize, prevent, and treat complications whether at the bedside, in the outpatient department, or by telephone triage and support.

Symptoms are usually related to increased intracranial pressure (ICP), tumor location, medication effects and side effects or complications. Patients presenting with a variety of signs and symptoms that do not anatomically correlate with their tumor location may require further investigation for the possibility of leptomeningeal disease, distant spread, or the tumor appearing in another location in the brain or spine. Leptomeningeal disease occurs when malignant cells infiltrate the leptomeninges surrounding the brain and spinal cord *(14)*. Some of the more common symptoms managed by nurses are discussed below.

Quality-of-Life

Quality-of-life (QOL) is a concept that describes the impact of the disease and treatment on the patient *(15)*. Symptoms experienced by patients with HGG can have a devastating effect on the patient's and family's quality of life. For that reason, most symptom management is aimed at improving the patient's quality of life. Most patients are usually not able to function at the same level as previosuly, but the goal is to restore them to the maximum level of functionality possible. The impact of neurological deficits can be dramatic. Patients and families experience their disease in a larger way than their symptoms indicate and the impact is felt far beyond the physical signs and symptoms observed during routine clinic visits. Often, much to the chagrin of family members, patients are usually on their best behavior at office visits and put themselves in the best light possible especially when dealing with the professional team *(4)*. For that reason, it is important to assess the impact of symptoms on the patient's day-to-day life *(16)*. The quality of one's life can be measured from multiple perspectives and is difficult to measure on any one instrument or to capture the many factors that can affect a person's quality of life *(17)*. The definition can vary from patient to patient and often changes over the course of their illness and treatment and will directly impact on the goals of nursing care. The definition of quality of life can also vary widely between the patient and the caregivers and is best defined from the patient's perspective.

There are numerous definitions of QOL, including that QOL is the degree to which an individual succeeds in accomplishing their desires despite the constraints put upon them. QOL measures the difference at a particular period of time between the hopes and expectations of the individual and the individual's present experience *(18)*.

Ferrell *(18)* uses four domains to define QOL: (1) physical well-being, (2) psychological well-being, (3) social well-being, and (4) spiritual strength. Physical well-being includes the ability to maintain functional activities, self care, exercise tolerance, ability to work, appearance, overall physical health, degree of independence, sleep and rest, and symptom control. Psychological well-being provides a sense of control in the face of illness, altered life priorities, and fear of the unknown. Diagnosis can causes anxiety, depression, fear, stress, and mood swings. Psychological well-being includes enjoyment of life, intellectual function, adjustment to the disease as well as confidence, acceptance, and satisfaction with treatment. Social well-being includes family issues, adjustment of children, changes in roles and relationships, family stress, patient's social appearance, social isolation, ability to communicate, ability to work, and financial situation. Also included is sexual function, marital relationship, and the degree of social support resources available. Spiritual well-being includes religious beliefs, a sense of hopefulness, and having a purpose in life. Maintaining hope is an important intervention. Patients and families have the right to remain hopeful over the course of their illness. The multidisciplinary team must provide realistic hope and cautious optimism so that patients and families can set realistic goals. Hope is a crucial coping behavior that is beneficial to not only the patient but to the entire family.

Emotional Distress and Social Support Issues

Diagnosis of a malignant brain tumor is a stressful and traumatic event for patients and families with a wide range of responses from anger, withdrawal, isolation, guilt, anxiety depression, and hopefully, acceptance. Adjustment to the many changes can take a dramatic toll on patients, family and caregivers *(19)*. Patients require varying levels of support depending on the stage of their illness.

As care has been shifted from the hospital to the home, caregivers must master a range of tasks that they are often unprepared to assume *(5)*. Caregivers must often assume duties previously performed by the patient. Caregivers overwhelmingly describe the work of providing care as mentally and physically exhausting and expressed feeling angry, frustrated and guilty for losing patience with the care recipient *(20)*. They must build a support system, find community resources, understand insurance and financial benefits, and get legal affairs in order. Other tasks include identifying and reporting side effects and new symptoms, dispensing medications, completing forms, providing meals, and transportation, as well as maintaining the household, maintaining family activities, and paying bills. They are expected to provide emotional support and personal care for the patient, cope with behavioral and personality changes, handle medical emergencies and make decisions regarding treatment. All of this may create conflict between the patient's needs and their own needs. Initially, the patient may exhibit minimal to no deficits and family and friends are attentive, denial is high, and hope for cure is real *(4)*. Sooner or later major disabilities usually complicate the course. As the patient's condition deteriorates it becomes increasingly difficult to maintain equilibrium. Involvement of the family is essential for compliance and continuity of care. Unfortunately the health care system often does little to address their needs and concerns. Caregiving can be demanding, overwhelming, and stressful. It can erode the caregiver's physical and psychological well-being when they are most needed by the patient. The strains of caring for a family member with a HGG can increase the risk of mortality by 63% within 5 yr and is more profound than those seen in other forms of cancer *(5)*. Caregiver support groups and informal networking may provide some benefit. Some caregivers may require individual counseling. They should be urged to seek temporary respite care to allow them time to attend to their own personal needs. Caregivers need to ask for help and take advantage of offers of help without feeling guilty.

The diagnosis affects the entire family and presents special challenges when children are involved. Children require honest information in words that they can understand. Responses will vary with age and teachers and school counselors should also be informed of the diagnosis and possible impact on the children. It is helpful to keep their daily routine as normal as possible. Many of the brain tumor and cancer associations provide workshops and resources especially for children whose parents are seriously ill. Parents should be provided with these resources as well as any written resources available.

Depression

Patients with malignant gliomas often develop progressive neurobehavioral deficits caused by the disease itself as well as treatments such as radiation and chemotherapy *(19)*. Depression in brain tumor patients can be related to the stress of the diagnosis, treatment, loss of function, or medications. Almost all patients faced with a potentially terminal diagnosis will experience, at minimum, temporary grief and anxiety. Patients may benefit from counseling, psychotherapy, or medication. Some patients may resist but studies have shown that patients have an improvement in overall QOL when emotional distress is treated. One recent study showed that patients wanted and expected more support than they were receiving, especially psychological support. They wanted someone to talk to them and spend more time with them *(21)*. A combination of drugs is often necessary and should not be withheld but neither should they replace compassionate care (22). Stress reduction is essential. Cautious use of drugs for agitation, anxiety, depression, mood elevation, fatigue, and alertness can improve functioning and have a dramatic impact on the patient and family's quality of life.

Fatigue

Fatigue is prevalent and disturbing, but largely an ignored symptom because it is not life threatening *(23)*. Fatigue can cause severe disruption in the patient's ability to function and also affect multiple aspects of life. Fatigue can be mild to debilitating and is usually cummulative. It is often excessive in nature and is a whole body experience not relieved by sleep and is not always the result of activity. Fatigue is not predictable by tumor type, treatment, or stage of illness. High levels of fatigue impact on all aspects and correlate with impaired QOL *(24)*. Fatigue may be one of the significant factors that limit a patient's QOL. Interventions include energy conservation, maintaining normal sleep-wake cycles, learning not to fight the fatigue, flexibility, preplanning, and setting limits and priorities to balance and organizing activities. Interventions such as exercise, yoga, meditation, prayer, walking, rest, and decreasing stimuli may help. Psychostimulants have been used to enhance cognition and memory, modulate behavior, and increase wakefulness and participation in activities of daily living in brain injured patients *(19)*.

Pain

Head pain may be related to increased ICP or tumor location. One classic symptom triad of increased ICP includes papilledema, headaches, and vomiting. Headaches caused by increased ICP are usually present upon awakening and may be accompanied by nausea, vomiting, or both. These headaches are usually worse when lying down and may be relieved when the patient assumes an upright posture. Headaches are usually progressive in nature, unrelieved by over-the-counter medication and interfere with activities of daily living. They may be accompanied by other symptoms such as lethargy, visual symptoms, and other neurological changes. Headaches occurring in the initial postoperative period are expected and are generally related to incisional pain or temporary increases in ICP. They are managed initially with narcotics but within 5 to 7 d patients should attain sufficient relief from over-the-counter medications. Headaches resulting from temporary increased ICP resulting from treatment or in the face of tumor growth are usually best managed by the temporary use of steroids. Steroid management is discussed later in this chapter. Narcotic use is generally reserved for end-stage treatment or for headaches not relieved by high-dose steroids. Any reports of neck or back pain should be acted upon immediately with further investigation. Leptomeningeal disease, spinal metastases, or meningitis may cause neck or back pain and stiffness. Further investigations may include an MRI of the spine and lumbar spinal tap.

Seizures

Approximately a third of patients with brain tumors present with seizures and more than 50 to 70% of patients experience some type of seizure over the course of their disease *(25)*. The occurrence of a seizure can be psychologically devastating to the patient and family. However, initial presentation with a seizure is often a good prognostic sign because it leads to early detection and treatment. Anticonvulsants are initiated for many patients at diagnosis or when presenting with a seizure. Studies suggest that prophylactic use may be unnecessary in patients who have never experienced a seizure but this remains a subject of some controversy *(26)*.

Side effects of some anticonvulsant medications range from simple to serious side effects such as Steven–Johnson syndrome (characterized by a severe rash with skin sloughing.) Vasculitis and purple glove syndrome can occur with intravenous infusions of phenytoin with extravesation. Arthritis and shoulder and hand syndrome can occur with phenobarbital although this drug is rarely used for brain tumor related seizures. Agranulocytosis and hyponatremia can occur with cabamazapine; white blood counts and sodium levels should be routinely monitored on patients taking these drugs. Cognitive dysfunction can occur with most anticonvulsants. Whenever possible a dose reduction or an alternative drug may reduce these symptoms. Patients should be educated regarding signs of toxicity particularly with phenytoin and cabamazapine, which can cause diplopia, visual blurring, nystagmus, ataxia, and gait imbalance at higher levels. Patients generally report feeling drunk or over drugged.

Liver function tests can increase with any anticonvulsant drug with hepatic clearance and hepatic function should be monitored on these patients routinely. Valproic acid can cause hair loss and thinning, weight gain, and hand tremor, which can be particularly disturbing to patients. Valproic acid may also cause increased bleeding time and thrombocytopenia. Many anticonvulsants with hepatic clearance exhibit nonlinear kinetics in terms of their dosing so that even a small dose increase can lead to toxicity. Drug levels should be monitored closely, especially when a change in dose occurs or another medication is added, removed, or adjusted. Nurses should be cautious to treat the patient and their symptoms and not just the blood levels.

Therapeutic levels are only guidelines and many patients may achieve seizure control at lower levels whereas others may require toxic levels but lack any significant side effects. Patient teaching should focus on the expected outcome of anticonvulsant therapy as well as potential side effects and symptoms of toxicity. The goal of therapy is to be seizure free on monotherapy with no side effects, but that is not always achievable *(27)*. Patients and families should be taught to keep a seizure diary to record frequency, duration, and type of seizures they experience. Teaching should also focus on care of the patient experiencing a seizure. In most cases only supportive care is required and emergency room visits are unnecessary; however, the medical team should be contacted regarding any seizure occurrence. Prolonged seizures or seizures that result in loss of consciousness, increase in frequency, change in pattern, or result in postictal deficits can cause permanent neurologic damage and require immediate attention.

Drugs that increase the activity of the P450 system in the liver can interact with many medications such as coumadin, chemotherapy, and other medications. Patients should inform their medical team whenever other medications are added such as antibiotics or antilipid medications that can potentially alter anticonvulsant levels. Nurses must monitor therapeutic effects, prevent and manage side effects and potential reactions, and assess hepatic, renal, hemopoetic function with serial lab work. Patients should be taught seizure risk management and be educated regarding contributing factors such as lack of sleep, missed doses, alcohol use, erratic meals, increased activity, illness, stress, and the addition of other medications that may increase their risk of seizures.

A seizure disorder can impact on the patient's activities of daily living with regard to driving, employment, and recreational activities. Driving restrictions vary widely among states and it is imperative that nurses are knowledgeable regarding state laws, particularly when patients are from out of state. Some states may restrict driving for specified periods of time whereas others leave it to the physician's discretion. Some states require mandatory reporting of any drivers with a seizure disorder. Generally, any patient with a seizure may be advised to avoid other potentially dangerous activities such as using heavy equipment, power tools, climbing at heights, and recreational activities such as swimming, climbing, biking, or even bathing, especially if done alone. Conversations with the patient and family regarding any restrictions in their driving or other activities needs to be accurately documented in the medical record.

Deep Vein Thrombosis (DVT)

Patients with HGG are at high risk for thromboembolic events and one third will have a DVT at some point in the course of their illness *(28)*. DVT increases morbidity and mortality with the most dangerous complication being pulmonary embolus, which can often be fatal. Only 10 to 17% of patients with DVT exhibit classic symptoms *(28)*. Early detection is essential to prevent complications. Risk factors include advanced age, immobility including prolonged bedrest, and a delay in mobility postoperatively *(12)*. A previous history of thromboembolism is another risk factor to be considered. Patients with a leg weakness are eight times more likely to develop DVT postoperatively, particularly in the affected leg *(28)*. Nineteen percent of ambulatory patients and 37 to 60% of postoperative patients may experience the occurrence of DVT, especially if they are hemiparetic, not ambulatory, or immobile. Patients and families should be educated regarding the signs and symptoms and what constitutes a life threatening medical emergency. Symptoms generally include calf pain and tenderness, asymmetric pedal edema, or pleuritic-type chest pain. The symptoms are usually asymmetric and more commonly occur in the dependent limb. Concurrent steroid use may mask or aggravate the symptoms and patients with a sensory deficit may not always experience pain in the affected leg. A low threshold of suspicion is best and any patient presenting with even mild symptoms should be screened with Doppler ultrasound. The goal of therapy is to stop propagation, relieve symptoms, and prevent pulmonary embolus. The medical team determines treatment based on patient status and interval to surgical intervention. Patients with a high risk for intracranial bleed are generally treated with an inferior vena cava filter whereas most patients will be treated with subcutaneous or oral anticoagulants. Treatment with warfarin requires frequent labwork to monitor the international normalized ratio (INR) and dose adjustments are made based on this value. Prevention in the immediate postoperative period may include low-dose mini-heparin subcutaneous injections, pneumatic boots, support hose, exercise, and early ambulation.

Steroid Management

Corticosteroids are used throughout the course of the disease to decrease increased ICP and control cerebral edema but can have a significant toxicity profile. Up to 50% of patients will experience at least one period of steroid induced toxicity (25). Steroids may initially result in a dramatic improvement in appetite, mood, and may decrease symptoms but the undesirable side effects can be devastating to patients and affect their QOL. Side effects are usually dose and time related and increase at higher doses and with longer treatment periods but are highly individual among patients (12). Effective nursing interventions can minimize these adverse reactions. The aim is to use the lowest dose that will control symptoms and the challenge when using steroids is to find the most effective dose to improve patient functioning with minimal side effects (29). The risk-benefit ratio must be considered and the lowest effective dose used for the shortest interval possible. Nursing interventions focus on the numerous side effects and potential complications and are aimed at preventing, reducing, and managing these side effects. Patient and family education should focus on these side effects in order to promote early recognition and prevent unnecessary complications. Patients and families need to be empowered to become active participants in dosing and tapering schedules.

Steroid tapering is done on an individual basis. It generally takes 3 to 5 d to determine whether a lower dose will be tolerated. Major problems encountered during tapering are steroid withdrawal and steroid dependence. It is important that patients and families understand the many side effects and therefore can be more supportive of the patient during this time.

Steroids can create a ravenous appetite along with significant weight gain. It is important for patients and families to understand that this does not result from a lack of willpower on the part of the patient. The best defense is to have low-calorie snacks available.

Steroids can create significant problems with body image causing a temporary Cushingoid appearance with weight gain and redistribution of fat causing increased abdominal girth and moon facies. Patients may also develop fat accumulation at the posterior neck (buffalo hump), to the abdomen with bloating, to the retro-orbital space, and to the supraclavicular and anterior throat area. Teaching patients that these are expected side effects will reduce their concern that they may be developing new tumors. Skin changes are common with easy bruising, capillary fragility, hirtsutism, acne, and abdominal striae which can be quite distressing to the patient. The easy bruising can make patients unduly concerned about the potential for internal hemorrhaging.

Steroids can cause immunosuppression and increase the risk of opportunistic infections such as oral *candida* and PCP pneumonia. Screening for oropharyngeal thrush should be done routinely at all office visits. Patients often complain of a white coating on the tongue or other oral surfaces, a bad taste, altered taste, anorexia, and in severe cases difficulty swallowing. *Candida* can be treated with oral topicals such as antifungal mouthwashes or lozenges but more severe cases with pharyngeal involvement may require systemic antifungal treatment. Steroids can also mask developing infections and patients may not always exhibit the typical symptoms of infection. Poor wound healing is also a concern. Steroid doses may need to be increased during periods of stress or infection.

Steroids can cause glucose intolerance in some patients with new onset hyperglycemia and can increase blood glucose levels in patients with existing diabetes. Symptoms would include increased thirst and frequent urination. Diabetic patients will require close monitoring of blood glucose levels and increased doses of insulin are best managed with a sliding scale dosing. Patients with new steroid induced glucose intolerance will also require close monitoring and sliding scale insulin.

Other side effects include sodium retention with fluid retention, hypertension, and significant pedal edema. Hypertension may require temporary treatment with antihypertensives and pedal edema may require leg elevation, support stockings, and in severe cases diuretic medications. The challenge is to determine whether the pedal edema is simply a side effect of the steroids or a symptom of possible DVT. Pedal edema that is equal bilaterally without calf pain or positive Homan's sign is generally steroid induced but suspicion level should be high for possible DVT and Doppler ultrasound should be done if there is any doubt as to the cause of the edema.

Musculoskeletal side effects are common. Osteoporosis and joint pain can occur and are usually reversible especially in younger patients *(12)*. Avascular necrosis of the hips or other joints can occur in rare cases. These symptoms may be confused with spinal cord compression or peripheral neuropathy. Hip pain radiating down the anterior thigh to the knee or localized to buttock and groin that is exacerbated by walking is a common symptom. MRI scanning is most sensitive in detecting avascular necrosis. In severe cases, joint replacement may be necessary. Steroid myopathy is common with proximal muscle weakness and decreased muscle mass particularly in the thigh muscles. Patients will usually complain of difficulty rising from a sitting position and climbing stairs and if they fall they often have great difficulty getting back up. Myopathy can also be seen in the arm muscles with difficulty lifting. Generalized muscle and joint pain often accompany steroid myopathy. In some instances respiratory muscles may be affected and compromise breathing, resulting in shortness of breath that is often aggravated by the abdominal fat accumulation. Patients with myopathy may benefit from physical and occupational therapy as well as weight bearing exercises.

Gastrointestinal effects are common with gastric irritation, bleeding, and bowel perforation often exacerbated by constipation and sedentary life style. Steroids themselves may mask the symptoms. Patients with spinal cord involvement may be more prone. The risk increases with concurrent NSAID use and narcotics. Patients with pre-existing conditions, such as a history of ulcer, are also at higher risk. Prophylaxis with H2 blockers is highly recommended in all patients on steroid therapy. Intractable hiccoughs can also occur and are usually dose related. Whenever possible, dose reduction of the steroid should be considered. Several medications have been used for hiccoughs including Thorazine or oral liquid antacids. Some patients may experience a decreased sense of taste and smell with accompanying anorexia. This side effect is most commonly observed in patients undergoing radiation therapy.

Psychological side effects are also quite common and can include irritability, anxiety, insomnia, trouble concentrating, increased sensitivity to stimuli, euphoria, emotional lability, and depression. Psychosis, including paranoia and hallucinations, is less common and does not appear to be correlated with duration of treatment; it can follow a single dose and often resolves when the dose is decreased. Insomnia and other sleep disturbances can occur and may be decreased by limiting daytime sleeping and adjusting the dosing schedule with higher doses given in the morning and the last dose taken no later than supper. Nocturia is common with late night dosing and seems to be more common in males, especially those with pre-existing benign prostatic hypertrophy. Avoiding late evening dosing is often effective in reducing nocturia and subsequent sleep disturbance.

A unique side effect observed in hospital patients receiving intravenous boluses of steroids is severe anogenital itching and tingling. This side effect can often be reduced or eliminated by slow intravenous infusion. Some patients receiving steroids complain of visual blurring and long-term use can result in the formation of cataracts.

Interactions with other drugs, especially those requiring hepatic clearance, are common. Blood levels of anticonvulsant drugs can fluctuate significantly when steroid doses are adjusted resulting in toxicity or increased seizures. Close monitoring of anticonvulsant levels during any adjustment in steroid dosing can avoid undue side effects.

The process of tapering or weaning steroid medications requires close monitoring. Steroids may be tapered by reducing the pill strength or by reducing the number of daily doses. There is no one tapering schedule that will work for every patient. Patients who have been on steroids for a short period of time can be tapered quickly whereas patients who have been on steroids for a prolonged period of time may require weeks to months to taper and in some cases may not be able to completely taper off the medication. Patients should be cautioned never to decrease or stop their medication abruptly. Patients also must contact their health care provider if they are unable to take their medications orally as a result of nausea or vomiting. Acute adrenal insufficiency can result with fever, muscle and joint pain, nausea, anorexia, orthostatic hypotension, dizziness, fainting, and hypoglycemia often requiring hospitalization. Steroid withdrawal can occur at any point during a steroid taper and includes symptoms such as acute myalgia, arthralgia, or both. Headaches, lethargy, fever, nausea, anorexia, vomiting, postural hypotension, and increased symptoms can occur. Steroid withdrawal is generally treated with return to the previous dose and slowing down of the tapering process. Patients need to be counseled that the need to increase the medication does not mean their tumor is growing or that the patient has made a mistake in their tapering schedule. During tapering, nurses must be alert for any exacerbation of existing conditions or allergies. Most commonly patients are started on steroids and anticonvulsant medications concurrently at diagnosis. During taper it is not uncommon for allergic reactions to anticonvulsant medications or other medications to appear.

REFERRALS

Over the course of the patient's illness, nurses need to continually assess the need for referrals to supportive resources. A primary care doctor is necessary to treat other medical conditions unrelated to the tumor such as high blood pressure, hyperlipidemia, or diabetes. Patients with psychosocial impairments or cognitive impairments may benefit from referral to a neuropsychiatrist, psychologist, counseling, or cognitive therapy. Physical therapist can provide gait training, durable medical equipment, and assistive devices such as canes, walkers or braces. Physical therapy can improve weakness, loss of coordination, and endurance. Therapists are helpful in documenting the degree of disability, teaching families how to manage disabilities, and assess the potential to return home or to work. Occupational therapists assist the patient in performing activities of daily living through visual retraining, safety training, and cognitive retraining. Rehabilitation programs can perform an assessment of the patient's driving ability using either a simulator or actual road test under controlled conditions. Reaction time, attention to traffic, judgment of stopping distance, and depth perception are important factors in determining the ability to drive. Speech therapists can assist patients with impaired verbal communication or reading impairments as well as swallowing difficulties. Patients with visual deficits may benefit from a neuro-ophthalmology consult for baseline assessment and ongoing monitoring of their visual deficits. Social workers can provide assistance and information regarding home health aids, counseling, support groups, financial assistance programs, and guidance in negotiating the health care system. They also assist patients with medical forms, applying for disability, completing living wills, and durable power of attorney. Patients with malignant gliomas generate a steady stream of paperwork that must be completed such as leave of absence, medication assistance programs, authorization for tests and equipment, and insurance and disability papers; nurses often attend to these tasks. Patients and families should also be informed regarding community resources such as brain tumor or cancer focused organizations and support groups.

Decisions regarding returning to work or applying for disability are often difficult and are very individual depending the patient's abilities, the job description, and the family situation. Returning to work for some may be a positive experience but many patients may require frequent breaks, a shorter work schedule, or transfer to a different job role. Neuropsychological testing is a series of tests designed to examine the various aspects of brain function and may help to document limitations and assist in assessing a patient's ability to return to work. Patients should be knowledgeable of the American Disabilities Act and the resources available to them to be sure their employer treats them fairly and reasonable accommodations are made to allow the patient to return to their job if they chose to do so.

Spirituality and religion can be an important factor for patients with terminal illness and their caregivers and can have a profound influence on their ability to cope and quality of life (5). Referrals to pastoral care may provide spiritual counseling and guide the patient and family to address concerns and spiritual distress. Pastoral care often plays a strong role in end of life decisions.

Home care, rehabilitation services, palliative care, and hospice referrals may be needed at different points in the patient's illness. Home assessment is helpful to identify the need for durable equipment, home health aid, therapies, or modifications of the patient's environment to promote the ability of function and safety. Typically, at some point, there are no meaningful treatment options and referral to palliative care or hospice services is appropriate. Palliative care is a medical specialty with the goal of extending the principles of hospice care to a broader population that could benefit from this type of care earlier in the disease process (5). Both hospice and palliative care focus on maximizing quality of life and treating symptoms. Hospice services may vary but in general hospice allows patients to receive care for the symptoms when treatment options to cure or control the disease are not available or are no longer effective. When rendering end-of-life care, the team has an obligation to see that the patient and family has necessary support systems in place. Most terminally ill patients do not require hospitalization and prefer to die in the comfort of their own home (4). The health care team is responsible for recognizing the opportunity and initiating the discussion. Managing symptoms at the end-of-life is critical for the comfort of the patient and the family's peace of mind *(30)*.

NURSING ROLES

Nurses provide care to patients with HGG in many settings from initial diagnosis to death. Depending on the size of the facility and the number of patients, some roles may be filled by one or more nurses whereas in smaller facilities one nurse may fulfill several roles. Some of the unique roles available to neuro-oncology nurses are briefly discussed below.

Neurosurgical Nurse

The neurosurgical nurse sees the patient at onset of diagnosis and prepares the patient and their family for the surgical process. Education is focused on pre- and postoperative concerns. Significant emotional support is needed as patients are coping with the new diagnosis of a brain tumor and are often fearful of their upcoming surgical procedure. Neurosurgical nurses also participate in surgical clinical trials and special procedures. They are responsible for handling any changes in condition following discharge from the hospital including wound problems, high fevers, or any neurologic change.

Radiation Oncology Nurse

Radiation therapy provides an important role in the management of HGG. Nursing care provided by the radiation oncology nurse begins at the initial consult visit and continues into the early post-radiation phase. Patients and families must be educated regarding treatment schedules and expected effects and side effects. Options available to patients include conventional regional radiation, whole brain radiation, stereotactic radiosurgery such as gamma knife or photon beam, brachytherapy, and hyperthermia *(31)*. It is often difficult to assess if symptoms are being caused by the radiation therapy itself, tumor growth, or other concurrent therapies. Acute symptoms occur within the first few weeks to months and are usually self-limiting. These include nausea but rarely vomiting, anorexia, impaired taste, fatigue, increased seizures, increased neurologic deficits, skin changes, hair loss, and impaired wound healing. Some patients whose radiation fields lie near the ear can experience hearing loss, ear pain, discomfort, and in some cases otitis media. Being prepared for hair loss can make the experience easier and allow patients to prepare by finding a wig, hairpiece, cutting their hair, or buying scarves, turbans, hats, or other head coverings. Patients may desire a wig for the alopecia and a prescription can be written for a cranial prosthesis, which is usually reimbursed by most insurance companies. Increased symptoms may require a temporary increase in the steroid dose. Delayed effects such as memory impairment, hypopituitarism, and radiation necrosis can often be progressive over time and are usually managed by the neuro-oncology nurse.

The Gamma Knife Nurse

Centers offering gamma knife radiosurgery usually have at least one nurse whose sole responsibility is caring for patients undergoing this unique procedure. The gamma knife nurse is the patient liaison from the pretreatment to the follow up visit. Nurses in this setting educate the patient on the procedure, what to expect, time frames, and help to reduce anxiety over the course of the day-long treatment. Hands-on care may include head frame application and removal, transport to scanning, medication administration, and patient monitoring throughout the procedure. The nurse assists with coordinating the treatment. The gamma knife nurse also communicates with the patient's family. The nurse ensures patient comfort throughout the procedure, provides aftercare, and discharge instructions including pin site care and steroid therapy management.

Medical Oncology Nurse

The medical oncology nurse works along with the medical oncologist who is prescribing any chemotherapy the patient may be receiving. Medical oncology nurses provide patient education regarding the specific drug's effects and potential side effects. Nurses monitor labwork during therapy and manage the many complications of chemotherapy, such as myelosuppression, neutropenia, anemia, thrombocytopenia, nausea and vomiting *(32)*. Chemotherapy drugs interfere with cell division and the rapidly dividing cells in the body are often innocent bystanders including white blood cells, red blood cells, and platelets. Low white blood cells place the patient at risk of serious infection. Thrombocytopenia can increase the risk of bleeding. Nurses educate patients and families about potential side effects and teach them precautions to reduce side effects.

Centers that utilize special procedures for the delivery of radiation and chemotherapy such as blood–brain barrier disruption, intra-arterial chemotherapy, intrathecal chemotherapy, intratumoral chemotherapy or radiation, or radiation implants may have nurses responsible for educating and monitoring all patients undergoing those procedures.

Neuro-Oncology Nurse

The neuro-oncology nurse works along with the neuro-oncologist in the medical management of patients over the course of their illness from diagnosis to death. Neuro-oncology nurses assess patient and family needs during office visits, provide education, manage the multiple symptoms already discussed, and provide emotional support over the course of the illness.

Clinical Trial Nurses

Centers that offer multiple clinical trials may have nurses who are responsible for screening patients for eligibility requirements, providing education regarding the particular trial, expected effects and side effects, and for obtaining informed consent. Patients and families should be provided with adequate information regarding the trial and other alternative treatment options in order to make an informed decision. Education includes the concept of randomization, the meaning of various phases of trials, and that the potential benefit and/or toxicity are sometimes unknown but that information learned during the trial may help other patients in the future. Patients also need to be reassured that they can withdraw at any time.

Hospice and Home Care Nurses

Hospice and home care nurses provide care in the patient's home setting or sometimes at special facilities. The concept of hospice and home care is discussed previously under the referrals section.

CONCLUSION

The diagnosis of a malignant brain tumor is a stressful and traumatic event for patients and families. Patients and families face a difficult ongoing process of adjustment throughout all phases of the disease and face many losses over time. Management of patients with a malignant brain tumor requires a team effort, where nursing plays a unique role. Neuro-oncology nurses face special challenges when caring for patients with HGG. These nurses provide care to patients in a variety of settings from initial diagnosis to death and in a wide range of roles. Nurses are constantly attempting to recognize, prevent, and treat complications at the bedside, in the outpatient department, and by telephone triage and support. General nursing concerns for this patient population focus on the following: patient and family education, symptom management, and appropriate referrals. The focus of nursing care is to improve survival and maintain quality of life through recognition of symptoms and knowledgeable symptom control.

REFERENCES

1. Sheidler VR. Introduction. Sem Oncol Nurs 1998;14:1.
2. Stark-Vance V, Dubay ML. 100 Questions and Answers About Brain Tumors. Boston: Jones and Bartlett Publishers; 2003.
3. Murphy PW, Chesson AL, Berman SA, Arnold CL, Galloway G. Neurology patient education materials: Do our educational aids fit our patients' needs? J Neurosci Nurs 2001;33:99–104.
4. Smith PW, Lemons JG. The psychological care of the brain tumor patient and family. In: Morantz RA, Walsh JW, eds. Brain Tumors: A Comprehensive Text, New York: Marcel Dekker Inc.;1994:809–821.
5. Glajchen M. The emerging role and needs of family caregivers in cancer care. Support Oncol 2004;2:145–155.
6. Bohan E. Neurosurgical Management of Patients with Central Nervous System Malignancies. Semin Oncol Nurs 1998;14(1):8–17.
7. American Society of Anesthesiologists. What You Should Know About Herbal Use and Anesthesia; 1999.
8. Devroom H, Smith R, Mogensen K, Clancey J. Nervous system tumors. In: Bader MK, Littlejohns L, eds. AANN Core Curriculum for Neuroscience Nursing, 4th ed., St. Louis:Saunders, 2004:516–517; 524–525.
9. Hickey JV. Management of patients undergoing neurosurgical procedures. In: Hickey JV, ed. The Clinical Practice of Neurological and Neurosurgical Nursing, 4th ed., Philadelphia:Lippincott;1997:335.
10. Dempsey P, Calhoun R. Brain cancer and deep vein thrombosis: risks and prevention. The Brain Tumor Society July/Aug;2001:3.
11. Saris S. Multidisciplinary approach to malignant gliomas. Med Health 1996;79(6):210–213.
12. Posner JB. Supportive care agents and their complications. In: Posner JB, ed. Neurologic Complications of Cancer, Philadelphia:F.A. Davis Co.;1995;59–74.
13. Armstrong TS, Cohen MZ, Eriksen LR, Hickey JV. Symptom clusters in oncology patients and implications for symptom research in people with primary brain tumors. J Nurs Scholarsh 2004;36:3197–206.
14. Craig C. Current treatment approaches for neoplastic meningitis: Nursing management of patients receiving intrathecal DepoCyt. Oncol Nurs Forum 2000;27:1225–1232.
15. Lovely MP. Quality of life of brain tumor patients. Semin Oncol Nurs. 1998;14:73–80.
16. Fox S: Use of a quality of life instrument to improve assessment of brain tumor patients in an outpatient setting. J Neurosci Nurs 1998;30:322–325.
17. Jalowiec A. Issues in using multiple measures of quality of life. Semin Oncol Nurs 1990;6:271–277.
18. Grant M, Padilla GV, Ferrell BR, Rhiner M. Assessment of quality of life with a single instrument. Semin Oncol Nurs 1990;6:260–270.
19. Kajs-Wyllie M. Ritalin revisited: Does it really help in neurological injury? J Neurosci Nurs 2002;34:303–313.
20. Sherwood PR, Given BA, Doorehbas AZ, Given CW. Forgotten Voices: Lessons from bereaved caregivers of persons with a brain tumor. Int J Palliat Nurs. 2004;10(2):67–75.
21. Lepola I, Toljamo M, Aho R, Lovet T. Being a brain tumor patient: A descriptive study of patients' experience. JNN 2001;33(3):143–147.
22. Passik SD, Malkin MG, Breitbart WS, Horowitz S. Psychiatric and psychosocial aspects of neuro-oncology. J Psychosoc Oncol1994;12:101–122.
23. Ferrell BR, Dow KH. Quality of life among long-term cancer survivors. Oncology 1997;4:565–576.
24. Lovely MP, Miakowski C, Dodd M: Relationship between fatigue and quality of life in patients with glioblastoma multiformae. Oncol Nurs Forum 1999;26:921–925.
25. Rabbitt JE, Page MS. Selected complications in neuro-oncology patients. Semin Oncol Nurs 1998;14:53–60.
26. Bohan EM. Brain Tumors. In: Barker,E, ed. Neuroscience Nursing: A Spectrum of Care, 2nd Ed. St. Louis: Mosby, 2002:269–301.

27. Goldenberg LB. Beyond a single seizure. Adv Nurse Pract 2004;6:61–65.

28. Warbel A, Lewicki L, Lupica KL. Venous thromboembolism: Risk factors in the craniotomy patient population. J Neurosci nurs 1999;31:180–186.

29. Lupica K. Corticosteroids—Friend or Foe? Managing side effects in the neuro-oncology patient. J Neurosci Nurs 1998;30:367–368.

30. Armstrong T, Hancock C, Gilbert M. Symptom management of the patient with a brain tumor at the end of life. Oncol Nurs Forum 2000;;27(4):616.

31. Strohl RA. Radiation therapy in tumors of the central nervous system. Semin Oncol Nurs 1998;14:26–33.

32. Armstrong TS, Gilbert MR. Chemotherapy of astrocytomas: An overview. Semin Oncol Nurs 1998;14:18–25.

ADDITIONAL RESOURCES

American Brain Tumor Association
2720 River Rd Suite 146
Des Plaines, IL 60018
Phone: 847-827-9910
www.abta.org

National Brain Tumor Foundation
22 Battery Street, Suite 612
San Francisco, CA 94111-5520
1-800-934-2873
www.braintumor.org

The Brain Tumor Society
124 Watertown St. Suite 3H
Watertown, ME 02472-2500
www.tbts.org

American Cancer Society
1599 Clifton Rd. NE
Atlanta, GA 30329
www.CANCER.org

Musella Foundation for Brain Tumor Research and Information
www.virtualtrials.com

NeedyMeds
www.NeedyMeds.com

CancerCare
www.cancercare.org

CancerSource
www.CancerSource.com

National Center for Complementary and Alternative Medicine
P.O. Box 8218
Silver Spring, MD 20907
www.nccam.nih.gov

V CONTEMPORARY INVESTIGATIONAL TREATMENTS

18 Convection-Enhanced Delivery

Andrew A. Kanner

Summary

Drug delivery is thought to be one of the limitations of therapies for brain tumors. Systemic administration of potential drugs requires high dosages to achieve therapeutic levels within the tumor itself and in the surrounding brain tissue because of the limited/selective flow across the blood–brain barrier. In spite of high systemic dosages, however, some of these drugs not only fail to penetrate into the tumor and brain tissue, they cause undesirable systemic toxicity with little or no therapeutic effect.

Convection-enhanced delivery shows promise of effectively transporting drugs selectively to the tumor. It is a novel approach for delivering drugs into brain tumors and the surrounding brain, and is based on continuous infusion of drugs via intratumoral or intraparenchymal catheters, enabling convective distribution of high-drug concentrations over large tissue volumes while avoiding systemic toxicity.

Key Words: Glioma; convection-enhanced delivery; brain neoplasm; targeted therapy.

INTRODUCTION

Treatment of high-grade glioma (HGG) still represents an enormous challenge to neuro-oncologists. The standard therapies of surgery, radiotherapy, and adjuvant chemotherapy have not increased overall survival significantly over the past three to four decades. The aggressive and infiltrative nature of this disease and its resistance to traditional therapies have recently led to new strategies in the approach to malignant gliomas. Two major developments have contributed to the feasibility of these new approaches in the clinical setting.

The first involves the continuing advances in our understanding of the molecular genetics and, more importantly, of the pathological mechanism of cellular signal transduction in malignant cells that have led to the development of selective targeting compounds. Several drugs with the ability to down-regulate the growth and invasion of malignant gliomas are at various stages of testing. Most of these drugs focus on interfering with oncogenic and tumor survival pathways *(1)*. Examples of targeting molecules include inhibitors of tyrosine kinases, farnesyltransferases, and matrix metalloproteinases. These drugs are at different stages of testing and the final verdict on their effectiveness, either alone or in combination with other therapeutic modalities, will need to await the results of ongoing investigation.

Drug delivery is thought to be one of the major limitations of therapies for brain tumors *(2,3)*. Systemic administration of potential drugs requires high dosages to achieve therapeutic levels within the tumor itself and in the surrounding brain tissue because of the selective flow across the blood–brain barrier (BBB) and increased interstitial pressure within the tumor *(4,5)*.

From: *Current Clinical Oncology: High-Grade Gliomas: Diagnosis and Treatment*
Edited by: G. H. Barnett © Humana Press Inc., Totowa, NJ

In spite of high systemic dosages, however, some of these drugs not only fail to penetrate into the tumor and brain tissue, they cause undesirable systemic toxicity with little or no therapeutic effect.

The second major breakthrough followed the recognition of the above limitations and led to a number of novel drug delivery strategies that are currently under investigation. The goal of developing local delivery technologies is to maximize anti-tumor effects within the tumor and/or surrounding brain tissue while minimizing systemic side effects. These new approaches are designed to bypass the BBB and deliver the active compound more directly to the malignant cells. Established approaches include BBB disruption with hyperosmolar agents (mannitol) and novel investigational techniques using ultrasound or electrical stimulation of the vagal nerve or pterygopalatine gagli to influence cerebral blood flow (CBF) dynamics (2,6). Advancements of therapeutic approaches for brain tumors include drug delivery via impregnated polymer wafers, local injection, intracavitary instillation, and convection-enhanced delivery (CED) (7–9). The following chapter will focus on the basic principles and the preclinical and clinical experiences of CED.

PRINCIPLES OF CONVECTION-ENHANCED DELIVERY

CED, a novel approach for delivering drugs into brain tumors, is based on continuous infusion of drugs via intratumoral or intraparenchymal catheters, enabling convective distribution of high drug concentrations over large tissue volumes while avoiding systemic toxicity.

Terminology

Several terms for describing "microinfusion generating a positive pressure gradient for drug delivery into the brain" have appeared in the literature, the most common of which is convection-enhanced (drug) delivery (10,11). The others are high-flow microinfusion delivery (12), high-flow interstitial brain infusion (13), intraparenchymal controlled-rate infusion (14), and intracerebral clysis (15,16).

Diffusion vs Convection

One rationale for applying CED in glioma therapy is based on the limitations of other local delivery methods (injection or wafers) that rely on diffusion together with the fact that glioma cells are present throughout the adjacent and distant brain tissue. Diffusion in tissue depends on the free concentration gradient and the diffusivity of the particular compound or molecule (11). Factors that influence diffusivity are polarity, molecular weight, and metabolic clearance (17,18). It has been demonstrated that within brain tissue compounds diffuse at only one to a few millimeters from the source point over time and produce a steep concentration gradient between the point of infusion and the surrounding brain tissue (19–23). Convection, on the other hand, is based on a positive continuous pressure gradient and so, in contrast to other local delivery methods, such as polymer wafers or local injections, which depend solely on diffusion, CED can overcome this limitation. Convective transport through the extracellular space of the brain is a physiological and pathophysiological phenomenon, which is clearly evident in several conditions, among them brain edema (18,24). Both fluids and molecules move within the extracellular space either by diffusion or by bulk flow (17,18,25–27). These naturally existing hydrostatic and oncotic pressure gradients are responsible for all molecular movements (28). Applying the same principles, CED distributes molecules homogeneously over large distances by positive pressure infusion (10–12,28–33). In this way, the flow through the interstitial space is used as a vehicle to distribute the active agent(s) over large volumes of brain tissue without increasing tissue volume or intracranial pressure (ICP).

Oldfield et al. introduced CED for neuro-oncological applications *(10)*. This was followed by a series of preclinical and clinical studies to improve the understanding of the underlying mechanism of CED and to optimize relevant parameters for its clinical application in the treatment of malignant gliomas *(10)*. The theoretical advantages of CED include circumvention of the BBB and achieving drug delivery with high intratumoral and peritumoral concentrations over large tissue volumes while minimizing systemic side effects.

PARAMETERS INFLUENCING CONVECTION

Initial preclinical and a number of phase I/II clinical studies have addressed technical variables to determine their importance in the application of CED, looking at factors for improving and optimizing drug distribution. The following paragraph presents a general overview of these works.

Rate and Duration of Infusion. The rate of infusion, which is critical for successful induction of convection, is dictated by tissue resistance *(10)*. Differences of tissue resistance have been described for gray and white matter in preclinical studies *(11)*. Effective convection has been demonstrated with infusion rates of 0.5–5.0 µL/min in small animal models *(10,12)*. Lower rates of infusion limit the attainable volume of distribution at a specific concentration *(10)* whereas higher rates cause backflow along the needle or catheter tract, thus limiting convection efficacy *(10,12,32)*.

An infusion rate of 5.0 µL/min resulted in a less than 30% backflow of the infusate along the needle tract in small animal models *(12)*. Both intratumoral and peritumoral infusion using rates of up to 10 µL/min were used in clinical studies *(28,34)*. Higher flow rates (i.e., over 6.2 µL/min), however, more commonly caused backflow into the subarachnoid space, depending on the catheter tip placement. Although clinically well tolerated by the patient, leak into the subarachnoid space is associated with failure of the active compound to reach the targeted tissue and may be locally toxic.

Higher flow rates lead to direct tissue damage caused by the hydrostatic pressure, thereby limiting the upper range of safe infusion rates. Cavitation around the needle tip can be caused by high flow, which will result in loss of convection. Importantly, it was demonstrated that different profiles of CED increase the volume of distribution (V_D) 5- to 10-fold compared with diffusion alone *(12)*.

Volume of Distribution (V_D). The impact of different variables on V_D was subject to a number of preclinical studies. The V_D of a molecule in brain tissue during interstitial infusion is influenced by loss of the compound resulting from capillary reuptake, degradation, receptor binding/affinity and the tissue–extracellular space ratio of the infused volume. Extensive cellular binding (caused by high receptor density) or rapid metabolic drug inactivation during CED limited the effectiveness of certain compounds *(11,12)*.

The effect of different sizes of molecules and their distribution within brain tissue was studied by several investigators *(11,12)*. Bobo et al. measured the volume of distribution of small (^{14}C-sucrose, Mr 359) and large molecules (^{111}In-Transferrin, Mr 80,000) *(10)*. After initiating interstitial infusion, the flow rate was gradually increased from 0.5 µL/min to 4 µL/min and maintained at the higher level for 24 h. The V_D within brain tissue increased linearly with the volume of infusion (V_I) of both molecules, although ^{14}C-sucrose distributed faster and occupied a larger volume compared with ^{111}In-Transferrin. Importantly, there was no evidence of any increase of intracranial pressure during the infusion period *(10)*.

In addition to molecular size, Chen at al. studied the effects of rate of infusion, cannula size, infusate concentration, and tissue sealing time on V_D. In a series of experiments in a rat brain CED model, they infused ^{14}C-Albumin in order to compare various parameters of the above-mentioned variables *(32)*. They concluded that the rate of infusion and the cannula size significantly affected the convective V_D in their model. Specifically, higher rates of infusion and larger cannula sizes were associated with less distribution resultgin from increased back leak along the cannula tract, while various concentrations of ^{14}C-Albumin and the preinfusion sealing time (defined as the time after inserting the cannula until the start of infusion) had no influence on the V_D.

Kroll et al. confirmed findings that showed a linear increase of V_D proportional to increase in time, volume, and dose with a constant infusion rate and concentration *(13)*. They studied the pharmacokinetics of iron oxide nanocompound (MION) and CED characteristics in a rat brain model and found that increased doses of MION delivered at slower rates resulted in an improved V_D. From this they concluded that concentration, rather that convection, seemed to have the greatest influence. These findings are important because they show that extremely large complexes (similar to viruses) can successfully be administered by CED and that higher concentrations of a compound have a strong positive effect on overall V_D. Comparisons between ^{14}C-sucrose and cytone arabinoside delivery to the brain by intravenous, intraven-tricular, intrathecal, and CED in preclinical settings demonstrated significantly higher brain tissue levels: for example, the level via CED was more than 10,000 times higher than by intravenous delivery *(33,35)*. These findings emphasize the inability of such compounds to penetrate into the brain parenchyma, limited by the BBB. Long-term infusion into the primate brain demonstrated feasibility of delivering compounds covering large volumes of white matter, with perfusion of over one-third of the white matter of the infused hemisphere having been achieved *(28)*.

CONCEPTS OF CLINICAL TRIALS

Most clinical studies using CED as the delivery method use targeted immuno-toxins con-sisting of tumor cell selective ligands bound to polypeptide toxins *(3,4,36–38)*. The fact that unique or overexpressed receptors, which are not detectable (or detected in very low concen-tration) in normal brain tissue, were identified on the cell surface of tumor (glioma) cells led to the development of these targeting strategies *(39–41)*. Thus far, the infused receptor ligands that have been used in clinical trails include human transferrin (Tt), interleukin (IL)-13, and IL-4 *(30,34,38,40,41)*. These ligands have been attached to mutated bacterial toxins, such as diphtheria toxin (CRM107) and pseudomonas exotoxin (PE_A) *(30,34,38,40,41)*. Other drugs used in phase I/II clinical trials included conventional cytotoxic chemotherapeutics (Nimustine [ACNU], Paclitaxel ([Taxol]) and suicide genes (HSV-1-tk-gene) *(42–44)*.

Clinical studies were conducted with both intratumoral and intraparenchymal (tumor sur-rounding brain tissue) infusions. These two approaches highlight one of the difficulties in finding the optimal catheter placement and integrate two approaches of treatment. Feasibility and safety of both intratumoral and intraparenchymal infusion have already been demon-strated in a number of clinical studies. Results from a phase I/II study conducted in patients with high-grade glioma (HGG) *(34)* proved both the feasibility and safety of intratumoral CED of IL-4 coupled to PE-38 toxin. For catheter related factors, it also has become obvious that the insertion depth or the distance to the cavities, pial surface or subarachnoid space is crucial to avoid backflow related loss of drug. More importantly, the physical characteristics of catheters, including shape, diameter, and outlet configuration, are still under intensive investigation. Our understanding of tissue properties and related effects on CED is also improving. Initial tissue related parameters were studied in small animal models and almost exclusively in normal brain tissue. The clinical experience provided evidence that tissue characteristics of both tumor and tumor infiltrated brain tissue are extremely difficult to model *(12)*. However, several efforts are actually underway to do so.

Compounds tested in clinical studies that have accumulated the most experience and are in the most advanced stage of clinical testing include Tf-CRM107, IL-13PE38QQR *(40)*, IL-4 NBI3001, and Paclitaxel (Taxol). As of January 2005, open clinical trials enrolling patients in phase III studies include the following immuno-toxin compounds: IL-13PE38QQR (PRE-CISE study) and Tf-CRM107 (TransMid study).

Example of Compound Currently in a Phase III Clinical Trial

Tf-CRM107 is a ligand-targeted toxin comprised of Tf linked to a conjugated protein of diphtheria toxin with point mutation (CRM107) *(45)*. This conjugate exhibits potent cytotoxicity in vitro against mammalian cells expressing the Tf-receptor. Transferring receptors are expressed on all rapidly dividing cells including tumors with minimal expression in nondividing tissues, such as those of the normal brain *(46,47)*. Therefore, the use of transferring as a vehicle does not require a unique cell-surface antigen for each type of tumor. The clinical experience comprises data of phase I II studies involving a total of 72 patients with mostly HGG and metastatic brain tumors. All of these patients had failed previous conventional standard therapies prior to enrollment *(30)*. Anywhere from 1 to 3 intracerebral catheters were placed stereotactically directly into the tumor or in the peritumoral brain tissue, and each patient received 2 treatments 4 and 10 wk apart. In phase I, 28 patients (with 32 tumors) underwent a total of 65 infusions. The results showed that intratumoral infusion was feasible. Some patients suffered reversible cerebral edema. Cerebral injury occurred primarily at higher drug concentrations. A partial and complete radiological response (MRI) was demonstrated in 10 of 28 patients (36%) *(47a)*. [p11] No results of the ongoing Phase III trial are currently available.

Imaging Modalities

Monitoring the progression of convection is important for monitoring the effect of the treatment. Findings in phase I/II studies demonstrated that a considerable percentage of patients did not effectively receive the infused drug as a result of deficient convection. This emphasizes the need for clinically applicable imaging methods. Several imaging modalities, among them computed tomography (CT), magnetic resonance imaging (MRI), and single-photon emission CT (SPECT), have been studied *(48–50)* and different markers have been identified within each of them. A comparison between those surrogate markers revealed considerable discrepancies in terms of reflecting the true volume of convection, the V_D *(50a)*. The "edema" that is generated around the infusion catheter is thought to represent the front wave of the convection. This has been demonstrated on different MR sequences and SPECT studies. Comparing T2-weighted images and SPECT, however, showed an underestimation of the convection volume for the MR images *(50a)*.

Recent publications have demonstrated the use of surrogate markers, such as liposomes or macromolecules (albumin) traced with contrast agents, that are visible on images obtained using noninvasive techniques, such as iopanoic acid (IPA) for CT and Gd-diethylenetriamine pentaacetic acid (Gd-DTPA) for MRI *(48–50)*. These markers are co-infused with the therapeutic agent to enable real-time monitoring of the distributed drugs.

Table 1

Clinical Studies Using CED for Drug Delivery in HGG

Author	Yr	Compound	Phase	No. of patients	CED details/results
Laske DW (30)	1997	Tf-107 CRM (Diphteria toxin)	I	28	2 catheters intra-/peritumoral, infusion over 5–7 d with dose escalation, repeated after 4–10 wk Rand
RW (34)	2000	IL-4 PE38KDEL (Pseudomonas exotoxin)	I/II	9	Intratumoral infusion, 1–3 catheters over 4–8 d. Dose escalation. Tumor necrosis. One patient survived >18 mo.
Wakabayashi T (43)	2001	Nimustine (ACNU)	I/II	9	15 infusions in 9 patients.
Sampson JH (4)	2003	TP-38+TGF-α (Pseudomonas exotoxin)	I	20	Intratumoral infusion, 2 catheters, dose escalation 25–100 ng/mL. Median survival after treatment 23 wk. One responder survived >83 wk.
Weber FW (38)	2003	IL-4 NBI-3001 (Pseudomonas exotoxin)	I		Dose escalation. Medium survival 5.8 mo, 6-mo survival 48%. One responder survived >3 yr (53).
Voges J (42)	2003	HSV-1-tk-gene bearing liposome vector	I/II	8	Intratumoral catheters. 2 patients >50% tumor reduction.
Weaver M (45)	2003	Tf-107 CRM (Diphteria toxin)	II	44	2 catheters intra-/peritumoral, infusion over 5–7 d, repeated after 4–10 wk.
Kunwar S (37)	2003	IL-13PE38QQR	I	46	Intratumoral infusion with and without resection. Dose escalation. Preliminary results.
Lidar Z (44)	2004	Paclitaxel (Taxol)	I/II	15	Intratumoral catheters, 20 cycles. Response rate 73%, high treatment associated-toxicity.

Table 2
Preclinical Studies Using CED for Drug Delivery

Author	Yr	Model	Compound	CED details/results
Bruce JN (16)	2000	Rat C6 glioma	Nitrosourea	Intratumoral, C6 brain tumor, ICP monitoring during infusions.
Cunningham J (54)	2000	Rat	Adeno-associated virus thymidine kinase	Adeno-associated virus (AAV)-based vectors. Efficient delivery of vector by CED.
Kaiser MG (15)	2000	Rat C6 glioma	Topotecan	Efficient delivery of drug, wide distribution. Increased survival of treated C6 bearing rats.
Groothuis DR (35)	2000	Rat brain	^{14}C-cytosine arabinoside (Ara-C)	CED can achieve therapeutic levels of AraC in the brain compared to systemic delivery methods.
Heimberger AB (55)	2000	Athymic rat, D54 MG (human glioma)	Temozolomide (TMZ)	Comparing CED vs Intraperitoneal delivery. Increased survival compared with controls.
Yang W (56)	2002	Rat, EGFR+ glioma (F98 vs F98 wt)	Boronated EGF (radiolabeled ^{125}I)	CED more effective than intratumoral injection to deliver boronated EGF to EGFR (+) gliomas for boron neutron capture therapy.
Degen JW (57)	2003	Rat 9L glioma	Carboplatin or gemcitabine	CED of carboplatin or gemcitabine accomplished therapeutic concentrations to tumors, it is safe and has potent antitumor effects.
Saito R (58)	2004	U87 athymic rat model	TRAIL and TMZ	Survival advantage for combined treatment CED of TRAIL and TMZ, compared with controls and single therapies.

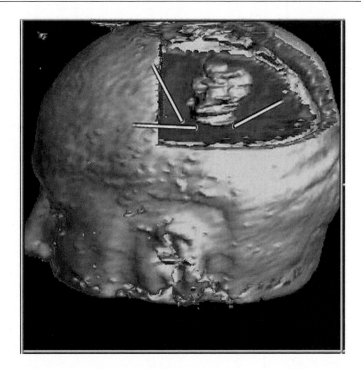

Fig. 1. Planning 3D MRI reconstruction of patient after resection of left temporal GBM and post resection insertion of three intracerebral infusion catheters.

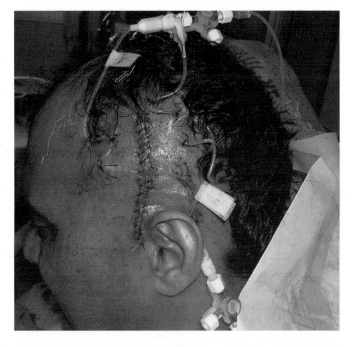

Fig. 2. Patient after insertion of three intracerebral infusion catheters.

Diffusion-weighted MRI (DWMRI) enables noninvasive characterization of biological tissues based on their water diffusion characteristics. It was shown that DWMRI might serve as a surrogate marker for assessing the propagation of the convective wave of Paclitaxel in brain tumors and for predicting tumor response in tumor volumes covered by convection *(44,51)*.

FUTURE CHALLENGES

CED is a relatively new approach for direct drug delivery into the brain, and one which depends on many physical and physiological parameters. The overall goal of local therapies should be to treat large volumes of tumor infiltrated brain with a selectively targeting agent. Such drugs should target the tumor cells with high selectivity and spare the normal brain tissue. This minimally invasive technique, however, still has multiple physical and patho-physiological variables that require extensive interdisciplinary research. In "optimal" conditions, CED has been shown to efficiently cover large volumes of brain tissue while concomitantly providing significantly high concentrations of marker compounds *(28)*. The accumulation of experience from clinical trails of different phases has narrowed down the important factors for creating "optimal" conditions. The variables that have been pointed out as having a significant impact on the volume of distribution are related to catheter character-istics and positioning, biophysical properties of the target tissue and parameters related to the infusate and to infusion. The success of continuous clinical research will depend on the progress in effectively creating and reproducing these "optimal" conditions in the clinical setting and on the identification of effective drugs to be delivered.

Important questions that have been addressed in some of the performed clinical studies but remain to be answered include the positioning and design of the catheter and defining the most favorable characteristics of the infused compound for achieving true convection. We also need better clinical applications of convection imaging (e.g., imaging modality, surrogate marker) to model and follow the drug distribution. Only a reproducible and reliable imaging method will provide us with the necessary information that will allow us to interpret the effects of individual compounds. Until one is available, it will remain unclear if treatment failure is due to ineffective drugs or inadequate delivery.

Currently under investigation are potential modifications of techniques that may enable CED of large particles, whereupon gene therapy-related products and liposomes may be suitable for distribution by CED *(50,52)*.

ACKNOWLEDGMENTS

The author would like to thank Yael Mardor, PhD and Zvi Ram, MD for the critical review of the manuscript and Esther Eshoo for her wonderful work in editing the manuscript.

REFERENCES

1. Tremont-Lukats IW, Gilbert MR. Advances in molecular therapies in patients with brain tumors. Cancer Control 2003;10(2):125–137.
2. Kroll RA, Neuwelt EA. Outwitting the blood-brain barrier for therapeutic purposes: osmotic opening and other means. Neurosurgery 1998;42(5):1083–99; discussion 99–100.
3. Hall WA. Targeted toxin therapy for malignant astrocytoma. Neurosurgery 2000;46(3):544–551; discussion 552.
4. Sampson JH, Akabani G, Archer GE, et al. Progress report of a Phase I study of the intracerebral microinfusion of a recombinant chimeric protein composed of transforming growth factor (TGF)-alpha and a mutated form of the Pseudomonas exotoxin termed PE-38 (TP-38) for the treatment of malignant brain tumors. J Neurooncol 2003;65(1):27–35.

5. Pardridge WM, Oldendorf WH, Cancilla P, Frank HJ. Blood-brain barrier: interface between internal medicine and the brain. Ann Intern Med 1986;105(1):82–95.

6. Henry TR, Votaw JR, Pennell PB, et al. Acute blood flow changes and efficacy of vagus nerve stimulation in partial epilepsy. Neurology 1999;52(6):1166–1173.

7. Brem H, Gabikian P. Biodegradable polymer implants to treat brain tumors. J Control Release 2001;74(1–3): 63–67.

8. Guerin C, Olivi A, Weingart JD, Lawson HC, Brem H. Recent advances in brain tumor therapy: local intracerebral drug delivery by polymers. Invest New Drugs 2004;22(1):27–37.

9. Kleinberg LR, Weingart J, Burger P, et al. Clinical course and pathologic findings after Gliadel and radiotherapy for newly diagnosed malignant glioma: implications for patient management. Cancer Invest 2004;22(1):1–9.

10. Bobo RH, Laske DW, Akbasak A, Morrison PF, Dedrick RL, Oldfield EH. Convection-enhanced delivery of macromolecules in the brain. Proc Natl Acad Sci USA 1994;91(6):2076–2080.

11. Lieberman DM, Laske DW, Morrison PF, Bankiewicz KS, Oldfield EH. Convection-enhanced distribution of large molecules in gray matter during interstitial drug infusion. J Neurosurg 1995;82(6):1021–1029.

12. Morrison PF, Laske DW, Bobo H, Oldfield EH, Dedrick RL. High-flow microinfusion: tissue penetration and pharmacodynamics. Am J Physiol 1994;266(1Pt 2):R292–R305.

13. Kroll RA, Pagel MA, Muldoon LL, Roman-Goldstein S, Neuwelt EA. Increasing volume of distribution to the brain with interstitial infusion: dose, rather than convection, might be the most important factor. Neurosurgery 1996;38(4):746–752; discussion 752–754.

14. Broaddus WC, Prabhu SS, Gillies GT, et al. Distribution and stability of antisense phosphorothioate oligonucleotides in rodent brain following direct intraparenchymal controlled-rate infusion. J Neurosurg 1998;88 (4):734–742.

15. Kaiser MG, Parsa AT, Fine RL, Hall JS, Chakrabarti I, Bruce JN. Tissue distribution and antitumor activity of topotecan delivered by intracerebral clysis in a rat glioma model. Neurosurgery 2000;47(6):1391–1398; discussion 1398–1399.

16. Bruce JN, Falavigna A, Johnson JP, et al. Intracerebral clysis in a rat glioma model. Neurosurgery 2000; 46(3):683–691.

17. Fenstermacher J, Kaye T. Drug "diffusion" within the brain. Ann N Y Acad Sci 1988;531:29–39.

18. Rosenberg GA, Kyner WT, Estrada E. Bulk flow of brain interstitial fluid under normal and hyperosmolar conditions. Am J Physiol 1980;238(1):F42–F49.

19. Kroin JS, Penn RD. Intracerebral chemotherapy: chronic microinfusion of cisplatin. Neurosurgery 1982; 010(3):349–354.

20. Sendelbeck SL, Urquhart J. Spatial distribution of dopamine, methotrexate and antipyrine during continuous intracerebral microperfusion. Brain Res 1985;328(2):251–258.

21. Morrison PF, Dedrick RL. Transport of cisplatin in rat brain following microinfusion: an analysis. J Pharm Sci 1986;75(2):120–128.

22. Jain RK. Delivery of novel therapeutic agents in tumors: physiological barriers and strategies. J Natl Cancer Inst 1989;81(8):570–576.

23. Blasberg RG, Patlak C, Fenstermacher JD. Intrathecal chemotherapy: brain tissue profiles after ventriculocisternal perfusion. J Pharmacol Exp Ther 1975;195(1):73–83.

24. Reulen HJ, Graham R, Spatz M, Klatzo I. Role of pressure gradients and bulk flow in dynamics of vasogenic brain edema. J Neurosurg 1977;46(1):24–35.

25. Cserr HF, Cooper DN, Milhorat TH. Flow of cerebral interstitial fluid as indicated by the removal of extracellular markers from rat caudate nucleus. Exp Eye Res 1977;25 Suppl:461–473.

26. Marmarou A, Takagi H, Shulman K. Biomechanics of brain edema and effects on local cerebral blood flow. Adv Neurol 1980;28:345–358.

27. Ohata K, Marmarou A. Clearance of brain edema and macromolecules through the cortical extracellular space. J Neurosurg 1992;77(3):387–396.

28. Laske DW, Morrison PF, Lieberman DM, et al. Chronic interstitial infusion of protein to primate brain: determination of drug distribution and clearance with single-photon emission computerized tomography imaging. J Neurosurg 1997;87(4):586–594.

29. Viola JJ, Agbaria R, Walbridge S, et al. In situ cyclopentenyl cytosine infusion for the treatment of experimental brain tumors. Cancer Res 1995;55(6):1306–1309.

30. Laske DW, Youle RJ, Oldfield EH. Tumor regression with regional distribution of the targeted toxin TF-CRM107 in patients with malignant brain tumors. Nat Med 1997;3(12):1362–1368.

31. Lonser RR, Gogate N, Morrison PF, Wood JD, Oldfield EH. Direct convective delivery of macromolecules to the spinal cord. J Neurosurg 1998;89(4):616–622.

32. Chen MY, Lonser RR, Morrison PF, Governale LS, Oldfield EH. Variables affecting convection-enhanced delivery to the striatum: a systematic examination of rate of infusion, cannula size, infusate concentration, and tissue-cannula sealing time. J Neurosurg 1999;90(2):315–320.

33. Groothuis DR, Ward S, Itskovich AC, et al. Comparison of 14C-sucrose delivery to the brain by intravenous, intraventricular, and convection-enhanced intracerebral infusion. J Neurosurg 1999;90(2):321–331.

34. Rand RW, Kreitman RJ, Patronas N, Varriccio F, Pastan I, Puri RK. Intratumoral administration of recombinant circularly permuted interleukin-4-Pseudomonas exotoxin in patients with high-grade glioma. Clin Cancer Res 2000;6(6):2157–2165.

35. Groothuis DR, Benalcazar H, Allen CV, et al. Comparison of cytosine arabinoside delivery to rat brain by intravenous, intrathecal, intraventricular and intraparenchymal routes of administration. Brain Res 2000;856(1–2):281–290.

36. Pastan I, FitzGerald D. Recombinant toxins for cancer treatment. Science 1991;254(5035):1173–1177.

37. Kunwar S. Convection enhanced delivery of IL13-PE38QQR for treatment of recurrent malignant glioma: presentation of interim findings from ongoing phase 1 studies. Acta Neurochir Suppl 2003;88:105–111.

38. Weber FW, Floeth F, Asher A, et al. Local convection enhanced delivery of IL4-Pseudomonas exotoxin (NBI-3001) for treatment of patients with recurrent malignant glioma. Acta Neurochir Suppl 2003;88:93–103.

39. Puri RK, Hoon DS, Leland P, et al. Preclinical development of a recombinant toxin containing circularly permuted interleukin 4 and truncated Pseudomonas exotoxin for therapy of malignant astrocytoma. Cancer Res 1996;56(24):5631–5637.

40. Husain SR, Puri RK. Interleukin-13 receptor-directed cytotoxin for malignant glioma therapy: from bench to bedside. J Neurooncol 2003;65(1):37–48.

41. Husain SR, Joshi BH, Puri RK. Interleukin-13 receptor as a unique target for anti-glioblastoma therapy. Int J Cancer 2001;92(2):168–175.

42. Voges J, Reszka R, Gossmann A, et al. Imaging-guided convection-enhanced delivery and gene therapy of glioblastoma. Ann Neurol 2003;54(4):479–487.

43. Wakabayashi T, Yoshida J, Mizuno M, Kajita Y. Intratumoral microinfusion of nimustine (ACNU) for recurrent glioma. Brain Tumor Pathol 2001;18(1):23–28.

44. Lidar Z, Mardor Y, Jonas T, et al. Convection-enhanced delivery of paclitaxel for the treatment of recurrent malignant glioma: a phase I/II clinical study. J Neurosurg 2004;100(3):472–479.

45. Weaver M, Laske DW. Transferrin receptor ligand-targeted toxin conjugate (Tf-CRM107) for therapy of malignant gliomas. J Neurooncol 2003;65(1):3–13.

46. Hall WA, Godal A, Juell S, Fodstad O. In vitro efficacy of transferrin-toxin conjugates against glioblastoma multiforme. J Neurosurg 1992;76(5):838–844.

47. Martell LA, Agrawal A, Ross DA, Muraszko KM. Efficacy of transferrin receptor-targeted immunotoxins in brain tumor cell lines and pediatric brain tumors. Cancer Res 1993;53(6):1348–1353.

47a. Patel S. Ann Oncol 2002;13: Abstract.

48. Lonser RR, Walbridge S, Garmestani K, et al. Successful and safe perfusion of the primate brainstem: in vivo magnetic resonance imaging of macromolecular distribution during infusion. J Neurosurg 2002;97(4):905–913.

49. Nguyen TT, Pannu YS, Sung C, et al. Convective distribution of macromolecules in the primate brain demonstrated using computerized tomography and magnetic resonance imaging. J Neurosurg 2003;98(3):584–590.

50. Saito R, Bringas JR, McKnight TR, et al. Distribution of liposomes into brain and rat brain tumor models by convection-enhanced delivery monitored with magnetic resonance imaging. Cancer Res 2004;64(7):2572–2579.

50a. Sampson JH et al. Abstract #TA-49. Neuro-Oncol 2004;6(4).

51. Mardor Y, Roth Y, Lidar Z, et al. Monitoring response to convection-enhanced taxol delivery in brain tumor patients using diffusion-weighted magnetic resonance imaging. Cancer Res 2001;61(13):4971–4973.

52. Mamot C, Nguyen JB, Pourdehnad M, et al. Extensive distribution of liposomes in rodent brains and brain tumors following convection-enhanced delivery. J Neurooncol 2004;68(1):1–9.

53. Rainov NG, Heidecke V. Long term survival in a patient with recurrent malignant glioma treated with intratumoral infusion of an IL4-targeted toxin (NBI-3001). J Neurooncol 2004;66(1–2):197–201.

54. Cunningham J, Oiwa Y, Nagy D, Podsakoff G, Colosi P, Bankiewicz KS. Distribution of AAV-TK following intracranial convection-enhanced delivery into rats. Cell Transplant 2000;9(5):585–594.

55. Heimberger AB, Archer GE, McLendon RE, et al. Temozolomide delivered by intracerebral microinfusion is safe and efficacious against malignant gliomas in rats. Clin Cancer Res 2000;6(10):4148–4153.

56. Yang W, Barth RF, Adams DM, et al. Convection-enhanced delivery of boronated epidermal growth factor for molecular targeting of EGF receptor-positive gliomas. Cancer Res 2002;62(22):6552–6558.

57. Degen JW, Walbridge S, Vortmeyer AO, Oldfield EH, Lonser RR. Safety and efficacy of convection-enhanced delivery of gemcitabine or carboplatin in a malignant glioma model in rats. J Neurosurg 2003;99(5):893–898.
58. Saito R, Bringas JR, Panner A, et al. Convection-enhanced delivery of tumor necrosis factor-related apoptosis-inducing ligand with systemic administration of temozolomide prolongs survival in an intracranial glioblastoma xenograft model. Cancer Res 2004;64(19):6858–6862.

19

Immunotoxins for Glioma Therapy*

Syed Rafat Husain and Raj K. Puri

Summary

Targeting cancer cells with an immunotoxin represents a novel therapeutic approach. Several immunotoxins composed of a ligand or antibody and truncated bacterial toxins are in clinical development to treat various cancers including glioblastoma multiforme (GBM). GBM is an infiltrative tumor that defies a "complete surgical resection" invariably recurring most often at the site of resection. A number of local therapies are being explored. One approach is to identify unique or over-expressed cell surface receptors on GBM cells and targeting them with a receptor-specific immunotoxin. We have identified over-expression of a receptor for an immune regulatory cytokine, interleukin-13 (IL-13) on human malignant glioma cell lines, primary brain tumor cell cultures, and tumor tissues. The targeting of IL-13 receptors (IL-13R) with a recombinant fusion protein composed of IL-13 and a mutated form of Pseudomonas exotoxin (IL13-PE38QQR or IL-13-PE38, referred to here as IL13-PE) demonstrated a potent and specific cell-killing of GBM cells in vitro. Normal brain cells, immune cells, and endothelial cells devoid of the unique IL-13R chain were not susceptible to immunotoxin cell killing activity. Direct injection of IL13-PE into subcutaneous (sc) or intracranial human GBM tumors in nude mice resulted in complete and durable regression of tumors. IL13-PE delivered through intravenous (iv) and intraperitoneal (ip) routes of administration also reduced sc tumor burden with fewer complete responses (CR). High doses of systemic (up to 50 μg/kg) or intracerebral (up to 100 μg/mL) IL13-PE were well tolerated in mice and rats, respectively without evidence of gross or microscopic necrosis.

Based on these encouraging preclinical results, four phase I and II clinical trials were initiated to investigate the safety, toxicity, and optimal convection-enhanced delivery (CED) of IL13-PE to patients with recurrent malignant gliomas; patients had already undergone standard therapy including surgery, radiation, and chemotherapy. CED uses a positive pressure to generate a pressure gradient that optimizes distribution of the macromolecule within tumor and peritumoral regions. A total of 97 patients were treated with IL13-PE in these studies. CED of IL13-PE into solid tumor component as well as the surrounding brain tissues felt to be at risk for residual infiltrating tumor before and after tumor resection, respectively was fairly well tolerated in terms of safety profile. Histological anti-tumor effects have been observed at drug concentrations of 0.5, 1.0 and 2.0 μg/mL without apparent increased antitumor activity at higher concentrations. Duration of infusions up to 7 d was fairly well tolerated. A randomized worldwide phase III clinical trial (PRECISE, phase III Randomized Evaluation of Convection Enhanced Delivery of IL13-PE38QQR with Survival Endpoint) is currently recruiting patients with recurrent supratentorial GBM at first recurrence to evaluate overall survival duration, safety, and quality-of-life of patients treated by tumor resection followed by peritumoral IL13-PE infusion vs Gliadel® Wafer placement.

Key Words: Glioma; immunotoxin; IL13-PE; chimeric fusion protein; xenograft; clinical trial.

---

*The views presented in this article do not necessarily reflect those of the Food and Drug Administration.

From: *Current Clinical Oncology: High-Grade Gliomas: Diagnosis and Treatment*
Edited by: G. H. Barnett © Humana Press Inc., Totowa, NJ

INTRODUCTION

Immunotoxins are potent cytotoxic agents that have emerged as an important therapeutic modality for cancer *(1)*. They are composed of toxins derived from plants or bacteria linked chemically or by recombinant engineering to antibodies or ligands that target cell surface molecules expressed on cancer cells. Plant toxins are either composed of catalytic and binding chains linked together through a disulfide bond or a catalytic chain alone. The bacterial toxins, *Pseudomonas* exotoxin (PE) and diphtheria toxin (DT) are made up of single-chain proteins containing binding and catalytic domains. Features common to fusion toxins include binding to cell surface molecules, internalization, translocation to the cytosol, and eventual catalytic inhibition of protein synthesis leading to cell death. The binding domains of natural toxins are either mutated or removed to prevent binding to normal cells and then fused to a ligand or antibody that specifically targets cancer cells *(2)*. The beneficial consequence of coupling a ligand to a truncated toxin is that binding to normal cells is diminished. Using this approach, several ligands and antibody fragments have been fused to toxins to exploit their therapeutic value in cancer therapy *(3–6)*.

These chemically conjugated or recombinant immunotoxins (also called cytotoxins) showed remarkable antitumor activity in vitro and in animal models of several human cancers *(7–13)*. Currently, several immunotoxins are being tested in the clinic. The immunotoxins, in which an antibody is linked to PE, ricin, or other toxic moieties have demonstrated encouraging results in the treatment of certain advanced tumors in patients *(14–19)*. In one of the earlier phase I clinical trials, Le^y antigen-binding MAb B3 was fused to PE38, a slightly smaller toxin molecule with deletions of unnecessary residues in domain 1b. The fusion product is designated LMB-1. Le^y antigen is found in 95% of colon cancers, over 50% of breast cancers, and in many epithelial malignancies. LMB-1 has produced several clinical responses including a complete response (CR) in a patient with breast cancer and partial response (PR) in a patient with colon cancer with extensive metastases *(20)*. Later, a recombinant anti-Tac(Fv)-PE38 (LMB-2) was developed as a single-chain immunotoxin to target CD25-expressing cells *(21)*. LMB-2 has produced clinical responses including 1 CR and 3 PRs in hairy cell leukemia and a PR in chronic lymphocytic leukemia, Hodgkin's disease and cutaneous T-cell lymphoma *(22)*. In contrast, another recombinant immunotoxin, LMB-7 in which the Fv portion of the B3 is fused to PE38 has elicited poor activity in a phase I trial. Single-chain Fv and single-chain immunotoxins were found to be unstable at 37°C because of their aggregation *(23)*. To overcome this problem, light- and heavy-chains were linked by a disulfide bond to improve the stability and the resulting immunotoxins were stable at 37°C for several days. BL22, a disulfide-linked immunotoxin in which the Fv portion of an anti-CD22 antibody is fused to PE38 showed remarkable activity in drug-resistant hairy cell leukemia *(24)*. Clinical trials involving recombinant antimesothelin immunotoxin, which targets mesothelin antigen expressed on mesothelioma, ovarian cancers and pancreatic cancers are also ongoing *(25)*.

Diphtheria toxin fused to IL-2 ($DAB_{389}IL-2$) also displayed remarkable antitumor activity in patients with cutaneous T-cell lymphoma and Hodgkin's lymphoma *(19)*. Based on promising clinical results, $DAB_{389}IL-2$ (Ontak®) was licensed for the treatment of cutaneous T-cell lymphoma *(26)*. In another DT based immunotoxin, epidermal growth factor (EGF) was fused to DAB_{389} for targeting of EGF receptor positive carcinoma and brain tumors *(27)*. EGF receptor-positive GBM cell lines were extremely sensitive (IC_{50} 0.4–50 pm) to a DT-EGF fusion protein (DAB_{389}-EGF) *(27)*. Several phase I and II clinical trials involving this fusion moiety have demonstrated tumor responsiveness in patients with non-small-cell lung cancer *(28,29)*.

Another immunotoxin in which an antibody targeting the CD33 antigen present in acute myelocytic leukemia (AML) cells was chemically conjugated to a bacterial antibiotic, calicheamicin *(30)*. This molecule (Mylotarg®) has been licensed for the treatment of AML *(31)*. In another phase I and II clinical trials, immunotoxins consisting of anti-CD25 or anti-CD30 monoclonal antibodies (MAbs) and deglycosylated ricin A chain were delivered intravenously (iv) to patients with refractory Hodgkin's lymphoma. Both immunotoxins showed moderate efficacy in the aggresively pretreated refractory patients *(32)*.

Several immunotoxins either attached to a MAb or ligand have also been tested on gliomas. Malignant gliomas, in particular GBM are the most insidious type of brain tumor and constitute the third leading cause of death with nearly 14,000 patients succumbing each year in the United States alone *(33)*. Because of their invading and migrating phenotype in surrounding brain parenchyma, the surgical resection is limited to the main tumor mass and the tumor eventually recurs. Development of targeted drugs, such as immunotoxins, along with recent advances in drug delivery have created some hope for patients with malignant brain tumors. For CNS tumors, Laske et al. observed potent antitumor activity of transferrin-diphtheria toxin (Tf-CRM107) in mammalian cells expressing the transferrin receptor. Phase I clinical trial results demonstrated that Tf-CRM107, delivered via a high-flow convection method utilizing stereotactically placed catheters, produced 2 CRs and 7 PRs in a group of 15 patients *(34–37)*. In a Phase II open-label single-arm trial, patients received continuous infusion of Tf-CRM107 (0.67 µg/mL) escalating to a delivery rate of 0.20 mL/h/catheter (a total of 0.40 mL/h for two catheters) for 4 to 5 d until a total volume of 40 mL was delivered. A second treatment was given 4 to 10 wk after initial infusion. A total of 5 CRs and 7 PRs were observed out of 44 enrolled patients in which 34 were evaluable in a Phase II open-label clinical trial *(36)*. Other cytotoxin targeting the EGF-R, transforming growth factor-α fused to PE (TGF-PE38) has shown increased survival in mice implanted with intracranial glioblastoma *(27,37)*. In a phase I clinical trial, TGF-PE38 (TP-38) was delivered by CED in patients with recurrent malignant brain tumors. Two of 15 patients with residual tumor at the time of receiving the therapy demonstrated radiographic responses. One patient treated at a 25 ng/mL concentration level experienced a complete response. Another patient, treated with a 100 ng/mL concentration, showed a PR characterized by a >50% shrinkage of tumor 34 wk after TP-38 therapy *(38)*. Diphtheria toxin (DT_{390}) attached to a urokinase-type plasminogen activator (uPA) has also been shown to decrease tumor burden in the subcutaneous (sc) implanted human glioblastoma in nude mice *(39,40)*.

In our own studies, we have identified over-expression of IL-4 receptors in human glioma cell lines, primary cell cultures, and GBM tissues prompting development of an IL4-PE that targets receptors for IL-4 in vitro and in vivo *(13)*. In a first Phase I clinical trial, IL-4-PE was well tolerated without apparent indication of incipient drug-related toxicity *(41)*. This trial showed objective tumor responses in patients with recurrent glioblastoma. In a follow-up open-label, dose escalation trial involving intratumoral administration of IL4-PE, a total of 31 patients with histologically verified supratentorial grade III and IV astrocytoma were treated. No systemic drug-related toxicity, as evidenced by a lack of hematological or serum chemical changes in blood, was noted in any patient. Treatment related adverse events were limited to the central nervous system (CNS). Grade III or IV toxicity was observed in 22% of patients at the MTD of 6 µg/mL × 40 mL. IL4-PE elicited tumor necrosis as evident by a change in gadolinium enhancement without systemic exposure of the drug *(42)*. A 27-yr-old male patient with recurrent malignant glioma treated with a single intratumoral infusion of IL-4-PE (9 µg/mL in 66 mL infusate) exhibited a long-term survival of 3 yr. The patient eventually died of

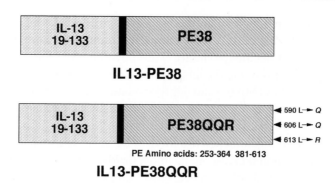

Fig. 1. Schematic diagram of IL13-*Pseudomonas* Exotoxin fusion proteins. In IL13-PE38, domain 1a (amino acid 1-252 and 365-380) of PE are deleted and replaced by IL-13. In IL13-PE38QQR, domain 1a is again replaced by IL-13. Lysine (K) residues at position 590 and 606 of PE38 are replaced by glutamine (Q) while lysine at position 613 is replaced by arginine (R) to yield PE38QQR.

local recurrence of the brain tumor. Though this response may be anecdotal, such clinical evolution subsequent to glioma therapy after a single round of immunotoxin is rather unusual suggesting that repeat courses of immunotoxin may be necessary for better tumor control *(43)*. A third Phase I/II clinical trial with IL4-PE was conducted, in which doses of IL4-PE and volume of infusion were optimized. In addition, all patients underwent surgical resection after IL4-PE infusion *(42)*. This study demonstrated that IL4-PE at a concentration of 1.5 μg/mL in a volume of 60 mL of fluid was well-tolerated with minimal neurological toxicities. Based on these clinical observations, IL4-PE should be further tested in a randomized controlled clinical trial to determine its efficacy. In addition, other drug delivery strategies should be explored with this promising antitumor agents because of the fact that IL-4R are over-expressed in most gliomas and other intracranial tumors.

IL-4 was found to be structurally and functionally related to a new cytokine discovered in 1993 termed IL-13. Not surprisingly, we found that IL-13R are also over-expressed in several human solid tumors including GBM cell lines, primary cell cultures, and tumors *(44,45)*. To exploit the presence of IL-13 receptors on tumor cells, we developed a fusion cytotoxin composed of IL-13 ligand and a mutated form of PE toxin (Fig. 1). Since the discovery of the IL-13 receptor on cancer cells almost a decade ago, we have been extensively engaged in studying the structure, function, and targeting of these receptors along with the toxicity and pharmacokinetics of IL13-PE associated with various routes of administration *(46)*. As a result of these studies, several clinical trials were initiated and currently on-going in patients with recurrent malignant glioma. In addition, a Phase I clinical trial in patients with renal cell carcinoma (RCC) has been completed *(47)*. Because of the limited scope of this chapter, we hereby focus the review on the development of IL 13-PE for malignant glioma therapy.

PRECLINICAL DEVELOPMENT OF IL13-PE

IL-13 Receptor on Glioma Cells

IL-13 is a pleiotropic cytokine sharing numerous biological activities with IL-4 in humans. Both cytokines are mainly produced by activated Th2 cells and mast cells *(48)*. These two cytokines can induce Ig class-switching, up-regulate expression of CD23 in B cells and monocytes *(48,49)*, inhibit the production of inflammatory cytokines in monocytes *(50)*, and

Table 1
IL-13 Receptor Expression on Glioma Cells and Their Sensitivity Toward IL13-PE

Cell line	Binding site[a]	Dissociation constant $(K_d)^a$ (nm)	IC_{50} (ng/mL)[b]
U251MG	28,000 (22,660)	2.1 (1.6)	0.2
A172	22,600	1.6	0.05
SNB19	17,600	1.4	0.05
U373	16,000	1.8	0.3
Hs683	ND	ND	0.4
DBTRG	ND	ND	<2.0
U87MG	3,000	ND	~600
T98G	550	1.0	300
G2 Explant	300,000	2.4	0.2

Notes: [a] Glioma cells (1×10^6) were incubated with 100 pM of radiolabeled IL-13 (^{125}I-IL-13) with or without increasing concentrations (up to 500 pM) of unlabeled IL-13. Binding sites and K_d were calculated from displacement curves and Scatchard analysis generated by LIGAND software program.

[b] In vitro cytotoxicity was performed by treating cells with varying concentration of IL13-PE using a protein synthesis inhibition assay *(44)*. The concentration of IL13-PE at which 50% protein synthesis (IC_{50}) occurred was calculated.

enhance the growth and differentiation of B cells, monocytes, and endothelial cells *(48,50–52)*. In contrast to IL-4, IL-13 does not exert direct effect on T cells *(48)*. IL-13 exerts its action by binding to IL-13R expressed on target cells *(51)*. The action of IL-13 in hematopoietic cells is well understood, but this is not the case with nonhematopoietic cells.

Based on our prior knowledge of IL-4R overexpression on a variety of human solid tumor cells including RCC cells, we were the first to observe that human RCC cells express large numbers of IL-13R *(53)*. As an extension of our search, we were pleasantly surprised to note that other types of tumor cells *(46)* including human glioma cells also expressed IL-13R in over-abundance *(44)*. We targeted these over-expressed receptors for anti-tumor therapy using IL13-PE immunotoxin. A detailed description of IL13-PE is described in sections below. Radiolabeling studies performed using glioma cell lines showed that most GBM cells expressed a large number of IL-13R with high to intermediate affinity. No difference in affinity of IL-13 for its receptor was noted among tumor cell lines or cells derived from primary culture, although one G2 explant cell was found to express a high density of IL-13R (Table 1). In contrast to glioma cells, human immune cells—including B cells, monocytes, and T lymphocytes, and nonimmune cells such as endothelial cells—either do not express or express a very low level of IL-13R *(53,54)*. Though the significance of IL-13R over-expression on tumor cells is not known, nonetheless we have extensively studied the structure of IL-13R on tumor cells, including glioma cells.

Structure of IL-13 Receptor

Receptor binding studies revealed that radiolabeled IL-13 cross-linked to a single 60- to 70-kDa protein on human RCC cells *(53)*. Based on these studies, we proposed that IL-13R was a dimeric protein comprised of 65-70 kDa subunit chains *(54,55)*. During the same period, two of the IL-13R chains, IL-13Rα1 and IL13Rα2 were cloned *(56–58)*. The murine and human

IL-13Rα1 chain was cloned first *(57,58)*. We and others showed that the IL-13Rα1 chain forms a functional complex with IL-4Rα, a primary IL-4 binding subunit, for signal transduction *(56,59)*. The second chain, IL-13Rα2, was cloned first from a human RCC line *(60)* and later from a human glioma cell line *(61)*. The IL-13Rα2 chain (65-kDa) binds to IL-13 with an affinity about 50 times greater than binding to the IL-13Rα1 chain *(60,62)*. We later demonstrated that the subunit structure of the IL-13R varies in different types of cells *(55,63)* and have proposed the existence of three different types of IL-13R *(63,64)*. In type I IL-13R, all three chains (IL-13Rα1, IL-13Rα2 and IL-4Rα) are present. IL-13 binds to all three chains, whereas IL-4 binds to IL-4Rα and IL-13Rα1 chains. Type I IL-13R are expressed on brain tumor cells, RCC, and AIDS-associated Kaposi's sarcoma cells *(10,59)*. Type II IL-13R containing IL-13Rα1 and IL4Rα chains are expressed on Colo 201, A431, Cos-7, HT-29, pancreas, breast, prostate tumor cells, and endothelial cells *(59,65–67)*. In type III IL-13R, an additional component of IL-2R complex (common γchain, γc) is also present. Type III IL-13R are expressed on B cells, monocytes, and TF-1 erythroleukemia cells *(48,55,68)*. The proposed IL-13R model was confirmed by reconstitution studies in CHO-K1 cells. We demonstrated that the IL-13Rα1 chain but not the IL-13Rα2 chain forms a functional complex with the IL-4Rα chain. The IL-13Rα2 chain inhibited IL-13 induced signal transduction induced by binding to IL-13Rα1 and IL-4Rα chains *(69)*.

Glioma Cells Express Type I IL-13R

We recently demonstrated that primary brain tumor cell cultures established from tumor specimens resected from patients expressed three chains of the IL-13R complex, IL-13Rα1, IL-13Rα2 and IL-4Rα and have classified them as type I IL-13R. The IL-13Rα2 chain was expressed at both the mRNA and protein level in 72% of samples; however, all specimens expressed both IL-13Rα1 and IL-4Rα chains *(45,70)*. Normal human astrocytes (NHAs), brain cells, or brain tissue samples had low levels of IL-13Rα2 mRNA. Other normal brain cell lines derived from normal human oligodendrocytes, NT-2 neuronal cell lines, and two cortex tissue-derived cell lines either did not express mRNA for IL-13Rα2 or had levels that were undetectable. Further studies confirmed that the IL-13Rα2 chain is overexpressed in adult human glioma samples and serves as a primary binding subunit target for IL13-PE to exert its antitumor activity *(64,70)*. In addition, we recently demonstrated that glioma cells not expressing IL-13R on their cell surface can be sensitized following IL-13Rα2 gene transfer. Interestingly, the introduction of IL-13Rα2 into the T98G cell line possessing undetectable levels of IL-13R resulted in an increased sensitivity (IC$_{50}$ from >1000 ng/mL to 0.7 ng/mL) to IL13-PE *(71,72)*. This clearly suggested that the IL-13Rα2 chain, a primary binding subunit of the IL-13R complex, is required to bind to IL13-PE in order for immunotoxin to exert its cytotoxicity. In addition, we proposed that IL-13Rα2 chain may serve as a biomarker for malignant glioma and may be useful in anticipating response to therapy or for monitoring disease recurrence.

Function of IL-13 Receptor

The significance of IL-13R overexpression on tumor cells including glioma cells is not known. Sequencing and single strand conformation polymorphism (SSCP) studies conducted in 19 GBM cell lines have not demonstrated any mutations in IL-13Rα2 chain. Although a single nucleotide polymorphism in the transmembrane domain of IL-13Rα1 was detected, this mutation did not result in a change of amino acid or charge. IL-13R on glioma cells were functional as IL-13 modulated the expression of VCAM-1 in one cell line. These results indicated that

IL-13R on GBM cell lines were not rearranged but appeared to be functional (61). The role for IL-13R on GBM cells in instigating tumorigenic processes has not been ruled out.

Production of Recombinant IL13-PE

PE is one of the pathogenic proteins secreted by *Pseudomonas aeruginosa* bacteria and is made up of three major domains (23,73). The N-terminal domain Ia is a cell-binding domain that binds ubiquitous receptors present on eukaryotic cells. To achieve the specific binding, domain 1a was replaced with IL-13 so the resulting toxin binds only to IL-13R positive cells. Joshi et al. in our laboratory cloned a mature form of human IL-13 from human peripheral blood mononuclear cells (PBMCs). IL-13 gene was subcloned into YR39 or pRKL438QQR to yield pBJIL13PE38 or pRPL13PE38QQR, respectively (74). IL13-PE38 or IL13-PE38QQR were expressed from these plasmids in *Escherichia coli* and purified chimeric proteins were obtained in high yields by size-exclusion and ion-exchange chromatography (74). As shown in Fig. 1, domain Ia amino acid 1-252 and amino acids 365 to 380 were deleted, and lysine (K) residues at position 590 and 606 were replaced by glutamine (Q) whereas lysine at position 613 was replaced by arginine (R) in IL13-PE38QQR (74). In IL13-PE38, domain 1a was deleted, but no amino acid substitutions were introduced (Fig. 1). It was initially believed that mutations in domain III would improve anti-tumor activity against tumor cells, consequently IL13-PE38QQR was developed (75). However, later in vitro studies indicated that both IL13-PE38QQR and IL13-PE38 molecules were equally cytotoxic (74). Because most of the initial anti-glioblastoma preclinical studies were performed with IL13-PE38QQR (referred herein as IL13-PE), it was selected for the clinical studies as well.

Targeting of IL-13 Receptors

The mechanism of cytotoxicity of IL13-PE includes binding of IL-13 to its receptor. The ligand–receptor complex undergoes receptor-mediated internalization to allow toxin processing. Domain II of PE is a site for proteolytic cleavage that catalyzes the translocation of the toxin into the cytosol. Domain III, located at C-terminus, possesses an adenosine diphosphate (ADP) ribosylation activity that inactivates elongation factor 2 leading to cell death (73). Because immunotoxins differ greatly from chemotherapy in their mode of action, tumor specificity and toxicity profile, we believe IL13-PE will play a major role in future brain tumor therapy.

In Vitro Targeting

Results from protein synthesis inhibition assays showed that picomolar concentrations of IL13-PE (<20 PM) effectively kill glioma cells (Table 1). Cell-killing blockage by excess of IL-13 indicated the specificity of the toxin (76). The cytotoxic assay by clonogenic method further confirmed the remarkable sensitivity of brain tumor cells to IL13-PE (46). The noninvasive *S*-type neuroblastoma cell line was less sensitive to IL13-PE. The presence of toxin-targeted receptors on normal tissues has always been a major impediment to the development of immunotoxins. Because of the fact that IL-13R are expressed either at low or undetectable levels on normal brain tissues, the toxin did not exert cytotoxic effect on NHAs (45). Similar to NHAs, normal endothelial and immune cells expressed undetectable levels of IL-13Rα2 (53,54). These findings suggested that our toxin would not exert deleterious effects on normal cells thereby offering a favorable potential therapeutic window. Encouraging in vitro results led us to further explore the efficacy of IL13-PE in xenograft models of GBM.

Efficacy in Xenograft Models

The therapeutic efficacy of IL13-PE was tested in athymic nude mice models of human U251MG and U87MG glioblastoma tumors *(46,76)*. Intravenous injections of IL13-PE (25 or 50 µg/kg for 5 d) into mice bearing subcutaneous U251 tumors reduced average tumor size by 65 and 75%, respectively, compared with controls. Even though the half- life of IL13-PE in nude mice is short ($t_{1/2}\alpha = 9$ min and $t_{1/2}\beta = 75$ min), it resulted in 20% CR at each dose. IL13-PE at a dose of 100 µg/kg × 5 d was toxic to animals *(10)*; however, tolerated doses induced tumor regression in a dose-dependent manner. Mice treated with twice daily (bid) intraperitoneal (ip) doses of 25 or 50 µg/kg of IL13-PE for 5 successive days reduced tumor burden by 36 and 54% along with durable 20 and 40% CRs, respectively. Similar ip injections of 50 µg/kg IL13-PE in the U87MG xenograft model resulted in tumor regression by 50%; no CR was observed *(76)*.

The MTD of 50 µg/kg given bid × 5 d ip administration could be increased to 100 µg/kg when IL13-PE was infused for 7 d using ip mini-osmotic pumps. The infusion regimen was better tolerated and more efficacious than ip bolus administration. U251MG tumors were reduced by 86% with 5 of 8 (63%) mice showing CRs. The lower doses, 25 and 50 µg/kg/d, also caused tumor regression by 50 and 72%, respectively. A higher dose of IL13-PE (250 µg/kg/d) was toxic to animals and 3 of 5 mice died within 7 d of pump-implantation *(77)*. Mice treated with MTD doses tolerated therapy well without any visible signs of toxicity.

GBM being a loco-regional disease, an attempt was made to treat with direct drug delivery to the tumor to bypass the blood–tumor barrier. Intratumoral delivery of IL13-PE (50 or 100 µg/kg × 5) into U251MG xenografts resulted in 80 and 100% CRs, respectively. More IL13-PE could be delivered at the tumor site as compared with iv or ip delivery *(10,76)*. Because U87MG tumors express lower number of IL-13R, a relatively higher dose of IL13-PE (250 µg/kg × 3 d) on alternate days (qod) was necessary to eliminate tumors in 100% of tumor xenografts. A total of 750 µg/kg IL13-PE was required to achieve 100% CRs in U87MG model compared to U251MG model, where 500 µg/kg (100 µg/kg × 5 d) resulted in all CRs. It was quite evident that a higher drug accumulation by intratumoral route yielded in a better efficacy. Surprisingly, a slightly higher dose of IL13-PE (250 µg/kg × 5 d) was able to eradicate even larger tumors (75 mm^2) in 33% of treated mice, which is an indication that IL13-PE may be utilized in a patient population even with a heavy tumor burden.

Pharmacology and Toxicity

Systemic Toxicity

In some instances, targeted receptors/antigens are present on normal cells and immunotoxins may cause undesirable side effects. Because the human IL-13 binds to murine IL-13R *(78)*, toxicity studies conducted in mice may provide an appropriate model for estimating a toxicity profile of IL13-PE in humans. To evaluate the toxicity profile, 3 doses (25, 50, and 75 µg/kg, qod) of IL13-PE were injected iv. Mice experienced a weight loss at the highest dose more prominently in female than male. Three out of five female mice died at the highest dose. A moderate zonal hepatic necrosis was observed. Hepatic transaminases (ALT and AST) were elevated more in female than male mice. The lower doses (up to 50 µg/kg) caused no significant changes in AST and ALT. None of the treated mice showed hematological toxicity or vascular leak syndrome. The chronic toxicity studies with MTD dose, 50 µg/kg, qod × 9 d caused transient weight loss more notable in female mice than male mice. The ALT and AST values were elevated in female, but not in male mice. Repeated injections of IL13-PE at lower doses (12.5 and 25 µg/kg) did not cause hepatic toxicity similar to those observed in the acute toxicity study *(79)*. Hepatic toxicity appears to be related to non-specific uptake of IL13-PE by hepatocytes.

Similar studies in cynomolgus monkeys with iv. bolus injections of IL13-PE (12.5 or 50 µg/kg/d × 5 d) caused moderate dose-related elevation of hepatic transaminases, maximal on days 5 through 8 returning to baseline by days 15 through 22. Transient depression of serum cholesterol was noted in high-dose treated animals. Elevation of creatinine kinase was also noted on day 3, with subsequent decline to normal. IL13-PE did not cause hematological toxicities. Body weight remained stable in all monkeys *(79)*.

INTRACEREBRAL TOXICITY

The injections of IL13-PE (0.1–100 µg/mL) into right frontal lobe (caudate nucleus) of Sprague-Dawley rats did not produce cytologic evidence of acute neuroglial cell toxicity at 96 h. Small regions of hemorrhage were noted at the site of injection for doses ≥ 1 µg/mL with rarefaction attributable to injection of fluids and/or a minimal inflammatory reaction. The hemorrhage may be related to drug toxicity but appears more consistent with inoculation track injury. In a similar intracerebral toxicity study with IL13-PE (0, 100, 500, 1000, 2000 µg/mL), no changes in behavior, weight, hematology or chemistry values were detected. No systemic detectable drug levels were observed. However, a single dose of $=500$ µg/mL of IL13-PE caused severe liquefactive necrosis surrounded by degenerating neurons and edema *(79)*. Inflammatory reaction was minimal.

PHARMACOKINETICS

Pharmacokinetics studies of IL13-PE (50 µg/kg, iv) conducted using CD2F1 mice revealed a serum half-life ($t_{1/2}\beta$) for the drug of 1.39 h with the C_{max} of 717 ng/mL, and an area under the curve (AUC) of 219 ng/h/mL. Serum half life in monkeys injected with 5 doses of 50 µg/kg of IL13-PE was 4.4 h with a C_{max} of 474 ng/mL, and an AUC of 582 ng/h/mL *(79)*.

CLINICAL TRIALS

IL13-PE provided promising results in preclinical studies and appeared to have a favorable therapeutic window for regional therapy to treat malignant gliomas. Consequently, four multi-center phase I/II clinical trials were initiated in patients with recurrent supratentorial glioma using CED technique. A total of 97 patients were treated with IL13-PE in these studies. These trials IL13-PEI-001, IL13-PEI-002, IL13-PEI-103, and IL13-PEI-105 are summarized below.

IL13PEI-001 Study

The primary objective of the phase I component of this study was to determine the safety and tolerability of IL13-PE administered by an intratumoral infusion into malignant gliomas in the supratentorial region over 96-h period without planned resection and repeat infusion 8 wk later *(80–82)*. This study is being undertaken by the National Cancer Institute (NCI)/New Approaches to Brain Tumor Therapy (NABTT) consortium.

Eligibility criteria for this study requires a prior diagnosis of supratentorial malignant glioma, recurrence after radiotherapy (RT), measurable disease (1–5 cm in diameter), and a stereotaxic biopsy confirming malignant glioma at the study entry. IL13-PE was administered by micro-infusion via one or two intratumoral catheters at 400 µL/h/all catheters for 96 h (total 38.4 mL). A maximum of two infusions of 96 h at weeks 1 and 9 were planned. IL13-PE concentration was increased in each cohort of three patients to determine the MTD in terms of systemic or CNS toxicity based on WHO toxicity criteria. Cohorts were expanded to six patients if one dose limiting systemic or CNS toxicity (DLT) was observed. At the initial concentration level (0.125 µg/mL), the cohort was expanded to six patients as one of the first three patients developed cerebral edema and symptoms of mass effect shortly after completion of the first infusion that responded rapidly to corticosteroid. No other DLTs were observed at the initial concentration. A second infusion at week 9 was given to three patients and was well tolerated. After the initial concentration, cohorts of 3 patients each received escalating concentrations of 0.25, 0.5, 1.0, 2.0, and 4.0 µg/mL of IL13-PE. One patient in the 4.0 µg/mL cohort had a DLT including a seizure associated with imaging histopathologic changes consistent with nonspecific necrosis of tumor-infiltrated and possibly normal brain parenchyma. Three additional patients have been treated at 4.0 µg/mL and are being followed. A total of 24 patients were treated in this study *(82)*. In general, drug-related adverse events of grade II included headache, and CNS events such as hemiparesis, aphasia, brain edema, ataxia, confusion, and seizures. After implementation of pre- and post-treatment corticosteroid guidelines in cohort 1, a reduction in neurological adverse events resulted to mass effects from the volume of infusate. Overall, 2 histopathologic (0.125 and 0.5 µg/mL) and 2 radiographic (0.125 and 1.0 µg/mL) responses were observed. Histopathologic responses were identified at the time of the surgery for debulking as 2 patients developed symptoms of mass effect accompanied by radiographic changes suggesting tumor progression. Overall median survival from time of treatment was 39 wk ranging from 8 to 183+ wk.

IL13PEI-002 Study

This study examined a novel treatment design consisting of pre- and postoperative infusion of IL13-PE in recurrent supratentorial malignant glioma and surrounding brain at risk for residual infiltrating tumor *(83–86)*. The primary objectives of this study were to determine the histologically effective concentration (HEC) of IL13-PE, the tolerability and toxicities of intratumoral and peritumoral IL13-PE administration, the tolerability of longer durations of infusion, and the feasibility of postoperative deferred catheter placement. Histologic efficacy was defined as geographic necrosis adjacent to tip of the catheter caused by loss of cellular integrity with eosinophilic staining or by complete cell loss. The finding of 90% necrotic cells in a radial distribution at least 1 cm from the catheter tip in the postinfusion specimen compared with the preinfusion biopsy defined the histologic evidence of the drug. This four-stage study is being conducted at the University of California, San Francisco, Memorial Sloan Kettering Cancer Center, NY, MD Anderson Cancer Center, TX and Yale University, CT. Eligibility criteria included prior histologically confirmed diagnosis of supratentorial grade III or IV malignant glioma including anaplastic astrocytoma, GBM, or malignant oligoastrocytoma. In stage I, after biopsy and placement of one catheter, IL13-PE was given over a 48 h period at 400 µL/h. Tumor was resected about 1 wk later and evaluated for necrosis adjacent to the catheter. Stage II of the study included the placement of 2 or 3 catheters into brain adjacent to operative site followed by a peritumoral infusion of IL13-PE at 750 µL/h/all catheters. Escalation of intratumoral and peritumoral concentrations, starting at 0.25 µg/mL, were performed separately (Table 2). After an HEC was identified in stage I, the intratumoral administration was omitted, and escalation of IL13-PE concentration using only a post-resection peritumoral infusion continued up to the identified MTD. Stage III of the study assessed the safety and toxicity of increasing duration (5 and 6 d) of a postresection peritumoral infusion of IL13-PE at a fixed concentration determined in stage II. Finally, in stage IV, the 2 highest peritumoral concentrations determined safe in stage II (0.25 and 0.5 µg/mL) with a 96-h infusion was used to assess the feasibility of post-operative deferred catheter placement

Table 2
IL13-PEI-002 Study Design[a]

Stage I: Pre- and Postresection infusion of IL-13-PE

| Dose level | Preresection/intratumoral | | Postresection/peritumoral | |
	Concentration (µg/mL)	Total dose (µg)	Concentration (µg/mL)	Total dose (µg)
1	0.25	4.8	0.25	18.0
2	0.5	9.6	0.25	18.0
3	1.0	19.2	0.25	18.0
4	2.0	38.4	0.25	18.0

Stage II: Postresection infusion only

	Concentration (µg/mL)	Total dose (µg)
1	0.5	36
2	1.0	72

Stage III: Postresection infusion only

	Duration (d)	Volume (mL)
1	5	90
2	6	108

Stage IV: Postresection infusion only, with catheter placement on day 3 after resection

	Concentration (µg/mL)	Total dose (µg)
1	0.5	36.0
2	0.25	18.0

Notes: [a] The study was designed to determine the histologically effective concentration, tolerability and toxicities of intratumoral and peritumoral IL13-PE administration, the tolerability of longer duration of infusion, and feasibility of postoperative catheter placement in patients with recurrent supratentorial malignant glioma.

Stage I: After biopsy and placement of one catheter, IL13-PE was infused over 48 h at a rate of 400 µL/h. Tumor was resected 1 wk later.

Stage II: Two or three catheter were placed into brain adjacent to operative site followed by a peritumoral infusion of IL13-PE at 750 µL/h/all catheters.

Stage III: Postresection peritumoral IL13-PE was infused at a fixed concentration determined in stage 2 for either for 5 or 6 d.

Stage IV: Two highest peritumoral concentrations of IL13-PE determined safe in stage II (0.25 and 0.5 µg/mL) were infused for 96 h to assess the feasibility of postoperative catheter placement.

compared to intraoperative placement immediately after tumor resection in stages I, II, and III. A total of 42 patients were treated in this phase I study (15 patients in stage I, 9 in stage II, 6 in stage III, and 12 in stage IV) (Table 2).

In 15 patients who received intratumoral IL13-PE in stage I, good evidence of drug-induced tumor necrosis at a concentration of 0.5, 1.0, and 2.0 µg/mL was observed. However, no increasing dose response was observed across those concentrations. All 15 patients received a peritumoral infusion at 0.25 µg/mL IL13-PE38QQR with no observation of DLT. Dose escalation of peritumoral infusion concentration began at 0.5 µg/mL in stage II. Among all 9 patients treated with a peritumoral infusion, 6 received 0.5 µg/mL and 3 received 1.0 µg/mL

Table 3
IL13-PEI-103 Study Design[a]

Stage I: Escalation of infusion duration at a constant concentration of IL13-PE

Dose level	Concentration (μg/mL)	Duration (d)	Total Dose (μg)
1	0.5	4	25.9
2	0.5	5	32.4
3	0.5	6	38.9
4	0.5	7	45.4

Stage II: Escalation of IL13-PE concentration at a constant infusion duration

Dose level	Concentration (μg/mL)	Duration (d)	Total Dose (μg)
5	1.0	7	90.7
6	2.0	7	181.9
7	3.0	7	272.9
8	4.0	7	362.8

Notes:[a] In this multicenter study, patients with recurrent supratentorial malignant glioma underwent stereotactic biopsy followed by the placement of one or two catheters.

Stage I: IL13-PE was infused at a fixed concentration (0.5 μg/mL) and a fixed infusion rate of 540 μL/h/all catheters. The infusion duration was escalated from 4 d (25.9 μg) to 7 d (45.4 μg) to identify a MTD based on infusion duration.

Stage II: The concentration of IL13-PE was escalated from 1.0 μg/mL to a maximum of 4.0 μg/mL at a fixed infusion rate of 540 μL/h to identify tolerability and MTD based on concentration.

of IL13-PE. As two patients at 1.0 μg/mL of IL13-PE experienced DLT consisting of nonspecific drug toxicity to normal brain parenchyma resulting in imaging changes associated with neurological symptoms, 0.5 μg/mL concentration was considered to be the MTD for stage II. In stage III, the duration of infusion of IL13-PE was 5 and 6 d without any evidence of toxicity. Subsequently, 12 patients were enrolled in stage IV. The data available from those patients showed that the procedure was feasible and well tolerated. In addition, the placement of catheters 24 to 48 hafter resection appears to have improved the accuracy of catheter placement, with approx 90% of the catheters having been optimally positioned compared to 50% with intraoperative catheter placement. In general drug-related adverse events of grade II included headache and CNS events such as hemiparesis, sensory disturbance, aphasia, facial weakness, amnesia, seizure, dysarthria, and ataxia as well as fatigue. Overall, median patient survival through January 13, 2004 was 51.7, ranging from 8 to 169+ wk in this study, which included a great majority of GBM.

Several abstracts have summarized the findings of this study *(83–90)*.

IL13-PEI-103 Study

This multicenter study evaluated the safety, tolerability, and the maximum tolerated duration and concentration of IL13-PE38QQR administered with an intratumoral infusion followed by resection of recurrent supratentorial malignant glioma *(87,91)*. This trial was conducted at the University Hospital Eppendorf and University Hospital Kiel, Germany, the Chaim Sheba Medical Center and Tel Aviv Sourasky Medical Center, Israel; Cleveland Clinic and University of Colorado. Eligibility criteria required that patients have histologically-confirmed supratentorial grade III or IV recurrent or progressive resectable tumor (<5.0 cm) with standard radiation therapy completed 12 wk prior to study entry. Patients underwent stereotactic biopsy for histopathological confirmation. One or two catheters were placed into the contrast-enhancing component of the tumor. As shown in Table 3, in the first stage, patients received infusion of IL13-PE at a fixed concentration of 0.5 µg/mL and at a fixed infusion rate of 540 µL/h/all catheters. The infusion duration was escalated from 4 d (51.8 mL equivalent to 25.9 µg as total dose) to a maximum of 7 d (90.7 mL, total dose 45.4 µg) to identify a MTD based on infusion duration. Fourteen days later, a resection of tumor was performed and anti-tumor drug effect was determined by histopathology. In stage II, the concentration of IL13-PE was escalated from 1.0 µg/mL to a maximum of 4.0 µg/mL to identify the tolerability and MTD based on concentration at a fixed infusion rate of infusion of 540 µL/h. A total of 25 patients were treated; 13 in stage I and 9 in stage II. In addition, 3 patients were treated using the design of stage IV of study IL13PEI-002 as a single institution amendment part of study IL13-PEI-103 to assess the feasibility of deferred postoperative catheter placement. Duration of infusion up to 7 d was well tolerated. The most frequent grade II drug-related adverse events were similar to those experienced in studies IL13PEI-001 and -002. Median overall survival was 40.8 wk, ranging from 13 to 96+ wk.

IL13-PEI-105 Study

This was a pilot imaging study, which utilized ^{123}I-Human Serum Albumin (^{123}I-HSA) as a surrogate tracer to assess the distribution of IL13-PE38QQR in patients with recurrent, resectable, supratentorial malignant glioma. This study was initiated on July 2003 at Duke University Medical Center, Durham, NC. In stage I of the study, drug distribution was evaluated for both intratumoral and peritumoral infusion, whereas in stage II, only a peritumoral distribution was performed. Four patients in stage I, and three in stage II, have been treated in the biodistribution study (92). The major findings include that intratumoral infusion does not appear to result in a significant peritumoral distribution and that catheter positioning significantly influences distribution of imaging surrogate tracer supporting the treatment design with only a peritumoral infusion following gross total resection of the tumor and deferred postoperative catheter placement (92).

Design of Phase 3 Study Protocol

The results from phase I/II studies were used to determine for the treatment design of the phase III study (Fig. 2). This study "Phase III Randomized Evaluation of Convection Enhanced Delivery of IL13-PE38QQR compared to Gliadel® Wafer with Survival Endpoint" (PRECISE Study) in GBM patients at first recurrence has been recently initiated. It will compare the overall survival of patients treated with a post-resection, peritumoral infusion of IL13-PE with the overall survival of patients treated with Gliadel® Wafer at the time of surgery. Secondary and tertiary objectives of this study include the assessment of safety and toxicity, and health related quality-of-life parameters, respectively in these patients. In the IL13-PE arm, histopathological confirmation of viable glioma consistent with recurrent/progressive will be determined from frozen section of resected tumor. Tumor resection will be followed by placement of 2 to 4 peritumoral catheters in a separate procedure 2 to 7 d later. A continuous peritumoral infusion of IL13-PE will be administered at a concentration of 0.5 µg/mL and a total flow rate (all catheters) of 750 µL/h for 96 h (Fig. 3). A total of 36.0 µg in a total volume of 72 mL is to be administered (Fig. 2). In a GLIADEL® Wafer arm, the tumor will be resected and confirmed for viable glioma followed by postresection placement of up to eight Wafers (3.85% carmustine, or 7.7 mg carmustine/Wafer). Patients will be assigned

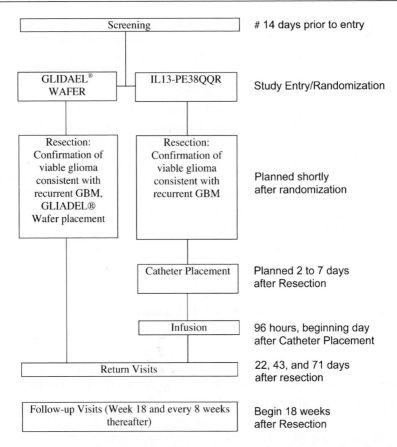

Fig. 2. Treatment scheme of phase 3 (PRECISE) study protocol. After screening, the eligible patients will be randomized and assigned either to the IL13-PE or GLIADEL® wafer arm in 2:1 ratio. In IL13-PE arm, 2 to 4 peritumoral catheters will be placed followed by infusion of IL13-PE at a concentration of 0.5 μg/mL and a flow rate of 750 μL/h/all catheters for 96 h. In GLIADEL® Wafer arm, up to 8 Wafers (7.7 mg Carmustine/Wafer) will be placed after resection of tumor.

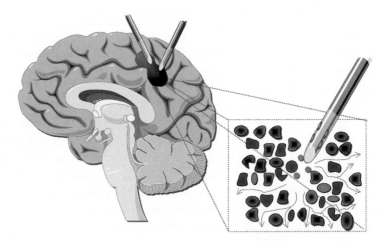

Fig. 3. CED of IL13-PE. The human brain diagram displays the placement of two catheters in to tumor mass (shown in blue color). IL13-PE is microinfused into brain tissues using pressure gradients. The enlarged area displays the regional distribution of the drug near the tip of the catheter. The homogeneity of drug distribution may be affected by interstitial fluid flow and hydrostatic pressure gradients.

either to the IL13-PE or GLIADEL® Wafer treatment group in a 2:1 ratio via central randomization. A total of 270 patients will be enrolled to evaluate efficacy of IL13-PE. Approximately 50 centers worldwide are expected to participate in the study. All AEs will be collected until disease progression, and then only SAEs related to study drug.

Immunogenicity and Serum Level

In a study to assess immunogenicity, 21% of patients possessed IgG antibody to IL13-PE prior to drug administration as determined by qualitative enyme-linked immunosorbent assay. Two of 7 (29%) and 11 of 15 (73%) evaluable patients in the IL13PEI-002 and IL13PE-103 studies, respectively developed IgG Ab to IL13-PE following drug administration. The IgG Ab produced in response to IL13-PE was specific for PE and not to the IL-13 portion of the molecule. The higher frequency of antibody development in IL13PEI-103 study patients may be related to the intratumoral delivery exposing the humoral immune system to the drug either through blood–tumor barrier disruption or local lymphocytic infiltration.

IL13-PE was not detected in the serum of any patient immediately after CED of the drug in either study. The lower limit of quantification for the cell-based cytotoxicity assay was <20 ng/mL.

CONCLUSION

Expression of IL-13R at a high density (relative to normal cells) provided a potential therapeutic target for IL13-PE38QQR. IL-13R were over-expressed on glioma cell lines and primary explants of malignant gliomas. IL-13R on glioma cells were composed of two IL-13 binding proteins; IL-13Rα1 and IL-13Rα2. IL-13Rα2 chain, the primary binding subunit of IL-13R complex binds to IL-13 with high affinity. We recently demonstrated that IL-13Rα2 chain is internalized after binding to IL-13 but did not induce signal transduction through the STAT6 pathway (64). Gene transfer of IL-13Rα2 chain into glioma cells that lack this chain can sensitize naive cells to the cytotoxic effect of IL13-PE (71,72). Furthermore, reverse-transcriptase polymerase chain reaction analyses and immunofluorescence studies confirmed that IL-13Rα2 chain is over-expressed in a majority of malignant gliomas and can serve as a biomarker for targeting immunotoxin or may act as tumor-associated antigen for specific immunotherapy (45,93). It is encouraging to note that IL13-PE38QQR kills only IL-13R positive cells, but not normal brain cells (46), which express either a low number of receptors or no receptors (45). This selective binding may provide a relative therapeutic window for targeting glioma cells versus normal cells.

The remarkable in vitro cytotoxicity of IL13-PE translated well into GBM animal models. Subcutaneous GBM tumors in mice regressed completely in response to local delivery of IL13-PE in absence of unintended toxicity. It is known that toxin moieties of immunotoxins, including PE, diphtheria toxin, and ricin kill cells not only by inhibition of protein synthesis but also by concomitant induction of apoptosis (94). We demonstrated that intratumoral delivery of IL13-PE38QQR caused induction of proapoptic molecules such as caspase-3, -8 and -9; cleavage of pro-caspase-3 and poly(ADP-ribose) polymerase; and release of cytochrome-c from mitochondria to cytoplasmic compartment. These two major apoptotic pathways appeared to play a role, at least in part, in the regression of tumors in xenograft models (95).

Our phase I/II clinical studies in recurrent supratentorial malignant glioma patients demonstrated that IL13-PE may be delivered safely using CED, bypassing the blood–brain barrier and minimizing systemic exposure. A higher concentration of IL13-PE can then be achieved within the tumor, as well as the brain parenchyma surrounding resection cavity, containing infiltrating tumor cells. Symptoms related to edema and local mass effect in IL13-PEI-001 protocol were minimized by implementation of pre- and post-treatment corticosteroid use guidelines. IL13-PE peritumoral infusion was well tolerated in part because overall tumor mass effect and edema was reduced by tumor resection. The evidence of regional necrosis at a concentration of 0.5, 1.0 and 2.0 µg/mL indicate the histological effects of the drug on tumor cells. There was no apparent increased histopathological effect with increasing concentration across these concentration levels (85). However, a postresection peritumoral MTD with a drug concentration of 0.5 µg/mL was identified in stage II of IL13PEI-002. Longer duration infusion (up to 7 d) at the fixed concentration of IL13-PE (0.5 µg/mL) in studies IL13PEI-002 and IL13-PEI-103 was also well tolerated in all patients. Although phase I studies are typically designed to assess safety and toxicity of study drug, encouraging patient survival in several subjects was observed in all three studies suggesting IL13-PE effect on tumor control.

The proposed IL13-PE concentration (0.5 µg/mL) for phase III is based upon HEC and peritumoral maximum tolerated infusion concentration determined in study IL13PEI-002. A concentration of 0.5 µg/mL is at least three log units higher than the IC_{50} of most glioma cells (Table 1) but is well below the no effect level (NOEL) of 100 µg/mL obtained in rodent safety evaluations for acute toxicity (76). For phase III, a fixed volume (72 mL, 18.0 mL/d) of infusion was selected to standardize the procedure and because supratentorial gliomas have an invasive and migrating phenotype and often infiltrate a large portion of a cerebral hemisphere despite their confined appearance on imaging studies. Other clinical trials using CED for malignant glioma have used infusion for as long as 16 d (34). There may be no benefit of continuing CED for a 16-d duration for 2 reasons: (1) a steady state of convection may occur after a number of days and (2) additional volume of infusion will not result in a significant expansion of the diameter of the volume of distribution. Another major consideration is the risk of infection associated with externalized catheters, which starts to increase on average 6 d after the device placement (96). A duration of infusion of 96 h and a 24- to 48-h period of observation will allow catheter removal in less than 6 d to reduce the risk of infection.

The ongoing phase III multicenter trial will determine whether efficacy of IL-13-PE in patients with GBM can be found at first recurrence. Several issues such as distribution of drug within tumor mass as well as to infiltrating tumor cells surrounding brain parenchyma, location of catheters, catheter configuration have been or are being addressed. As GBM is a heterogenous tumor that expresses several different types of receptors, a combination therapy using immunotoxins targeting different receptors, may be another approach for optimal treatment of these tumors.

ACKNOWLEDGMENTS

We would like to thank Drs. Donald Fink and Koji Kawakami for reviewing the manuscript. We acknowledge the contributions of Drs. Bharat Joshi, Koji Kawakami, Mariko Kawakami, Mitomu Kioi, Nicholas Obiri, and Ms. Pamela Dover of Laboratory of Molecular Tumor Biology, CBER and Drs. Aquilur Rahman, Prafulla Gokhle, and Usha Kasid of Georgetown University, Washington, DC for manufacturing of IL13-PE and its preclinical studies. The studies presented herein were conducted as part of a collaboration between the Food and Drug Administration and NeoPharm Inc, Lake Forest, IL, under a Cooperative Research and Development Agreement (CRADA). We thank the New Approaches to Brain Tumor Therapy (NABTT), CNS Consortium, Baltimore MD, especially Drs. Stuart Grossman and Jon Weingart for their leadership in the first NCI-sponsored clinical trial. Acknowledgments are given to Drs. Michael Prados, Sandeep Kunwar, and Mitchell Berger of University of California San Francisco, Joseph Piepmeier of Yale University, Philip Gutin and Jeffrey Raizer of Memorial Sloan-Kettering, NY, Ken Aldape, Frederick Lang, and Alfred Yung of MD Anderson Cancer Center, TX for conducting the second trial at their centers. We also thank Dr. Zvi Ram of the Chaim Sheba Medical Center in Israel, Drs. Gene Barnett and Michael Vogelbaum of the Cleveland Clinic, Dr. Shlomo Constantini of the Dana Hospital in Israel, Dr. Kevin Lillehei of the University of Colorado Health Sciences Center, Dr. Maximilian Medhorn of the University Hospital Kiel in Germany, and Dr. Manfred Westphal of the University Hospital of Eppendorf in Germany for supervising the third clinical trial and John Sampson and his colleagues at Duke University for conducting the fourth clinical trial. We are extremely grateful to Dr. Jeffrey Sherman, Dr. Theodora Cohen, Dr. David Croteau, Amy Grahn, Dr. Imran Ahmad, Jim Hussey, John Kapoor, and Greg Young of NeoPharm, Inc. for their unwavering support in the development of IL13-PE.

Note added to the proof: At the time of the review of the proofs, the Phase 3 (PRECISE) was completed. A total of 288 patients were enrolled. These patients are being monitored for clinical responses.

REFERENCES

1. Kawakami K, Aggarwal BB, Puri RK. eds. Cytotoxins and Immunotoxins for Cancer Therapy: Clinical Applications. New York:Taylor and and Francis CRC Press; 2004.
2. Kreitman, RJ. Immunotoxin in cancer therapy. Curr Opin Immunol 1999;11:570–578.
3. Brandes AA, Basso U, Pasetto LM, Ermani B. New strategy developments in brain tumor therapy. Curr Pharm Design 2001;7:1553–1580.
4. Basso U, Ermani B, Vastola F, Brandes AA. Non-cytotoxic therapies for malignant glioma. J Neuro-Oncol 2002;58:57–69.
5. Amlot PL, Stone MJ, Cunnigham D, Fay J, Newman J, Collins R, May R, McCarthy M, Richardson J, Ghetie V, Ramilo O, Thorpe PE, Uhr JW, Vitetta ES. A phase I study of anti-D22-deglycosylated Ricin A chain immuno- toxin in the treatment of B-cell lymphomas resistant to conventional therapy. Blood 1993;82:2624–2633.
6. Reiter Y. Recombinant immunotoxins in targeted cancer therapy. Adv Cancer Res 2001;81:93–124.
7. Laske DW, Ilercil O, Akbasak A, Youle RJ, Oldfield E H. Efficacy of direct intratumoral therapy with targeted protein toxins for solid human gliomas in nude mice. J Neurosurg 1994;80:520–526.
8. Husain SR, Behari N, Kreitman RJ, Pastan I, Puri RK. Complete regression of established human glioblastoma tumor xenograft by interleukin-4 toxin therapy. Cancer Res 1998;58:3649–3653.
9. Husain SR, Kreitman RJ, Pastan I, Puri RK. Interleukin-4 receptor directed cytotoxin therapy of AIDS-associated Kaposi's sarcoma tumors in xenograft model. Nature Med 1999;5:817–822.
10. Husain SR, Puri RK. Interleukin-13 fusion cytotoxin as a potent targeted drug for AIDS-Kaposi's sarcoma xenograft. Blood 2000;95:3506–513.
11. Vallera DA, Li C, Jin N, Panoskaltsis-Mortari A, Hall WA. Targeting urokinase-type plasminogen activator receptor on human glioblastoma tumors with diphtheria toxin fusion protein DTAT. J Natl Cancer Inst 2002;94:597–606.
12. Li C, Hall WA, Jin N, Panoskaltsis-Mortari A, Vallera DA. Targeting glioblastoma multiforme with an IL-13/diphtheria toxin fusion protein in vitro and in vivo in nude mice. Protein Eng 2002;15:419–427.
13. Kawakami M, Kawakami K, Puri RK, Interleukin-4-Pseudomonas exotoxin chimeric protein for malignant glioma therapy. J Neuro-Oncol 2003;65:15–25.
14. Pai LH, Wittes R, Setser A, Willingham MC, Pastan I. Treatment of advanced solid tumors with immunotoxin LMB-1:An antibody linked to Pseudomonas exotoxin. Nature Med 1996;2:350–353.
15. Kreitman RJ, Wilson WH, White JD. Stetler-Stevenson M, Jaffe E, Waldman TA, Pastan I. Phase I trial of recombinant immunotoxin Anti-Tac(Fv)-PE38 (LMB-2) in patients with hematologic malignancies. J Clin Oncol 2000;8:1622–1636
16. Kreitman RJ, Wilson WH, Robbins D. Margulis I, Stetler-Stevenson M, Waldman TA, Pastan I. Responses in refractory hairy cell leukemia to a recombinant immunotoxin. Blood 1999;94:3340–3348.
17. Stone MJ, Sausville EA, Fay JW, et al. A phase I study of bolus versus continuous infusion of the anti-CD19 immunotoxin, IgG-HD37-dgA, in-patients with B-cell lymphoma. Blood 1996;88:1188–1197.
18. Hesketh P, Caguioa P, Koh H, et al. Clinical activity of a cytotoxic fusion protein in the treatment of cutaneous T-cell lymphoma. Blood 1993;11:1682–1690.

19. LeMaistre CF, Saleh MN, Kuzel, TM, et al. Phase 1 trial of ligand fusion-protein (DAB$_{389}$IL-2) in lymphomas expressing the receptor for interleukin-2. Blood 1998;91:399–405.

20. Pai LH, Wittes R, Setser A, Willingham MC, Pastan I. Treatment of advanced solid tumors with immunotoxin LMB-1: an antibody linked to *Pseudomonas* exotoxin. Nature Med 1996;2:350–353.

21. Chaudhary VK, Queen C, Junghans RP, Waldmann TA, Fitzgerald DJ, Pastan I. A recombinant immunotoxin consisting of two antibody variable domains fused to *Pseudomonas* exotoxin. Nature 1989;339:394–397.

22. Kreitman RJ, Pastan I. Targeting *Pseudomonas* exotoxin to hematological malignancies Semin Cancer Biol 1995;6:297–306.

23. Pastan I. Immunotoxins containing *Pseudomonas* exotoxin A: a short history. Cancer Immunol Immunother 2003;52:338–341.

24. Kreitman RJ, Wilson WH, Bergeron K, et al. Efficacy of the anti-CD22 recombinant immunotoxin BL22 in chemotherapy resistant hairy-cell leukemia. N Eng J Med 2001;345:241–247.

25. Chawdhury PS, Viner JL, Beers R, Pastan I. Isolation of high affinity stable single chain Fv specific for mesothelin from DNA-immunized mice by phage display and construction of a recombinant immunotoxin with anti-tumor activity. Proc Natl Acad Sci USA 1998;95:669–674.

26. Olsen E, Duvic M, Frankel A, et al. Pivotal phase III trial of two dose levels of denileukin diftitox for the treatment of cutaneous T-cell lymphoma. J Clin Oncol 2001;19:376–388.

27. Liu TF, Chen KA, Ramage JG, Willingham MC, Thorburn AM, Frankel AE. A diphtheria toxin-epidermal growth factor fusion protein is cytotoxic to human glioblastoma multiforme cells. Cancer Res 2003;63:1834–1837.

28. Foss FM, Saleh MN, Kruger JG, Nicholas JC, Murphy JR Diphtheria toxin fusion proteins. In: Frankel AE, ed. Berlin:Springer-Verlag. Clinical Applications of Immunotoxins. Curr Topics Microbiol Immunol 1998;234:63–81.

29. Lorimer IA, Keppler-Hafkemeyer A, Beers RA, Pegram CN, Bigner DD, Pastan I. Immunotoxins that target an oncogenic mutant epidermal growth factor receptor expressed in human tumors. Clin Cancer Res 1995;1:859–864.

30. Piccaluga PP, Martinelli G, Rondoni M, Malagola M, Gaitani S, Visani G, Baccarani M.First experience with gemtuzumab ozogamicin plus cytarabine as continuous infusion for elderly acute myeloid leukaemia patients. Leukemia Res 2004;28:987–990.

31. Sievers EL. Antibody-targeted chemotherapy of acute myeloid leukemia using gemtuzumab ozogamicin (Mylotarg). Blood Cells Molecules Diseases 2003;31:7–10.

32. Schnell R, Borchmann P, Staak JO, Ghetie V, Vitetta ES, Engert A. Clinical evaluation of ricin A-chain immunotoxins in patients with Hodgkin's lymphoma. Ann Oncol 2003;14:729–736.

33. National Center for Health Statistics for the United States, 1994. Washington, DC: Public Health Service; 1997.

34. Laske DW, Youle RJ, Oldfield EH. Tumor regression with regional distribution of the targeted toxin TF-CRM107 in patients with malignant brain tumors. Nature Med 1997;3:1362–1368.

35. Oldfield E H, Youle RJ. Immunotoxin for brain tumor therapy. Curr Opin Microbiol 1998;234:9–114.

36. Weaver M, Laske DW. Transferrin receptor ligand-targeted toxin conjugate (TfCRM107) for therapy of malignant gliomas. J Neuro-Oncol 2003;65:3–14.

37. Phillips PC, Levow C, Caterall M, Colvin OM, Pastan I, Brem H. Transforming growth factor-α-*Pseudomonas* exotoxin fusion protein (TGF-PE38) treatment of subcutaneous and intracranial human glioma and medulloblastoma xenografts in athymic mice. Cancer Res 1994;54:1008–1015.

38. Sampson JH, Akabani G, Archer GE, et al. Progress report of a Phase I study of the intracerebral microinfusion of a recombinant chimeric protein composed of transforming growth factor (TGF)-α and a mutated form of the *Pseudomonas* exotoxin termed PE38 (TP-38) for the treatment of malignant brain tumors. J Neuro-Oncol 2003;65:27–35.

39. Rustamzadeh E, Li CB, Doumbia S, Hall WA, Vallera DA. Targeting the over-expressedurokinase-type plasminogen activator receptor on glioblastoma multiforme. J Neuro-Oncol 2003;65:63–75.

40. Todhunter DA, Hall WA, Rustamzadeh E, Shu YQ, Doumbia SO, Vallera DA. A bispecific immunotoxin (DTAT13) targeting human IL-13 receptor (IL-13R) and urokinase-type plasminogen activator receptor (uPAR) in a mouse xenograft model. Protein Engg Design Select 2004;17:157–164.

41. Rand RW, Kreitman RJ, Patronas N, Varricchio F, Pastan I, Puri RK. Intratumoral administration of recombinant circularly permuted interleukin-4-*Pseudomonas* exotoxin inpatients with high grade glioma. Clin Cancer Res 2000;6:2157–2165.

42. Weber F, Asher A, Bucholz R, et al. Safety, tolerability, and tumor response of IL-4-*Pseudomonas* exotoxin (NBI-30010) in patients with recurrent malignant glioma J.Neuro-Oncol 2003;64:125–137.

43. Rainov NG, Heidecke V. Long term survival in a patient with recurrent malignant glioma treated with intratumoral infusion of an IL4-targeted toxin (NBI-3001). J Neuro-Oncol 2004;66:197–201.

44. Debinski W, Obiri NI, Powers SK, Pastan I, Puri RK. Human glioma cells overexpress receptors for interleukin 13 and are extremely sensitive to a novel chimeric protein composed of interleukin 13 and *Pseudomonas* exotoxin. Clin Cancer Res 1995;1:1253–1258.

45. Joshi BH, Plautz GE, Puri RK. Interleukin-13 receptor α chain: a novel tumor-associated transmembrane protein in primary explants of human malignant gliomas. Cancer Res 2000;60:1168–1172.

46. Husain SR, Puri RK. Interleukin-13 receptor-directed cytotoxin for malignant glioma therapy: from bench to bedside. J Neuro-Oncol 2003;65:37–48.

47. Kuzel T, Smith II J, Urba W, Fox B, Moudgil T, Strauss L, Joshi B, Puri R. IL13-PE38QQR cytotoxicity in advanced renal cell carcinoma (RCC): phase 1 and pharmacokinetics study. San Francisco:American Society of Clinical Oncology (ASCO); 2002.

48. Zurawski G, De Vries JE. Interleukin 13, an interleukin 4-like cytokine that acts on monocytes and B cells, but not on T cells. Immunol Today 1994;15:19–26.

49. Punnonen J, Aversa G, Cocks BG, et al. Interleukin 13 induces interleukin 4-independent IgG4 and IgE synthesis and CD23 expression by human B cells. Proc Natl Acad Sci USA 1993;90:3730–3734.

50. Minty A, Chalon P, Derocq J-M, et al. Interleukin-13 is a new human lymphokine regulating inflammatory and immune responses. Nature 1993;362:248–250.

51. Defrance T, Carayon P, Billian G, et al. Interleukin-13 is a B cell stimulatory factor. J Exp Med 994;179: 135–143.

52. Herber J-M, Savi P, Laplace MC, et al. IL-4 and IL-13 exhibit comparable abilities to reduce pyrogen-induced expression of procoagulant activity in endothelial cells and monocytes. FEBS Lett 1993;328: 268–270.

53. Obiri NI, Debinski W, Leonard WJ, Puri RK. Receptor for interleukin 13. Interaction with interleukin 4 by a mechanism that does not involve the common γ chain shared by receptors for interleukin 2, 4, 7, 9, and 15. J Biol Chem 1995;270:8797–8804.

54. Husain SR, Obiri NI, Gill P, et al. Receptors for interleukin 13 on AIDS-associated Kaposi's sarcoma cells serves as a new target for a potent *Pseudomonas* exotoxin-based chimeric toxin protein. Clin Cancer Res 1997; 3:151–156.

55. Obiri NI, Leland P, Murata T, Debinski W, Puri RK. The IL-13 receptor structure differs on various cell types and may share more than one component with IL-4 receptor complex. J Immunol 1997;158:756–764.

56. Miloux B, Laurent P, Bonnin O, Luker J, Caput D, Vita N, Ferrara P. Cloning of the human IL-13Ralpha1 chain and reconstitution with the IL-4R alpha of functional IL-4/IL-13 receptor complex. FEBS Lett 1997;401:163–166.

57. Hilton DJ, Zhang, JG, Metcalf D, Alexander WS, Nicola NA, Wilson TA. Cloning and characterization of binding subunits of the interleukin 13 receptor that is also a component of the interleukin 4 receptor. Proc Natl Acad Sci USA 1996;93:497–501.

58. Aman MJ, Tayebi N, Obiri NI, Puri RK, Modi WS, Leonard W. cDNA cloning and characterization of the human interleukin 13 receptor α chain. J Biol Chem 1996;271:29,265–29,670.

59. Murata T, Obiri NI, Puri RK. Structure and signal transduction through interleukin-4 and interleukin-13 receptors, Int J Mol Med 1998;1:551–557.

60. Caput D, Laurent P, Kaghad M, et al. Cloning and characterization of a specific interleukin (IL)-13 binding protein structurally related to IL-5 receptor α chain. J Biol Chem 1996;271:16,921–16,926.

61. Kawakami M, Leland P, Kawakami K, Puri RK. Mutation and functional analysis of IL-13 receptors in human malignant glioma cells. Oncol Res 2001;12:459–467.

62. Donaldson DD, Whitters MJ, Fitz LJ, et al. The murine IL-13 receptor α2: Molecular cloning, characterization, and comparison with murine IL-13 receptor α1. J Immunol 1998;161:2317–2324.

63. Murata T, Obiri NI, Debinski W, Puri RK. Structure of IL-13 receptor: analysis of subunit composition in cancer and immune cells. Biochem Biophys Res Comm 1997;238:90–94.

64. Joshi BH, Husain SR, Puri RK. Preclinical studies with IL-13PE38QQR for therapy of malignant glioma. Drug News Perspect 2000;13:599–605.

65. Schnyder B, Lugi S, Fenf N, et al. Interleukin-4 (IL-4) and IL-13 bind to a shared heterodimeric complex on endothelial cells mediating vascular cell adhesion molecule-1 induction in the absence of the common γ chain. Blood 1996;87:4286–4295.

66. Kawakami K, Kawakami M, Snoy P, Husain SR, Puri RK. In vivo overexpression of IL-13 receptor α2 chain inhibits tumorigenicity of human breast and pancreatic tumors in immunodeficient mice. J Ex Med 2001;196:1743–1754.

67. Kawakami K, Husain SR, Bright RK, Puri RK. Gene transfer of interleukin 13 receptor α2 chain dramatically enhances the antitumor effect of IL-13 receptor-targeted cytotoxin in human prostate cancer xenografts. Cancer Gene Ther 2001;8:861–868.

68. Vita N, Lefort S, Laurent P, Caput D, Ferrara P. Characterization and comparison of the interleukin 13 receptor with the interleukin 4 receptor on several cell types. J Biol Chem 1995;270:3512–3517.

69. Kawakami K, Taguchi J, Murata T, Puri RK. The interleukin-13 receptor α2 chain: an essential component for binding and internalization but not interleukin-13-induced signal transduction through the STAT6 pathway. Blood 2001;97:2673–2679.

70. Joshi BH, Husain SR, Leland P, Puri RK. Interleukin-13 receptors and development of IL-13-*Pseudomonas* exotoxin for human cancer therapy. In: Aggarwal BB, Kawakami K, Puri RK, eds. Cytotoxins and Immunotoxins for Cancer Therapy: Clinical applications. New York: Taylor and Frances CRC Press; 2004:45–69.

71. Kawakami K, Joshi BH, Puri RK. Sensitization of cancer cells to interleukin-13-Pseudomonas exotoxin-induced cell death by gene transfer of interleukin-13 α chain. Hum Gene Ther 2000;11:1829–1835.

72. Kawakami K, Kawakami M, Puri RK. Cytokine receptor as a sensitizer for targeted cancer therapy. Anticancer Drugs 2002;13:693–699.

73. Pastan I, Chaudhary VK, FitzGerald D. Recombinant toxins as novel therapeutic agents. Annu Rev Biochem 1992;61:331–354.

74. Joshi BH, Kawakami K, Leland P, Puri RK. Heterogeneity in interleukin-13 receptor expression and subunit structure in squamous cell carcinoma of head and neck: Differential sensitivity of to chimeric fusion proteins comprised of interleukin-13 and a mutated form of *Pseudomonas* exotoxin. Clin Cancer Res 2002;8:1948–1956.

75. Debinski W, Obiri NI, Pastan I, Puri RK. A novel chimeric protein composed of interleukin 13 and *Pseudomonas* exotoxin is highly cytotoxic to human carcinoma cells expressing receptors for interleukin 13 and interleukin 4. J Biol Chem 1995;270:16,775–16,780.

76. Husain SR, Joshi, BH, Puri RK. Interleukin-13 Receptors as a unique target for anti-glioblastoma therapy. Int J Cancer 2001;92:168–175.

77. Husain SR, Kawakami M, Kawakami K, Snoy PJ, Puri RK. Continuous intraperitoneal infusion increases the efficacy and safety of IL-13 toxin in elimination of established human glioblastoma tumor xenografts. Proc Amer Assn Cancer Res 2001;42:777.

78. Zurawski SM, Chomarat P, Djossou O, et al. The primary binding subunit of the human interleukin-4 receptor is also a component of the interleukin-13 receptor. J Biol Chem 1995;270:13,869–13,878.

79. Husain SR, Oshima Y, Gokhale PC, Kasid UN, Puri RK. Pre-clinical safety evaluation of recombinant interleukin 13-pseudomonas exotoxin (IL13-PE38) for targeted cancer therapy. Proc Amer Assoc Cancer Res 2003;44(1st Ed.):1257 and 44(2nd Ed.):1092.

80. Weingart J, Grossman SA, Bohan E, Fisher JD, Strauss L, Puri, RK. Phase I/II study of interstitial infusion of IL13-PE38QQR cytotoxin in recurrent malignant glioma. Washington, DC: First Quadrennial meeting—World Federation of Neuro-Oncology. November 15–17, 2001.

81. Weingart J, Strauss LC Grossman SA, Markett J, Tatter S, Fisher JD, Fleming CK, Puri RK. Phase I/II study: Intra-tumoral infusion of IL13-PE38QQR cytotoxin for recurrent supratentorial malignant glioma. Neuro-oncology 2002;4:379.

82. Weingart J, Markert J, Tatter S, et al. Determination of toxicities and maximum tolerated dose (MTD) of intra-tumoral infusion of IL13-PE38QQR cytotoxin in patients with recurrent supratentorial malignant glioma: a phase I/II study. Proc Am Soc Clin Oncol 2003;22:101.

83. Prados, MD, Lang FF, Strauss L, et al. Intratumoral and intracerebral microinfusion of IL13-PE38QQR cytotoxin: Phase I/II study of pre- and post-resection infusions in recurrent resectable malignant glioma. Proc Am Soc Clin Oncol 2002;21(2):69b.

84. Lang F, Kunwar S, Strauss L, et al. A clinical study of convection-enhanced delivery of IL13-PE38QQR cytotoxin pre- and post-resection of recurrent GBM. Chicago: American Society of Neuro-Oncologists; April, 2002.

85. Prados MD, Lang FF, Sherman JW, et al. Convection-enhanced delivery (CED) by positive pressure infusion for intra-tumoral and peri-tumoral administration of IL13-PE38QQR a recombinant tumor-targeted cytotoxin in recurrent malignant glioma. Neuro-oncology 2002;4:S78.

85. Prados MD, Lang FF, Strauss LC et al. Pre- and Post- resection interstitial infusion of IL13-PE38QQR cytotoxin: Phase I study in recurrent resectable malignant glioma. Washington, DC: Quadrennial Meeting of the World Federation of Neuro-Oncology; Nov 15–18, 2001.

86. Kunwar S. Convection enhanced delivery of IL13-PE38QQR for treatment of recurrent malignant glioma: presentation of interim findings from ongoing phase 1 studies. In: Westphal M, Tonn JC, Ram, ed. New York: Springer Wien. Local therapies for glioma: present status and future development, Acta Neurochir Suppl 2003;88:105–111.

88. Kunwar S, Prados MD, Lang FF, et al. Intratumoral and peritumoral convection-enhanced delivery of IL13-PE38QQR, a recombinant tumor-targeted cytotoxin in a recurrent malignant glioma phase I trial. J Neurosurg 2003;98:697.
89. Kunwar S, Prados M, Lang F, et al. Intracerebral convection-enhanced delivery (CED) of IL13-PE38QQR, a recombinant tumor-targeted cytotoxin, in recurrent malignant glioma: a phase I trial. Neuro-oncology 2003;5:387.
90. Kunwar S, Prados M, Lang F, et al. Pre- and post-operative infusion of IL13-PE38QQR cytotoxin by convection-enhanced delivery (CED) in recurrent malignant glioma: a phase I study. Proc Am Soc Clin Oncol 2003;22:119.
91. Ram Z, Barnett G, Vogelbaum M, et al. Pre-operative infusion of IL13-PE38QQR cytotoxin by convection-enhanced delivery (CED) in recurrent malignant glioma: a phase I/II study. Proc Am Soc Clin Oncol 2003;22:101.
92. Sampson JH, Friedman AH, Reardon DA, et al. Convection Enhanced Delivery of IL13-PE38QQR in Malignant Glioma: Effect of Catheter Placement on Drug Distribution. Orlando, FL: American Association of Neurological Surgeons Annual Meeting; 2004.
93. Kawakami M, Kawakami K, Abe M, Puri RK. Analysis of interleukin-13 receptor α2 expression in human pediatric brain tumors. Cancer 2004;101:1036–1042.
94. Brinkmann U, Keppler-Hafkemeyer A, Hafkemeyer P. Recombinant immunotoxins for cancer therapy. Exp Opin Biol Ther 2001;1:693–702.
95. Kawakami M, Kawakami K, Puri RK. Intratumor administration of interleukin 13 receptortargeted cytotoxin induces apoptotic cell death in human malignant glioma tumor xenografts. Mol Cancer Ther 2002;1:999–1007.
96. Kim DK, Uttley B, Bell BA, Marsh HT, Moore AJ. Comparison of rates of infection of two methods of emergency ventricular damage. J Neurol Neurosurg Psych 1995;58:444–446.

20 Small Molecule Agents

Michael Vogelbaum and Tina Thomas

Summary

The prognosis for patients with malignant gliomas remains poor despite investigation of multiple novel therapies. Ongoing discovery of many of the genetic alterations associated with the transformed phenotype has permitted the development of new therapeutic approaches focused specifically on attacking these changes in neoplastic cells. Targeted therapies can be divided into three categories: (1) monoclonal antibodies (MAbs), (2) antisense oligonucleotides, and (3) small molecule drugs (SMDs). SMDs target growth factors and their receptors, downstream signaling signal transduction cascades, cell–cycle control molecules, and modulators of apoptosis, or invasion factors. This chapter focuses on the rationale for using small molecule targeted therapy for the treatment of malignant gliomas, and on progress made in the development of this class of drugs for clinical use. In the future, molecular profiling of gliomas will provide a basis for individualized "tailored therapy" using targeted molecules along with traditional cytotoxic therapies.

Key Words: Glioma inhibitors; growth factors; high-grade glioma (HGG); small molecule drugs (SMDs); targeted therapy; tyrosine kinase inhibitors.

BACKGROUND

The prognosis for patients with malignant gliomas remains poor despite active investigation of multiple new types of chemotherapy. Despite the lack of clinical progress, there has been significant progress in elucidating many of the specific genetic defects associated with high-grade gliomas (HGG). Overexpression or amplification of oncogenes (e.g., EGF/EGFR, PDGF/PDGFR, CDK4, MDM-2, Ras, Akt) as well as mutation or deletion of tumor suppressor genes (e.g., PTEN, TP53, Rb, p16INK4, p14ARF) are a few of the defects that have been implicated in the development and resistance to therapy of these tumors *(1–4)*. Oncogenes are involved in membrane-related and internal signal-transduction pathways that affect cell proliferation and growth potential, whereas tumor suppressor genes are negative regulators of the cell cycle or inhibit signal-transduction pathways *(2)*. These genetic changes have profound effects on the activation states of cellular signal-transduction pathways, which results in the transformed phenotype. Cancer cells may become dependent on these altered pathways for survival, unlike normal cells which can usually compensate for inhibition of one pathway by activation of redundant, parallel pathways. This new understanding has permitted the development of new therapeutic approaches focused specifically on attacking these alterations found only in cancer cells *(5,6)*.

From: *Current Clinical Oncology: High-Grade Gliomas: Diagnosis and Treatment*
Edited by: G. H. Barnett © Humana Press Inc., Totowa, NJ

Signal Transduction and New Targeted Therapies

Unlike conventional cytotoxic chemotherapies, targeted therapies are intended to be more specific for cancer cells and, consequently, to have less toxicity *(7,8)*. At the present time, targeted therapies can be divided into three categories: (1) monoclonal antibodies (MAbs), (2) antisense oligonucleotides, and (3) small molecule drugs (SMDs).

ANTIBODY-BASED THERAPIES

Antibody-based therapies involve the use of MAbs directed against a specific target, which is usually extracellular. These antibodies block initiation of receptor-mediated signaling by attaching to the extracellular domain of cell surface receptors, thereby impeding interactions with ligand and/or blocking receptor dimerization *(9,10)*. They may also initiate immune responses, including complement-mediated or antibody-dependent cell-mediated cytotoxicity, and cause receptor downregulation or internalization *(10,11)*. Examples of these are trastuzumab (Herceptin), which is directed against HER2, and cetuximab (C225), which is directed against epidermal growth factor receptor (EGFR). A newer approach uses "armed antibodies" by conjugating immunotoxins, fusion proteins, radionuclides, or immunoliposomes to the antibody to create additional cytotoxic effects *(5,10)*. This approach is of limited utility in central nervous system (CNS) malignancies because of the inability of these agents to cross the blood–brain barrier (BBB) *(12)*. In addition, some mutant receptors present in glioblastoma multiforme (GBM) have an altered or missing extracellular domain *(9)*.

ANTISENSE OLIGONUCLEOTIDES

Antisense oligonucleotides are short sequences of nucleotides that bind with high affinity to complementary messenger RNA (mRNA) and prevent translation by either steric blocking of the ribosome complex or by causing mRNA cleavage by RNase H *(13–15)*. They may be used to block synthesis of gene products that are involved in signal transduction, such as growth factor receptors. Because of their short half-life, they must be administered by continuous intravenous (iv) infusion. Furthermore, their highly negative charge and high molecular-weight impede their penetration of the intact BBB *(13)*.

SMALL MOLECULE INHIBITORS OF PROTEIN SIGNALING

Small molecule inhibitors of protein signaling pathways, which will be the focus of this chapter, are low-molecular-weight, non-immunogenic compounds designed to interfere with the growth and invasion of neoplastic cells *(5)*. SMDs can be engineered to attack specific targets of choice. Small molecule inhibitors of signal transduction target the three distinct levels of cell signal transduction: the input layer, composed of ligands (e.g., growth factors); the receptor level (e.g., EGFR); and the output level, composed of secondary signaling events (e.g., Ras/Raf/MEK/MAPK pathway). Other SMDs target matrix metalloproteinases, proteasomes, as well as pro-apoptotic and anti-apoptotic proteins. Because of their small size, these drugs have a theoretical advantage over their traditional large molecule counterparts because of more effective penetration into cells and tissues. The most extensively studied SMDs have been the quinazolines or pyrazolo/pyrrolo/pyrido pyrimidines, which compete with adenosine triphosphate (ATP) for binding to the intracellular domain of growth factor receptors ("adenine mimicry") and thus block their activation and subsequent signal transduction *(2,16)*.

TARGETING STRATEGIES

Cellular targets for cancer therapy may be divided into four broad categories:

1. Growth factors (mitogens) and their receptors, such as EGF/EGFR, PDGF/PDGFR, and VEGF/VEGFR. Rationales for the targeting of these factors include:
   a. These factors modulate cell division, proliferation and differentiation.
   b. Their receptors are overexpressed on tumor cells.
   c. The structure of these targets is known and they can be manipulated genetically or chemically in order to improve binding affinity, reduce immune complications, and disrupt the molecular pathways they normally employ (5).
2. Signal transduction cascades, such as the Ras/Raf/MEK/MAPK and PI3K/Akt pathways.
3. Cell cycle control molecules and modulators of apoptosis such as INK4a (inhibitor of CDK4), CDK4, pRB, Arf, MDM-2, p53, the proteasome, and the pro- and anti-apoptotic proteins (17).
4. Invasion factors, such as matrix metalloproteinases.

HER-Kinase (EGFR) Axis

The HER (human EGF-like receptors) kinase axis includes EGFR (HER1), HER2, HER3, and HER4. The EGF receptor seems to be the most implicated in the genesis of cancers, including HGG (7,9). In fact, the most common gene amplification event in high-grade astrocytomas involve the EGFR gene (9). Interaction of this receptor with its ligands (EGF, TGF-α, β-celluline, neuregulins, heregulins) activates downstream pathways including Ras/Raf/MEK/MAPK, PI3K/Akt (PKB), PLC-γ/PKC, JAK-STAT pathways and Src, Shc, Grb2, and Stress-activated protein kinases (2,7,9). Activation can aso occur in a ligand-independent fashion in the setting of certain EGFR mutations or with high-level wild-type receptor overexpression. This activation results in stimulation of transcriptionl processes to accelerate cell division, resist apoptosis, cause tumor invasion, and promote angiogenesis (7).

EGFR has been studied extensively in many types of cancer including gliomas. There is amplification of wild-type EGFR in 40 to 50% of de novo (primary) GBMs (1,2,18,19). This results in increased membrane density of EGFR and inappropriate activation of its signaling pathway. Higher-grade tumors have a higher level of EGFR expression (5). In addition, these tumors may simultaneously secrete ligand for EGFR (EGF and TGF-α), resulting in autocrine and paracrine loops, which affect the secreting tumor cell, surrounding tumor cells, and other neighboring cells (4,19). EGFRvIII (ΔEGFR) is a mutant form of the receptor caused by an in-frame deletion of exons 2 to 7 in its mRNA (1,4,17). This results in truncation of the extracellular domain, resulting in a fragment which can no longer bind ligand (9,19). This molecule is constitutively phosphorylated, and has continuous low-level kinase activity (18,19). It also has an extended half-life and is invulnerable to downregulation by the endosome-lysosome pathway (1). ΔEGFR is present in 67% of EGFR-positive gliomas (2,5,20). There are also other mutant forms of EGFR with abnormally increased receptor activity (2). Constitutive kinase activity of ΔEGFR causes increased activity of Ras protein, constitutively active levels of PI3K, and c-Jun N-terminal kinase (a stress-activated protein kinase belonging to the MAPK family), and upregulation of Bcl-xL (anti-apoptotic factor) expression, which protects neoplastic cells from apoptosis (1,2,18,21). The c-jun N-terminal kinase pathway may be important in GBM cell migration and motility (9). Moreover, tumor cells with EGFR mutations demonstrate upregulation of matrix metalloproteinases and serine proteases. These cells are consequently more invasive with increased cell scatter, motility, and infiltrative capacities (2). Presence of ΔEGFR seems to be associated with worse prognosis, including shorter time to progression and shorter overall survival *(22)*. In addition, upregulation of EGFR activity interferes with cytotoxic treatments *(7)*.

Interestingly, EGFR activity may also mediate radiation resistance in gliomas *(4)*. Response of GBM to radiation therapy is inversely proportional to EGFR immunoreactivity *(23)*. Radiation exposure causes phosphorylation and activation of EGFR as if by ligand, which results in activation of downstream kinases that inhibit apoptotic response (e.g., MAPK, Akt). In addition, Rao and colleagues have shown that transfection of human glioma cell lines with dominant negative EGFR mutants causes radiosensitization *(4)*. Inhibition of EGFR by C225 anti-EGFR MAb or by CI-1033 tyrosine kinase inhibitor also sensitizes cells to radiation *(4)*.

Small molecule inhibitors of EGFR compete with ATP for binding to the intracellular tyrosine kinase domain of the EGFR receptor *(2)*. Gefitinib (Iressa, ZD1839) and erlotinib (Tarceva, OSI-774, CP-358, 774) are examples of these specific, reversible EGFR inhibitors *(24)*. Gefitinib has shown efficacy (increased median survival) in several human tumor xenograft models with or without upregulation of EGFR signaling *(2,25,26)*. Clinical antitumor efficacy has been demonstrated using gefitinib as single-agent therapy in patients with advanced cancers *(26)*. Erlotinib causes cell cycle arrest and apoptosis in multiple cell types *(26,27)*. In human tumor xenografts, it inhibits EGFR-specific tyrosine phosphorylation and growth inhibition and regression *(26)*. Erlotinib also has additive or "supra-additive" effects in vivo in combination with standard cytotoxic agents and irradiation, without increased toxicity *(7,26)*. CI-1033 (PD183805) is an irreversible inhibitor of EGFR *(24)*. It inhibits human tumor xenografts with weekly instead of daily dosing. A single dose eliminated EGFR phosphorylation in tumor cells for more than 72 h. It also has favorable effects when combined with cytotoxic agents *(26)*.

PDGFR

PDGF-α and PDGF-β are the two isotypes of PDGF receptors. Binding of ligand (PDGF-A, PDGF-B, PDGF-C, PDGF-D) to these receptors results in activation of multiple second messengers such as Src, Shc, Grb2, Nck, PasGAP, PI3K, Janus kinases (JAK), signal transducers and activators of transcription (STATs), and phospholipase C (PLC)-γ *(2,9)*. These signaling cascades result in tumor cell proliferation and in angiogenesis. PLC-γ seems to be equally involved in tumor cell migration *(9)*.

The PDGFR gene is overexpressed in many gliomas, especially in oligodendrogliomas *(17)*. All four PDGF ligands are expressed in gliomas *(10)*. In addition, glial tumors co-express PDGFR and its ligand, PDGF *(7,18,19,28–33)*. Overexpression is most pronounced in malignant tumors *(1)*. There have been no identified rearrangements or amplification of the PDGF or PDGFR genes. This fact points to a possible autocrine growth-stimulatory loop for their role in neoplasia, as described for EGFR *(1,5,16,18,34)*. Activation of PDGFR stimulates Ras, MAPK, and Akt(PKB) pathways, resulting in cell proliferation, resistance to apoptosis, cellular motility, and angiogenesis *(10)*. PDGF-A is expressed in tumor cells, which coexpress PDGFR-α. In contrast, PDGF-B is expressed by hyperplastic glioma endothelial cells which coexpress PDGFR-β *(19,29,30,35)*. This finding suggests that PDGF-A and PDGFR-α participate in tumor cell proliferation, whereas PDGF-B and PDGFR-β participate in angiogenesis *(19,28,29,36,37)*. The mechanism for promotion of angiogenesis by PDGF may be through induction of VEGF-A expression during neo-angiogenesis *(16,38)*. Evidence that PDGF autocrine stimulation results in glioma formation in neonatal mice further supports the role of PDGF signaling pathways in gliomagenesis *(39)*.

Transfection of dominant negative mutants of PDGF ligand has been shown to reverse the malignant phenotype in human glioma cell lines *(4)*. Insertion of truncated, inactive PDGFR-β into rat glioma cells decreases their growth rate *(4)*. Anti-PDGF treatment (e.g., MAbs and suramin or trapidil) decreases malignancy of glioma cells by decreasing DNA synthesis, inhibiting tumor colony growth, and reversing the transformed phenotype *(40,41)*.

Small molecule inhibitors of PDGFR are also ATP-competitive inhibitors for the tyrosine kinase domain of the receptor. Leflunomide (SU 101) has been shown to block entry of PDGF-stimulated cells into the *S*-phase and to inhibit growth of intracerebral glioma xenografts *(1)*. Imatinib mesylate (Gleevec, STI-571) is a bcr-Abl and c-kit inhibitor, which is also highly active against PDGFR. It has been used clinically for the treatment of chronic myeloid leukemia with excellent results *(26,42–44)*. Treatment of glioma cell lines which have PDGF-mediated autocrine growth properties inhibits their growth in vitro *(2,4,5)*. It also inhibits growth of GBM xenografts in an in vivo model of brain tumors *(3,42,45)*.

VEGFR

Another targeting strategy consists of blocking neoangiogenesis, a process essential to tumor proliferation, particularly in gliomas, which are reputed for their microvascular proliferation *(16)*. Interest in this strategy stems from:

1. The ease of drug delivery to endothelial cells and pericytes in tumor-associated vessels.
2. The expression of several growth factor receptors in tumor vasculature, in distinction to normal vessels, which allows for specific targeting of tumor-related cells.
3. The stability of genomes in these non-transformed cells (which decreases the likelihood of development of resistance).
4. The indirect control of tumor cell growth independent of tumor growth fraction and heterogeneity.
5. The amplification effect (since each capillary network may supply hundreds of tumor cells).
6. Minimal toxicity to the host *(5,10,46,47)*.

Angiogenesis is regulated by three principal mechanisms: (1) integrin-mediated signaling, (2) cell surface interactions between integrins and matrix metalloproteinases, and (3) the VEGF/ VEGFR tyrosine kinase pathway *(16)*. The most important of these is the VEGF/VEGFR pathway, which is also involved in the regulation of lymphangiogenesis, vascular permeability, and inflammation *(16)*.

There are three types of VEGF receptors: VEGFR-1 *(flt-1)*, VEGFR-2 (Flk-1, KDR), and VEGFR-3 (Flt-4). VEGFR-2 (KDR) is the primary subtype through which VEGFs exert their mitogenic, chemotactic, and vascular permeabilizing effects *(26,44,48–50)*. VEGFR is expressed in hyperplastic endothelial cells in GBM, but not in normal brain endothelium *(19)*. VEGFRs are activated by interaction with their ligands VEGF-A,-B, -C, and -D. VEGF-A and-B are implicated in hemangiogenesis and types-C and -D in lymphangiogenesis *(16,44)*. VEGFR uses many of the same signaling pathways as EGFR, EGFRvIII, and PDGFR (i.e., PI3K/Akt, Ras/MAPK and PLC/PKC) to modulate nuclear transcription factors *(7)*.

VEGFR-1 and -2 are upregulated in a tumor stage-specific manner in glioma endothelial cells; the highest levels are found in GBM, particularly in regions of cell palisading *(3,5, 10)*. VEGF itself is expressed in low levels in normal brain and levels are increased in proportion to tumor grade *(5,7,19)*. Upregulation of VEGF expression may occur via EGFR upregulation or PTEN mutations, two abnormalities that are common in GBM. In particular, VEGF-A is overexpressed by gliomas; its level of expression correlates directly with vascularity and grade of the tumor and indirectly with prognosis *(16)*. It stimulates endothelial cell proliferation through its effect on the Raf/MEK/MAPK pathway. Endothelial cell survival is promoted by activation of PI3K/AKT (PKB).

PTK787 is an anilinophthalazine small molecule inhibitor of all three VEGFRs, which also has inhibitory effects on PDGFR-β and *c-kit (26)*. It has been shown to inhibit VEGFR-2 autophosphorylation, therefore inducing endothelial cell apoptosis and decreasing density of tumor microvessels in animal models *(51,52)*. Semaxanib (SU5416) is a quinazoline selective inhibitor of VEGFR-1,-2, and-3, as well as of c-Kit and flt-3 kinases and PDGFR *(3,26,53)*. It has been shown to inhibit endothelial cell proliferation as well as growth of glioma xenografts *(3,54)*. ZD6474 is another quinazoline that inhibits VEGFR-2 *(49)*. ZD4190 is a quinazoline that inhibits VEGFR-2 and *flt-1*. It inhibits capillary invasion of cartilage and growth of human tumor xenografts *(50)*. All of these VEGFR inhibitors are ATP-competitive and bind to the ATP pocket of the receptor's kinase domain, thus inhibiting its activation *(46)*.

It is thought that VEGFR inhibitors may also reduce radioresistance in malignant cells by inhibiting the endothelial rise in VEGF-A that is the normal response to radiation exposure *(16)*. Combined treatment of U87 glioma cell lines with radiation and anti-VEGF antibody resulted in supra-additive effects in one study *(55)*. Another study showed that combined radiotherapy with SU5416 caused enhanced apoptosis of endothelial cells and reversal of radioresistance in a GL261 GBM model *(56)*. An additional rationale for the use of VEGFR inhibitors in combination with cytotoxic therapy is that glioma neovessels are abnormally permeable and are unable to maintain normal gradients between vascular and interstitial pressures, leading to interstitial hypertension *(57)*. This causes impaired flow of oxygen and of other molecule. Normalization of vessels with anti-angiogenic therapy could theoretically restore normal flow dynamics for better delivery of oxygen and of cytotoxic drugs, resulting in potentiation of radiotherapy and chemotherapy *(57,58)*.

PI3K/AKT Inhibitors

Phosphatidylinositol 3-kinase (PI3K) is activated by growth factor receptors including EGFR, ΔEGFR, PDGFR, and VEGFR. It generates second messengers PIP2 and PIP3, which in turn activate Akt(PKB) and PKC *(1,8,17)*. Akt activates mTOR and p70S6 kinase, which promote cell cycling and transcription. Akt also activates the FKHR (forkhead) transcription factor, endothelial nitric oxide synthase, and BAD, which promote angiogenesis, DNA repair, and apoptosis *(59,60)*. It also stabilizes cyclin D by inhibition of glycogen synthase kinase-3, which promotes cell proliferation *(60)*.

Seventy to 90% of GBM have LOH of chromosome 10q, which is the site of PTEN, a dual-specific phosphatase which acts in opposition to PI3K by dephosphorylating PIP2 and PIP3 *(1,7,9,17,18)*. Loss of all or part of chromosome 10 is the most common genetic change observed in GBM, and is seen with increased frequency with increasing tumor grade *(1,18)*. PTEN-deficient glioma cells have increased PIP3 levels, which activate the Akt-mediated cell growth and survival pathway and contribute to chemotherapy resistance *(61,62)*. Eighty percent of human GBM express activated Akt *(9)*. This is likely caused both by loss of functional PTEN and by overexpression of EGFR *(9,17,18)*.

2-(4-Morpholinyl)-8-phenylchromone (LY294002) is a specific inhibitor of PI3K, which induces growth inhibition through apoptosis and/or G1 arrest in carcinoma cells in vitro and in vivo *(63–67)*. It also suppresses attachment, migration and invasiveness and increases susceptibility to anticancer drugs *(60,68–71)*. LY294002 was shown to induce G1 cell-cycle arrest in U87MG cells and cause apoptosis in four tested malignant cell lines *(60,72)*. It also enhances cytotoxicity induced by etoposide, BCNU, and cisplatin in human malignant glioma cells in vitro *(60)*. However, there has been no association demonstrated between PTEN status and response to LY294002 *(60)*.

Other strategies to downregulate the PI3K pathway have targeted downstream molecules. PKC inhibitors include calphostin, byrostatin, and staurosporine. Akt inhibitors have been difficult to develop but are being actively studied *(73)*. MTOR inhibitors and CDK inhibitors are discussed in the following sections.

MTOR Inhibitors

Mammalian target of rapamycin (MTOR) is a non-receptor kinase that is a downstream target of the PI3K and Akt pathways *(74)*. It functions as a regulator of translation through regulation of S6K1 protein and 4E-BPs (eukaryotic initiation factor 4E (eIF4E) binding proteins) *(7,74,75)*. 4E-BPs promote translation of mRNAs encoding cyclin D1 and ornithine decarboxylase *(74)*. The MTOR pathway also regulates translation initiation of survival factors (c-MYC, hypoxia-inducible factor 1α, and VEGF) *(74)*. It also regulates cyclin A, CDK 1/2, CDKIs (p21Cip1 and p27Kip1), Rb protein, RNA polymerases, and protein phosphatases PP2A, PP4, and PP6 *(74)*. It therefore plays a crucial role in the control of cell growth, size, proliferation, and survival. So far, no activating mutations or overexpression have been demonstrated as primary events in transformation. However, activation of signaling pathways proximal and distal to MTOR is frequently seen *(74)*. For example, with loss of PTEN, there is constitutive activation of Akt and subsequent upregulation of MTOR pathways *(12,74)*. As explained above, abnormalities in growth factor receptors EGFR and PDGFR are known to be present in GBM and cause upregulation of this pathway.

Rapamycin forms a complex with immunophilin FKB12, which binds to MTOR and inhibits its kinase activity. It generally has a cytostatic effect, causing cell arrest in G1 *(74)*. CCI-779 is an ester analog of rapamycin which has the same mechanism of action and also inhibits the G1-S transition. *(7,74,75)*. Both of these molecules inhibit GBM in cell culture and in xenograft models *(3,76)*. Rapamycin can also induce apoptosis, although this is not thought to be its primary mechanism of action *(7)*. PDGF stimulation of GBM line T98G was inhibited by treatment with CCI-779 *(77)*. In addition, PTEN deletion is associated with increased sensitivity to CCI-779, which is promising for the treatment of GBM, which, as mentioned previously, have a high frequency of this mutation *(3,7,74–76)*. CCI-779 also induces apoptosis under certain conditions. This fate may be decided by p53 tumor suppressor status of the cell (i.e., apoptosis may be induced in the absence of functional p53) *(74)*. Treatment of p53-mutant cells with MTOR inhibitors causes activation of ASK1 (apoptosis signal-regulating kinase 1), which leads to sustained activation of c-JUN and subsequent apoptosis *(74)*.

RAS Inhibitors

Ras is a family composed of four isoforms of small membrane-associated GTPases, which transmit signals from growth factor receptors (e.g., EGFR, EGFRvIII, PDGFR, FGF, IGF-1, TGF-α, IL-2, and IL-3) *(2,59)*. They enhance cell proliferation, differentiation, survival, transformation, and angiogenesis *(59,78)*. Ras is synthesized as proRas, an inert cytosolic propeptide, which must be modified by post-translational addition of a farnesyl group to the C-terminal amino acid group by the enzyme farnesyl transferase (FTase) *(59)*. This allows Ras to attach to the plasma membrane, where it is active. Ras is situated at a "hub" of intracellular signaling pathways: many external signals converge to activate it, and its activation in turn initiates several signaling cascades (59). One of these is the Ras/Raf/MEK/ERK pathway, which is critical for cell proliferation and tumor invasion. Another is the MAPK pathway, which activates the E2F transcription factor. The overall outcome of Ras signaling is to promote cell-cycle progression beyond the G1/S restriction point (3). Ras or MAPK signaling is also known to result in expression of intermediate-early genes that are rapidly and transiently expressed by modification of pre-existing factors, and have a role in the G0–G1 phase of the cell cycle. These include ternary complex factor, serum response factor (SRF), c-JUN, c-fos, and the AP-1 transcription factor (59). Inhibition of Ras causes cell-cycle arrest in G1 and prevents exit of growth factor-stimulated cells from G0 (59). Thirty percent of all human cancers have at least one mutation of the Ras gene.

GBM do not have actual Ras mutations, but can have constitutive activation through aberrant EGFR, ΔEGFR, PDGFR, FGFR, and IGF-1R signaling (1–3,9,11). This leads to increased activation of CDK-4/cyclin D, resulting in transition to S-phase and mitosis (9). This is the rationale for therapeutic targeting of Ras.

Farnesyltransferase inhibitors (FTIs) impair processing of proRas and thus block Ras-mediated signaling. They also prevent anchorage-independent growth, cytoskeletal alterations, and morphological transformation of cells in vitro (2). L-744, 832 causes decreased S-phase entry and accumulation of cells in G2/M as well as induction of pro-apoptotic proteins Bax and Bak (1). Lonafarnib (SCH66336) inhibits viability, anchorage-independent growth, and cell cycling in glioma cell lines (3,79). It also decreases in vitro proliferation of astrocytic cell lines with arrest in G1 or G2-M, and inhibits the growth of xenograft models (3,7,78). In addition, lonafarnib has a synergistic effect with certain cytotoxic drugs and with imatinib mesylate (3). Tipifarnib (R115777) radiosensitizes glioma cell lines in vitro (81). EGFR overexpression may be associated with increased sensitivity to FTIs (73).

It is interesting to note that tumors with endogenous Ras activation are more radioresistant (4,82–84). Inhibition of Ras in these cells by the FTI tipifarnib (R115777) sensitizes them to the cytotoxic effects of radiation in vitro and in vivo (4,7). Lovastatin, which also inhibits Ras farnesylation and inhibits cell proliferation and migration, has also been shown to sensitize tumor cells to radiation (4).

RAF

The Raf kinase family is composed of ARAF, BRAF, and Raf-1 (c-Raf). Raf is a downstream effector of Ras signaling (Ras/Raf/MAPK(ERK) (78). Raf kinase is at the head of several protein kinase signaling cascades, and initiates a signaling cascade which ultimately leads to activation of nuclear factors and expression of cell-growth-promoting genes (59). The Raf pathway also suppresses integrin expression, which may relate to decreased cell-matrix adhesion and increased metastatic potential (59). BRAF and Raf-1 have also been implicated in endothelial cell survival (85–87).

In gliomas, overexpression of the EGFR, PDGFR, and PDGFR RTKs upregulates the Ras/Raf pathway, as previously mentioned. BAY 43-9006 is an inhibitor of Raf-1 both in vitro and in vivo (78). It has also been shown to inhibit BRAF, VEGFRs-2 and-3, and PDGFR-β. It targets tumor cell proliferation and tumor angiogenesis (87). BAY 43-9006 has been shown to inhibit Raf-1 and in vitro tumor cell proliferation, as well as xenograft tumor growth (87–89). It has an effect on angiogenesis as well, with both decreased tumor microvessel area and microvessel density in treated tumor (non-glioma) xenografts (87).

CDK Inhibitors

Cell-cycle transition is regulated by two main clases of regulatory molecules: (1) cyclin-dependent kinases (CDKs) (e.g., cdk4 and cdk6), which phosphorylate other proteins in order to activate or inactivate them, and (2) phosphatases, which dephosphorylate proteins. CDKs are themselves regulated by two classes of molecules. Cyclins (e.g., D-cyclins) activate them and thus facilitate G0-to-G1 and G1-to-S transitions. Cyclin-dependent kinase inhibitors (CKIs) (e.g., INK4 [inhibitors of cdk4] proteins) perform opposite functions. An example of such a regulatory circuit is the retinoblastoma protein (pRB). Hypophosphorylated pRB binds to the E2F family of transcription factors, and prevents activation of genes for entry into *S*-phase *(17)*. Cdk4 or cdk6 phosphorylate pRB, resulting in release of E2F proteins and increased transcription of genes for DNA synthesis (dihydrofolate reductase, thymidine kinase, thymidylate synthase, and DNA polymerase-α).

A small but significant percentage of high-grade astrocytomas have CDK4 amplifications which seem to favor proliferation of astrocytes and diminish apoptosis *(18)*.

Flavopiridol (NSC 649890, L86-8275, HMR 1275) inhibits CDKs 1, 2, and 4, producing cell-cycle arrest at G1/S and G2/M checkpoints and enhances caspase-mediated apoptosis induced by cytotoxic agents *(11,90–92)*. Other CDK inhibitors include UCN-01 (7-hydroxy-staurosporine, NSC 638850, KW-2401), CTC202 (R-roscovitine, Cyclacel), and BMS-387032.

Matrix Metalloproteinase Inhibitors

Metalloproteinases include matrix metalloproteinases (MMPs), adamalysin-like proteinases with both metalloproteinase and disintegrin-like domains, and astacins. They are enzymes that exist in secreted and membrane-bound forms and function extracellularly *(5)*. They are involved in proteolytic degradation or activation of cell surface and extracellular-matrix proteins, basement membranes, growth factors, and adhesion molecules, thus enhancing or reducing their biological effects and modulating cell–cell and cell–extracellular matrix interactions *(3,5)*. MMPs influence cell differentiation, migration, proliferation, and survival *(93)*. Under normal physiological conditions, endogenous tissue inhibitors of metalloproteinases (TIMPs) and MMPs exist in a balance that prevents overactivity of MMPs *(7,93)*.

MMPs are implicated in tumor growth, invasion, extravasation into distant sites, and angiogenesis *(7)*. MMP expression, in particular MMP-2 and -9, is increased in most cancers, including gliomas *(3,7)*.

The goal of MMP inhibition is to alter the balance of metalloproteinases to TIMPs in order to limit the tissue invasion and neovascularization required for tumor growth. Studies have shown that upregulation of TIMPs or or downregulation of MMP-9 inhibits tumor growth and invasion *(7)*. The most well studied MMP inhibitor (MMPI) to date is marimastat (MRM, BB-251), a synthetic pseudo-peptide that mimics structural components of MMP substrates and chelates the Zn^{2+} ion at the active site of MMPs *(3,7)*. In vitro studies have shown cytostatic effects *(7)*. Animal models have shown efficacy in preventing growth and vascularization of pre-malignant tumors, with relative lack of effect for advanced cases *(93)*. Most clinical trials have not shown survival benefit for GBM patients *(7)*. However, most of these trials have been of single-agent therapy for patients with advanced cancers *(93)*. One trial that looked at MRM in combination with temozolamide showed a 6-mo progression-free survival of 39%, compared with 18 to 21% with temozolamide alone *(7)*. Survival benefits have been shown with MRM in phase II trials with advanced pancreatic cancer and phase III trials with gastric cancer *(94,95)*. Prinomastat (AG3340) is a lipophilic MMPI, which crosses the BBB, making it promising for the treatment of glioma *(3)*.

The proteasome is an enzyme complex expressed in the nucleus and cytoplasm of all eukaryotic cells *(96)*. It is the primary component of the fundamental protein degradation pathway of the cell and functions to degrade proteins such as signaling molecules, tumor suppressors, cell-cycle regulators, transcription factors, inhibitory molecules, and anti-apoptotic proteins *(3,97)*. Proteasome inhibition interferes with the ordered degradation of cell-cycle proteins including p53, mdm2, p21, p27, Rb, cyclins A, B, and E, IκB, NF-κB, Bcl-2, Bax, and caspase-3 *(3,96)*. Complete blockade of proteasome activity induces apoptosis, possibly through altered ratios of anti-apoptotic to pro-apoptotic proteins, with transformed cells being much more sensitive than quiescent or differentiated cells *(96–99)*.

The proteasome is intimately involved in mechanisms of carcinogenesis and of metastasis, including cell-cycle regulation, apoptosis, and angiogenesis *(100)*. It plays a direct role by degrading cell-cycle regulatory proteins and an indirect role by regulation the availability of transcriptional activators such as NF-κB *(100)*.

Preclinical studies have shown selective cytotoxicity towards transformed cells, additive effects with other antineoplastic therapies, sensitization of cells to radiotherapy and to chemotherapy, and apoptosis induction in Bcl-2 overexpressing cells *(100)*.

Bortezomib (PS-341, Velcade) is a low-molecular-weight drug that has shown potent anticancer activity in vitro through inhibition of proteolysis of long-lived proteins, inhibition of cell growth with arrest in G2-M, and induction of apoptosis *(3,97,101)*. Its mechanism of action is linked to blockage of NF-κB, which is constitutively activated in certain cancers, causing increased tumor cell survival and decreased efficacy of anticancer therapy. In normal situations, NF-κB is bound to the IκB inhibitory protein, which renders it inactive and sequesters it in the cytoplasm *(96,100)*. In stress situations (including chemotherapy and radiation-induced stress), IκB is degraded by the proteasome, which permits translocation of NF-κB to the nucleus where it initiates transcription of genes encoding stress-response enzymes, cell-adhesion molecules, pro-inflammatory cytokines, and anti-apoptotic proteins such as Bcl-2 *(96,98,100)*. Many types of cancer have constitutive activation of NF-κB, which leads to drug resistance *(99,102)*. Furthermore, it has been shown that NF-κB has a consensus binding site in the first intron of the human mdr1 gene, where NF-κB complexes bind and may regulate gene expression and subsequent drug resistance *(103)*. Proteasome inhibition blocks chemotherapy-induced activation of NF-κB in vitro, resulting in increased chemosensitivity and increased apoptosis in mice tumor xenografts *(104)*. It also increases radiation-induced apopotosis *(105)*. This suggests that NF-κB activity induced by chemotherapy or radiotherapy-related stress is downregulated by proteasome inhibition, which are findings that may provide a rationale for combination therapy *(99)*.

Inhibitors of Bcl-2 Family

A relatively new area of development in SMIs involves targeting of the Bcl-2 family of pro-apoptotic and anti-apoptotic proteins. Proteins in this family include the Bax, Bak, Bid, and Bad pro-apoptotic proteins, as well as the Bcl-2 and Bcl-XL anti-apoptotic proteins. Bcl-2 and Bcl-XL have BH1 (Bcl-2 homology-1), BH2, and BH3 domains, which form a hydrophobic binding pocket into which the Bax, Bak, Bid, or Bad BH3 domains bind to form heterodimers *(106)*. Most conventional chemotherapeutic regimens target DNA integrity or replication, with the aim of triggering apoptosis. However, most human cancers overexpress Bcl-2, Bcl-XL, or both. These molecules function at the mitochondrial level by preventing the release of cytochrome C and subsequent initiation of the caspase cascade and apoptosis. Overexpression of these proteins renders cells resistant to chemotherapy and radiation *(106)*. Furthermore, whereas Bcl-2 and Bcl-XL are overexpressed in cancer cells, only low levels are found in normal cells *(106)*. This suggests that cancer cells may be dependent on these proteins for survival, whereas normal cells are not. Therefore, this type of targeted therapy may be expected to have good specificity and decreased side effects.

There is upregulation of Bcl-2 expression in multinucleated giant cells of otherwise Bcl-2 negative GBMs, in reactive astrocytes, and in proliferating capillary endothelial cells of malignant astrocytomas *(15)*. Bcl-2 expression increases with increasing grade of tumor. Overproduction of Bcl-2 also seems to be associated with resistance to chemotherapy *(15)*. Human GBM and oligodendroglioma-derived cell lysates have increased expression of both Bcl-2 and Bcl-xL compared with non-neoplastic glial cells *(107,108)*. Furthermore, downregulation of these molecules by antisense oligonucleotides causes cell death, which is mediated by caspase 6 and caspase 7 *(15,108,109)*. Exposure of oligodendroglioma cell lines to BCNU causes downregulation of Bcl-xL and Bcl-2, which is correlated with increased cell death *(107)*. Nevertheless, the role of Bcl-2 in the pathogenesis and progression of glial tumors has yet to be demonstrated *(15)*. Bcl-xL has been implicated in resistance to cisplatin in EGFRvIII-expressing GBM cells *(105)*.

One of the molecules studied to date is HA14-1, which competitively binds to Bcl-2 and inhibits binding to Bak *(106)*. It has been shown to produce apoptosis in human acute myelogenous leukemia cells overexpressing Bcl-2, with decreased mitochondrial membrane potential and activation of caspases 9 and 3. Unfortunately, the molecules studied to date have only moderate binding affinity to Bcl-2 and Bcl-XL, and their limited inhibition of cell growth has impeded their clinical applicability *(106)*.

FUTURE DIRECTIONS: ISSUES FACED BY SMALL MOLECULE DRUGS FOR BRAIN TUMORS

Reversible vs Irreversible SMIs

As mentioned in the discussion of EGFR inhibitors, SMIs may be either reversible or irreversible in their binding to target. Reversible inhibition (e.g., gefitinib, erlotinib) leads to a need to maintain plasma concentrations at high levels for long periods *(10,26)*. In contrast, irreversible inhibitors (e.g., CI-1033) are less likely to require prolonged exposure to drug and their "absolute finality" may prove advantageous for antitumor efficacy *(10,26,110)*. It is not clear, yet, whether irreversible inhibitors will have the same toxicity profile as exhibited by the reversible inhibitors.

Promiscuity vs Specificity

The signaling pathways previously described are, in reality, not linear; there exists significant cross-communication, convergence, and divergence between many of them. Thus, inhibition of one pathway at a single level may be compensated by the activity of related, parallel pathways, thereby producing decreased therapeutic efficacy. In addition, unlike many hematologic malignancies, gliomas are characterized by multiple genetic abnormalities, as well as by a heterogeneous cell population. By contrast, chronic myelogenous leukemia (CML) is a disease caused by a single genetic abnormality, which produces the Bcr-Abl fusion gene/protein responsible for driving this form of cancer. In this situation, single-agent targeted therapy with the Bcr-Abl inhibitor imatinib (Gleevec) has shown excellent results *(26)*.

These considerations have lead to the dilemma of balancing *specificity* of therapeutic molecules and "*promiscuity*." Should targeted therapies be engineered for extreme specificity for one kinase or, rather, to affect other related kinases for more widespread effects *(10)*? The second option could theoretically entail increased efficacy against tumor cells at the expense of a greater impact on normal cell populations and increased systemic toxicity *(10)*.

Blood–Brain Barrier

Drug delivery to the brain has been a great challenge in neuro-oncology because of several physiological barriers to the CNS penetration of systemically delivered molecules. These barriers include the BBB, the blood–cerebrospinal barrier (BCSFB), and the blood–tumor barrier (BTB).

The first and most well known barrier is the BBB, which is composed of brain capillary endothelial cells and astrocytic foot processes *(10,111)*. Its 5000-fold greater surface area than the BCSF barrier makes it the principal source for uptake of substances into the CNS parenchyma *(112,113)*. The endothelial layer is characterized by tight junctions, large amounts of degradative enzymes and mitochondria, as well as high concentrations of P-glycoprotein, a drug efflux transporter protein in the luminal membrane of these cells which actively removes the drug before its entry into the brain *(113,114)*. Brain capillaries also lack intercellular clefts, fenestrae, and pinocytotic vesicles *(113,114)*.

The BCSFB is formed by the choroid epithelium and the arachnoid membrane, which are again joined by tight junctions. Choroid plexus capillaries, however, do not contain tight junctions *(111,114)*.

The BBB and BCSFB are further aided by efflux transport systems that actively eliminate drugs *(112)*. The ABC transporters are characterized by a cytoplasmically located ATP-binding cassette (which acts as a catalytic domain for ATP hydrolysis) and by unidirectional efflux to the outside of cells *(115)*. Human P-glycoprotein (P-gp) and the multidrug resistance-associated protein-1 (MRP1) are members of this family. P-gp exists in the brain as the product of the MDR1 gene. It is a transporter with broad substrate specificity for molecules (e.g., vinca alkaloids, etoposide, methotrexate, rapamycin, glucocorticoids, and phemytoin). The MDR phenotype allows a cancer cell exposed to a single agent to become simultaneously resistant to both that drug and to other drugs of unrelated structure or function. P-gp is expressed on the luminal membrane of brain capillary endothelial cells in the BBB and sub-apically on choroid epithelial cells in the BCSFB, where it actually transports in an opposite direction than in the BBB (i.e., towards the CSF) *(111)*. P-gp is present in malignant brain tumor and associated endothelial cells, and its expression level increases with tumor grade *(113)*. MRP1 is an organic anion transporter that transports anionic drugs as well as neutral drugs conjugated to acidic ligands and confers mutlidrug resistance to doxorubicin, daunorubicin, epirubucin, vincristine, and etoposide *(112)*. It also confers resistance to methotrexate *(113)*. MRP is expressed on the basal membrane of choroid plexus, but its presence on the BBB has not yet been established *(112,113)*. It is likely involved in the elimination of harmful compounds from the CSF *(111,113)*. MRP mRNA levels are associated with the degree of cellular resistance to etoposide, adriamycin, and vincristine in in vitro glioma cells. MRP1 expression, like P-gp expression is increased with tumor grade *(111)*.

The BTB is assumed by many clinicians to be "open" as demonstrated by the uptake of intravenous contrast agents on computed tomography (CT) or magnetic resonance imaging (MRI). However, this is a misconception; there remains a barrier to the transport of many therapeutic compounds into brain tumors, as evidenced by the low concentrations found for most chemotherapeutic agents in brain tumors *(111)*. BBB breakdown associated with malignant tumors is typically local and heterogeneous *(10,114)*. In addition, despite morphological abnormalities in inter-endothelial tight junctions and increased number of pinocytotic vesicles in glioma-associated vessels, tight junctions have been shown to be present, fenestrations are rare, even in GBMs, and peritumoral capillaries are ultrastructurally normal *(111)*. Furthermore, there is a functional barrier produced by the BTB as a result of heterogeneous distribution of vessels in the tumor interstitium, decreased vascular surface area and increased intracapillary distance with tumor growth, and high interstitial pressure in tumor and adjacent edematous areas *(10,114)*. On the other hand, in the infiltrated areas that characterize gliomas, the widely dispersed tumor cells within the normal parenchyma are actually protected by an intact BBB *(2,10)*. This has been well demonstrated with MAbs, which failed to increase survival in animals with intracerebral tumors because of the lack of penetration into brain parenchyma *(9)*. Finally, both the BTB and the tumor cells themselves express P-gp and other efflux transport pumps.

The development of methods to overcome these barriers has been a major goal in neurooncology. It is well known that in order to traverse the BBB molecules must be lipophilic, have low-molecular-mass, or benefit from facilitated delivery *(10,113)*. Large or charged molecules do not cross over into the brain *(10,112)*. Tyrosine kinase inhibitors, despite their small size, are for the most part charged molecules and may not be effectively delivered to brain tumors *(10)*. There is also reason to suspect that many of these molecules are substrates for the active transport pumps, which further reduce CNS penetration of these drugs. Presently, there is lack of data concerning the ability of SMIs to cross the BBB; however, data from our laboratory, presented at the 2003 AACR-NCI-EORTC Molecular Therapeutics Meeting suggests brain tumor levels of one EGFR SMI to be approx 40% of serum levels *(4,116)*.

Methods to overcome the BBB include direct infusion into surgical cavities, transient BBB disruption, convection-enhanced delivery into the brain parenchyma, specialized vehicles such as immunoliposomes, modulation of interstitial fluid pressure, and engineering of compounds to improve their penetration, as in the case of SMIs *(114)*.

Drug Resistance

Potential mechanisms of cellular resistance to targeted antineoplastic therapies include: (1) amplification of the target to increase signal; (2) mutation of the target to prevent inhibitor binding; (3) compensatory upregulation of parallel signaling pathways to bypass blockade; (4) loss of the tumor suppressor pathway which mediated the inhibitory effects of the kinase inhibitor, and (5) upregulation of drug efflux pumps *(6)*.

ZD 1839 (Iressa) resistance was studied in an in vitro model of glioma with EGFR expression *(117)*. Treatment of glioma cells with Iressa resulted in significant suppression of EGFR autophosphorylation with low levels of drug; however, significantly higher levels were required for full inhibition of its downstream targets in the PI3K/Akt and MAPK/ERK pathways. This demonstrates a differential resistance in target effect with respect to drug levels.

The most well known example of resistance to SMIs is the case of Gleevec for treatment of CML *(118)*. Ninety five percent of CML cases have a single genetic defect, a 9:22 translocation resulting in the Bcr-Abl fusion protein, which is a constitutively active protein tyrosine kinase *(6)*. Imatinib (Gleevec) is an inhibitor of this kinase (as well as of Kit and PDGFR) *(118,119)*. Phase I studies showed 95% complete hematologic remission with Gleevec treatment *(119)*. Durable responses have been obtained in patients in the chronic phase of CML, but resistance has been shown mainly in patients in the accelerated or blast crisis phases of the disease *(6)*. The principal mechanism of this resistance is a mutation in the catalytic Abl kinase domain of Bcr-Abl, which sterically blocks imatinib binding to Abl *(10,120,121)*. This is thought to result from selective outgrowth of pre-existing subclones of CML cells *(6)*. Thus, a single mutation can lead to resistance to therapy. Other putative mechanisms of resistance include Bcr-Abl gene amplification, activation of an alternative tyrosine kinase, and Mdr-1 P-glycoprotein expression *(119)*.

Preclinical studies have shown that resistance of glioma cell lines to EGFR inhibitors is associated with activation of IGF1/PI3K/Akt *(10)*. Thus, cells treated with one type of tyrosine kinase inhibitor may regrow with increased expression of another growth factor *(10)*.

Combination Therapy

Combination therapy entails the use of SMIs in association with other SMIs or with cytotoxic treatments such as traditional chemotherapy or radiotherapy. There are several reasons for considering combination therapy for gliomas. First, most SMIs have demonstrated cytostatic effects as opposed to chemotherapy or radiation therapy, which are cytoreductive treatments *(6)*. Second, gliomas are a heterogeneous group of tumors, which show evidence of aberrant activity at multiple levels, including extracellular growth factors or growth factor receptors, signal transduction cascades, and cell-cycle control molecules *(10,17)*. Most gliomas have abnormalities at all three of these levels *(17)*. Third, as discussed previously, these pathways are highly redundant and inter-related *(2)*. Finally, one tumor can show molecular heterogeneity in different geographic areas *(2,10)*. All of these facts seem to mandate simultaneous targeting of multiple signaling pathways and/or targeting of downstream effectors common to multiple upstream mutations (e.g., Akt activation by PTEN deletion or by EGFR/ EGFRvIII) *(7,10)*. Eventually, "tailored therapies" based on a tumor's specific molecular abnormalities may be feasible *(4)*. This strategy may be limited, however, by the intrinsic genetic instability associated with HGG.

Combinations have been attempted in the case of CML *(119)*. Imatinib with the FTI lonafarnib (SCH66336) demonstrated enhanced antiproliferative effects against Bcr-Abl-expressing cells *(122)*. This combination also inhibited hematopoietic colony formation by primary human CML cells and induced apoptosis in imatinib-resistant Bcr-Abl-expressing cells *(122,123)*. Imatinib in combination with wortmannin (a PI3K inhibitor) showed synergy against Bcr-Abl cell lines *(124)*.

Active trials of small molecule inhibitors in glioma, as of October 2004, are listed in Table 1 *(125)*.

CONCLUSIONS

It is likely that successful development of SMIs will require a focus on markers of therapeutic efficacy and on determination of actual target delivery.

In most past clinical trials of cytotoxic agents, the only endpoints examined were response (defined as complete or partial tumor shrinkage) and survival. Clinical trials involving cytostatic agents, such as SMIs, will also need to look at other measures of efficacy including time-to-progression, progression-free survival, tumor response (including stabilization of disease), and identification of molecular determinants of drug sensitivity (i.e., decreased levels of activated downstream effectors) *(10)*. These trials could also be stratified based on molecular inclusion criteria (via use of microarray or gene chip technology), because differences in molecular profiles between tumors may actually translate to different biological behavior and could mask a high response to therapy in a subset of patients if all are grouped together *(6,126)*. The strategy would be to identify subgroups, for example, of primary and secondary GBM and to establish predictive markers or profiles to guide therapy *(7,42)*. Dose selection may eventually be based on maximal inhibition of target rather than on maximal tolerated dose (MTD),

Table 1
SMI Clinical Trials Recruiting Patients as of October 2004 (126)

Drug	Type	Phase	Protocol ID	Study population
Erlotinib (OSI-774, Tarceva)	EGFR inhibitor	I/II	NABTC-0103	Recurrent/progressive malignant glioma or meningioma
Erlotinib		I	NCI-04-C-0256	Recurrent/refractory solid tumors, including all brain tumors
Erlotinib		I	CDR0000069170	Solid tumors, including gliomas with hepatic/renal dysfunction
Erlotinib		II	CDR0000380835	Adult GBM
Erlotinib		II	EORTC-26034-16031	Recurrent GBM
Erlotinib		II	CDR0000270723	Recurrent/progressive GBM
Erlotinib		I/II	NCCTG-N0177	GBM, gliosarcoma, other grade IV astrocytoma variants
Gefitinib (ZD1839, Iressa)	EGFR inhibitor	II	PBTC-007	Newly diagnosed brain stem gliomas or incompletely resected supratentorial malignant gliomas
Gefitinib		II	NABTC-0001	Recurrent/progressive supratentorial maliganant gliomas and brain/spinal meningiomas
Gefitinib		I	NCI-03-C-0062	Solid cancers in children
Gefitinib		I/II	CDR0000370826	Progressive/recurrent GBM in combination with everolimus
Imatinib mesylate (STI571, Gleevec)	PDGFR inhibitor	I/II	PBTC-006	Newly diagnosed/poor prognosis brain stem glioma or recurrent high grade glioma with/without radiotherapy
Imatinib mesylate		I/II	NABTC-9908	Recurrent/progressive/unresectable glioma or meningioma
Imatinib mesylate		I/II	NCCTG-N0272	Recurrent oligodendroglioma/mixed oligoastrocytoma
AP23573	mTOR inhibitor	I	AP23573-02-101	Refractory/advanced malignancy
Lonafarnib (SCH66336, Sarasar)	FTI	I	EORTC-16027	Recurrent/progressive primary supratentorial gliomas in combination with temozolamide
Lonafarnib		II	DM01-258	Recurrent/progressive supratentorial GBM in combination with temozolamide
Tipifarnib (R115777, Zarnestra)	FTI	II	COG-ACNS0226	Recurrent/progressive high-grade glioma, medulloblastoma/PNET, or brain stem/visual pathway/hypothalamic glioma
Tipifarnib		I/II	PBTC-014	Newly diagnosed diffuse intrinsic brain stem glioma in combination with radiotherapy
Tipifarnib		I	NABTC-0202	Newly diagnosed GBM/gliosarcoma in combination with radiotherapy
Tipifarnib	FTI	I/II	ID02-126	Recurrent/progressive GBM
Bortezomib (PS-341, Velcade)	Proteasome inhibitor	I	NABTT-9910	Recurrent/progressive malignant glioma

351

as with cytotoxic drug development in order to establish an "optimal biological dose" (OBD) based on target modulation *(6,127)*. However, whether these drugs should be dosed based upon MTD or OBD remains an open question. Trial design will also need to compensate for the effects of enzyme (P450)-inducing agents such as phenytoin, carbamazepine, and phenobarbital that are commonly employed in this patient population by using two-arm trials *(10)*. Increased dosing may be needed for SMIs that are metabolized by the cytochrome P450 (e.g., CCI-779, erlotinib), which may lead to prohibitive side effects prior to the achievement of an effective tumor tissue concentration *(75)*.

Pathological studies will need to provide data on cell-surface receptors on tumor tissue, as well as on the activation state of signal-transduction pathways in paraffin-embedded tumor tissue. Biomarkers could be measured on tissue at initial diagnosis, after a short trial of therapy (e.g., short-term pretreatment with a kinase inhibitor before surgery), or at tumor recurrence *(10)*. They could also be measured in surrogate tissue (e.g., circulating lymphocytes or on skin biopsy samples) in order to provide a less invasive measurement of efficacy *(10)*. Patients may also eventually be divided into cohorts by looking at gene expression and signaling pathway activation profiles using phosphorylation status-specific antibodies that allow for the detection of activated signaling molecules in biopsy tissue *(10)*. Thus, molecular profiling of gliomas is gaining new clinical relevance with the ultimate goal of providing a scientific basis for tailored therapy.

REFERENCES

1. Besson A, Yong VW. Mitogenic signaling and the relationship to cell cycle regulation in astrocytomas. J Neuro-Oncology 2001;51:245–264.
2. Newton HB. Molecular neuro-oncology and development of targeted therapeutic strategies for brain tumors. Part 1: Growth factor and Ras signaling pathways. Expert Rev Anticancer Ther 2003;3:595–614.
3. Tremont-Lukats IW, Gilbert MR. Advances in molecular therapies in patients with brain tumors. Cancer Control 2003;10:125–137.
4. Rao RD, Uhm JH, Krishnan S, James CD. Genetic and signaling pathway alterations in glioblastoma: relevance to novel targeted therapies. Front Biosci 2003;1:e270–e280.
5. Samoylova TI, Morrison NE, Cox NR. Molecular markers of glial tumors: current targeting strategies. Curr Med Chem 2003;10:831–843.
6. Laird AD, Cherrington JM. Small molecule tyrosine kinase inhibitors: clinical development of anticancer agents. Expert Opin Investig Drugs 2003;1:51–64.
7. Jendrossek V, Belka C, Bamberg M. Novel chemotherapeutic agents for the treatment of glioblastoma multiforme. Expert Opin Investig Drugs 2003;12:1899–1924.
8. Harris TK. PDK1 and PKB/Akt: ideal targets for development of new strategies to structure-based drug design. IUBMB Life 2003;55:117–126.
9. Kapoor GS, O'Rourke DM. Mitogenic signaling cascades in glial tumors. Neurosurgery 2003;52:1425–1435.
10. Rich JN, Bigner DD. Development of novel targeted therapies in the treatment of malignant glioma. Nat Rev Drug Discov 2004;3:430–446.
11. Fischer OM, Streit S, Hart S, Ullrich A. Beyond herceptin and gleevec. Curr Opin Chem Biol 2003;7:490–495.
12. Kapoor GS, O'Rourke DM. Receptor tyrosine kinase signaling in gliomagenesis: pathobiology and therapeutic approaches. Cancer Biol Ther 2003;2:330–342.
13. Avgeropoulos NG, Batchelor TT. New treatment strategies for malignant gliomas. Oncologist 1999;4:209–224.
14. Campbell JW, Pollack IF. Growth factors in gliomas: antisense and dominant negative mutant strategies. J Neuro-Oncology 1997;35:275–285.
15. Julien T, Frankel B, Longo S, et al. Antisense-mediated inhibition of the Bcl-2 gene induces apoptosis in human malignant glioma. Surg Neurol 2000;53:360–369.
16. Jansen M, deWitt Hamer PC, Witmer AN, Troost D, vanNoorden JF. Current perspectives on antiangiogenesis strategies in the tretment of malignant gliomas. Brain Res Rev 2004;45:143–163.
17. Lassman AB. Molecular biology of gliomas. Curr Neurol Neurosci Rep 2004;4:228–233.
18. Konopka G, Bonni A. Signaling pathways regulating gliomagenesis. Curr Mol Med 2003;3:73–84.

19. Weiner HL. The role of growth factor receptors in central nervous system development and neoplasia. Neurosurgery 1995;37:179–194.

20. Wikstrand CJ, McLendon RE, Friedman AH, Bigner DD. Cell surface localization and density of the tumor-associated variant of the epidermal growth factor receptor, EGFRvIII. Cancer Res 1997;57:4130–4140.

21. Nagane M, Levitzki A, Gazit A, Cavanee WK, Huang HJS. Drug resistance of human glioblastoma cells conferred by a tumor-specific mutant epidermal growth factor receptor through modulation of Bcl-XL and caspase-3-like proteases. Proc Natl Acad Sci USA 1998;95:5724–5729.

22. Feldkamp MM, Lala P, Lau N, Roncari L, Guha A. Expression of activated epidermal growth factor receptors, ras-guanosine triphosphate and mitogen-activated protein kinase in human glioblastoma multiforme specimens. Neurosurgery 1999;45:1442–1453.

23. Barker FG, Simmons SM, Chang SM, et al. EGFR overexpression and radiation response in glioblastoma multiforme. Int J Radiat Oncol Biol Phys 2001;51:410–418.

24. Gross ME, Shazer RL, Agus DB. Targeting the HER-kinase axis in cancer. Semin Oncol 2004;31:9–20.

25. Ciardiello F, Caputo R, Bianco R, et al. Antitumor effect and potentiation of cytotoxic drugs activity in human cancer cells by ZD-1839 (Iressa), an epidermal growth factor receptor-selective tyrosine kinase inhibitor. Clin Cancer Res 2000;6:2053–2063.

26. Morin MJ. From oncogene to drug: development of small molecule tyrosine kinase inhibitors as anti-tumor and anti-angiogenic agents. Oncogene 2000;19:6574–6583.

27. Moyer JD, Barbacci EG, Iwata KK, et al. Induction of apoptosis and cell cycle arrest by CP-358,774, an inhibitor of epidermal growth factor receptor tyrosine kinase. Cancer Res 1997;57:4838–4848.

28. Fleming TP, Saxena A, Clark WC, et al. Amplification and/or overexpression of platelet-derived growth factor receptors and epidermal growth factor receptor in human glial tumors. Cancer Res 1992;52:4550–4553.

29. Hermanson M, Funa K, Hartman M, et al. Platelet-derived growth factor and its receptors in human glioma tissue: expression of messenger RNA and protein suggests the presence of autocrine and paracrine loops. Cancer Res 1992;52:3213–3219.

30. Maxwell M, Naber SP, Wolfe HJ, et al. Coexpression of platelet-derived growth factor (PDGF) and PDGF-receptor genes by primary human astrocytomas may contribute to their development and maintenance. J Clin Invest 1990;86:131–140.

31. Shamah SM, Stiles CD, Guha A. Dominant-negative mutants of platelet-derived growth factor revert the transformed phenotype of human astrocytoma cells. Mol Cell Biol 1993;13:7203–7212.

32. Guha A, Dashner K, Black PM, Wagner JA, Stiles CD. Expression of PDGF and PDGF receptors in human astrocytoma operation specimens supports the existence of an autocrine loop. Int J Cancer 1995;60:168–173.

33. Takeuchi H, Kanzawa T, Kondo Y, Kondo S. Inhibition of platelet-derived growth factor signalling induces autophagy in malignant glioma cells. Br J Cancer 2004;90:1069–1075.

34. Vassbotn FS, Ostman A, Langeland N, et al. Activated platelet-derived growth factor autocrine pathway drives the transformed phenotype of a human glioblastoma cell line. J Cell Physiol 1994;158:381–389.

35. Plate KH, Breier G, Welch HA, Risau W. Vascular endothelial growth factor is a potential tumor angiogenesis factor in human gliomas in vivo. Nature 1992;359:845–848.

36. Hermanson M, Funa K, Hartman M, et al. Platelet-derived growth factor and its receptors in human glioma tissue: expression of messenger RNA and protein suggests the presence of autocrine and paracrine loops. Cancer Res 1992;52:3213–3219.

37. Leon SP, Zhu J, Black PM. Genetic aberrations in human brain tumors. Neurosurgery 1994;34:708–722.

38. Guo P, Hu B, Gu W, et al. Platelet-derived growth factor-B enhances glioma angiogenesis by stimulating vascular endothelial growth factor expression in tumor endothelia and by promoting pericyte recruitment. Am J Pathol 2003;162:1083–1093.

39. Uhrbom L, Hesselager G, Nister M, Westermark B. Induction of brain tumors in mice using a recombinant platelet-derived growth factor B-chain retrovirus. Cancer Res 1998;58:5275–5279.

40. Vassbotn FS, Andersson M, Westermark B, Heldin CH, Ostman A. Reversion of autocrine transformation by a dominant negative platelet-derived growth factor mutant. Mol Cell Biol 1993;13:4066–4076.

41. Kuratsu J, Ushio Y. Antiproliferative effect of trapidil, a platelet-derived growth factor antagonist, on a glioma cell line in vitro. J Neurosurg 1990;73:436–440.

42. Mischel PS, Cloughesy TF. Targeted molecular therapy of GBM. Brain Pathol 2003;13:52–61.

43. Druker BJ. Perspectives on the development of a molecularly targeted agent. Cancer Cell 2002;1:31–36.

44. Druker BJ. Efficacy and safety of a specific inhibitor of the BCR-ABL tyrosine kinase in chronic myelogenous leukemia. N Engl J Med 2001;344:1031–1037.

45. Kilic T, Alberta JA, Zdunek PR, et al. Intracranial inhibition of platelet-derived growth growth factor-mediated glioblastoma cell growth by an orally active kinase inhibitor of the 2-phenylaminopyridine class. Cancer Res 2000;60:5143–5150.

46. Underiner TL, Ruggeri B, Gingrich DE. Development of vascular endothelial growth factor receptor (VEGFR) kinase inhibitors as anti-angiogenic agents in cancer therapy. Curr Med Chem 2004;11:731–745.
47. Kirsch M, Schackert G, Black PM. Anti-angiogenic treatment strategies for malignant brain tumors. J Neurooncol 2000;50:149–163.
48. Plate KH, Breier G, Welch HA, Mennel HD, Risau W. Vascular endothelial growth factor and glioma angiogenesis: coordinate induction of VEGF receptors, distribution of VEGF protein and possible in vivo regulatory mechanisms. Int J Cancer 1994;59:520–529.
49. Wedge SR, Ogilvie DJ, Dukes M, et al. ZD4190: an orally active inhibitor of vascular endothelial growth factor signaling with broad-spectrum antitumor efficacy. Cancer Res 2000;60:970–975.
50. Wedge SR, Ogilvie DJ, Dukes M, et al. ZD6474 inhibits vascular endothelial growth factor signaling, angiogenesis, and tumor growth following oral administration. Cancer Res 2002;62:4645–4655.
51. Wood JM, Bold G, Buchdunger E, et al. PTK787/ZK 222584, a novel and potent inhibitor of vascular endothelial growth factor receptor tyrosine kinases, impairs vascular endothelial growth factor-induced responses and tumor growth after oral administration. Cancer Res 2000;60:2178–2189.
52. Drevs J, Muller-Driver R, Wittig C, et al. PTK787/ZK 222584, a specific vascular endothelial growth factor-receptor tyrosine kinase inhibitor, affects the anatomy of the tumor vascular bed and the functional vascular properties as detected by dynamic enhanced magnetic resonance imaging. Cancer Res 2002;62:4015–4022.
53. Fong TAT, Shawver LK, Sun L, et al. SU5416 is a potent and selective inhibitor of the vascular endothelial growth factor receptor (Flk-1/KDR) that inhibits tyrosine kinase catalysis, tumor vascularization, and growth of multiple tumor types. Cancer Res 1999;59:99–106.
54. Mendel DB, Laird AD, Smolich BD, et al. Development of SU5416, a selective small molecule inhibitor of VEGF receptor tyrosine kinase activity, as an anti-angiogenesis agent. Anti-Cancer Drug Design 2000;15:29–41.
55. Lee CG, Heijn M, diTomaso E, et al. Anti-vascular endothelial growth factor treatment augments tumor radiation response under normoxic or hypoxic conditions. Cancer Res 2000;60:5565–5570.
56. Geng L, Donnelly E, McMahon G, et al. Inhibition of vascular endothelial growth factor receptor signaling leads to reversal of tumor resistance to radiotherapy. Cancer Res 2001;61:2413–2419.
57. Jain RK. Normalizing tumor vasculature with anti-angiogenic therapy: a new paradigm for combination therapy. Nat Med 2001;7:987–989.
58. Tong RT, Boucher Y, Kozin SV, Winkler F, Hicklin DJ, Jain RK. Vascular normalization by vascular endothelial growth factor receptor 2 blockade induces a pressure gradient across the vasculature and improves drug penetration in tumors. Cancer Res 2004;64:3731–3736.
59. Nottage M, Siu LL. Rationale for Ras and Raf-1 kinase as a target for cancer therapeutics. Curr Pharm Des 2002;8:2231–2242.
60. Shingu T, Yamada K, Hara N et al. Growth inhibition of human malignant glioma cells induced by the PI3K-specific inhibitor. J Neurosurg 2003;98:161–200.
61. Cantley LC, Neel BG. New insights into tumor suppression: PTEN suppresses tumor formation by restraining the phospho-inositide 3-kinase/AKT pathway. Proc Natl Acad Sci USA 1999;96:4240–4245.
62. Ciechomska I, Pyrzynska B, Kazmierczak P, Kaminska B. Inhibition of Akt kinase signaling and activation of Forkhead are indispensable for upregulation of FasL expression in apoptosis of glioma cells. Oncogene 2003;22:7617–7627.
63. Carson JP, Kulik G, Weber MJ. Antiapoptotic signaling in LNCaP prostate cancer cells: a survival signaling pathway independent of phosphatidylinositol 3-kinase and Akt/protein kinase B. Cancer Res 1999;59:1449–1453.
64. Curnock AP, Knox KA. LY294002-mediated inhibition of phosphatidylinositol 3-kinase activity triggers growth inhibition and apoptosis in CD40-triggered Ramos-Burkitt lymphoma B cells. Cell Immunol 1998;187:77–87.
65. Hu L, Zaloudek C, Mills GB. In vivo and in vitro ovarian carcinoma growth inhibition by a phosphatidylinositol 3-kinase inhibitor (LY294002). Clin Cancer Res 2000;6:880–886.
66. Moore SH, Rintoul RC, Walker TR, et al. The presence of a constitutively active phosphoinositide 3-kinase in small cell lung cancer cells mediates anchorage-independent proliferation via a protein kinase B and p70S6K-dependent pathway. Cancer Res 1998;58:5239–5247.
67. Vlahos CJ, Matter WF, Hui KY et al. A specific inhibitor of phosphatidylinositol 3-kinase, 2-(4-morpholinyl)-8-phenyl-4H-1-benzopyran-4-one (LY 294002). J Biol Chem 1994;269:5241–5248.
68. Kubiatowski T, Jang T, Lacyankar MB, et al. Association of increased phosphatidylinositol 3-kinase signaling with increased invasiveness and gelatinase activity in malignant gliomas. J Neurosurg 2001;95:480–488.
69. Ling J, Liu Z, Wang D, Gladson CL. Malignant astrocytoma cell attachment and migration to various matrix proteins is differentially sensitive to phopshoinositide 3-OH kinase inhibitors. J Cell Biochem 1999;73:533–544.

70. O'Gorman DM, McKenna SL, McGahon AJ et al. Sensitization of HL60 human leukaemic cells to cytotoxic drug-induced apoptosis by inhibition of PI3-kinase survival signals. Leukemia 2000;14:602–611.

71. Toretsky JA, Thakar M, Eskenazi AE, Frantz CN. Phosphoinositide 3-hydroxide kinase blockade enhances apoptosis in the Ewing's sarcoma family of tumors. Cancer Res 1999;59:5745–5750.

72. Li DM, Sun H. PTEN/MMAC1/TEP1 suppresses the tumorigenicity and induces G1 cell cycle arrest in human glioblastoma cells. Proc Natl Acad Sci USA 1998;95:15,406–15,411.

73. Mischel PS, Nelson SF, Cloughesy TF. Molecular analysis of glioblastoma: pathway profiling and its implications for patient therapy. Cancer Biol Ther 2003;2:242–247.

74. Huang S, Bjornsti MA, Houghton PJ. Rapamycins: mechanism of action and cellular resistance. Cancer Biol Ther 2003;2:222–232.

75. Knobbe CB, Merlo A, Reifenberger G. PTEN signaling in gliomas. Neuro-oncol 2002;4:196–211.

76. Neshat MS, Mellinghoff IK, Tran C, Stiles B, Thomas G, Petersen R, Frost P, Gibbons JJ, Wu H, Sawyers CL. Enhanced sensitivity of PTEN-deficient tumors to inhibition of FRAP/mTOR. Proc Natl Acad Sci USA 2001;98:10,314–10,319.

77. Dancey JE. Clinical development of mammalian target of rapamycin inhibitors. Hemat Oncol Clin North Am 2002;16:1101–1114.

78. Lowinger TB, Riedl B, Dumas J, Smith RA. Design and discovery of small molecules targeting Raf-1 kinase. Curr Pharm Des 2002;8:2269–2278.

79. Glass TL, Liu TJ, Yung WK. Inhibition of cell growth in human glioblastoma cell lines by farnesyltransferase inhibitor SCH66336. Neuro-oncol 2000;2:151–158.

80. Guha A, Feldkamp MM, Lau N, Boss G, Pawson A. Proliferation of human malignant astrocytomas is dependent on Ras activation. Oncogene 1997;15:2755–2765.

81. Delmas C, Heliez C, Cohen-Jonathan E. Farnesyltransferase inhibitor R115777, reverses the resistance of human glioma cell lines to ionizing radiation. Int J Cancer 2002;100:43–48.

82. Gupta AK, Bakanauskas VJ, Cerniglia GJ, Cheng Y, Bernhard EJ, Muschel RJ, McKenna WG. The Ras radiation resistance pathway. Cancer Res 2001;61:4278–4282.

83. Gupta AK, Bakanauskas VJ, McKenna WG, Bernhard EJ, Muschel RJ. Ras regulation of radioresistance in cell culture. Methods Enzymol 2001;333:284–290.

84. Bernhard EJ, Stanbridge EJ, Gupta S, et al. Direct evidence for the contribution of activated N-ras and K-ras oncogenes to increased intrinsic radiation resistance in human tumor cell lines. Cancer Res 2000;60:6597–6600.

85. Alavi A, Hood J, Frausto R, Stupack DG, Cheresh D. Role of Raf in vascular protection from distinct apoptotic stimuli. Science 2003;301:94–96.

86. Hood JD, Bednarski M, Frausto R, et al. Tumor regression by targeted gene delivery to the neovasculature. Science 2002;296:2404–2407.

87. Wilhelm SM, Carter C, Tang L, et al. BAY 43-9006 exhibits broad spectrum oral antitumor activity and targets the RAF/MEK/ERK pathway and receptor tyrosine kinases involved in tumor progression and angiogenesis. Cancer Res 2004;64:7099–7109.

88. Wilhelm S, Chien DS. BAY 43-9006: preclinical data. Curr Pharm Des 2002;8:2255–2257.

89. Lyons JF, Wilhelm S, Hibner B, Bollag G. Discovery of a novel Raf kinase inhibitor. Endocr Relat Cancer 2001;8:219–225.

90. Dai Y, Grant S. Small molecule inhibitors targeting cyclin-dependent kinases as anticancer agents. Curr Oncol Rep 2004;6:123–130.

91. Kim KS, Sack JS, Tokarski JS, et al. Thio- and oxoflavopiridols, cyclin-dependent kinase 1-selective inhibitors: synthesis and biological effects. J Med Chem 2000;43:4126–4134.

92. Motwani M, Delohery TM, Schwartz GK. Sequential dependent enhancement of caspase activation and apoptosis by flavopiridol on paclitaxel-treated human gastric and breast cancer cells. Clin Cancer Res 1999;5:1876–1883.

93. Baker AH, Edwards DR, Murphy G. Metalloproteinase inhibitors: biological actions and therapeutic opportunities. J Cell Science 2002;115:3719–3727.

94. Evans JD, Stark A, Johnson CD, et al. A phase II trial of marimastat in advanced pancreatic cancer. Br J Cancer 2001;85:1865–1870.

95. Bramhall SR, Hallissey MT, Whiting J, et al. Marimastat as maintenance therapy for patients with advanced gastric cancer: a randomised trial. Br J Cancer 2002;86:1864–1870.

96. Adams J. Development of the proteasome inhibitor PS-341. Oncologist 2002;7:9–16.

97. Adams J. The proteasome: structure, function, and role in the cell. Cancer Treat Rev 2003;29(suppl 1):3–9.

98. Adams J. Proteasome inhibitors as new anticancer drugs. Curr Opin Oncol 2002;14:628–634.

99. Adams J. The proteasome: a suitable antineoplastic target. Nat Rev Cancer 2004;4:349–360.

100. Adams J. The development of proteasome inhibitors as anticancer drugs. Cancer Cell 2004;5:417–421.

101. Shah SA, Potter MW, McDade TP, et al. 26S proteasome inhibition induces apoptosis and limits growth of human pancreatic cancer. J Cell Biochem 2001;82:110–122.

102. Karin M, Cao Y, Greten FR, Li ZW. NF-KB in cancer: from innocent bystander to major culprit. Nature Rev Cancer 2002;2:301310.

103. Bentires-Alj M, Barbu V, Fillet M, et al. NF-KB transcription factor induces drug resistance through through MDR1 expression in cancer cells. Oncogene 2003;22:90–97.

104. Cusack JC, Liu R, Houston M, et al. Enhanced chemosensitivity to CPT-11 with proteasome inhibitor PS-341: implications for systemic nuclear factor kappa B inhibition. Cancer Res 2001;61:3535–3540.

105. Russo SM, Tepper JE, Baldwin AS, et al. Enhancement of radiosensitivity by proteasome inhibition: implications for a role of NF-KB. Int J Radiat Oncol Biol Phys 2001;50:183–193.

106. Wang S, Yang D, Lippman ME. Targeting Bcl-2 and Bcl-XL with nonpeptidic small-molecule antagonists. Semin Oncol 2003;30:133–142.

107. Lytle RA, Jiang Z, Zheng X, Rich KM. BCNU down-regulates anti-apoptotic proteins Bcl-xL and Bcl-2 in association with cell death in oligodendroglioma-derived cells. J Neuro Oncol 2004;68:233–241.

108. Jiang Z, Zheng X, Rich KM. Down-regulation of Bcl-2 and Bcl-xL expression with bispecific antisense treatment in glioblastoma cell lines induce cell death. J Neurochem 2003;84:273–281.

109. Guensberg P, Wacheck V, Lucas T, Monia B, Pehamberger H, Eichler E, Jansen B. Bcl-xL antisense oligonucleotides chemosensitize human glioblastoma cells. Chemotherapy 2002;48:189–195.

110. Fry DW. Site-directed irreversible inhibitors of the erbB family of receptor tyrosine kinases as novel chemotherapeutic agents for cancer. Anti-Cancer Drug Design 2000;15:3–16.

111. deLange ECM. Potential role of ABC transporters as a detoxification system at the blood-CSF barrier. Adv Drug Deliv Rev 2004;56:1793–1809.

112. Kusuhara H, Sugiyama Y. Efflux transport systems for drugs at the blood-brain barrier and blood-cerebrospinal fluid barrier (part 1). Drug Discov Today 2001;6:150–156.

113. Regina A, Demeule M, Laplante A, Jodoin J, Dagenais C, Moghrabi A, Beliveau R. Multidrug resistance in brain tumors: roles of the blood-brain barrier. Cancer Metastasis Rev 2001;20:13–25.

114. Misra A, Ganesh S, Shahiwala A, Shah SP. Drug delivery to the central nervous system: a review. J Pharm Pharm Sci 2003;6:252–273.

115. Kusuhara H, Sugiyama Y. Efflux transport systems for organic anions and cations at the blood-CSF barrier. Adv Drug Deliv Rev 2004;56:1741–1763.

116. Vogelbaum MA, Nelms JL, Daneshvar H, Cutter CT, Gill S. Evaluation of tissue penetration of Erlotinib (OSI-774) in a rat xenograft brain tumor model. Proceedings of the AACR-NCI-EORTC International Conference on Molecular Targets and Cancer Therapeutics Discovery, Biology, and Clinical Applications; Boston, Massachusetts: American Association for Cancer Research; Nov 17–21, 2003.

117. Li B, Chang CM, Yuan M, McKenna WG, Shu HKG. Resistance to small molecule inhibitors of epidermal growth factor receptor in malignant gliomas. Cancer Res 2003;63:7443–7450.

118. Krystal GW. Mechanisms of resistance to imatinib (STI571) and prospects for combination with conventional chemotherapeutic agents. Drug Resist Updat 2001;4:16–21.

119. Weisberg E, Griffin JD. Resistance to imatinib (Glivec): update on clinical mechanisms. Drug Resist Updat 2003;6:231–238.

120. Gorre ME, Mohammed M, Ellwood K. Clinical resistance to STI-571 cancer therapy caused by BCR-ABL gene mutation or amplification. Science 2001;293:876–880.

121. Huron DR, Gorre ME, Kraker AJ, Sawyers CL, Rosen N, Moasser MM. A novel pyridopyrimidine inhibitor of abl kinase is a picomolar inhibitor of Bcr-abl-driven K562 cells and is effective against STI571-resistant Bcr-abl mutants. Clin Cancer Res 2003;9:1267–1273.

122. Nakajima A, Tauchi T, Sumi M, Bishop WR, Ohyashiki K. Efficacy of SCH66336, a farnesyl transferase inhibitor, in conjunction with imatinib against BCR-ABL-positive cells. Mol Cancer Ther 2003;2:219–224.

123. Hoover RR, Mahon FX, Melo JV, Daley GQ. Overcoming STI571 resistance with the farnesyl transferase inhibitor SCH66336. Blood 2002;100:1068–1071.

124. Klejman A, Rushen L, Morrione A, Slupianek A, Skorski T. Phosphatidylinositol-3 kinase inhibitors enhance the anti-leukemia effect of STI571. Oncogene 2002;21:5868–5876.

125. ClinicalTrials.gov website. A service of the National Institutes of Health developed by the National Library of Medicine. Available at: http://www.clinicaltrials.gov. Accessed October 20, 2004.

126. Cloughesy TF, Filka E, Kuhn J, Nelson G, Kabbinavar F, Friedman H, Miller LL, Elfring GL. Two studies evaluating irinotecan treatment for recurrent malignant glioma using an every-3-week regimen. Cancer 2003;97(9 Suppl):2381–2386.

127. Goel S, Mani S, Perez-Soler R. Tyrosine kinase inhibitors: a clinical perspective. Curr Oncol Rep 2002;4:9–19.

21

Cytokine Immuno-Gene Therapy for Malignant Brain Tumors

Roberta P. Glick, Terry Lichtor, Henry Lin, and Edward P. Cohen

Summary

The prognosis for patients with malignant glioma is poor. Conventional treatments such as surgery, radiation therapy, and chemotherapy have done little to affect long-term survival, and new methods of treatment are urgently needed. In this report, approaches involving cytokine gene therapy in treatment of malignant brain tumors are reviewed and contrasted with a strategy developed in this laboratory involving the use of allogeneic cells which have been genetically modified to secrete cytokines. In our studies, mice with an intracerebral glioma, melanoma, or breast carcinoma treated solely by intratumoral injections with allogeneic cells genetically modified to secrete interleukin-2 were found to survive significantly longer than mice in various control groups. The anti-tumor response was mediated predominantly by T-cell subsets (CD8+ and NK/LAK cells). The injections resulted in the killing of only the neoplastic cells; non-neoplastic cells were unaffected. Experiments involving treatment of animals with intracerebral tumor using subcutaneous injections of cytokine secreting allogeneic cells in the presence of tumor antigens demonstrated no effect in prolonging survival in spite of the development of a vigorous system antitumor immune response. Of special interest, mice injected intracerebrally with the cytokine-secreting allogeneic cells alone exhibited no neurologic defect and there were no adverse effects on survival. The injection of cytokine-secreting allogeneic cells into the microenvironment of an intracerebral tumor may induce an anti-tumor immune response capable of prolonging survival. This preclinical animal data directly translates into clinical treatments for patients with a malignant intracerebral tumor. Based upon data from our laboratory and from other Neuro-Oncologists, it is time to think about including immunotherapy in the treatment paradigm for malignant gliomas as a possible means of delaying recurrence.

Key Words: Immuno-gene therapy; glioma, IL-2; tumor vaccine.

INTRODUCTION

The current prognosis for patients with malignant brain tumors remains poor *(1)*. Malignant gliomas are the most common primary brain tumor. Despite treatment with surgery, radiation, and chemotherapy, the 2-yr survival remains less than 20%. One emerging strategy in the treatment of tumors involves stimulation of an immunologic response against the neoplastic cells. The hope is that the immune system can be called into play to destroy malignant cells. However, in most instances, proliferating tumors do not provoke anti-tumor cellular immune responses. The precise mechanisms that enable antigenic neoplasms to escape host immunity are not completely understood. The cells appear to escape recognition by the immune system in spite of the fact that neoplastic cells form weakly immunogenic tumor associated antigens (TAAs).

From: *Current Clinical Oncology: High-Grade Gliomas: Diagnosis and Treatment*
Edited by: G. H. Barnett © Humana Press Inc., Totowa, NJ

Tumor cells may evade immune responses by losing expression of antigens or major histocompatiblity complex (MHC) molecules or by producing immunosuppressive cytokines. In addition, T cells that recognize self-antigens may differentiate into suppressor or regulatory cells, which inhibit the activation and/or functions of effector cells. The inhibitory effects of suppressor cells may be mediated by cytokines. In particular interleukin-10 and TGF-β are two examples of such cytokines. Successful methods to induce immunity to TAAs could lead to tumor cell destruction and prolong the survival of cancer patients.

A variety of strategies have been used to increase the immunogenetic properties of vaccine therapies for brain tumors. The immune response can be augmented by genetic modification of tumor cells to secrete cytokines including IL-2, granulocyte macrophage-colony stimulating factor (GM-CSF) and interferon-γ. One can also alter the MHC of the tumor cells to express allogeneic determinants. Finally, one can genetically modify the tumor cells to express co-stimulatory molecules such as B7. In some instances, objective evidence of tumor regression has been observed in patients receiving immunizations only with tumor cell immunogens, suggesting the potential effectiveness of this type of immunotherapy for malignant neoplasms. In addition, modification of delivery techniques to treat intracerebral tumors has included intrathecal, intralymphatic, subcutaneous and intratumoral injections of treatment cells. We have utilized many of these techniques to enhance the immune response in the development of our cellular vaccine, as discussed below.

Recent advances in our understanding of the biology of the immune system have led to the identification of numerous cytokines that modulate immune responses (2–4). These agents mediate many of the immune responses involved in anti-tumor immunity. Several of these cytokines have been produced by recombinant DNA methodology and evaluated for their anti-tumor effects. In experimental clinical trials, the administration of cytokines and related immunomodulators has resulted in objective tumor responses in some patients with various types of neoplasms (4–6).

Interleukin-2 (IL-2) is an important cytokine in the generation of anti-tumor immunity (5). In response to tumor antigens, the helper T-cell subset of lymphocytes secretes small quantities of IL-2. This IL-2 acts locally at the site of tumor antigen presentation to activate cytotoxic T-cells and natural killer cells that mediate systemic tumor cell destruction. Intravenous, intralymphatic, or intralesional administration of IL-2 has resulted in clinically significant responses in several types of cancer (5–9). However, severe toxicities (hypotension and edema) limit the dose and efficacy of intravenous and intralymphatic IL-2 administration (6,8). The toxicity of systemically administered cytokines is not surprising as these agents mediate local cellular interactions, and they are normally secreted in quantities too small to have systemic effects. To circumvent the toxicity of systemic IL-2 administration, several investigators have examined intralesional injection of IL-2 (9,10). This approach eliminates the toxicity associated with systemic IL-2 administration. However, multiple intralesional injections are required to optimize therapeutic efficacy (9,10). These injections will be impractical for many patients without potential significant morbidity, particularly when tumor sites are not accessible for direct injection.

Cytokine gene transfer has resulted in significant anti-tumor immune responses in several animal tumor models (11–14). In these studies, the transfer of cytokine genes into tumor cells has reduced or abrogated the tumorigenicity of the cells after implantation into syngeneic hosts. The transfer of genes for IL-2 (11,12), γ interferon (IFN-γ) (13), and IL-4 (14) significantly reduced or eliminated the growth of several different histological types of murine tumors. Other cytokines capable of producing similar results include GM-CSF (15) and interleukin-12 *(16)*. In the studies employing IL-2 gene transfer, the treated animals also developed systemic anti-tumor immunity and were protected against subsequent tumor challenges with the unmodified parental tumor *(11,12)*. Similar inhibition of tumor growth and protective immunity were also demonstrated when immunizations were performed with a mixture of unmodified parental tumor cells and genetically modified tumor cells engineered to express the IL-2 gene. No toxicity associated with expression of the cytokine transgenes was reported in these animal tumor studies *(11–14)*. An alternative strategy is to genetically modify tumor cells to express an antisense gene to TGF-β, which is a cytokine highly expressed in glioma cells that acts to inhibit the function of cytotoxic T cells *(17)*.

Previous immunotherapy strategies have utilized classical immunologic cell types including activated lymphocytes and LAK cells. More recently, a variety of cells have been investigated for their usefulness in tumor oncology, including tumor cells themselves (syngeneic or allogeneic), dendritic cells, or fibroblasts (syngeneic or allogeneic). Although syngeneic tumor cells have the advantage that they express most of the appropriate antigens needed for targeted therapy, many types of tumors are difficult to establish in culture. In addition, cytokine gene therapies requiring the transduction of autologous tumor cells may not be practical for many cancer patients. Modification of neoplastic cells taken directly from tumor-bearing patients may be difficult. In particular, a primary tumor cell line required for retroviral modification has to be established. An alternative cell type that can be used for therapeutic immunizations is the dendritic cell (DC), which is a specialized antigen-presenting cell (APC). Preclinical studies have indicated that immunizing either mice or rats with DC pulsed using tumor cell antigens can stimulate a cytotoxic T-cell response that is tumor-specific and that engenders protective immunity against central nervous system (CNS) tumor in the treated animals *(18,19)*. It is also conceivable that a subpopulation of the primary tumor, selected for its capacity to grow in vitro, may not reflect the tumor cell population as a whole especially because tumors such as glioma are known to be heterogeneous.

We have chosen an allogeneic fibroblast cell line as an "off-the-shelf" cellular vaccine for a number of reasons. Fibroblasts obtained from established allogeneic fibroblast cell lines may be readily cultured in vitro and genetically modified to express and secrete cytokines *(20–24)*. The cells can be genetically modified to secrete cytokines and subsequently injected directly into the tumor bed. The use of allogeneic rather than syngeneic cells was initially based upon evidence that allogeneic MHC determinants augment the immunogenic properties of the tumor vaccine *(22–24)*. Application of genetically modified fibroblasts in therapeutic vaccines facilitates titration of single or multiple cytokine doses independent of tumor cell doses. Like other allografts, the allogeneic cytokine-secreting cells are rejected. Furthermore, the number of cells can be expanded as desired for multiple rounds of therapy. In addition, the slow continuous release of cytokines and the eventual rejection of the allograft may be a useful advantage in the treatment of brain tumors where long-term secretion of high concentrations of certain cytokines may be associated with increased morbidity. Thus, an allogeneic cytokine secreting vaccine is readily available, easily expanded, possibly less toxic, and more immunogenic. These considerations provide the rationale for examining the use of allogeneic fibroblasts genetically modified to secrete cytokines in our studies as a means of enhancing anti-tumor immune responses in treatment of malignant intracerebral tumors *(20–26)*. We will review our studies investigating the use of this cellular vaccine not only as a treatment vaccine for an existing malignant glioma but also as a protective vaccine for the possibility of delaying recurrence of gliomas.

MATERIALS AND METHODS

Cell Lines and Experimental Animals

Gl261 is a malignant glial tumor syngeneic in C57BL/6 mice. The tumor was originally obtained from Dr. J. Mayo (DCT, DPT, National Cancer Institute, Frederick, MD); it was maintained by serial transfer in histocompatible C57BL/6 mice. LM cells, a fibroblast cell line of C3H/He mouse origin, were from the American Type Culture Collection (Manassas, VA). The LM cells were maintained at 37°C in a humidified 7% CO_2/air atmosphere in Dulbecco's modified Eagle's medium (DMEM) (Life Technologies, Grand Island, NY) supplemented with 10% fetal bovine serum (FBS) (Sigma, St. Louis, MO) and antibiotics (Life Technologies) (growth medium).

The animals used were 8- to 10-wk-old pathogen-free C57Bl/6 (H-2^b) or C3H/He (H-2^k) mice obtained from Charles River Breeding Laboratories (Portage, MI). The mice were maintained in the animal care facilities of the University of Illinois, according to National Institutes of Health (NIH) Guidelines for the Care and Use of Laboratory Animals. They were 8- to 12-wk-old when used in the experiments.

Intracerebral Injection of Mice

A cannula system, which we developed and previously described, was modified for injection of tumor cells and the modified fibroblasts (26). Small screws (0–80 × 1/16; 1.6 mm in length) were obtained from Plastics One (Roanoke, VA) and a .022 µmdiameter hole was subsequently drilled through the center of the screw. Mice were anesthetized and a small burr hole was placed with a D#60 drill bit (Plastics One, Roanoke, VA) over the right frontal lobe in the region of the coronal suture. The screws bearing a central hole were subsequently secured into the small burr hole using Elmer's Super Glue Gel. The mice were allowed to recover and on specified days injections were made using a Hamilton syringe containing a 26-gage needle with a small piece of solder placed 5 mm from the tip of the needle to maintain a uniform depth of injection. The total injection volume was between 5 and 10 µL.

Preparation of Cytokine (IL-2 and/or IFN-γ) Secreting Mouse Fibroblasts

IL-2 secreting mouse fibroblasts were prepared as described previously (27). The gene for IL-2 was transduced into LM fibroblasts with a retroviral plasmid (pZipNeoSV-IL-2) (obtained originally from T. Taniguchi, Institute for Molecular and Cellular Biology, Osaka University, Japan) (28). The plasmid contains a human IL-2 cDNA and a gene (neo^r) that confers resistance to the aminoglycoside antibiotic, G418 (29) used for selection.

To prepare the IL-2/IFN-γ double cytokine-secreting cells, the IL-2 secreting cells were co-transfected (lipofectin-mediated; Gibco BRL, Grand Island, NY) with DNA from pZipNeo SVIFN-γ (obtained from M. K. L. Collins, Institute of Cancer Research, London, England) along with DNA from pHyg (obtained from L. Lau, University of Illinois, Chicago, IL), as previously described (30). The plasmid confers resistance to hygromycin (31) used for selection.

IFN-γ single cytokine-secreting cell-lines were prepared by co-transfection of LM cells with DNA from pZipNeoSVIFN-γ along with DNA from pHyg, as previously described (30). The cells were maintained for 14 d in growth medium containing 300 g/mL hygromycin. To maintain cytokine-secretion, every third passage the cells were routinely placed in the relevant selection medium.

Modification of LM or LM-IL-2 Fibroblasts (H-2^k) to Express H-2K^b Class I-Determinants (Eemi-Allogeneic/Syngeneic Cells)

A plasmid (pBR327H-2K^b from Biogen Research Corp, Cambridge, MA) encoding MHC H-2K^b determinants was used to modify LM or LM-IL-2 fibroblasts to express H-2K^b determinants. Ten μg of PBR327H-2K^b and 1 μg of pBabePuro was mixed with Lipofectin (Gibco BRL), according to the supplier's instructions. The plasmid pBabePuro (obtained from M. K. L. Collins, University College, London, England) conferring resistance to puromycin, was used for selection. The plasmid-mixture was added to 1×10^6 LM or LM-IL-2 cells in 10 mL of DMEM, without FBS. For use as a control, an equivalent number of LM or LM-IL-2 cells were transfected with 1 μg of pBabePuro alone. The cells were incubated for 18 h at 37°C in a CO$_2$/air atmosphere, washed with DMEM, followed by the addition of growth medium. After incubation for 48 h, the cell cultures were divided and replated in growth medium supplemented with 3.0 μg/mL puromycin (Sigma; St. Louis, MO) followed by incubation at 37°C for an additional 7 d. The surviving colonies were pooled and tested by staining with specific fluorescein isothiocyanate (FITC)-conjugated antibodies for the expression of H-2K^b-determinants. One hundred percent of nontransfected fibroblasts maintained in growth medium containing puromycin died during the 7-d period of incubation.

Assays for Cytokine Secretion

LIL-2 secretion by the G418-resistant cells was assayed with the use of the IL-2-dependent cell-line CTLL-2, as previously described *(32)*. One unit of IL-2 gave half-maximal proliferation of CTLL-2 cells under these conditions *(32)*. IL-2 and IFN-g secretion by the transfected cells were assayed by the use of a human IL-2 or a mouse IFN-g enzyme-linked immunosorbent assay (ELISA) kit (Genzyme, Cambridge, MA).

The Detection of mRNAs Specifying IL-2 or IFN-γ by Transfected LM Cells by the Reverse Transcription-Polymerase Chain Reaction

Reverse-transcriptase polymerase chain reaction (RT-PCR) was used as a further confirmation of the expression of the transferred cytokine genes. Total cellular RNA was prepared from the relevant cell types, according to the method described by Chomczynski et al. *(33)* and then transcribed into cDNA and amplified, as previously described *(30)*.

Histopathologic Examination of the Tumors

Animals from each group were sacrificed near death (animal unable to feed) for histologic examination

Spleen Cell-Mediated Cytotoxicity by ^{51}Cr-Release Assay

Mononuclear cells from the spleens of C57BL/6 mice immunized with the various cell constructs were used as sources of effector cells for the cytotoxicity studies using a standard 4-h cromium release assay, as previously described *(30)*.

In Vitro Determination of the Classes of Effector Cells Activated for the Anti-Glioma Cytotoxicity

The effect of monoclonal antibodies (MAbs) for T-cell subsets or NK/LAK cells on the anti-tumor response was used to identify the predominant cell-types activated for anti-tumor cytotoxicity in mice immunized with the cytokine-secreting cells.

Statistical Analysis

Student's *t*-test was used to determine the statistical differences between the survival of mice in various experimental and control groups. A *p* value below 0.05 was considered significant.

RESULTS

Simultaneous Intracerebral Injection of Glioma and Cytokine Secreting Allogeneic Cells

We measured the survival of C57Bl/6 mice injected intracerebrally (ic) with a mixture of Gl261 glioma cells and cytokine secreting LM cells. Gl261 cells are a glioma cell-line of C57Bl/6 mouse origin (H-2^b). LM fibroblasts are derived from C3H/He mice and express H-2^k determinants. We initially evaluated the immunotherapeutic effects of single cytokine-secreting LM-IL-2 cells and double cytokine-secreting LM-IL-2/interferon-γ cells in mice bearing an ic glioma. A mixture of G1261 cells and the single or double cytokine-secreting cells were injected ic into the right frontal lobe of C57BL/6 mice, syngeneic with G1261 cells (Fig. 1). Mice injected ic with the mixture of glioma and LM-IL-2 cells survived significantly longer (*p* < 0.025) than control mice injected ic with an equivalent number of glioma cells alone. Somewhat more dramatic results were obtained for mice injected ic with a mixture of glioma cells and LM-IL-2/interferon-γ double cytokine-secreting cells. In addition, the survival of this group was statistically prolonged relative to either untreated mice with glioma or those animals injected with Gl261 cells and LM-IL-2 cells. The survival time of mice injected with a mixture of glioma cells and LM-Interferon-γ cells was not significantly different from that of mice injected with glioma cells alone (*p* > 0.1). Of special interest, mice injected ic with an equivalent number of LM-IL-2 cells alone lived for more than 3 mo and showed no evidence of ill effects or neurologic deficit. Immunocytotoxic studies demonstrated a significantly elevated cromium release from Gl261 cells co-incubated with spleen cells from mice injected ic with glioma cells and the cytokine secreting fibroblasts (Table 1).

Thus, therapy with an immunogen that combined the expression of allogeneic antigens and the secretion of cytokines led to the most significant benefit in mice with an intracerebral glioma.

Specificity of the Immune Response

The specificity of the immunocytotoxic response was evaluated against a variety of tumor cell lines (Table 2). Only spleen cells from immunized animals demonstrated an immunocytotoxic response. The response, although somewhat nonspecific when tested against a variety of tumor cell lines, was markedly enhanced when tested against the same tumor cells with which the animal was initially injected.

Intracerebral Survival and Toxicity of the Cytokine-Secreting Allogeneic Cells

The toxicity of the allogeneic cell based cytokine gene therapy for tumors is likely to depend in part on the ability of the genetically modified cells to survive in the CNS. The intracerebral distribution and survival of the cytokine secreting cells was investigated using both allogeneic C57BL/6 and syngeneic C3H/He mice. As a means of assessing survival of the allogeneic cells in the CNS, PCR analysis was performed to identify the presence of the neomycin gene in the brain sections at various time intervals (2–60 d). In brief, high-molecular-weight DNA was isolated using techniques described previously *(32)*. PCR amplification of the DNA was subsequently performed in a reaction mixture consisting of 0.4 μ*M* of primer

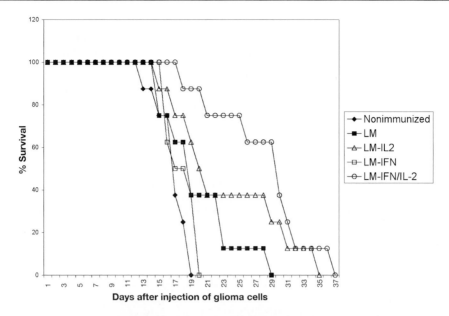

Fig. 1. Graph showing the survival rate of mice injected ic with a mixture of glioma cells and fibroblasts (LM cells) engineered to secrete cytokines. The C57Bl/6 mice (8/group) were injected ic with a mixture of 10^6 cells of one of the cell types and 10^5 Gl261 glioma cells. The median lengths of survival were as follows (in days): mice with nonimmunized glioma cells, 16.9 ± 1.9; glioma plus LM cells, 20.0 ± 4.5; glioma plus LM-IL-2 cells, 23.4 ± 6.8; glioma plus LM-IFN-γ cells, 18.0 ± 1.8; glioma plus LM-IL-2/IFN-γ cells, 28.1 ± 5.8. Probability values were: nonimmunized vs LM-IL-2, $p < 0.025$; nonimmunized or LM vs LM-IL-2/IFN-γ, $p < 0.005$; LM-IL-2 vs LM-IL-2/IFN-γ , $p < 0.05$.

Table 1
The Effect of MAbs Against T-Cell Subsets of NK/LAK Cells on the Anti-Glioma
Cytotoxic Activities of Spleen Cells From C57BL/6 Mice Injected
IC With a Mixture of Glioma and the Cytokine(s)-Secreting Cells

Cell-types for immunization[a]	MAb-treatment	% cytolysis at E:T ration of 100:1
Glioma	—	3.6 ± 1.2
	Anti-Lyt-2.2	-1.4 ± 2.5
	Anti-asialo GM1	-7.1 ± 2.8
Glioma + LM	—	5.8 ± 2.8
	Anti-Lyt-2.2	-1.9 ± 4.2
Glioma + LM-I-2	Anti-asialo GM1	-7.8 ± 1.8
	—	17.7 ± 0.7[b,c]
	Anti-Lyt-2.2	5.2 ± 2.0
	Anti-asialo GM1	-6.6 ± 2.3
Glioma + LM-IL-2/IFN-γ	—	38.3 ± 4.4[c,d,e]
	Anti-Lvt-2.2	20.4 ± 11.9

Notes:[a] C57BL/6 mice received a single ic injection of (10^5) glioma cells together with one of the modified fibroblast cell-types (10^6 cells). Three weeks after the injection, mononuclear cells from the spleens of the immunized mice obtained through Ficoll-Hypaque centrifugation were used for the ^{51}Cr-release assay. All values represent the mean ± SD of triplicate determinations.

[b] $p < 0.005$ relative to ^{51}Cr release for spleen cells from animals immunized with glioma.

[c] $p < 0.05$ relative to ^{51}Cr release for spleen cells from animals immunized with glioma + LM cells.

[d] $p < 0.025$ relative to ^{51}Cr release for spleen cells from animals immunized with glioma.

[e] $p < 0.05$ relative to ^{51}Cr release for spleen cells from animals immunized with glioma + LM-IL-2 cells.

Table 2
Cytotoxicity Toward Various Tumor Cell-Types in Spleen Cells From C57BL/6 Mice
Injected IC With a Mixture of Glioma and the Cytokine(s)-Secreting Cells

Cell type[a]	% cytolysis at E:T ration of 100:1		
	Nonimmunized	LM-IL-2	LM-IL-2/IFN-γ
Γ1261	2.2 ± 2.9	44.6 ± 0.8	63.3 ± 7.2
B16F1	-0.2 ± 2.0	14.9 ± 1.2	15.4 ± 1.3
EL4	4.1 ± 1.3	46.3 ± 4.8	37.8 ± 1.5
LI/2	10.1 ± 1.0	19.3 ± 1.4	15.1 ± 1.4

Notes: [a] C57BL/6 mice received a single ic injection of (2.0×10^5) Gl261 glioma cells together with one of the modified fibroblast cell-types (10^6 cells). Two weeks after the injection, mononuclear cells from the spleens of the immunized mice obtained through Ficoll-Hypaque centrifugation were used for the ^{51}Cr-release assay using 4 different ^{51}Cr-labeled cell types as tumor targets including Gl261 glioma, B16F1 melanoma, EL-4 lymphoma,, and LL/2 Lewis lung carcinoma cells. All tumor cells are of C57Bl/6 origin (H-2^b haplotype). All values represent the mean ± SD of triplicate determinations.

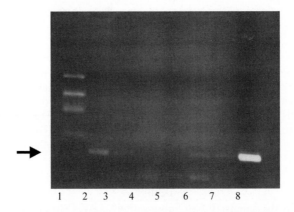

Fig. 2. PCR anaylsis for the survival of modified fibroblasts in the CNS. PCR analysis was performed for the presence of the neomycin resistance gene in brain sections taken at various time intervals (0–60 d) after implantation of modified fibroblasts into the CNS in allogeneic and syngeneic mice. DNA sequences for the neomycin resistance gene were observed on days 8 and 14 but not on days 28 or 60 after implantation in allogeneic mice, and up to 55 d in syngeneic mice. *Lane 1*, low-mass molecular marker (Life Technologies); *lane 2*, 8 d after injection into allogeneic mice; *lane 3*, 14 d after injection into allogeneic mice; *lane 4*, 28 d after injection into allogeneic mice; *lane 5*, 60 dafter injection into allogeneic mice; *lane 6*, 55 d after injection into syngeneic mice; *lane 7*, 10^3 LM-IL-2 cells; *lane 8*, pZipNeo plasmid. *Arrow* indicates the location of the 249-base pair *Neo*[r] gene.

for the *Neo*[r] gene, 3–5 µL of the DNA samples, 1.5 m*M* MgCl$_2$, 0.5 m*M* of each deoxynucleotide triphosphate (dNTP), and 2.0 U Taq plymerase (Gibco). The sequences of the *Neo* gene primers are as follows: 5' primer, 5'-GCTGTGCTCGACGTTGTCAC-3'; 3' primer, 5'-CTCT TCGTCCAGATCATCCTG-3'. The reactions were run for 38 cycles of 94°C for 1 min, 55°C for 1 min, 72°C for 1 min using a Perkin-Elmer Cetus thermal cycler. After amplification, 5 µL of the reaction mixture was removed and analyzed by electrophoresis in a 2.0% agarose gel. DNA sequences specific for the neomycin gene were found in DNA isolated from allogeneic mice on days 8 and 14, but were no longer detected on days 28 and 60 (Fig. 2). Similar experiments in syngeneic mice detected DNA sequences specific for the neomycin gene at 55

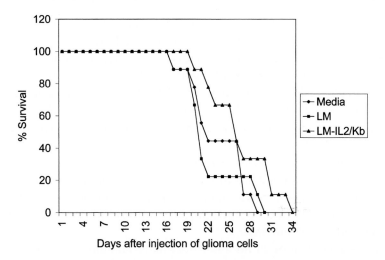

Fig. 3. Treatment of an established glioma with IL-2 secreting cells. C57Bl/6 mice (nine animals/ group) were injected ic through a cannula with 5.0×10^4 Gl261 cells followed 2 d later by the first of three weekly injections of 1.0×10^6 LM-IL-2/K^b cells. As controls, animals received an equivalent number of tumor cells followed by treatment with either LM cells or media alone at the same time intervals as described previously. MST (d): media alone, 23.4 ± 4.1; LM, 22.3 ± 4.3; LM-IL-2/K^b, 26.7 ± 4.6. p values: media alone vs LM-IL-2/K^b, $p < 0.05$; LM vs LM-IL-2/K^b, $p < 0.025$.

d. DNA sequences specific for the neomycin gene were not found in control mice injected with LM (noncytokine secreting) fibroblasts (data not shown). Thus, modified allogeneic cells fail to survive in the CNS beyond 14 d as evidenced by PCR. The animals implanted with the genetically modified cells were observed daily for evidence of neurologic deficit and other morbidity or mortality for over 60 d, and at no time did the mice exhibit neurologic deficits or adverse effects on survival.

Evaluation of the Therapeutic Benefits of LM Cells Modified to Secrete Interleukin-2 in Mice with an Established Pre-Existing Glioma

To determine if the cytokine secreting cells could be effective in treating a clinically relevant model of mice with an established glioma, naïve C57Bl/6 mice bearing cannulas were first injected with Gl261 glioma followed two days later with injection of either non-IL-2-secreting allogeneic LM fibroblasts or syngeneic/allogeneic LM-IL-2/K^b cells. The animals received two more injections of the same type of cells as first injected through the cannulas at weekly intervals for a total of three injections. The animals with an established glioma treated with IL-2 secreting syngeneic/allogeneic fibroblasts survived significantly longer in comparison to either untreated animals ($p < 0.05$) or animals treated with allogeneic LM fibroblasts ($p < 0.025$) (Fig. 3). This experiment was repeated with similar results.

Intracerebral vs Subcutaneous Immunization With Allogeneic Fibroblasts Genetically Engineered to Secrete Interleukin-2 in the Treatment of Central Nervous System Tumor

The purpose of this study was to determine the optimal route of delivery of gene therapy for an intracerebral tumor. Systemic delivery of gene therapy is of significant clinical interest.

In this study, allogeneic fibroblasts engineered to secrete interleukin-2 were administered either subcutaneously (in the presence or absence of Gl261 cells) or intracerebrally to C57Bl/6 mice with ic glioma. The results indicate a significant prolongation of survival in mice with ic glioma treated intracerebrally with LM-IL-2 cells, relative to the survival of mice with ic glioma treated subcutaneously with LM-IL-2 cells (either alone or mixed with Gl261 cells) or untreated mice with glioma ($p < 0.05$). The specific release of isotope from ^{51}Cr-labeled glioma cells co-incubated with spleen cells from animals treated either subcutaneously or intracerebrally with LM-IL-2 cells was significantly greater than the release of isotope from glioma cells co-incubated with spleen cells from nonimmunized mice ($p < 0.005$). Direct ic administration of fibroblasts genetically engineered to secrete IL-2 was more effective in prolonging survival than peripheral subcutaneous administration in the treatment of mice with ic glioma even though both treatments stimulated a strong antiglioma immune response (data not shown).

Histopathological evaluation of tumors from treated and untreated mice was performed on all animals at the time of cromium release studies (2 wk) and at the time of death (3–4 wk). The most extensive lymphocytic infiltration was in mice treated with the ic IL-2 secreting cells.

Pretreatment of Mice With Allogeneic Cytokine Secreting Cells Protects Against the Development of an Intracerebral Glioma

We previously found that the survival of C57Bl/6 mice injected with Gl261 glioma cells mixed with allogeneic IL-2 secreting fibroblasts is significantly prolonged in comparison with various control groups. In addition, in previous studies we also found that allogeneic LM-IL-2 fibroblasts modified to express H-2K^b determinants (syngeneic in C57Bl/6 mice) to form semiallogeneic LM-IL-2/K^b cells (semi-allogeneic/syngeneic) are more effective than IL-2-secreting fibroblasts that express allogeneic determinants alone in treating mice with Gl261 glioma. In order to investigate the mechanism involved in using these genetically engineered cells for protecting against the development of an intracerebral tumor, cannulas were placed into the right frontal lobe of the mice. The animals were treated two times at weekly intervals with LM-IL-2/K^b cells injected through the cannulas prior to injection of glioma cells. The tumor cells were mixed with the vaccine and introduced through the cannulas 1 wk following the second injection. The results demonstrate a significant delay in the development of glioma ($p < 0.005$) in the animals treated with either nonsecreting cells or IL-2-secreting syngeneic/allogeneic fibroblasts (Fig. 4).

Six animals in the IL-2 treated group that survived for over 3 mo were then re-challenged with an ic injection into the same site as the previous injections of 5×10^4 Gl261 glioma cells alone to determine if a long-term resistance toward glioma had been established in these animals. The results demonstrated a significant prolongation of survival ($p < 0.01$) for those animals that had been previously injected with a mixture of tumor and LM-IL-2/K^b cells in comparison to the naïve animals injected with glioma cells alone (Fig. 5). There were four long-term survivors (> 90 d) of the six total animals in the group previously treated with LM-IL2/K^b cells after receiving a second tumor challenge. These results suggest that a long-term immunity was established at the injection site in the animals that underwent multiple ic injections of LM-IL-2/K^b cells prior to tumor injection. Whether or not a more generalized systemic immunity against glioma was established in these animals has not been determined.

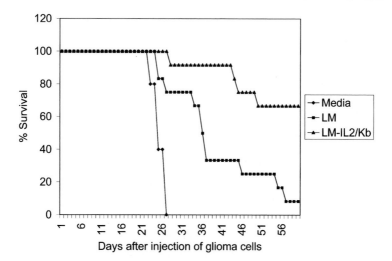

Fig. 4. Pretreatment with allogeneic fibroblasts prevents the development of a glioma. C57Bl/6 mice (12 animals/group) were injected with 1.0×10^6 LM-IL-2/K^b cells through a cannula on 2 occasions separated by 1 wk. One week following the second injection the animals were injected a third time with a mixture of 1.0×10^6 LM-IL-2/K^b cells and 5.0×10^4 Gl261 cells. As controls, animals were injected through the cannula with either 1.0×10^6 LM cells or media at the same time points along with an equivalent number of Gl261 cells at the time of the third injection. MST (d): media alone, 25.4 ± 1.6; LM, 39.6 ± 12.2; LM-IL-2/K^b, 53.9 ± 10.3. p values: media alone vs LM, $p < 0.005$; media alone vs LM-IL-2/K^b, $p < 0.0005$; LM versus LM-IL-2/K^b, $p < 0.005$.

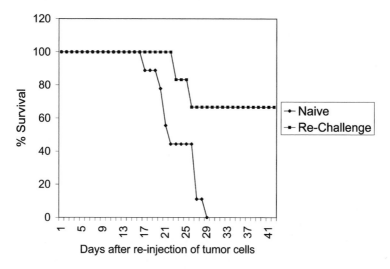

Fig. 5. Long-term immunity in mice with glioma that survived prior treatment with IL-2 secreting allogeneic fibroblasts. Six C57Bl/6 mice surviving 90 d after prior injection of Gl261 cells and LM-IL-2/K^b fibroblasts were injected through the same right frontal burr hole a second time with 5.0×10^4 Gl261 cells alone. As a control, eight naïve C57Bl/6 mice were injected ic with an equivalent number of Gl261 cells alone. MST for the untreated naïve animals injected with tumor cells was 23.4 ± 4.1 d, and 36.2 ± 7.2 for the animals that had previously been vaccinated with LM-IL-2/K^b cells and re-challenged with tumor cells. The four animals that were still alive at the conclusion of this experiment all of which had previously been treated with LM-IL2/K^b cells survived for longer than 90 d without evidence of any neurologic deficit. $p < 0.01$ for the difference in survival of mice in the two groups.

DISCUSSION

The efficacy of active tumor immunotherapy with cytokine-transduced syngeneic or allo-geneic fibroblasts has been reviewed in this paper. Intracerebral injections with IL-2 trans-duced allogeneic fibroblasts generated systemic anti-tumor immunity capable of eradicating brain tumors. In particular we constructed a cellular vaccine with enhanced anti-tumor effec-tiveness by transducing LM cells, a mouse fibroblast cell-line expressing defined MHC-determinants (H-2^k), with a modified retroviral vector that specified the gene for IL-2. C57BL/ 6 mice (H-2^b) injected ic with a mixture of Gl261 glioma cells and LM cells (H-2^k) modified for IL-2 secretion (LM-IL-2) survived significantly longer than mice in various other treat-ment groups. The anti-tumor immune responses in the tumor-bearing mice were mediated predominantly by CD8$^+$ and NK/LAK cells. This cellular vaccine was effective in treating a pre-existing tumor and in protecting against the development of a malignant glioma when vaccine is administered intracerebrally. Of special interest, mice injected ic with the cytokine-secreting allogeneic cells alone exhibited no neurologic deficit and there were no adverse effects on survival. The injection of cytokine-secreting allogeneic cells into the microenviron-ment of an intracerebral tumor is hypothesized to induce an anti-tumor immune response capable of prolonging survival.

The toxic effects of cytokines in the CNS may limit the quantity that can be administered *(34–36)*. Neurologic effects have been seen in animals injected intracranially with syngeneic cytokine-secreting cells. The co-implantation into the rat brain of syngeneic (RG-2) glioma cells and RG-2 cells modified by retroviral transduction to secrete IL-2 or IFN-γ resulted in short-term cell mediated anti-glioma responses. However the survival of the tumor bearing rats was not prolonged, and the animals died from secondary effects including severe cerebral edema *(37)*. The toxicity of a cellular-based cytokine gene therapy for tumors is likely to depend in part on the survival of the genetically modified cells in the CNS. We investigated the survival of an allogeneic IL-2 secreting vaccine in the CNS by two different means: PCR and bioassay *(38)*. We found that the survival of allogeneic cells in the CNS was less than 28 d. The cells like other allografts were rejected. The cells were well tolerated, and the animals did not demonstrate any significant neurologic or systemic toxicity. This suggests that cytokine-secreting allogeneic cells may serve as a useful vehicle for the safe delivery of cytokines into brain tumors, and supports the possibility and safety of using a monthly retreatment schedule in a clinical protocol. Most of the systemic toxicities of IL-2 therapy should be avoided by the introduction of the gene for IL-2 directly into the tumor mass, resulting in primarily local concentrations of the cytokine. This form of treatment is particularly attractive in the treatment of primary gliomas, since these tumors usually only recur locally and are rarely metastatic.

More recently, the use of a small ic cannula enables one to inject the treatment cells directly into the tumor bed on numerous occasions *(26)*. This allows us to investigate both "protective" vaccine strategies using pretreatment via the cannula prior to tumor injection as well as the effect of the vaccine on the treatment of an established tumor. One of the major concerns related to the immunologic treatment of brain tumors is the effect of the blood–brain barrier (BBB) on the development of a host immune response in the CNS. Studies using IL-4 secreting plasmacytoma cells implanted into the brains of nude mice along with human glioma cells demonstrated a dramatic eosinophilic infiltrate in regions of necrotic tumor, suggesting that an immune response can take place against a tumor of the CNS *in situ*. The response, however, was non-T-cell dependent *(26)*. We found that a specific and significant systemic immuno-cytotoxic response (by [51]cromium release assay) was present in animals with an ic glioma treated with allogeneic IL-2 secreting fibroblasts administered intracerebrally *(25,40)*. Thus the secretion of IL-2 by the cellular immunogen, or an immunogenic derivative of the cells, may have altered the BBB, enabling the immunogen to reach the spleen and lymph nodes in the periphery (41,42).

Although preclinical studies with cytokine gene therapy appear promising (15,26,43–46), clinical trials for brain tumors have been limited. Some of these trials have involved immunization with tumor cells modified with the IL-2 gene (21), the IL-4 gene (47), or TGF-β2 antisense gene (48). A number of different vaccination strategies are also currently being evaluated (49,50). The approaches to vaccination with TAAs include those based on: (1) defined antigens or antigenic peptides, (2) tumor cell lysates or lysate fractions, and (3) whole irradiated tumor cells or apoptotic tumor cell bodies. Vaccines prepared using TAAs or TAA-derived epitopes presented by APCs or fed to dendritic cells (DCs) are in early clinical trials for patients with gliomas (51–54). Many investigators use vaccines composed of defined tumor antigens. However, defined antigens have to be identified and purified, a tremendous effort requiring an "antigen discovery" approach. The quantity of purified antigen must be increased, to enable multiple immunizations of the cancer patient. Whereas new TAAs are being discovered, the question of which TAA to be used in the vaccine is uncertain and extensively debated. The choice of TAA is not a trivial decision. Not only are isolation and purification of TAAs or antigenic peptide highly labor intensive, but it remains uncertain whether or not TAA/peptide based vaccines are superior to tumor-cell vaccines. Selection of the immunizing antigen is generally based on its abundant expression in the tumor and lack of expression in normal tissues. Few antigens meet this criterion, and those that do may not always be immunogenic. The heterogeneity of antigen expression in the tumor cell population is likely to be a concern. Some tumor cells may not express the antigen chosen for therapy. de Vries, for example (55) found that expression of known tumor antigens such as gp100 and tyrosinase was variable in different melanoma lesions in the same patient. Not all the malignant cells in the patient's neoplasm expressed these determinants. Since the tumor cell population is heterogeneous, tumor cells that fail to express the defined antigen chosen for therapy are likely to escape destruction by the activated immune system. They could be the source of recurrent tumor.

The use of tumor lysates, lysate fractions or apoptotic tumor bodies for vaccination overcomes some of these limitations. However, preparation of the vaccine requires the availability of autologous tumor, often in substantial quantities. Vaccines have been prepared by culturing patient-derived DCs, and then pulsing or "feeding" the cells tumor lysates or apoptotic bodies. However, DC-based vaccines are laborious and costly to prepare. Their efficacy in generating anti-tumor immune responses capable of tumor rejection remains unproven. In all cases, the optimal adjuvant, protein or peptide concentration, the ratios of DCs or apoptotic bodies, and routes of delivery as well as immunization schedules remain undefined. They may be critical for success. Immunization by injection of "naked" plasmid DNA or RNA encoding a tumor antigen is also currently under evaluation. However, as for immunization with defined antigens, there is a danger that the antigen specified by the polynucleotide chosen may not be the most appropriate for CTL or helper T-cell generation. Anichini et al. found (56) that CTLs in melanoma patients are not always directed toward known melanoma antigens, such as Melan-A/Mart-1, MAGE-3, gp100, or tyrosinase. The implication is that there are multiple other tumor antigens, in addition to those previously identified that are expressed by different cells that comprise the malignant cell population. Only certain of these TAAs are able to induce tumor specific immune responses. The identification of the most "clinically relevant" tumor antigen cannot always be accomplished a priori, without extensive preclinical studies. Even then, subsequent validation in the patient may not confirm that these are "tumor rejection" antigens.

Another strategy involves preparation of vaccines by transfer of tumor DNA into nonmalignant fibroblast. The major advantage of this approach is that TAAs do not have to be purified or produced in large quantities. DNA-based vaccines are able to elicit robust and long-lasting activation of the immune system, which results in tumor rejection *(57,58)*. In comparison with protein vaccines, DNA-based vaccines provide prolonged expression and direct presentation of tumor antigens. This offers an opportunity for the development of effector as well as memory immune responses to many different epitopes encoded by the tumor-derived DNA. From a practical point of view, these vaccines are easy and relatively inexpensive to prepare. Unlike other strategies, vaccines can be prepared from only a limited quantity of tumor-derived DNA, which can be obtained from small surgical specimens. Furthermore, the recipient fibroblasts can be selected to meet the requirement for rapid expansion in culture and MHC restriction. The DNA-based vaccines offer a number of important advantages, which greatly encourage their further development for cancer immunotherapy.

In summary, our studies suggest that Immuno-Gene therapy using IL-2 secreting fibroblasts as a cellular vaccine can be useful as a new therapeutic approach in treatment of a primary or metastatic intracerebral tumor especially when the tumor burden is small or at the time of tumor resection. The use of cytokine secreting tumor vaccines as a "protective treatment" introduced following tumor resection hopefully will play an important role in delaying tumor recurrence. We believe that this is where immunotherapy is most promising.

REFERENCES

1. Mahaley MS, Mettlin C, Natarajan N, Laws ER, Peace BB. National survey of patterns of care for brain-tumor patients. J Neurosurg 1989;71:826–836.
2. Gabrilove JL, Jakubowski A. Hematopoietic growth factors: biology and clinical application. Monogr J Natl Cancer Inst 1990;10:73–77.
3. Kelso A. Cytokines: structure function and synthesis. Curr Opin Immunol 1989;2(2):215–225.
4. Borden EC, Sondel PM. Lymphokines and cytokines as cancer treatment. Immunotherapy realized. Cancer 1990;65(3 Suppl):800–814.
5. Rosenberg SA, Lotze MT, Mule JJ. New approaches to the immunotherapy of cancer. Ann Intern Med 1988;108:853–864.
6. Lotze MT, Chang AE, Seipp CA, Simpson C, Vetto JT, Rosenberg SA. High-dose recombinant interleukin-2 in the treatment of patients with disseminated cancer: responses, treatment-related morbidity and histologic findings. JAMA 1986;256:3117–3124.
7. Pizza G, Viza D, DeVince C, Vichi-Pascuuchi JM, Busutti L, Bergami T. Intralymphatic administration of interleukin-2 (IL-2) in cancer patients: a pilot study. Cytokine Research 1988;7:45–48.
8. Sama G, Collins J, Figlin R, Robertson P, Altrock B, Abels R. A pilot study of intralymphatic interleukin-2. II Clinical and biological effects. J Biol Resp Mod 1990;9:81–86.
9. Gandolfi L, Solmi L, Pizza GC, et al. Intratumoral echo-guided injection of interleukin-2 and cytokine-activated killer cells in hepatocellular carcinoma. Hepato-Gastroenterology 1989;36:352–356.
10. Bubenik J, Viotenok NN, Kieler J, et al. Local administration of cells containing an inserted IL-2 gene and producing IL-2 inhibits growth of human tumors in nu/nu mice. Immunol Lett 1988;19:279–282.
11. Fearon ER, Pardoll DM, Itaya T, et al. Interleukin-2 production by tumor cells bypasses T helper function in the generation of an anti-tumor reponse. Cell 1990;60:387–403.
12. Gansbacher B, Zier K, Daniels B, Cronin K, Bannedi R, Gilboa E. Interleukin-2 gene transfer into tumor cells abrogates tumorigenicity and induces protective immunity. J Exp Med 1990;172:1217–1223.
13. Watanabe Y, Kuribayashi K, Miyatake S, et al. Exogenous expression of mouse interferon gamma cDNA in mouse neuroblastoma C1300 cells results in reduced tumorigenicity by augmented anti-tumor immunity. Proc Natl Acad Sci USA 1989;86: 9456–9460.
14. Tepper RI, Pattengale PK, Uder P. Murine interleukin-4 displays potent anti-tumor activity in vivo. Cell 1989; 57:503–512.
15. Yu JS, Burwick JA, Dranoff G, Breakefield XO. Gene therapy for metastatic brain tumors by vaccination with granulocyte-macrophage colony-stimulating factor-transduced tumor cells. Human Gene Therapy 1997;8: 1065–1072.

16. Ehtesham M, Kabos P, Kabosova A, Neuman T, Black KL, Yu JS. The use of interleukin 12-secreting neural stem cells for the treatment of intracranial glioma. Cancer Res 2002;62:5657–5663.

17. Fakhrai H, Dorigo O, Shawler DL, et al. Eradication of established intracranial rat gliomas by transforming growth factor β antisense gene therapy. Proc Natl Acad Sci USA 1996;93:2909–2914.

18. Ashley DM, Faiola B, Nair S, Hale LP, Bigner DD, Gilboa E. Bone marrow-generated dendritic cells pulsed with tumor extracts or tumor RNA induce antitumor immunity against central nervous system tumors. J Exp Med 1997;186:1177–1182.

19. Heimberger AB, Archer GE, Crotty LE, et al. dendritic cells pulsed with a tumor-specific peptide induce long-lasting immunity and are effective against murine intracerebral melanoma. Neurosurgery 2002;50: 158–164.

20. Fakhrai H, Shawler DL, Gjerset R, et al. Cytokine gene therapy with interleukin-2 transduced fibroblasts: effects of IL-2 dose on anti-tumor immunity. Human Gene Therapy 1995;6:591–601.

21. Sobol RE, Fakhrai H, Shawler DL, et al. Interleukin-2 gene therapy in a patient with glioblastoma. Gene Therapy 1995; 2:164–167.

22. Kim TS and Cohen EP. Interleukin-2-secreting mouse fibroblasts transfected with genomic DNA from murine melanoma cells prolong the survival of mice with melanoma. Cancer Res 1994;54(10):2531–2535.

23. Kim TS, Russell SJ, Collins MKL, Cohen EP. Immunity to B 16 melanoma in mice immunized with IL-2- secreting allogeneic mouse fibroblasts expressing melanoma-associated antigens. Int J Cancer 1992;51(2):283–289.

24. Tahara H, Zeh HJ 3rd, Storkus WJ, et al. Fibroblasts genetically engineered to secrete interleukin 12 can suppress tumor growth and induce antitumor immunity to a murine melanoma in vivo. Cancer Res 1994; 54(1):182–189.

25. Lichtor T, Glick PP, Kim TS, Hand R, Cohen EP. Prolonged survival of mice with glioma injected intracerebrally with double cytokine-secreting cells. J Neurosurg 1995;83:1038–1044.

26. Lichtor T, Glick RP, Tarlock K, Moffett S, Mouw E, Cohen EP. Application of interleukin-2 secreting syngeneic/allogeneic fibroblasts in the treatment of primary and metastatic brain tumors. Cancer Gene Therapy 2002;9:464–469.

27. Kim TS, Russell SJ, Collins MKL, Cohen EP. Immunity to B 16 melanoma in mice immunized with IL-2- secreting allogeneic mouse fibroblasts expressing melanoma-associated antigens. Int J Cancer 1992;51: 283–289.

28. Yamada G, Kitamura Y, Sonoda H, et al. Retroviral expression of the human IL-2 gene in a murine T cell line results in a cell growth autonomy and tumorigenicity. EMBO J 1987;6:2705–2709.

29. Colbere-Garapin F, Horodniceanu F, Kouritsky P, Garapin AC. A new dominant hybrid selective marker for higher eukaryotic cells. J Mol Biol 1981;150:1–14.

30. Kim TS, Xu WS, Cohen EP. Immunization with interleukin-2/interferon-γ double cytokine-secreting allogeneic fibroblasts prolongs the survival of mice with melanoma. Melanoma Res 1995;5: 217–227.

31. Sugden B, Marsh K, Yates J. A vector that replicates as a plasmid and can be efficiently selected in B-lymphoblasts transformed by Epstein–Barr virus. Mol Cell Biol 1985;5:410–413.

32. Gillis S, Ferm MM, Ou W, Smith KA. T cell growth factors: parameters of production and a quantitative microassay for activity. J Immunol 1978;120:2027–2032.

33. Chomczynski P, Sacchi N. Single step method of RNA isolation by acid guanidinium-thiocyanate-phenol-chloroform extraction. Anal Biochem 1987;162:156–159.

34. Robinson WA, Lobe K, Stevens R. Central nervous system metastases in malignant melanoma. Cancer Treat Res 1987;35:155–163.

35. Kim H, Rosenberg SA, Steinberg SM, Cole DJ, Weber JS. A randomized double blind comparison of the antiemetic efficacy of ondansetron and dropidol in patients receiving high dose interleukin-2. J Emphasis Tumor Immunol 1994;16: 60–65.

36. Birchfield GR, Rodgers GM, Girodias KW, Ward JH, Samlowski WE. Hypoprothrobinemia associated with interleukin-2 therapy. J Immunother 1992;11: 71–75.

37. Tjuvajev J, Gansbacher B, Desai R, et al. RG-2 glioma growth attenuation and severe brain edema caused by local production of interleukin-2 and interferon-γ . Cancer Res 1995;55:1902–1910.

38. Griffitt W, Glick RP, Lichtor T, Cohen EP. Survival and toxicity of an allogeneic cytokine-secreting fibroblast vaccine in the central nervous system. Neurosurgery 1998;42:335–340.

39. Yu JS, Wei MX, Chiocca A, Martuza RL, Tepper RI. Treatment of glioma by engineered interleukin-4-secreting cells. Cancer Res 1993;53:3125–3128.

40. Glick RP, Lichtor T, Kim TS, Ilangovan S, Cohen EP. Fibroblasts genetically engineered to secrete cytokines suppress tumor growth and induce antitumor immunity to a murine glioma in vivo. Neurosurgery 1995;36: 548–555.

41. Watts RG, Wright JL, Atkinson LL, Merchant RE. Histopathological and blood-brain barrier changes in rats induced by intracerebral injection of human recombinant interleukin-2. Neurosurgery 1989;25: 202–208.

42. Zhang RD, Price JE, Fujimaki T, Bucana CD, Fidler IJ. Differential permeability of the blood brain barrier in experimental brain metastases produced by human neoplasms implanted into nude mice. Am J Pathol 1992; 141:1115–1124.

43. Sampson, JH, Ashley DM, Archer GE, et al. Characterization of a spontaneous murine astrocytoma and abrogation of its tumorigenicity by cytokine secretion. Neurosurgery 1997;41:1365–1372.

44. Giezeman-Smits, KM, Okada H, Brissette-Storkus CS, et al. Cytokine gene therapy of gliomas: induction of reactive CD4+ T cells by interleukin-4-transfected 9L gliosarcoma is essential for protective immunity. Cancer Res 2000;60:2449–2457.

45. Okada H, Villa L, Attanucci J, et al. Cytokine gene therapy of gliomas: effective induction of therapeutic immunity to intracranial tumors by peripheral immunization with interleukin-4 transduced glioma cells. Gene Therapy 2001;8:1157–1166.

46. Natsume A, Mizuno M, Ryuke Y, Yoshida J. Antitumor effect and cellular immunity activation by murine interferon-beta gene transfer against intracerebral glioma in mouse. Gene Therapy 1999;6:1626–1633.

47. Okada H, Pollack IF, Lotze MT, et al. Gene therapy of malignant gliomas: a phase I study of IL-4-HSV-TK gene-modified autologous tumor to elicit an immune response. Hum Gene Thery 2000;11:637–653.

48. Fakhrai H, Mantil J, Gramatikova S, et al. Gene therapy of human gliomas with TGF-β2 antisense gene modified autologous tumor cells. A Phase I trial. Proc Am Assoc Cancer Res 2000;41:543.

49. Nestle FO, Alijagic S, Gilliet M, et al. Vaccination of melanoma patients with peptide-or-tumor lysate-pulsed dendritic cells. Nature Med 1998;4:328–332.

50. Tighe H, Corr M, Roman M, Raz E. Gene vaccination: plasmid DNA is more than just a blue print. Immunol Today 1998;19:89–97.

51. Yu JS, Wheeler, CJ, Zeltzer PM, et al. Vaccination of malignant glioma patients with peptide-pulsed dendritic cells elicits systemic cytotoxicity and intracranial T-cell infiltration. Cancer Res 2001;61:842–847.

52. Yamanaka R, Tsuchiya N, Yajima N, et al. Induction of an antitumor immunological response by an intratrumoral injection of dendritic cells pulsed with genetically engineered Semliki Forest virus to produce interleukin-18 combined with the systemic administration of interleukin-12. J Neurosurg 2003;99:746–753.

53. Kikuchi T, Akasaki Y, Irie M, Homma S, Abe T, Ohno T. Results of a phase I clinical trial of vaccination of glioma patients with fusions of dendritic and glioma cells. Cancer Immunol Immuother 2001;50:337–344.

54. Okada H, Pollack IF, Lieberman F, et al. Gene therapy of malignant gliomas: a pilot study of vaccination with irradiated autologous glioma and dendritic cells admixed with IL-4 transduced fibroblasts to elicit an immune response. Hum Gene Ther 2001;12:575–595.

55. de Vries TJ, Fourkour A, Wobbes T, Verkroost G, Ruiter DJ, van Muijen GNP. Heterologous expression of immunotherapy candidate proteins gp100, MART-1 and tyrosinase in human melanoma cell lines and in human melanocytic lesions. Cancer Res 1997;57:3223–3229.

56. Anichini AR, Mortarini C, Maccalli P, et al. Cytotoxic T cells directed to tumor antigens not expressed on normal melanocytes dominate HLA-A2.1-restricted immune repertoire to melanoma. J Immunol 1996;156:208–217.

57. Lichtor T, Glick RP, O-Sullivan I, Cohen EP. DNA-based vaccine for treatment of intracerebral neoplasms. Gene Ther Mol Biol 2004;8:395–402.

58. Lichtor T, Glick RP, Lin H, O-Sullivan I, Cohen EP. Intratumoral injection of IL- secreting syngeneic/allogeneic Fibroblasts transfected with DNA from breast cancer cells prolongs the survival of mice with intracerebral breast cancer. Cancer Gene Ther 2005;12:708–714.

22 Monoclonal Antibodies

Abraham Boskovitz, David A. Reardon,
Carol J. Wikstrand, Michael R. Zalutsky,
and Darell D. Bigner

Summary

Over the last decades, progress has been made in diagnostic imaging, surgical techniques, radiotherapy, and chemotherapy for the treatment of tumors of the central nervous system. However, the outcome for patients with high-grade gliomas (HGG) has remained essentially unchanged. The use of monoclonal antibodies (MAbs), either unarmed or armed, to target and kill HGG cells has appeared as a prospective adjuvant therapeutic option. The potential of this approach is being investigated in a large number of clinical trials currently in progress for patients with HGG; the encouraging results of some of these phase I/II trials will be summarized here.

In this chapter, we review the critical components for the safe, efficient, and practical implementation of MAb-based immunotherapy for HGG patients as well as the current and future targetable antigens and their corresponding monoclonal antibodies.

Key Words: Glioma; glioblastoma; anaplastic astrocytoma (AA); tumor antigen; monoclonal antibody (MAb); radioisotope; radiotherapy; immunotoxin; clinical study.

INTRODUCTION

High-grade gliomas (HGG) remain resistant to current standard treatments including aggressive surgical resection, external beam radiotherapy, and cytotoxic chemotherapy. The use of monoclonal antibodies (MAbs) has emerged as a potential adjuvant therapeutic modality with the additional advantages of specifically and more effectively targeting and killing tumor cells than conventional adjuvant treatments (radiotherapy, chemotherapy) which are self-limited by cytotoxicity to normal tissues. Although the principle of an antibody-based tumor immunotherapy was published more than 60 yr earlier *(1,2)*, glioma patients were not enrolled in clinical studies until the early 1960s when iv-administered ^{131}I-labeled polyclonal antibodies were used to target human glioblastoma multiforme (GBM) *(3,4)* or fibrinogen on intracranial tumors, including gliomas *(5)*. In these studies, the radiation dose that was conveyed to the tumor was sufficient for imaging but not for therapy. It was only with the development of new technology to obtain MAbs with defined affinity and specificity for a tumor-associated antigen *(6)* (Ag) that the use of antibody-mediated therapy could be realistically envisioned.

From: *Current Clinical Oncology: High-Grade Gliomas: Diagnosis and Treatment*
Edited by: G. H. Barnett © Humana Press Inc., Totowa, NJ

The use of MAbs to localize within a tumor in vivo or to function as an immunotherapeutic agent require that several critical factors are met, including: Ag accessibility (external surface of the cell membrane or extracellular localization); Ag stability (lack of shedding; internalization), and sufficient density within the tumor; high specificity, affinity and stability of the targeting MAb; and reasonable MAb transport kinetics within the tumor (dependent on tumor vascularity, vascular permeability, extracellular fluid dynamics, interstitial pressure). The route of administration is also important as the limited permeability of the blood–brain (BBB) and blood–tumor (BTB) barriers restricts the use of systemic injection *(7)*.

In this chapter, we first address the nature of existing MAb constructs, their cytotoxic mechanisms including those that are intrinsic (unarmed MAb) or acquired (armed MAb), and the various administration routes available to optimize target reactivity, as these are some of the most critical components that determine whether a MAb will effectively interact with a targeted tumor. We then review the various targetable HGG Ags and their corresponding MAbs.

ESSENTIAL CRITERIA IN THE PREPARATION OF MONOCLONAL ANTIBODY-BASED THERAPY
Selection of the Monoclonal Antibody Format

The MAb molecular format must be compatible with the biology and macroscopic appearance (size, shape) of the targeted tumor as well as the characteristics of the possible radioactive or toxic conjugate, and the intended administration route *(7)* (Fig. 1).

Murine Monoclonal Sntibodies

Murine MAbs currently constitute the reference standard. The vast majority of MAbs investigated for immunotherapeutic purposes are murine immunoglobulins despite the fact that their clinical use is potentially affected by human anti-mouse antibody (HAMA) formation following systemic injection. Immune complexes consequently accelerate Mab clearance from the circulation, thus lessening their therapeutic potential. More radical responses such as hypersensitivity or allergy are also possible *(8,9)*. MAb-based treatment of high-grade gliomas is, however, frequently approached on a compartmental administration basis. As MAbs eventually find their way into the systemic circulation, the HAMA-induced systemic clearance may confer more advantageous compartment-to-blood and/or tumor-to-blood ratios, which is critical from a therapeutic standpoint *(7)*.

Chimeric Human/Mouse, Humanized, and Fully Human Monoclonal Antibodies

Chimeric human/mouse MAbs have been engineered to be less immunogenic in humans as only the antigen-binding variable regions are of murine origin *(10,11)*. Chimeric MAbs containing human constant regions of the IgG2 or IgG4 sub-class are more appropriate for MAb-based immunotherapy as Fc-receptor binding is diminished. In consequence, nonspecific binding (i.e., liver, spleen, bone marrow) and activation of antigen-dependent cytotoxicity (ADC) and complement-dependent cytotoxicity (CDC) are decreased *(12,13)*. Moreover, IgG2 chimeric MAbs benefit from the stiffness of the human IgG2 hinge region which enhances the stability of the MAb and, in comparison with murine counterparts, translates into better in vivo tumor localization *(14–16)*. Nonetheless, the presence of murine domains is sufficient to trigger an immune response from the treated host *(17,18)*. Thus, humanized MAbs have been engineered with the aim of further limiting the presence of potentially immunogenic regions. The humanization process consists of the insertion of the murine complementarity-determin-

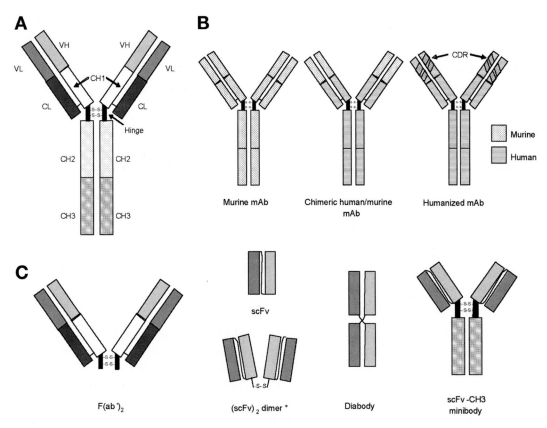

Fig. 1. (A) Structure and legend of an intact IgG MAb. **(B)** Structure of a murine MAb, a chimeric human/ murine MAb construct with hybridization of domains of murine and human origin, and a humanized MAb with murine CDRs grafted within a human Ig. **(C)** Schematic structure of various fragment MAbs (legend: see **A**); covalently-bound scFvs after C-terminal incorporation of cysteine residue; peptide linker version not represented.

ing regions (CDRs), which are responsible for binding to the antigenic epitope, into a human IgG framework *(19–21)*. In recent studies, fully human MAbs have been generated using mice genetically-engineered (XenoMouse®) to produce human IgGs[22] or from scFv and Fab fragment MAbs produced by human naïve phage display libraries *(23)*.

MONOCLONAL ANTIBODY FRAGMENTS

MAb fragments can present a range of advantageous features such as decreased immunogenicity, lack of immunogenic and cell-receptor binding Fc region, more prompt systemic clearance, and better diffusion into the tumor tissue *(7)*.

F(ab')$_2$ MAb fragments (110 kDa) retain divalent binding capacity and F(ab')$_2$ fragments of chimeric IgG2 MAbs benefit also from the rigid IgG2 hinge region as the rate of in vivo inter-chain cleavage is reduced *(24)*. Single-chain scFv fragments are monovalent 26 kDa molecules containing only one heavy- and one light-chain variable domain *(25)*. Affinity for the antigenic epitope is reduced as they have a single binding site *(9,26)* but fragments with very high affinity can be isolated using phage display *(27)*, and affinity-maturation processes have also significantly enhanced this decisive aspect of the Ag-MAb binding dynamic *(25)*.

Because of their small size, a more widespread and homogenous tumor tissue penetration can be expected *(28)*. However, systemic clearance is expedited *(9,26)*, which may restrict the use of scFvs for MAb-based targeted radiotherapy because of rapid renal irradiation, unless scFvs are labeled with short half-life radionuclides such as 7.2-h astatine-211 (^{211}At) *(7)*. Starting from the basic scFv unit, divalent diabodies and (scFv)$_2$ dimers, and multivalent scFvs all have been engineered *(9,12,29)*.

MINIBODIES

Minibodies consist of two scFvs joined by genetic fusion to a human IgG1 hinge region and CH3 domain *(30,31)*. As a consequence of their intermediate molecular weight (80 kDa) and divalent nature, they have the attractive capability of minimizing many of the disadvantages that the larger entire MAbs and the smaller monovalent scFv fragments display *(7)*.

Selection of the Mechanism to Achieve Tumor Cell Toxicity

Many MAbs can intrinsically kill targeted tumor cells to which they attach. When this is not the case, advantage can be taken of their Ag-binding capability in order to convey a radioactive or toxic load to the tumor cell.

UNARMED MONOCLONAL ANTIBODIES

Possibly the most interesting model of unarmed MAb cell killing is provided by the anti-epidermal growth factor receptor (EGFR) MAbs, whose mechanism of action interferes with cellular biomolecular and signaling activity as cells are set on an apoptotic course or vital cellular pathways are shut down *(32)*. Anti-EGFRvIII MAbs also display the capacity to prevent tumor cell proliferation in in vitro experiments and, in vivo, to extend the survival of mice previously inoculated subcutaneously or intracranially with EGFRvIII-expressing xenografts, after administration via either the systemic or intratumoral route *(33)*.

RADIOLABELED MONOCLONAL ANTIBODIES

Radionuclides are characterized by the type of particle emitted, amount of energy transferred, half-life, and radiation range. These are critical criteria to take into consideration when targeting a tumor of a particular size, geometry, and localization. A summary of the characteristics, advantages, and drawbacks of the most important radionuclides for the targeted radioimmunotherapy of HGG is provided in Table 1. Other important factors for radioimmunotherapy include the clinical pharmacokinetics of the carrier moiety it is labeled to, as well as the strength of the conjugation linkage, which can vary with the labeling technique employed *(7,34)*.

Radioisotopes most commonly used for targeted radiotherapy of HGG are iodine-131 (^{131}I) and yttrium-90 (^{90}Y), both β-particle emitters. ^{131}I, with its 910 μm radiation range in tissue, is optimal for radiotherapy of small lesions. However, clinical use of ^{131}I is complicated by the emission of medium-energy γ-rays, which requires additional protective measures for the patient's surroundings *(34)*. The longer-range (3900 μm) ^{90}Y is an exclusive β-particle emitter routinely available and best suited to target a larger tumor bed area. Its main drawback is the lack of γ-emissions which complicates the ability to image its biodistribution in preclinical and clinical investigations *(34)*. A third β-particle emitter of promise for radiotherapy of HGG is lutetium-177 (^{177}Lu). Its short-range β-particle radiation (670 μm) is most effective for targeted radiotherapy of smaller tumors, for instance post-surgical resection tumor residues or micro-metastasis, while γ-ray emissions permit the tracking and imaging of the radiolabeled MAb *(34)*. Another radionuclide of noteworthy

Table 1

Characteristics, Clinical Indications, Advantages, and Drawbacks of the Radionuclides[34] Most Relevant to the Targeted Radioimmunotherapy of HGG Using Specific MAbs

Radionuclide	β-energy (mean; keV)	Radiation range (mean; in μm)	Half-life (d)	Other emissions	Optimal targeted tumor	Advantage	Drawback
131I	182	910	8.1	Mid-energy γ-ray (364 keV)	Small tumor/postoperative residue	Commercially available and inexpensive	Not optimal for in vivo imaging; Radioprotection of surroundings
90Y	935	3900	2.7	—	Large tumor bed	Commercially available and inexpensive	In vivo imaging not possible
177Lu	133	670	6.7	Mid-energy γ-ray (208 keV)	Micro-metastasis	Commercially available and inexpensive	In vivo imaging feasible
	α-energy (MeV)	Radiation range (mm)	Half-life (h)				
211At	5.87 + 7.44*	55–70	7.2	α-recoil nuclei X-ray (77-92 keV)	Micro-metastasis, residual tumor margin, thin-sheeted lesion, disseminated or circulating/free-floating tumor cell	High LET at max. relative biological effectiveness; not dependent on cellular oxygenation level	Availability
	Electron emission	Radiation range	Half-life (d)				
125I / 123I	Auger, Coster Kronig	Subcellular <0.1	60/0.6	—	Individually targetable and accessible tumor cell	High LET, relative biological effectiveness when localized within cell DNA	Internalization close/within nucleus required; 125I half-life too long

Abbr: LET: linear energy transfer.
Notes: *α-particle emission by 211Po daughter.

377

interest for treatment of micro-metastasis, disseminated or thin-sheeted tumors such as neoplastic meningitis, or a residual tumor margin is the 7.2-h half-life α-particle emitter ^{211}At. The very high decay energy combined with the short range of tissue over which it is distributed (55–70 µm) confer on ^{211}At a linear energy transfer (LET) of about 97 keV/µm. In comparison, the LET of the β-particles emitted by ^{90}Y is 0.22 keV/µm *(34)*. Moreover, when an ^{211}At-labeled MAb is internalized within the nucleus of a targeted tumor cell, additional lethal damage can be inflicted to the cell by emission of α-particle recoil nuclei *(35)*.

IMMUNOTOXINS

An immunotoxin is the product of the conjugation, chemical or genetic, of a toxin to a MAb. Although the mechanism of action may vary with the toxin, internalization is always a prerequisite and inhibition of protein synthesis is the lethal end result. If internalization can be achieved, uptake of one immunotoxin molecule can suffice to effectively kill the targeted cell *(36,37)*. With the exception of ligand-based immunotoxins or "fusion" toxins, such as Tf-CRM107 (a transferrin-receptor ligand conjugated to a diphtheria toxin mutant) or TP-38 (TGF-α, an EGFR ligand, conjugated to a variant of the *Pseudomonas* exotoxin PE-38), no MAb-based immunotoxin is involved at this time in clinical trials for patients with HGG *(7)*. In preclinical investigations, however, the modified *Pseudomonas* exotoxin PE38 conjugated to an anti-EGFRvIII scFv showed encouraging results in an animal model of EGFRvIII-expressing neoplastic meningitis; following intrathecal administration, long-term survivors were observed and median survival was dramatically increased *(38)*.

Selection of the Administration Route

SYSTEMIC ADMINISTRATION

The efficacy of MAb-based targeted therapy of HGG using the vascular injection route, whether intravenous (iv) or intracarotid (ic), has repeatedly been limited by the relative impermeability of the BBB and BTB. Clinical studies have shown that, after systemic administration, only a small fraction of the injected dose of radiolabeled intact MAbs and F(ab')$_2$ fragments can be found within the intracranial tumor (0.001–0.005% ID/g) which is insufficient for therapeutic purposes *(39,40)*. Targeting tumor Ags that are not sequestrated from the systemic circulation by the BBB and BTB, such as the vascular endothelial growth factor receptor (VEGFR), may improve the relative tumor localization of systemically administered MAbs *(7)*. Furthermore, the bradykinin analogue RMP-7 has been intensely investigated to disrupt the BBB. Following ic injection in rats previously inoculated intracranially with glioma cells, penetration of dextran (70 kDa) within the intracranial tumor was augmented by RMP-7 *(41)*. Thus, mechanisms to disrupt the BBB and BTB may eventually permit the effective use of the systemic route for MAb-based immunotherapy of central nervous system (CNS) tumors such as HGG.

COMPARTMENTAL ADMINISTRATION

Compartmental administration of tumor-targeting MAbs represents a strong alternative to the systemic route as it limits nonspecific systemic exposure, allowing for higher treatment dose injection, and bypasses the BBB and BTB, increasing the amount of MAb localizing to the targeted tumor. The most commonly used injection route for patients with HGG is intralesional, whether intratumoral for large lesions, or intracavitary for cystic gliomas or when a tumor resection cavity is surgically-created (SCRC).

Intratumoral injection and diffusion thereafter into the tumor tissue or brain parenchyma is restricted by the diffusion capacity of the therapeutic compound. The latter is determined by the size of the compound, its concentration gradient, and the rate of physiological elimination *(42)*. Tumors often have an elevated interstitial pressure which constitutes an additional impeding factor to distant and homogenous diffusion of the MAb *(43)*. However, efficacy of intratumoral administration is greatly enhanced using convection-enhanced delivery (CED), discussed elsewhere in this book. The main objective of intracavitary injection following surgical-resection of the HGG is to eliminate residual tumor cells infiltrating the surrounding brain parenchyma, which are the probable cause of a majority of recurrences, regardless of post-operative adjuvant irradiation to the tumor bed *(44)*.

When tumor cells penetrate into the intrathecal and subarachnoid space and metastasize along the leptomeninges, the subsequent neoplastic meningitis carries a dramatically poor outcome despite chemotherapy and radiotherapy of the entire neuroaxis. MAbs administered into the intrathecal or intraventricular compartments circulate via the cerebrospinal fluid (CSF) stream along the brain and spine to the disseminated leptomeningeal tumor cells *(7)*. However, one must bear in mind that compounds injected in the lumbar area may not effectively reach the lateral ventricles because of a unidirectional flow pattern *(45)*.

HIGH-GRADE GLIOMA ANTIGENS AND CORRESPONDING MONOCLONAL ANTIBODIES

The majority of Ags initially targeted by antibodies were not tumor-specific but rather tumor-associated and therefore exhibited variable cross-reactivity with normal tissues. However, Ags expressed by a brain tumor but not the normal brain or spine can be considered tumor-specific, or operationally specific, within the CNS compartment. Effective tumor targeting can thus be achieved by administration of the corresponding MAb within the CNS compartment *(8)*. The current and most therapeutically pertinent molecules that have been exploited as HGG targets and their respective MAbs are discussed below. A summary of these and other MAbs involved in clinical trials for patients with malignant glioma is provided in Table 2.

Tenascin

Tenascin is a large extracellular matrix protein expressed in the normal adult kidney, liver, spleen, and papillary dermis *(46,47)* but not in the normal brain. Its expression is increased in malignant gliomas (>90%) as well as some carcinomas and mesenchymal tumors *(48,49)*. An increase in tenascin expression is observed in correlation with increasing glioma histopathological grade as well as angiogenesis *(50,51)*. The anti-tenascin MAbs BC-2 and BC-4 *(44)*, and 81C6 *(52)* have been investigated in numerous clinical trials for patients with HGG in Europe and the United States, respectively.

[131]I-labeled BC-2 and BC-4 have been investigated in large clinical trials after intracavitary administration via surgically-implanted catheters in patients with malignant glioma. The catheters were placed following maximal tumor resection during which a SCRC was created, if possible. In these trials, median survival was increased to 23, >46, and 19 mo for patients with anaplastic oligodendroglioma (AO), anaplastic astrocytoma (AA) and GBM, respectively, and no significant toxicity was observed *(53)*. In an ongoing study, involving a similar patient population treated with intracavitary ^{90}Y-labeled BC-4, patients with GBM have a median survival of 17 mo and 85% of those with AA were alive after 5 yr *(44)*. BC-4 has also been introduced in a phase I/II trial for patients with recurrent malignant glioma using the

Table 2
Clinical Trials With MAbs for Patients With HGG[†]

MAb	Targeted antigen	IgG format	Conjugate	Targeted tumor	Injection route	Trial phase	Reference
81C6 *	Tenascin	Murine	^{131}I	Leptomeningeal tumor/ brain tumor with SCRC - subarachnoid communication	IT	I	Brown et al., 1996
		Murine	^{131}I	Malignant glioma	SCRC	II	Reardon et al., 2002
		Chimeric	^{131}I	Malignant glioma	SCRC	I	Reardon et al., (unpublished data)
		Chimeric	^{211}At	Recurrent malignant glioma	SCRC	I	Zalutsky et al., 2002
		Chimeric F(ab')$_2$	^{131}I	Recurrent malignant glioma	SCRC	I	Boskovitz et al., 2004
BC-1 (AS1405) *	(B+)-fibronectin	Murine	^{111}In/^{90}Y	Recurrent GBM	SCRC	I	www.antisoma.com
BC-2/BC-4 *	Tenascin	Murine	^{131}I	Malignant glioma	ITum/SCRC	II	Riva et al. 2000
BC-4 *		Murine	^{90}Y	Malignant glioma	ITum/SCRC	II	Goetz et al., 2003
Biotinylated BC-4 *		Murine	^{90}Y-Biotin	Recurrent malignant glioma	IV	I/II	Paganelli et al., 1999
chTNT-1 (Cotara®)*	H1/DNA	Murine	^{90}Y-Biotin	Malignant glioma	IV	Pilot	Grana et al., 2002
		Chimeric	^{131}I	Recurrent GBM and AA	ITum CED	I/II	*www.peregrineinc.com*
		Chimeric	^{131}I	Recurrent GBM	ITum CED	Registration	*www.peregrineinc.com*
ERIC-1	NCAM	Murine	^{131}I	Malignant glioma	SCRC/ICyst	Pilot	Papanastassiou et al., 1993
Mab 425 (EMD55900) *	EGFR wt	Murine	Unarmed	Malignant glioma / recurrent mal. glioma	IV	I/II	Stragliotto et al., 1996
		Murine	Unarmed	GBM	ITum	I/interrupted	Wersall et al., 1997
		Murine	^{125}I	High grade glioma	IV/(IC)	II	Quang et al., 2004
Mel-14	GP240	Murine	^{131}I	Glioma/melanoma n oplastic meningitis	IT	Pilot/I	Coakham et al., 1998
		Murine F(ab')$_2$	^{131}I	Glioma/melanoma n oplastic meningitis	IT	I	Cokgor et al., 2001
Trastuzumab (Herceptin®)*	HER2	Humanized	Unarmed	Recurrent GBM	IV	I/II	*www.virtualtrials.com*

Notes:* Active in clinical trials at time of publication.
Abbr: IC, intracarotid; ICyst, intracystic; IT, intrathecal; ITum, intratumoral; IV, intravenous; SCRC, surgically-created tumor resection cavity; CED, convection-enhanced delivery;
[†]Reprinted with permission from ref. 7.

three-step pretargeted antibody-guided radioimmunotherapy (PAGRIT) systemic approach. The purpose of this method is to limit the nonspecific radioisotope binding. Thus, a cold, biotinylated MAb is initially administered. Taking advantage of the high-affinity and specificity of biotin-avidin binding, avidin and streptavidin are injected within 24 to 36 ho, followed, less than 24 h later, by ^{90}Y-labeled biotin. Results were encouraging as systemic toxicity was found acceptable and a therapeutic effect was detected *(54)*. In a subsequent pilot study, selected patients with newly-diagnosed malignant glioma treated with PAGRIT following surgery and conventional radiotherapy had an increased median survival; however a randomized trial is necessary to determine the true potential of this promising treatment approach *(55)*. The high immunogenicity of streptavidin is a major concern as multiple treatment cycles would most likely have to be avoided *(54)*.

81C6 is a murine IgG2b MAb that recognizes a tenascin isoform created by alternate splicing within the FN III-like CD region *(48)*. This isoform is abundantly expressed by most primary human gliomas, human glioma cell lines, and glioma xenografts in nude mice and rats but not by normal adult or fetal brain *(48,56,57)*. ^{131}I-labeled 81C6 has been investigated in patients with malignant gliomas via injection into the SCRC. Phase I studies identified the maximal tolerated dose (MTD) to be: 120 mCi for patients with newly diagnosed and previously untreated HGG; 100 mCi for those with recurrent malignant glioma previously treated with conventional radiotherapy; and 80 mCi for patients with a SCRC communicating with the CSF or after administration in the intrathecal space *(7)*. A phase II trial with ^{131}I-labeled 81C6 (120 mCi) followed by conventional radiotherapy and chemotherapy in patients with newly diagnosed and previously untreated malignant gliomas achieved a median survival of 86.7 and 79.4 wk for all patients and those with GBM, respectively *(7,52)*. In Fig. 2, serial brain images of a patient from this series in whom long-term disease control was achieved are illustrated. Irreversible neurotoxicity developed in 15% of patients, but only occurred in patients where the SCRC was contiguous with, or immediately adjacent to, eloquent areas or motor cortex *(7,52)*. Of note, only one patient required surgical resection of radiation necrosis. In comparison, other strategies to boost radiation to the resection perimeter, such as radiosurgery or interstitial brachytherapy, are complicated by radionecrosis requiring resection in 30 to 64% of cases *(58)*.

Extensive analysis of dosimetry performed during phase I studies with ^{131}I-labeled 81C6 revealed a quantitative relationship between the absorbed dose and dose rate to the 2-cm SCRC shell and clinical as well as histopathological outcome (Fig. 3). The delivery of 44 Gy to the 2-cm SCRC shell was calculated to maximize tumor control and minimize damage to the normal brain *(59)*. Thus, a phase II study incorporating administration of ^{131}I-labeled 81C6 to deliver 44 Gy to the 2-cm margin of the SCRC has been initiated. In addition, phase I trials have determined the MTD of ^{131}I-labeled human/mouse chimeric 81C6 (ch81C6) to be 80 mCi when administered into the SCRC of patients with newly diagnosed or recurrent malignant glioma. ch81C6 exhibits greater intracavitary retention compared with its murine parent and therefore may be associated with greater anti-tumor activity. However, it also exhibits a longer systemic clearance half-life, contributing to greater hematologic toxicity (Reardon et al.; unpublished data). A phase II study with ^{131}I-labeled ch81C6 is nearing completion and will better define its potential therapeutic benefit as well as its toxicity. A F(ab')$_2$ MAb fragment of ch81C6 has been developed which, when compared with the intact chimeric MAb, demonstrated similar affinity for the antigenic epitope of tenascin. After iv injection in subcutaneous tenascin-expressing tumor-bearing mice, tumor localization was comparable for 24 h although systemic elimination of the F(ab')$_2$ fragment was accelerated *(24)*. A phase I study with

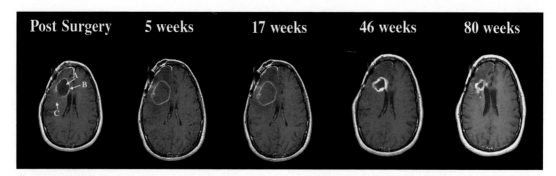

Fig. 2. Postoperative serial magnetic resonance imaging (MRI) analysis of the brain from a patient with a newly diagnosed right frontal lobe glioblastoma. Images taken immediately after the surgery show the presence of a **(A)** SCRC with **(B)** a signal-enhancing rim and **(C)** significant surrounding edema. Patient was thereafter treated with SCRC injection of 120 µCi of ^{131}I-labeled anti-tenascin 81C6 MAb, conventional radiotherapy, and chemotherapy; serial MRI images taken at 5, 17, 46, and 80 wk demonstrate shrinkage of the remaining enhancing region and regression of the edema (Reprinted with permission from ref. *52*).

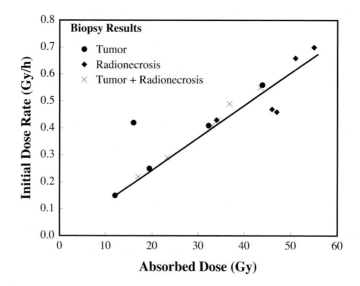

Fig. 3. Based on the histopathological examination of biopsy specimen obtained from patients treated for HGG with maximal surgical resection and injection of ^{131}I-labeled 81C6 into the SCRC, a qualitative relationship was shown between absorbed dose and dose rate to the 2-cm SCRC shell and the clinical and histopathological outcome. An absorbed dose of 44 Gy was determined as optimal to minimize the risks for both tumor recurrence and radiation-induced damage to the normal brain (Reprinted with permission from ref. *59*).

SCRC injection of ^{131}I-labeled ch81C6 F(ab')$_2$ for patients with recurrent HGG has been initiated. In another phase I trial performed in a similar patient population, the SCRC administration of ^{211}At-labeled ch81C6 is being investigated *(60)*. As the half-life of ^{211}At is only 7.2 h and the chimeric construct exhibits excellent in vivo stability, an estimated 98.2% of the decays occur in the SCRC. In addition, because of its shorter irradiation range, the SCRC interface-to-normal brain dose ratio of ^{211}At is increased by 150-fold compared with that observed in this setting for murine 81C6 labeled with ^{131}I *(61)*. No dose-limiting toxicities have been observed and the MTD for intracavitary ^{211}At-labeled 81C6 has yet to be determined.

Epidermal Growth Factor Receptor and its Variant III Form

The EGFR is involved in signal transduction mechanisms critical to cell differentiation, proliferation, motility, and invasion as well as angiogenesis *(62)*. EGFR expression is found in a large number of normal tissues *(63)* as well as in numerous malignancies. With regard to expression in brain tumors, 27 to 57% of astrocytomas, 71 to 94% of AA, and 60 to 90% of GBM express the EGFR protein *(51)*. The EGFR-encoding gene is amplified in 37 to 58% of GBMs and its amplification has been correlated with an increasing tumor grade *(64,65)*. However, the EGFR protein was overexpressed without genetic amplification in 12 to 38% of GBM, indicating that additional translational and post-translational processes may increase EGFR expression *(32)*.

Numerous anti-EGFR MAbs have been produced, among them the MAb 425 (EMD55900), which has been introduced in a phase I trial where it is administered using the intratumoral route in patients with primary or recurrent GBM. The study was discontinued as a result of severe local inflammatory reaction and tumor necrosis in some cases *(66)*. No significant toxicity was observed after iv injection of MAb 425 in patients with malignant glioma. However, no therapeutic effect was found either in a phase I/II trial for patients with recurrent HGG *(67,68)*.

Radiolabeled anti-EGFR MAbs were involved in the first targeted radioimmunotherapy trials via systemic injection in patients diagnosed with glioma *(69–71)*. Phase II clinical trials using iv or ic ^{125}I-labeled MAb 425 following surgery and conventional radiotherapy for patients with HGG showed an improvement in median survival with this treatment *(72)*, prompting the continuation of the study using the iv injection route *(7)*.

The EGFR variant III (EGFRvIII) protein lacks part of the extracellular domain of the wild-type (wt) EGFR as a result of genetic rearrangements of the EGFR encoding region *(73)*. Because it is expressed exclusively in tumors, EGFRvIII is a more attractive therapeutic epitope than its full-length parent. EGFRvIII protein expression is found in 58 to 67% of GBM *(74,75)* although more recent studies reported a lower incidence of 21 to 43% *(73)*. Other HGG, such as AA, express EGFRvIII at a significantly lower rate *(73)*. Of note, EGFRvIII expression has also been suggested as a negative prognosis factor for GBM *(75,76)*. Subcutaneous and intracranial EGFRvIII-expressing tumor-bearing mice survived longer after intraperitoneal and intratumoral injection, respectively, of the EGFRvIII-specific Y10 MAb *(33)*. Other important anti-EGFRvIII MAbs include L8A4, which has been produced in both murine and chimeric human/murine formats *(77)*. The anti-EGFRvIII scFv fragments MR1 and its affinity-matured analogue MR1-1 also have been generated *(25)*. Despite encouraging results from in vivo preclinical investigations *(7)*, none of these EGFRvIII-specific MAbs have reached the clinical investigation stage at this date, although an investigational new drug (IND) permit should be filed imminently for MR1-1dsFvPE38KDEL, a recombinant immunotoxin composed of a disulfide-stabilized (dsFv) version of MR1-1 and the genetically engineered *Pseudomonas* exotoxin, PE38KDEL.

Of note, a phase I/II trial using iv injection of trastuzumab (Herceptin®), which specifically recognizes the human transmembrane protein HER2 (also known as EGFR-2 or Erbb-2), has been initiated for patients with recurrent HER2/neu-positive GBM *(7)*.

Histone/DNA Complex

Necrotic foci are frequently found within certain tumors such as HGG, but not within normal tissues. Both normal and tumor cells contain histone/DNA complexes. However, as an abnormal contact interface exists between the contents of necrotic cells and the extracellular milieu, histone/DNA complexes can become visible to specific MAbs. The ability to localize immunotherapeutic compounds specifically within a necrotic focus constitutes the basis of the tumor necrosis treatment (TNT) strategy *(78)*. Phase I and II trials have been initiated using Cotara®, the ^{131}I-labeled form of the anti-H1/DNA complex chimeric MAb chTNT-1/B, administered intralesionally with the CED microinfusion system in patients with recurrent AA and GBM. Subsequently, a registration trial for patients with recurrent GBM was approved by the Food and Drug Administration *(7)* (*www.peregrineinc.com*).

(B⁺)-Fibronectin

Fibronectins are high-molecular-weight glycoproteins located in body fluids and the extracellular matrix of tissues. High levels of expression of the (B⁺)-fibronectin isoform are found in fetal tissues but remain practically undetected in adult tissues, with the exception of the regenerating endometrium. This molecule is also expressed in tumors, particularly in the vicinity of developing blood vessels and a responsibility in the angiogenic process has been suggested. As malignant gliomas are highly vascularised lesions, the (B⁺)-fibronectin may represent an attractive target for MAb-based immunotherapy *(79,80)*. Patients with recurring GBM are being enrolled in a phase I study that evaluates the therapeutic efficacy of the (B⁺)-fibronectin-specific murine IgG1 MAb BC-1. Following maximal surgical resection, ^{111}In-labeled BC-1 is administered into the SCRC to confirm the integrity of the cavity prior to the injection of ^{90}Y-labeled BC-1 (AS1405) *(7,80)* (*www.antisoma.com*).

GP240

GP240 is a cell-surface high-molecular-weight chondroitin sulfate proteoglycan expressed by a majority of gliomas, melanomas, neuroblastomas, and medulloblastomas. The anti-GP240 murine IgG2a MAb Me1-14[81] was involved in the first targeted radioimmunotherapeutic trials using the intrathecal route for patients with melanoma or glioma neoplastic meningitis *(82)*. In another phase I trial, intrathecal administration of escalating doses (40–100 mCi) of ^{131}I-labeled Me1-14 F(ab')₂ MAb fragment in patients with neoplastic meningitis of various primary origins, including HGG, was evaluated *(8)*. Of note, in one of the cases of neoplastic meningitis of melanoma origin, the patient was alive more than 7 yr following ^{131}I-labeled Me1-14 F(ab')₂ injection *(83)*.

Prospective Antigens

As mentioned earlier, the systemic administration section of this chapter, the vascular endothelial growth factor receptor (VEGFR) has the significant advantage of being readily accessible by MAbs following systemic administration *(84)*. In vivo preclinical investigations of the DC101 Mab, which binds to the VEGFR-2 (Flk-1) receptor, indicated that neovascularization and tumor growth are inhibited after systemic treatment of mice bearing intracranial human GBM xenografts *(85)*. DC101 has not been involved yet in clinical trials for patients with HGG.

Gangliosides are glycosphingolipids expressed on the surface of normal cells prior to being internalized in lipid rafts *(86,87)*. Both lacto-series gangliosides 3'-isoLM1 and 3',6'-isoLD1 have been detected in gliomas. Despite the fact that they are also expressed in normal brain during the late fetal period and early after birth, they are generally not detectable after 2 yr age *(88)*. Additionally, 3'-isoLM1 is expressed for the most part on the edge of invasive GBM as well as on remote tumor cells that have infiltrated the brain parenchyma *(89)*. Thus, effective targeting of these cells may possibly help eliminate the most important source of recurrence. However, despite the production of specific IgM MAbs *(88)*, no anti-3'-isoLM1 or 3',6'-isoLD1 MAb of the IgG class is available at this time.

Recently, two additional proteins have been identified as possible targets for MAb-based immunotherapy of HGG *(7)*. GPNMB is a transmembrane glycoprotein whose encoding gene is expressed in malignant gliomas (64%) but not in normal tissues, including the brain *(90)*. Furthermore, an association between GPNMB and invasive and metastatic tumor patterns has been observed *(91)*. The multidrug resistance protein 3 (MRP3) is a complex transmembrane protein expressed in a majority of HGG (>80%) as well as in various normal tissues but not in the brain *(92,93)*. Efforts to generate MAbs targeting cell surface or extracellular domains of GPNMB or MRP3 are ongoing *(7)*.

CONCLUSIONS

The prognosis for patients with HGG has remained unchanged for more than 25 yr and continues to be grim. Despite the use of current multimodality therapy incorporating surgery, external beam radiotherapy, and systemic chemotherapy, the failure to eradicate local tumor growth is a major factor contributing to this poor outcome. However, during that same period of time, MAb therapy has emerged from a speculative approach to a realistic potential adjuvant treatment as illustrated by the number of existing immunotherapy clinical trials. In several studies, the administration of specific MAbs, most often radiolabeled, increased the survival of patients with HGG and was associated with lower toxicity than non-MAb based adjuvant therapies.

Ongoing efforts are focused on further improving these immunotherapeutic procedures to make them more effective, less toxic to normal tissues, and more convenient. Preclinical research is attempting to optimize all the individual aspects of immunotherapy. As a result, MAb-based targeted therapy is gradually being better matched to the characteristics of the patient and his tumor, so that ultimately the use of an individualized combination of MAbs, based on the immunoreactive profile of the targeted tumor, may become a realistic approach.

REFERENCES

1. Ehrlich P. Collected Studies on Immunity. New York: Wiley, 1906.
2. Hericourt J, Richet C. Traitement d'un cas de sarcome par la serotherapie. CR Hebd Seances Acad Sci 1895; 120:948–950.
3. Day ED, Lassiter S, Woodhall B, Mahaley JL, Mahaley MS, Jr. The localization of radioantibodies in human brain tumors. I. Preliminary exploration. Cancer Res 1965;25:773–778.
4. Mahaley MS, Jr., Mahaley JL, Day ED. The localization of radioantibodies in human brain tumors. II. Radioautography. Cancer Res 1965;25:779–793.
5. Marrack D, Kubala M, Corry P, et al. Localization of intracranial tumors. Comparative study with 131-I-labeled antibody to human fibrinogen and neohydrin-203Hg. Cancer 1967;20:751–755.
6. Kohler G, Milstein C. Continuous cultures of fused cells secreting antibody of predefined specificity. Nature 1975;256:495–497.
7. Boskovitz A, Wikstrand C, Kuan CT, Zalutsky M, Reardon DA, Bigner DD. Monoclonal antibodies for brain tumor treatment. Expert Opin Biol Ther 2004;4(9):1453–1471.
8. Wikstrand CJ, Zalutsky MR, Bigner DD. Radiolabeled antibodies for therapy of brain tumors. In: Liau LM, Becker DP, Cloughesy TF, Bigner DD, eds. Brain Tumor Immunotherapy. Totowa, NJ: Humana Press, 2001:205–229.

9. Batra SK, Jain M, Wittel UA, Chauhan SC, Colcher D. Pharmacokinetics and biodistribution of genetically engineered antibodies. Curr Opin Biotechnol 2002;13:603–608.

10. Morrison SL, Johnson MJ, Herzenberg LA, Oi VT. Chimeric human antibody molecules: mouse antigen-binding domains with human constant region domains. Proc Natl Acad Sci USA 1984;81:6851–6855.

11. Boulianne GL, Hozumi N, Shulman MJ. Production of functional chimaeric mouse/human antibody. Nature 1984;312:643–646.

12. Colcher D, Pavlinkova G, Beresford G, Booth BJ, Choudhury A, Batra SK. Pharmacokinetics and biodistribution of genetically-engineered antibodies. Q J Nucl Med 1998;42:225–241.

13. Shin SU. Chimeric antibody: potential applications for drug delivery and immunotherapy. Biotherapy 1991;3: 43–353.

14. Reist CJ, Bigner DD, Zalutsky MR. Human IgG2 constant region enhances in vivo stability of anti-tenascin antibody 81C6 compared with its murine parent. Clin Cancer Res 1998;4:2495-502.

15. Batra SK, Niswonger ML, Wikstrand CJ, et al. Mouse/human chimeric Me1-14 antibody: genomic cloning of the variable region genes, linkage to human constant region genes, expression, and characterization. Hybridoma 1994;13:87–97.

16. Zalutsky MR, Archer GE, Garg PK, Batra SK, Bigner DD. Chimeric anti-tenascin antibody 81C6: increased tumor localization compared with its murine parent. Nucl Med Biol 1996;23:449–458.

17. He X, Archer GE, Wikstrand CJ, et al. Generation and characterization of a mouse/human chimeric antibody directed against extracellular matrix protein tenascin. J Neuroimmunol 1994;52:127–137.

18. Khazaeli MB, Saleh MN, Liu TP, et al. Pharmacokinetics and immune response of 131I-chimeric mouse/human B72.3 (human gamma 4) monoclonal antibody in humans. Cancer Res 1991;51:5461–5466.

19. Jones PT, Dear PH, Foote J, Neuberger MS, Winter G. Replacing the complementarity-determining regions in a human antibody with those from a mouse. Nature 1986;321:522–525.

20. Riechmann L, Clark M, Waldmann H, Winter G. Reshaping human antibodies for therapy. Nature 1988; 332:323–327.

21. Vaughan TJ, Osbourn JK, Tempest PR. Human antibodies by design. Nat Biotechnol 1998;16:535–539.

22. Foon KA, Yang XD, Weiner LM, et al. Preclinical and clinical evaluations of ABX-EGF, a fully human anti-epidermal growth factor receptor antibody. Int J Radiat Oncol Biol Phys 2004;58:984–990.

23. Powers DB, Marks JD. Monovalent phage display of Fab and scFv fusions. Antibody fusion proteins. New York:Wiley Liss, John Wiley & Sons; 1999:151–188.

24. Boskovitz A, Akabani GH, Pegram CN, Bigner DD, Zalutsky MR. Human/murine chimeric 81C6 F(ab')(2) fragment: preclinical evaluation of a potential construct for the targeted radiotherapy of malignant glioma. Nucl Med Biol 2004;31:345–55.

25. Kuan CT, Wikstrand CJ, Archer G, et al. Increased binding affinity enhances targeting of glioma xenografts by EGFRvIII-specific scFv. Int J Cancer 2000;88:962–969.

26. Colcher D, Bird R, Roselli M, et al. In vivo tumor targeting of a recombinant single-chain antigen-binding protein. J Natl Cancer Inst 1990;82:1191–1197.

27. Schier R, McCall A, Adams GP, et al. Isolation of picomolar affinity anti-c-erbB-2 single-chain Fv by molecular evolution of the complementarity determining regions in the center of the antibody binding site. J Mol Biol 1996;263:551–567.

28. Yokota T, Milenic DE, Whitlow M, Schlom J. Rapid tumor penetration of a single-chain Fv and comparison with other immunoglobulin forms. Cancer Res 1992;52:3402–408.

29. Todorovska A, Roovers RC, Dolezal O, Kortt AA, Hoogenboom HR, Hudson PJ. Design and application of diabodies, triabodies and tetrabodies for cancer targeting. J Immunol Methods 2001;248:47–66.

30. Hu S, Shively L, Raubitschek A, et al. Minibody: A novel engineered anti-carcinoembryonic antigen antibody fragment (single-chain Fv-CH3) which exhibits rapid, high-level targeting of xenografts. Cancer Res 1996;56: 3055–3061.

31. Yazaki PJ, Wu AM. Construction and characterization of minibodies for imaging and therapy of colorectal carcinomas. Methods Mol Biol 2003; 207:351–364.

32. Kuan CT, Wikstrand CJ, Bigner DD. EGF mutant receptor vIII as a molecular target in cancer therapy. Endocr Relat Cancer 2001;8:83–96.

33. Sampson JH, Crotty LE, Lee S, et al. Unarmed, tumor-specific monoclonal antibody effectively treats brain tumors. Proc Natl Acad Sci USA 2000;97:7503–7508.

34. Zalutsky M. Radionuclide therapy. In: Vertes A, Nagy S, Klencsar Z, eds. Handbook of Nuclear Chemistry, Vol. 4. Dordrecht, Netherlands: Kluwer Academic; 2003:315–348.

35. Zalutsky MR, Vaidyanathan G. Astatine-211-labeled radiotherapeutics: an emerging approach to targeted alpha-particle radiotherapy. Curr Pharm Des 2000;6:1433–1455.

36. Hall WA, Fodstad O. Immunotoxins and central nervous system neoplasia. J Neurosurg 1992;76:1–12.

37. Rustamzadeh E, Low WC, Vallera DA, Hall WA. Immunotoxin therapy for CNS tumor. J Neurooncol 2003; 64:101–116.

38. Archer GE, Sampson JH, Lorimer IA, et al. Regional treatment of epidermal growth factor receptor vIII-expressing neoplastic meningitis with a single-chain immunotoxin, MR-1. Clin Cancer Res 1999;5:2646–2652.

39. Zalutsky MR, Moseley RP, Benjamin JC, et al. Monoclonal antibody and F(ab')2 fragment delivery to tumor in patients with glioma: comparison of intracarotid and intravenous administration. Cancer Res 1990;50:4105–4110.

40. Schold SC, Jr., Zalutsky MR, Coleman RE, et al. Distribution and dosimetry of I-123-labeled monoclonal antibody 81C6 in patients with anaplastic glioma. Invest Radiol 1993;28:488–496.

41. Bartus RT, Elliott PJ, Dean RL, et al. Controlled modulation of BBB permeability using the bradykinin agonist, RMP-7. Exp Neurol 1996;142:14–28.

42. Sampson JH, Akabani G, Archer GE, et al. Progress report of a Phase I study of the intracerebral microinfusion of a recombinant chimeric protein composed of transforming growth factor (TGF)-alpha and a mutated form of the Pseudomonas exotoxin termed PE-38 (TP-38) for the treatment of malignant brain tumors. J Neurooncol 2003;65:27–35.

43. Jain RK, Baxter LT. Mechanisms of heterogeneous distribution of monoclonal antibodies and other macromolecules in tumors: significance of elevated interstitial pressure. Cancer Res 1988;48:7022–7032.

44. Goetz C, Riva P, Poepperl G, et al. Locoregional radioimmunotherapy in selected patients with malignant glioma: experiences, side effects and survival times. J Neurooncol 2003;62:321–328.

45. Groothuis DR. The blood–brain and blood–tumor barriers: a review of strategies for increasing drug delivery. Neuro-oncol 2000;2:45–59.

46. Erickson HP. Tenascin-C, tenascin-R and tenascin-X: a family of talented proteins in search of functions. Curr Opin Cell Biol 1993;5:869–876.

47. Jones FS, Jones PL. The tenascin family of ECM glycoproteins: structure, function, and regulation during embryonic development and tissue remodeling. Dev Dyn 2000;218:235–259.

48. Bourdon MA, Wikstrand CJ, Furthmayr H, Matthews TJ, Bigner DD. Human glioma-mesenchymal extracellular matrix antigen defined by monoclonal antibody. Cancer Res 1983;43:2796–2805.

49. Bourdon MA, Matthews TJ, Pizzo SV, Bigner DD. Immunochemical and biochemical characterization of a glioma-associated extracellular matrix glycoprotein. J Cell Biochem 1985;28:183–195.

50. Zagzag D, Friedlander DR, Dosik J, et al. Tenascin-C expression by angiogenic vessels in human astrocytomas and by human brain endothelial cells in vitro. Cancer Res 1996;56:182–189.

51. Wikstrand CJ, Fung KM, Trojanowski JQ, McLendon RE, Bigner DD. Antibodies and molecular immunology: immunohistochemistry and antigens of diagnostic significance. In: Bigner DD, McLendon RE, Bruner JM, eds. Russell and Rubinstein's Pathology of the Nervous System. New York: Oxford University Press; 1998:251–304.

52. Reardon DA, Akabani G, Coleman RE, et al. Phase II trial of murine (131)I-labeled antitenascin monoclonal antibody 81C6 administered into surgically created resection cavities of patients with newly diagnosed malignant gliomas. J Clin Oncol 2002;20:1389–1397.

53. Riva P, Franceschi G, Riva N, Casi M, Santimaria M, Adamo M. Role of nuclear medicine in the treatment of malignant gliomas: the locoregional radioimmunotherapy approach. Eur J Nucl Med 2000;27:601–609.

54. Paganelli G, Grana C, Chinol M, et al. Antibody-guided three-step therapy for high grade glioma with yttrium-90 biotin. Eur J Nucl Med 1999;26:348–357.

55. Grana C, Chinol M, Robertson C, et al. Pretargeted adjuvant radioimmunotherapy with yttrium-90-biotin in malignant glioma patients: a pilot study. Br J Cancer 2002;86:207–212.

56. Zagzag D, Shiff B, Jallo GI, et al. Tenascin-C promotes microvascular cell migration and phosphorylation of focal adhesion kinase. Cancer Res 2002;62:2660–2668.

57. Zalutsky MR, Moseley RP, Coakham HB, Coleman RE, Bigner DD. Pharmacokinetics and tumor localization of 131I-labeled anti-tenascin monoclonal antibody 81C6 in patients with gliomas and other intracranial malignancies. Cancer Res 1989;49:2807–2813.

58. Shrieve DC, Alexander E, 3rd, Wen PY, et al. Comparison of stereotactic radiosurgery and brachytherapy in the treatment of recurrent glioblastoma multiforme. Neurosurgery 1995;36:275–282; discussion 282–284.

59. Akabani G, Cokgor I, Coleman RE, et al. Dosimetry and dose-response relationships in newly diagnosed patients with malignant gliomas treated with iodine-131-labeled anti-tenascin monoclonal antibody 81C6 therapy. Int J Radiat Oncol Biol Phys 2000;46:947–958.

60. Zalutsky M, Reardon DA, Akabani G, et al. Astatine-211 labeled human/mouse chimeric anti-tenascin monoclonal antibody via surgically created resection cavities for patients with recurrent glioma: Phase I study (abstract). Neuro-oncol 2002;4:103.

61. Akabani G, Reist CJ, Cokgor I, et al. Dosimetry of 131I-labeled 81C6 monoclonal antibody administered into surgically created resection cavities in patients with malignant brain tumors. J Nucl Med 1999;40: 631–638.

62. Vanhoefer U, Tewes M, Rojo F, et al. Phase I study of the humanized antiepidermal growth factor receptor monoclonal antibody EMD72000 in patients with advanced solid tumors that express the epidermal growth factor receptor. J Clin Oncol 2004;22:175–184.

63. Pimentel E. Peptide growth factors. In: Pimentel E, ed. Handbook of growth factors. London: CRC;1994:104–185.

64. Bigner SH, Wong AJ, Mark J, et al. Relationship between gene amplification and chromosomal deviations in malignant human gliomas. Cancer Genet Cytogenet 1987;29:165–170.

65. Wikstrand CJ, Reist CJ, Archer GE, Zalutsky MR, Bigner DD. The class III variant of the epidermal growth factor receptor (EGFRvIII): characterization and utilization as an immunotherapeutic target. J Neurovirol 1998;4:148–158.

66. Wersall P, Ohlsson I, Biberfeld P, et al. Intratumoral infusion of the monoclonal antibody, mAb 425, against the epidermal-growth-factor receptor in patients with advanced malignant glioma. Cancer Immunol Immunother 1997;44:157–164.

67. Faillot T, Magdelenat H, Mady E, et al. A phase I study of an anti-epidermal growth factor receptor monoclonal antibody for the treatment of malignant gliomas. Neurosurgery 1996;39:478–483.

68. Stragliotto G, Vega F, Stasiecki P, Gropp P, Poisson M, Delattre JY. Multiple infusions of anti-epidermal growth factor receptor (EGFR) monoclonal antibody (EMD 55,900) in patients with recurrent malignant gliomas. Eur J Cancer 1996;32A:636–640.

69. Kalofonos HP, Pawlikowska TR, Hemingway A, et al. Antibody guided diagnosis and therapy of brain gliomas using radiolabeled monoclonal antibodies against epidermal growth factor receptor and placental alkaline phosphatase. J Nucl Med 1989;30:1636–645.

70. Brady LW, Miyamoto C, Woo DV, et al. Malignant astrocytomas treated with iodine-125 labeled monoclonal antibody 425 against epidermal growth factor receptor: a phase II trial. Int J Radiat Oncol Biol Phys 1992; 22:225–230.

71. Epenetos AA, Courtenay-Luck N, Pickering D, et al. Antibody guided irradiation of brain glioma by arterial infusion of radioactive monoclonal antibody against epidermal growth factor receptor and blood group A antigen. Br Med J (Clin Res Ed) 1985; 290:1463–1466.

72. Quang TS, Brady LW. Radioimmunotherapy as a novel treatment regimen: 125I-labeled monoclonal antibody 425 in the treatment of high-grade brain gliomas. Int J Radiat Oncol Biol Phys 2004;58:972–975.

73. Aldape KD, Ballman K, Furth A, et al. Immunohistochemical detection of EGFRvIII in high malignancy grade astrocytomas and evaluation of prognostic significance. J Neuropathol Exp Neurol 2004;63:700–707.

74. Wikstrand CJ, McLendon RE, Friedman AH, Bigner DD. Cell surface localization and density of the tumor-associated variant of the epidermal growth factor receptor, EGFRvIII. Cancer Res 1997;57:4130–4140.

75. Feldkamp MM, Lala P, Lau N, Roncari L, Guha A. Expression of activated epidermal growth factor receptors, Ras-guanosine triphosphate, and mitogen-activated protein kinase in human glioblastoma multiforme specimens. Neurosurgery 1999; 45:1442–1453.

76. Shinojima N, Tada K, Shiraishi S, et al. Prognostic value of epidermal growth factor receptor in patients with glioblastoma multiforme. Cancer Res 2003;63:6962–6970.

77. Reist CJ, Batra SK, Pegram CN, Bigner DD, Zalutsky MR. In vitro and in vivo behavior of radiolabeled chimeric anti-EGFRvIII monoclonal antibody: comparison with its murine parent. Nucl Med Biol 1997;24: 639–647.

78. Khawli LA, Mizokami MM, Sharifi J, Hu P, Epstein AL. Pharmacokinetic characteristics and biodistribution of radioiodinated chimeric TNT-1, -2, and -3 monoclonal antibodies after chemical modification with biotin. Cancer Biother Radiopharm 2002;17:359–370.

79. Mariani G, Lasku A, Pau A, et al. A pilot pharmacokinetic and immunoscintigraphic study with the technetium-99m-labeled monoclonal antibody BC-1 directed against oncofetal fibronectin in patients with brain tumors. Cancer 1997;80:2484–489.

80. Ravic M. Intracavitary treatment of malignant gliomas: radioimmunotherapy targeting fibronectin. Acta Neurochir Suppl 2003;88:77–82.

81. Carrel S, Accolla RS, Carmagnola AL, Mach JP. Common human melanoma-associated antigen(s) detected by monoclonal antibodies. Cancer Res 1980;40:2523–2528.

82. Coakham HB, Kemshead JT. Treatment of neoplastic meningitis by targeted radiation using (131)I-radiolabelled monoclonal antibodies. Results of responses and long term follow-up in 40 patients. J Neurooncol 1998; 38:225–232.

83. Cokgor I, Akabani G, Friedman HS, et al. Long term response in a patient with neoplastic meningitis secondary to melanoma treated with (131)I-radiolabeled antichondroitin proteoglycan sulfate Mel-14 F(ab')(2): a case study. Cancer 2001;91:1809–1813.

84. Lamszus K, Kunkel P, Westphal M. Invasion as limitation to anti-angiogenic glioma therapy. Acta Neurochir Suppl 2003;88:169–77.

85. Kunkel P, Ulbricht U, Bohlen P, et al. Inhibition of glioma angiogenesis and growth in vivo by systemic treatment with a monoclonal antibody against vascular endothelial growth factor receptor-2. Cancer Res 2001;61:6624–6628.

86. Pelkmans L, Helenius A. Endocytosis via caveolae. Traffic 2002;3:311–320.

87. Dykstra M, Cherukuri A, Sohn HW, Tzeng SJ, Pierce SK. Location is everything: lipid rafts and immune cell signaling. Annu Rev Immunol 2003;21:457–481.

88. Wikstrand CJ, Fredman P, Svennerholm L, Bigner DD. Detection of glioma-associated gangliosides GM2, GD2, GD3, 3'-isoLM1 3',6'-isoLD1 in central nervous system tumors in vitro and in vivo using epitope-defined monoclonal antibodies. Prog Brain Res 1994;101:213–223.

89. Hedberg KM, Mahesparan R, Read TA, et al. The glioma-associated gangliosides 3'-isoLM1, GD3 and GM2 show selective area expression in human glioblastoma xenografts in nude rat brains. Neuropathol Appl Neurobiol 2001;27:451–464.

90. Kuan CT, Wikstrand C, Wakiya K, Riggins GJ, Bigner DD. Expression of GPNMBwt/GPNMBsv mRNA and protein in human high-grade gliomas (abstract). Neuro-oncol 2003;5:387.

91. Rich JN, Guo C, McLendon RE, Bigner DD, Wang XF, Counter CM. A genetically tractable model of human glioma formation. Cancer Res 2001;61:3556–3560.

92. Wikstrand C, Wakiya K, Kuan CT, Riggins GJ, Bigner DD. Expression of multidrug resistance protein 3 (MRP3) by human gliomas: detection and determination of incidence with polyclonal and monoclonal antibodies (MAbs) (abstract). Proc Am Assoc Cancer Res 2003;44:424.

93. Wakiya K, Kuan CT, Riggins GJ, Wikstrand C, Bigner DD. MRP3: a potential target for glioma therapy (abstract). Neuro-oncol 2003;5:401.

23 Clinical Trials of Oncolytic Viruses for Gliomas

E. Antonio Chiocca and M. L. Lamfers

Summary

There has been resurgent interest in the use of mutant or genetically engineered strains of viruses for the local treatment of gliomas. The clinical status of these agents is reviewed and further progress in this area with new agents is detailed. Safety in glioma patients has been shown, but anticancer efficacy needs additional refinements in the technologies employed.

Key Words: Oncolytic virus; gene therapy; brain tumor; clinical trial; adenovirus; herpes simplex virus.

INTRODUCTION

Despite progress made in understanding the pathogenesis and molecular characteristics of malignant gliomas, successful treatment options for these tumors have not been established. The survival for these patients has not changed during the past several decades. One alternative that has received considerable attention involves the use of viral therapy. Historically, scientific and clinical examples on the use of viruses to treat a variety of cancers have been published, but the seminal study by Martuza et al. provided a resurgence in interest for this type of research *(1)*. This has progressed into attempts to study safety and effectiveness in clinical trials. Herein, we will review these trials and attempt to derive some insight into how this modality may evolve in the future.

BASIC PRINCIPLES

Viruses have evolved to efficiently infect human cells, usurp the cellular machinery, and replicate themselves into multiple progenies, which can, in turn, go on to infect other cells in the body. Advances in molecular virology have shown that these processes require an exquisite and carefully coordinated interaction between viral proteins and cellular proteins. For example, once inside the cell, the virus expresses proteins that interfere with cellular processes (e.g., to prevent apoptosis or induce cell–cycle progression). This ensures robust viral replication and viral protein production, which eventually causes lysis of the infected cell and release of progeny virus that can infect neighboring cells, upon which the cycle is repeated. In this way, the virus is capable of disseminating throughtout solid tumor mass.

The terminology "oncolytic virus" refers to viruses, which preferentially replicate in tumor cells as compared with normal cells (Fig. 1). Some naturally attenuated oncolytic viral strains

From: *Current Clinical Oncology: High-Grade Gliomas: Diagnosis and Treatment*
Edited by: G. H. Barnett © Humana Press Inc., Totowa, NJ

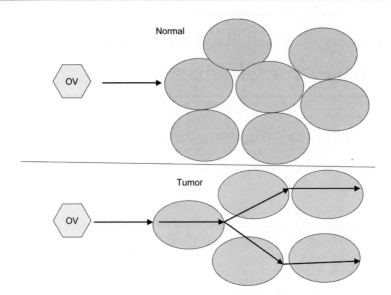

Fig. 1. An oncolytic virus will infect and replicate in tumor cells but not in normal cells.

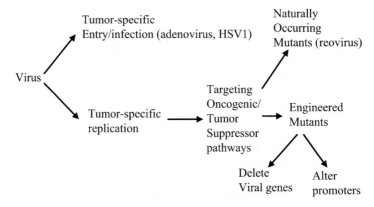

Fig. 2. How are oncolytic viruses generated? A wild-type virus can be genetically re-engineered so that its tropism for normal cells is re-directed towards tumor cells. This has been done for adenovirus and HSV1. It can also be re-engineered so that its replication inside a cell occurs preferentially if the cell is neoplastic. This is performed naturally by some viruses, such as reovirus, but most times genetic re-engineering is needed so that viral replication occurs in cells with defects in tumor suppressor pathways. Another avenue to ensure viral replication in tumor cells is to use tumor-specific promoters to drive expression of viral genes. In addition, anticancer cDNAs can be added to the mutant oncolytic viral genome to increase its cancer selectivity.

exist that appear to replicate more efficiently in cancer cells than in normal tissue, whereas others acquire oncolytic qualities through genetic engineering (such as herpes simplex virus [HSV] and adenovirus) (Fig. 2). The tumor selectivity of oncolytic viruses occurs either during infection or replication. Oncolytic viral vectors based on adenovirus, herpes virus, poliovirus, and reovirus have all been described as therapeutic agents for malignant glioma *(1–12)*. Current research in this field is mainly focused on improving the tumor selectivity and oncolytic potency of these agents.

Table 1
Potential Advantages and Disadvantages of HSV1 as an Oncolytic Virus

Potential advantages of HSV1 as an oncolytic virus
- Can be genetically re-engineered to improve cancer selectivity
- Can rapidly kill tumor cells (within 12–18 h) and produce 500–1000 progeny viruses
- Can deliver/express in tumors multiple anticancer transgenes
- Does not randomly insert into the cellular genome, minimizing the risk for additional mutagenesis events
- Effective antitherpetic agents can be used to abort viral infection/replication, if necessary
  Has been used in human clinical trials for gliomas

Theoretical disadvantages of HSV1 as an oncolytic virus
- Pre-existing an innate immunity may limit the extent of tumor infection
- Some of the more attenuated and less toxic mutants are difficult to produce to very high titers
- Encephalitis, meningitis and inflammation are likely dose-limiting toxicities in humans
- The mutant viral genome could recombine with wild-type HSV1 and added transgenes could be passed onto a wild-type HSV-1
- The mutant viral genome could change after multiple passages.

LOCAL DELIVERY OF HERPES SIMPLEX VIRUS INTO GLIOMAS

Herpes simplex virus type I (HSV-1) is an enveloped, double-stranded, linear DNA virus with a genome of 152 kb which encodes more than 80 genes. About one half of the genes are essential for viral replication whereas the other (nonessential) genes encode proteins which support the viral life cycle within the host cell. The major advantages and disadvantages of HSV-1 for tumor oncolysis are illustrated in Table 1.

Several different strategies have been applied to generate tumor-selective HSV-1 vectors, as first shown by Martuza et al. It appears that most oncolytic viruses may ultimately be targeting cells, which have altered signal-transduction pathways that promote tumorigenesis. This can occur spontaneously as is the case for reovirus *(10–12)* or can occur by genetic re-engineering. In the latter case, mutations or deletions in the viral genome are commonly introduced to eliminate the expression of specific viral proteins, which renders the mutant vector dependent on the tumor cells for viral propagation. Some of these viral proteins are also associated with neurotoxicity and a dual beneficial effect is obtained by mutating these genes. One of these mutants (designated 1716) has progressed to phase 1 clinical trial in 2 studies which include 21 patients altogether *(13,14)*. In both studies patients with recurrent malignant glioma, refractory to conventional therapy, were treated. The HSV-1 vector was well tolerated at doses up to 10^5 infectious particles after stereotactic intratumoral injection, and no adverse events were reported. In the first trial, multiple injections of a 1-mL total volume were performed. No viral DNA was detected by polymerase chain reaction (PCR) in serum and buccal swab samples taken from five patients. Four out of nine patients were alive at 14 mo after the treatment *(13)*. In the second trial, patients were injected with virus followed by tumor resection after 4 to 9 d, which showed virus replication in the tumor tissue. In some patients the amount of recovered virus exceeded the input dose *(14)*. 1716 has also been clinically tested for advanced melanoma *(15)*. In three patients receiving multiple intranodular injections, histopathological analyses revealed tumor necrosis and HSV-antigen presence in the tumor only.

Table 2
Potential Advantages and Disadvantages of AAd as an Oncolytic Virus

Potential advantages of Ad as an oncolytic virus
- Can be genetically re-engineered to render it selective for specific tumor-suppressor pathways
- Can take 24–48 h to kill tumor cells, but can produce several thousand progeny viruses
- Can deliver/express in tumors 1 or 2 additional anticancer transgenes.
- Does not randomly insert into the cellular genome, minimizing the risk for additional mutagenesis events
- Has been used in human clinical trials for gliomas

Theoretical disadvantages of Ad as an oncolytic virus
- Some of the more attenuated and less toxic mutants are difficult to produce to very high titers
- Encephalitis, meningitis, and inflammation are likely dose-limiting toxicities in humans
- The mutant viral genome could recombine with wild-type adenovirus and added transgenes could be passed onto a wild-type Ad
- There are no effective antiadenoviral agents for aborting viral infection/replication, if necessary
- The adenoviral receptor (CAR) is poorly expressed in gliomas, thus limiting efficient infection.

Using a single mutant, HSV-1 vectors are potentially associated with the risk of restoring a wild-type phenotype *(16)*. Concern about this risk led to the design of an oncolytic virus with dual mutations: G207. G207 has been tested in a phase I clinical trial in patients with recurrent glioma *(17)*. Twenty-one patients were included and single injections of doses up to 3×10^9 infectious particles were administered. No adverse events were observed and the virus was well tolerated to the extent that no maximum tolerated dose was achieved. Promisingly, 2 patients were still alive 4 yr after the treatment.

LOCAL DELIVERY OF ADENOVIRUS INTO GLIOMAS

Adenoviruses are also attractive candidates as oncolytic viruses. Their potential advantages and disadvantages in tumor oncolysis are illustrated in Table 2. The life cycle and replication of wild-type adenovirus is very well understood. The primary attachment of the adenovirus particle to the surface of the host cell is via one of its surface proteins (fiberknob) to the coxsackie and adenovirus receptor (CAR). The CAR-docked viral particles also interact with α_v integrins at the cell surface, which promote virus internalization by endocytosis. In the cell the adenovirus escapes from the endosome and is transported toward the cell nucleus, during which the virus particle is partially broken down. In the nucleus, the viral DNA remains extrachromosomal and the program of viral gene expression begins. The Ad proteins encoded by the early (E) regions of the adenovirus genome are expressed first, upon which the adenoviral genome is replicated followed by expression of Ad proteins encoded by the late (L) regions. Progeny adenovirus particles are assembled and induction of cell death leads to the release of adenovirus progeny from the cell *(18–20)*.

The first oncolytic adenovirus to enter a clinical trial for malignant glioma was designated ONYX-015. This virus lacks the gene for E1B rendering it unable to bind to the cellular p53 protein *(3)*. When wild-type adenovirus infects a cell, the cell attempts to terminate efficient viral replication by increasing its p53 levels, thereby committing apoptosis (Fig. 1). The adenoviral gene product, E1B, prevents this by binding to p53 thus ensuring that the infected cell will live long enough to produce the several-thousands progeny Ads. It follows that a mutant E1B adenovirus will be able to replicate effectively only in cells with defects in the p53 tumor suppressor pathway, a common mutation in tumors, but will be restricted in replication in normal cells.

Controversy exists as to whether or not this is the sole mechanism by which ONYX-015 has selective replication capacity in malignant cells *(21,22)*. A recent report by the primary scientist involved in the engineering of ONYX-015 is now recognizing that tumor selectivity has little to do with p53 tumor suppressor pathway defects in tumor cells. Nevertheless, this oncolytic adenovirus has been tested in a wide range of preclinical models for various tumor types, including cervical carcinoma, laryngeal carcinoma, colorectal carcinoma, head and neck cancer, and glioma *(3,23–35)*. Based on these studies ONYX-015 rapidly entered phase I clinical trials and was the first such Ad to reach clinical testing. Multiple trials of ONYX-015 in over 300 cancer patients, using both intratumoral and intravascular delivery techniques, have established the safety of this approach and demonstrated selective activity of the virus within the malignant tissue *(26–28)*. However, despite biological activity of ONYX-015 clinical benefit was not seen in the majority of patients until the viral treatment was combined with chemotherapy in patients with head and neck cancer *(29)*.

ONYX-015 has also been injected in patients with recurrent malignant glioma. This phase I trial has involved the injection of escalating doses of the virus into the brain adjacent to a resected tumor cavity. Injected doses up to 10^{10} pfus have been well-tolerated. The trial thus demonstrated the relative safety of inoculating a replication-conditional virus into brain.

OTHER VIRUSES

Currently, a phase I trial of a reovirus strain into gliomas is being conducted in Canada. Reovirus has been shown to primarily replicate in cells with an overactive *ras* pathway, a signal transduction abnormality that is commonly observed in gliomas. Results of the trial are pending.

Several other types of viral mutants (e.g., poliovirus, Newcastle disease virus) are slowly making their way through various regulatory agencies in an attempt to get to clinical trials in humans. One strain of Newcastle disease virus has recently been reported to have been given to four humans with glioblastoma *(30)*. This does not appear to have been done as part of a formal clinical trial, although the authors report remarkable success.

AREAS OF ACTIVE RESEARCH

Retargeting of Infection Toward Tumor Cells

Some authors have emphasized that an important limitation for efficient adenoviral infection is the low levels of the adenovirus receptor (CAR) on malignant tumor cell membrane *(31–34)*. To overcome this possible barrier, it has been shown that Ad can be retargeted towards other molecules highly expressed on the glioma cell membranes, such as epidermal growth factor (EGFR) and α_v integrins. This concept was demonstrated using bispecific antibodies directed towards EGFR on one end and the Ad fiber knob on its other end. Preincubation of the adenoviral vector with the bispecific antibodies resulted in CAR-independent glioma cell infection and improved infection of primary glioma cell cultures obtained from tumor material *(31,33)*. In the context of replication-competent Ads, the use of bispecific antibodies to redirect adenoviral cell binding will only improve the first infection round, as the progeny adenoviruses will not have access to the bispecific antibody. This limitation was overcome by insertion of an expression cassette encoding the bispecific antibody, into the genome of the Ad, thereby allowing the progeny viruses to become retargeted. The EGFR-targeted adenoviral mutant efficiently killed primary human CAR-deficient brain tumor specimens that were refractory to the parent control virus *(35)*.

Another approach used to target the adenovirus to glioma cells involved the insertion of an integrin-binding peptide, arg-gly-asp (RGD), into the fiber of the virus, allowing the virus to make its primary attachment to integrins. Using replication-deficient adenoviral vectors encoding luciferase, it was demonstrated that the RGD modifications drastically enhanced infection efficiency of various tumor cells, including glioma *(31,36,37)*. An RGD-modified oncolytic Ad, demonstrated that improved infection efficiency translates to markedly enhanced oncolysis in (primary) glioma cells and impressive anti-glioma activity in subcutaneous and intracranial glioma xenografts *(32,38)*.

Retargeting of oncolytic adenovirus to glioma cells was also demonstrated by Shinoura et al. *(39)*. An increased cytopathic effect was found when ONYX-015 was modified with a stretch of 20 lysine residues at the C-terminal of the fiber, on glioma cells and in subcutaneous xenografts *(39)*. Alternative molecules that have been proven useful for redirecting adenoviral attachment and entry and which may be of potential interest to targeting glioma, are the fibroblast growth factor receptor *(40)*, folate receptor *(41)*, transferrin receptor *(42)*, and vascular endothelial growth factor receptor (VEGFR) *(43)*.

In summary, it is likely that retargeting of Ad will be required to improve its ability to destroy gliomatous tumors.

Interfering With the Immune Response Against the Virus

For the viral antitumor effect to succeed, viral replication must out-compete tumor proliferation. However, the fact that oncolytic viruses are attenuated in their replication and that they also provoke an intense immunogenic response may hinder efficient tumor spread and lysis. Therefore, one strategy to improve biologic efficacy may involve interfering with the immune response.

The immune response of the body to adenoviruses and HSVs follows a similar pattern consisting of an immediate innate response and a slower adaptive response. The nonspecific early occurring immune response contributes the largest effect to elimination of the viruses *(44)*. This innate response includes the activation of the complement cascade *(45)* and the recruitment and activation of macrophages, neutrophils, and natural killer cells which kill the infected cells either directly, or indirectly by secreting antiviral cytokines and chemokines *(46,47)*. In addition, the recruitment and activation of antigen-presenting cells (APCs) is essential for the development of an adaptive immune response *(48,49)*. The adaptive immune response is elicited when the viral antigens are presented to the T-helper cells, resulting in activation and secretion of cytokines by the T-helper cells and the maturing of B-cells into plasma cells. Plasma cells produce large amounts of high-affinity antibodies directed against the infected cells and the viral proteins. Together, these responses can result in a rapid inactivation of the oncolytic viruses and impede their therapeutic efficacy.

For this reason, several strategies have been developed to circumvent early inactivation of the virus by the immune system. Initially, these studies were performed using replication-deficient vectors in the interest of improving and prolonging transgene expression. Partial immune ablation using cytokines or CTL4A-Ig can lead to persistent adenoviral gene expression in mouse lung and liver *(50,51)*. The anti-cancer drugs etoposide and cyclophosphamide (CPA) were shown to enhance intratumoral transgene expression in immunocompetent mice *(52)*. The production of neutralizing antibodies to Ad and cytotoxic T-lymphocyte-mediated lysis of virally transduced cells were significantly suppressed in these animals. In a study using herpes vectors for gene transfer to neurons in the spinal cord, co-administration of cyclosporin A led to more persistent transgene expression in infected cells *(53)*. The inactivating role of the complement system was underscored by studies of Ikeda et al. *(55)* who demonstrated that rodent plasma inhibits cell transduction by adenoviral and herpes vectors. In vitro inactivation of complement with mild-heat treatment of the serum restored transduction efficiency. In vivo, complement depletion was achieved by administering cobra venom factor (CVF) prior to intra-arterial delivery of replication-conditional (oncolytic) HSV in a rat model for multiple intracerebral tumors. The complement inactivation led to a strong increase in the initial infection efficiency of the tumors *(54)*. In earlier reports, it had been demonstrated that administration of CPA enhanced the propagation of the oncolytic virus *(55)*. Combined treatment of oncolytic HSV with CVF and CPA inhibited both the innate and anti-HSV neutralizing antibody response, and their concerted action prolonged survival of rodents bearing intracerebral tumors *(54)*. More recently, cyclophosphamide was shown to inhibit the production of antiviral cytokines by peripheral blood mononuclear cells (PBMCs) as well as PBMC numbers even in the presence of active viral oncolysis *(56)*. This appears to suggest that PBMC responses may be limiting to viral oncolysis.

Combining Viral Oncolysis With Delivery of Anticancer Genes

Another approach to improving oncolysis by replicative viruses involves the insertion of therapeutic transgenes into the viral genome. Such "armed" replication-competent viruses allow the action of therapeutic proteins to be combined with the anti-tumor properties of the viral infection. This approach embodies several possible advantages. First, as a result of the amplification of the virus within the tumor, transgene production and spread are also highly increased as compared with infection with the replication-defective vector counterparts. This concept was demonstrated for adenovirus using the marker gene Luciferase *(57,58)* as well as for HSV using the β-galactosidase genne *(59–61)*. Marked increases in transgene expression were noted using the replication-competent compared with the replication-defective vectors. In addition, transgenes can be selected that have a nonoverlapping toxicity range with the viral-induced oncolytic effects in order to maximize their therapeutic benefit. Transgenes have been inserted that encode prodrug-converting enzymes, immunes stimulatory molecules, and apoptosis-enhancing proteins.

Several groups have constructed genetically engineered oncolytic viruses encoding a prodrug-converting enzyme. These enzymes convert nontoxic prodrugs into cytotoxic metabolites and are often soluble to allow for spreading within the tumor. Using this approach, a tumor-selective herpes virus was engineered encoding the rat cytochrome P450 (CYP2B1) transgene *(62)*. This liver enzyme activates the prodrug cyclophosphamide into an active anti-cancer and immunosuppressive metabolite *(63)*. Addition of cyclophosphamide potentiated oncolytic effects of this HSV mutant against cultured tumor cells and subcutaneous tumor xenografts established in athymic mice *(62)*.

Recently, an ONYX-015-based adenovirus was described encoding the prodrug converting enzyme carboxylesterase (CE), which converts the camptothecin derivative CPT-11 to the much more potent chemotherapeutic SN-38. Survival of tumor-bearing mice was strongly enhanced with the CE-expressing virus in combination with CPT-11 compared with controls *(64)*.

Multiple prodrug-activating gene therapies have also been used simultaneously in combination with oncolytic viruses. A replicating adenovirus with double enzyme/prodrug gene therapy containing the cytosine deaminase and HSV-Tk fusion gene markedly enhanced oncolysis relative to the isolated viral effect in cancer cells *(65)*. The combination of HSV-TK and CYP21 gene transfer mediated by an oncolytic HSV provided anti-tumor effects that were more significant than all other treatment combinations *(66)*.

The second type of transgenes that have been inserted into the oncolytic viruses, were selected to boost the immune response to the infected tumor cells by stimulating localized inflammatory and/or immune responses. In the context of Adses, this was first demonstrated using a tumor-selective virus engineered to express interferon (IFN) which strongly enhanced anti-tumor activity compared to relevant control adenovirus in immune-deficient mice bearing breast carcinoma xenografts *(9)*. Moreover, a number of replication-competent recombinant HSVs that encode immunostimulatory molecules have been constructed. Andreansky et al. *(67)* demonstrated that survival of immunocompetent mice bearing intracerebral tumors could be prolonged when treated with tumor-selective HSV encoding interleukin 4 (IL-4) compared to controls and immunohistochemical analysis demonstrated marked accumulation of inflammatory cells. Similarly, oncolytic HSV mutants expressing IL-12, IL-2, or the soluble B7-1 immunomodulatory molecule were found to produce survival benefit compared with control viruses in various tumor models including glioma in immunocompetent mice, by combining oncolytic and immunostimulatory effects *(68–71)*. Moreover, insertion of the potent immune stimulator granulocyte macrophage-colony stimulating factor (GM-CSF) into an oncolytic HSV backbone, improved shrinkage or clearance of tumors compared to control virus. These mice were also protected against re-challenge with tumour cells *(72)*. This suggests not only that expression of immunomodulatory molecules can potentiate oncolysis but may also induce a level of anti-tumor immunity.

Finally, insertion of transgenes may improve the oncolytic potential of the replication-competent virus itself. Opportunities for enhancing the anti-tumor potential of oncolytic viruses are at the final stage of the reproductive cycle that involves the lysis of the host cell and release of viral progeny *(73)*. Oncolysis of cancer cells when compared with lysis of the virus' natural host cells may be suboptimal as a result of cancer cell specific genetic alterations. These alterations mainly affect pro- and anti-apoptotic pathways that regulate the cell cycle. Coordinated and timely (over)expression of key players in these processes concomitant with the viral replicative cycle is expected to enhance the anti-tumor potential of the oncolytic virus. This concept was demonstrated using the AdΔ24 oncolytic adenovirus engineered to express p53 during late stages of viral replication and which exhibited up to >100-fold enhanced oncolytic potency on human cancer cell lines of various tissue origins *(74)*. In another study, expression of a dominant-negative I-κ B from a selectively replicating adenovirus sensitized tumor cells to recombinant human tumor necrosis factor α (TNF-α)-mediated apoptosis. Using this approach it could be demonstrated that induction of apoptosis during viral DNA replication compromised virus production, whereas apoptosis induced after virion assembly enhanced viral release from infected cells and dissemination *(75)*.

Combination treatment with conventional therapies may offer a number of advantages. First, enhanced therapeutic efficacy of dual treatments will allow administration of lower viral doses to achieve a certain therapeutic effect, which is important given the fact that sufficient virus delivery to tumors remains one of the major hurdles in clinical viral (gene) therapy strategies. Furthermore, combined treatment allowing lower viral doses may also lower toxic side-effects.

The first studies to describe the effects of dual treatment with an oncolytic virus and conventional therapy were performed with the ONYX-015 Ad. The efficacy of this agent combined with cisplatin and 5-fluorouracil was significantly greater than either agent alone in nude mouse tumor xenografts *(24)*. These results led to the design of a phase II trial using these agents in patients with squamous cell carcinoma of the head and neck *(29)*. The results of this study mirrored the preclinical data, including the frequent occurrence of complete remissions in patients treated with combination therapy. Synergy with the chemotherapeutic agents paclitaxel and docetaxel was demonstrated with the prostate cancer-specific oncolytic Ad, CV706, in a xenograft model of prostate cancer *(76)*.

Synergy with chemotherapeutic agents has also been described for HSV. The oncolytic effect of HSV-1716 in combination with mitomycin was synergistic in two of five nonsmall cell lung cancer cell lines in vitro and inhibited tumor growth more efficiently than either agent alone *(77)*. Combination treatment of the HSV mutant G207 and vincristine led to strongly enhanced in vitro cytotoxicity without affecting infection efficiency and replication of G207 in rhabdomyosarcoma cells. In vivo combination treatment of alveolar rhabdomyosarcoma using intravenous G207 and vincristine resulted in complete tumor regression without evidence of regrowth in five of eight animals whereas none of the animals receiving either monotherapy were cured *(78)*.

In the context of malignant brain tumors, the combination of oncolytic viruses with radiotherapy is perhaps more relevant than with chemotherapy considering the efficacy of standard treatments. Rogulski et al, *(79)* have studied the anti-tumor activity of ONYX-015 in combination with irradiation in colon carcinoma xenografts . ONYX-015 viral therapy combined with irradiation improved tumor control beyond that of either monotherapy. Studies with the prostate stimulating antigen (PSA) promoter-driven oncolytic Ad, CV706, in combination with radiotherapy demonstrated such an improvement in therapeutic response in prostate cancer xenografts without increasing toxicity, that a phase I study was initiated *(80,81)*. In glioma, synergistic oncolytic activity of ONYX-015 with radiotherapy was demonstrated in subcutaneous xenografts *(82)*. Also, the strong anti-tumor activity of Ad5-Δ24RGD, the integrin-targeted AdΔ24 variant, in malignant glioma could be further enhanced with low-dose irradiation such that the same therapeutic effect was achieved with a 10-fold lower viral dose *(32)*.

Combination therapy with oncolytic HSV and irradiation has produced varying results. Whereas a potentiating effect of irradiation on G207 viral oncolysis in cervical and colorectal cancer xenografts was found *(83,84)*, no enhancement of anti-tumor activity was seen when these treatment modalities were combined in subcutaneous tumor models of human and murine prostate cancer *(85)*. Spear et al. *(86)* also found complementary toxicity between irradiation and the oncolytic HSV-1 mutant for the ICP6, regardless of cell type, time, MOI, irradiation dose, or culture conditions, without evidence of augmented apoptosis or viral replication. In human glioma xenografts on the other hand, dual treatment with the HSV-1 γ34.5-mutant caused a significantly greater reduction in volume or total regression of tumors than either irradiation or infection alone. This enhanced oncolytic effect of the combined treatment correlated with two- to fivefold enhanced viral replication in irradiated tumor cells compared to tumors receiving virus only *(87)*. These results were extended to a second study in mice bearing intracerebral tumors which received γ34.5-mutant virus in combination with fractionated radiotherapy. Analysis of survival data revealed that the interaction between these treatment modalities was synergistic *(88)*.

In conclusion, the results from studies into combination therapy, demonstrating enhanced therapeutic efficacy of oncolytic viral therapy over single modality treatment, are very encouraging. Currently, investigators are successfully combining the above-described strategies with armed therapeutic viruses. A trimodal approach (i.e., lytic virus, double enzym/prodrug gene therapy, and irradiation) was found to be superior to any other combination in carcinoma xenografts. Significant tumor regression and ultimately 100% tumor cure were reported *(89)*.

CONCLUSIONS

Like a number of other translational disciplines of science (i.e., organ transplants, immunotoxin therapy, anti-angiogenesis), virotherapy is observing a historical waxing and waning interest because of results from initial clinical trials which have not always been as encouraging as the animal data. In spite of this, reasons for problems that have rendered its human use relatively nonefficacious are relatively understood. From this knowledge, solutions are beginning to emerge which could provide evidence for applications in neuro-oncology. A variety of newer generations of OV products are emerging. These will have to undergo testing in traditional phase I, and if promising, phase II and III trials. Understanding that gene therapy, like other therapeutics, can have dose-limiting toxicities in phase I trials and approaching such toxicities with the traditional tools of discovery, analysis, and finding of solutions that have defined the field of oncologic therapeutics should remain the regular course of action for these trials.

REFERENCES

1. Martuza RL, MalickA, MarkertJ.M, RuffnerKL, Coen DM. Experimental therapy of human glioma by means of a genetically engineered virus mutant. Science 1991;252:854–856.
2. Chiocca AE. Oncolytic viruses. Nat Rev Cancer 2002;2:938–950.
3. Bischoff JR, Kirn DH, Williams A, et al. An adenovirus mutant that replicates selectively in p53-deficient human tumor cells. Science 1996;274:373–376.
4. Boviatsis EJ, Park JS, Sena-Esteves M et al. Long-term survival of rats harboring brain neoplasms treated with ganciclovir and a herpes simplex virus vector that retains an intact thymidine kinase gene. Cancer Res 1994;54: 5745–5751.
5. Fueyo J, Gomez-Manzano C, Alemany R, et al. A mutant oncolytic adenovirus targeting the Rb pathway produces anti-glioma effect in vivo. Oncogene 2000;19:2–12.
6. Fulci G, Chiocca,EA. Oncolytic viruses for the therapy of brain tumors and other solid malignancies: a review. Front Biosci 2003;8:e346–360.
7. Gromeier M, Wimmer E. Viruses for the treatment of malignant glioma. Curr Opin Mol Ther 2001;3: 503–508.
8. Markert JM, Gillespie GY, Weichselbaum RR, Roizman B, Whitley RJ. Genetically engineered HSV in the treatment of glioma: a review. Rev Med Virol 2000;10:17–30.
9. Zhang JF, HuC, Geng Y, et al.Treatment of a human breast cancer xenograft with an adenovirus vector containing an interferon gene results in rapid regression due to viral oncolysis and gene therapy. Proc Natl Acad Sci USA 1996;93:4513–4518.
10. Yang WQ, Senger D, Muzik H, et al. Reovirus prolongs survival and reduces the frequency of spinal and leptomeningeal metastases from medulloblastoma. Cancer Res 2003;63:3162–3172.
11. Wilcox ME, Yang W, Senger D, et al. Reovirus as an oncolytic agent against experimental human malignant gliomas. J Natl Cancer Inst 2001;l93:903–912.
12. Coffey MC, Strong JE, Forsyth PA, Lee P.W. Reovirus therapy of tumors with activated Ras pathway. Science 1998;282:1332–1334.
13. Rampling R, Cruickshank G, Papanastassiou V, et al. Toxicity evaluation of replication-competent herpes simplex virus (ICP 34.5 null mutant 1716) in patients with recurrent malignant glioma. Gene Ther 2000;7: 859–866.
14. Papanastassiou V, Rampling R, Fraser M, et al. The potential for efficacy of the modified (ICP 34.5(-)) herpes simplex virus HSV1716 following intratumoural injection into human malignant glioma: a proof of principle study. Gene Ther 2002;9:398–406.
15. MacKie,RM, Stewart B, Brown SM. Intralesional injection of herpes simplex virus 1716 in metastatic melanoma. Lancet 2001;357:525–526.
16. Mohr I, Gluzman Y. AA herpesvirus genetic element which affects translation in the absence of the viral GADD34 function. Embo J 1996;15:4759–4766.

17. Markert JM, Medlock MD, Rabkin SD, et al. Conditionally replicating herpes simplex virus mutant, G207 for the treatment of malignant glioma: results of a phase I trial. Gene Ther 2000;7:867–874.
18. Philipson L, Pettersson U, Lindberg U. Molecular biology of adenoviruses. Virol Monogr 1975;14:1–115.
19. Marechal V, Piolot T. Lytic infection by double-strand DNA viruses and cell cycle alterations. Pathol Biol (Paris) 2000;48:289–300.
20. Nemerow GR., Cell receptors involved in adenovirus entry. Virology 2000;274:1–4
21. Hall AR, Dix BR, O'Carroll SJ, Braithwaite AW.,p53-dependent cell death/apoptosis is required for a productive adenovirus infection. Nat Med 1998;4:1068–1072.
22. Goodrum FD, Ornelles DA. p53 status does not determine outcome of E1B 55-kilodalton mutant adenovirus lytic infection. J Virol 1998;72:9479–9490.
23. Heise CC, Williams AM, Xue S, Propst M, Kirn DH. Intravenous administration of ONYX-015, a selectively replicating adenovirus, induces antitumoral efficacy. Cancer Res 1999;59:2623–2628.
24. Heise C, Sampson-Johannes A, Williams A, McCormick F, Von Hoff DD, Kirn DH. ONYX-015, an E1B gene-attenuated adenovirus, causes tumor-specific cytolysis and antitumoral efficacy that can be augmented by standard chemotherapeutic agents. Nat Med 1997;3:639–645.
25. Geoerger B, Grill J, Opolon P, et al. Oncolytic activity of the E1B-55 kDa-deleted adenovirus ONYX-015 is independent of cellular p53 status in human malignant glioma xenografts. Cancer Res 2002;62:764–772.
26. Post L E. Selectively replicating adenoviruses for cancer therapy: an update on clinical development. Curr Opin Investig Drugs 2002;3:1768–1772.
27. Reid T, Warren R, Kirn D. Intravascular adenoviral agents in cancer patients: lessons from clinical trials. Cancer Gene Ther 2002;9:979–986.
28. Kirn D. Clinical research results with dl1520 (Onyx-015), a replication-selective adenovirus for the treatment of cancer: what have we learned? Gene Ther 2001;8:89–98.
29. Khuri FR, Nemunaitis J, Ganly I, et al. A controlled trial of intratumoral ONYX-015, a selectively-replicating adenovirus, in combination with cisplatin and 5-fluorouracil in patients with recurrent head and neck cancer. Nat Med 2000;6:879–885.
30. Csatary LK, Gosztonyi G, Szeberenyi J, et al. MTH-68/H oncolytic viral treatment in human high-grade gliomas. J Neuro-oncol 2004;67:83–93.
31. Grill J, Van Beusechem,VW, Van Der Valk P, et al. Combined targeting of adenoviruses to integrins and epidermal growth factor receptors increases gene transfer into primary glioma cells and spheroids. Clin Cancer Res 2001;7:641–650.
32. Lamfers ML, Grill J, Dirven CM, et al. Potential of the conditionally replicative adenovirus Ad5-Delta24RGD in the treatment of malignant gliomas and its enhanced effect with radiotherapy. Cancer Res 2002;62:5736–5742.
33. Miller CR, Buchsbaum DJ, Reynolds PN, et al. Differential susceptibility of primary and established human glioma cells to adenovirus infection: targeting via the epidermal growth factor receptor achieves fiber receptor-independent gene transfer. Cancer Res 1998;58:5738–5748.
34. Fuxe J, Liu L, Malin S, Philipson L, Collins VP, Pettersson RF. Expression of the coxsackie and adenovirus receptor in human astrocytic tumors and xenografts. Int J Cancer 2003;03:723–729.
35. van Beusechem VMDC., van den Doel P, Lamfers MLM, et al.Conditionally replicative adenovirus expressing a targeting adapter molecule exhibits enhanced oncolytic potency on CAR-deficient tumors. Gene Therapy 2003;10:1982–1991.
36. Staba MJ, Wickham TJ, Kovesdi I, Hallahan DE.,Modifications of the fiber in adenovirus vectors increase tropism for malignant glioma models. Cancer Gene Ther 2000;7: 13–19.
37. Dmitriev I, Krasnykh V, Miller CR, et al. An adenovirus vector with genetically modified fibers demonstrates expanded tropism via utilization of a coxsackievirus and adenovirus receptor-independent cell entry mechanism. J Virol 1998;72:9706–9713.
38. Fueyo J, Alemany R, Gomez-Manzano C, et al. Preclinical characterization of the antiglioma activity of a tropism-enhanced adenovirus targeted to the retinoblastoma pathway. J Natl Cancer Inst 2003;95:652–660.
39. Shinoura N, Yoshida Y, Tsunoda R, et al. Highly augmented cytopathic effect of a fiber-mutant E1B-defective adenovirus for gene therapy of gliomas. Cancer Res 1999;59:3411–3416.
40. Gu DL, Gonzalez AM, Printz MA, et al. Fibroblast growth factor 2 retargeted adenovirus has redirected cellular tropism: evidence for reduced toxicity and enhanced antitumor activity in mice. Cancer Res 1999;59: 2608–2614.
41. Douglas JT, Rogers BE, Rosenfeld ME, et al. Targeted gene delivery by tropism-modified adenoviral vectors. Nat Biotechnol 1996;14:1574–1578.
42. Xia H, Anderson B, Mao Q, Davidson BL. Recombinant human adenovirus: targeting to the human transferrin receptor improves gene transfer to brain microcapillary endothelium. J Virol 2000:l74:11,359–11,366.

43. Fisher KD, Stallwood Y, Green NK, Ulbrich K, Mautner V, Seymour LW. Polymer-coated adenovirus permits efficient retargeting and evades neutralising antibodies. Gene Ther 2001;8:341–348.

44. Worgall S, Wolff G, Falck-Pedersen E, Crystal RG. Innate immune mechanisms dominate elimination of adenoviral vectors following in vivo administration. Hum Gene Ther 1997;8:37–44.

45. Da Costa XJ, Brockman MA, Alicot E, et al. Humoral response to herpes simplex virus is complement-dependent. Proc Natl Acad Sci USA 1999;96:12,708–12,712.

46. Wakimoto H, Johnson PR, Knipe DM, Chiocca EA. Effects of innate immunity on herpes simplex virus and its ability to kill tumor cells. Gene Ther 2003;10:983–990.

47. Ginsberg HS, Prince GA. The molecular basis of adenovirus pathogenesis. Infect Agents Dis 1994;3:1–8.

48. Guidotti LG, Chisari FV. Noncytolytic control of viral infections by the innate and adaptive immune response. Annu Rev Immunol 2001;19:65–91.

49. Horwitz MS, Sarvetnick N. Viruses, host responses, and autoimmunity. Immunol Rev 1999;169:241–253.

50. Kay MA, Holterman AX, Meuse L, et al. Long-term hepatic adenovirus-mediated gene expression in mice following CTLA4Ig administration. Nat Genet 1995;11:191–197.

51. Yang Y, Trinchieri G, Wilson J.M. Recombinant IL-12 prevents formation of blocking IgA antibodies to recombinant adenovirus and allows repeated gene therapy to mouse lung. Nat Med 1995;1:890–893.

52. Bouvet M, Fang B, Ekmekcioglu S, et al. Suppression of the immune response to an adenovirus vector and enhancement of intratumoral transgene expression by low-dose etoposide. Gene Ther 1998;5:189–195.

53. Mabon PJ, Weaver LC, Dekaban,GA. Cyclosporin A reduces the inflammatory response to a multi-mutant herpes simplex virus type-1 leading to improved transgene expression in sympathetic preganglionic neurons in hamsters. J Neurovirol 1999;5:268–279.

54. Ikeda,K, Wakimoto H, Ichikawa T, et al. Complement depletion facilitates the infection of multiple brain tumors by an intravascular, replication-conditional herpes simplex virus mutant. J Virol 2000;74:4765–4775.

55. Ikeda K, Ichikawa T, Wakimoto H, et al. Oncolytic virus therapy of multiple tumors in the brain requires suppression of innate and elicited antiviral responses. Nat Med 1999;5:881–887.

56. Wakimoto H, Fulci G, Tyminski E, Chiocca EA. Altered expression of antiviral cytokine mRNAs associated with cyclophosphamide's enhancement of viral oncolysis. Gene Ther 2004;11:214–223.

57. Nanda D, Vogels R, Havenga M, Avezaat CJ, Bout A, Smitt PS. Treatment of malignant gliomas with a replicating adenoviral vector expressing herpes simplex virus-thymidine kinase. Cancer Res 2001;61:8743–8750.

58. Grill J, Lamfers ML, van Beusechem VW, et al. The organotypic multicellular spheroid is a relevant three-dimensional model to study adenovirus replication and penetration in human tumors in vitro. Mol Ther 2002;6:609–614.

59. Ichikawa T, Chiocca EA. Comparative analyses of transgene delivery and expression in tumors inoculated with a replication-conditional or -defective viral vector. Cancer Res 2001;61:5336–5339.

60. Boviatsis EJ, Scharf JM, Chase M, et al. Antitumor activity and reporter gene transfer into rat brain neoplasms inoculated with herpes simplex virus vectors defective in thymidine kinase or ribonucleotide reductase. Gene Ther 1994;1:323–331.

61. Boviatsis EJ, Chase M, Wei MX, et al. Gene transfer into experimental brain tumors mediated by adenovirus, herpes simplex virus, and retrovirus vectors. Hum Gene Ther 1994;5:183–191.

62. Chas, M, Chung RY, Chiocca EA. An oncolytic viral mutant that delivers the CYP2B1 transgene and augments cyclophosphamide chemotherapy. Nat Biotechnol 1998;16:444–448.

63. Wei MX, Tamiya T, Rhee RJ, Breakefield XO, Chiocca EA. Diffusible cytotoxic metabolites contribute to the in vitro bystander effect associated with the cyclophosphamide/cytochrome P450 2B1 cancer gene therapy paradigm. Clin Cancer Res 1995;1:1171–1177.

64. Stubdal H, Perin N, Lemmon M, et al.A prodrug strategy using ONYX-015-based replicating adenoviruses to deliver rabbit carboxylesterase to tumor cells for conversion of CPT-11 to SN-38. Cancer Res 2003;63:6900–6908.

65. Freytag SO, Rogulski KR, Paielli DL, Gilbert JD, Kim JH. A novel three-pronged approach to kill cancer cells selectively: concomitant viral, double suicide gene, and radiotherapy. Hum Gene Ther 1998;9:1323–1333.

66. Aghi M, Chou TC, Suling K, Breakefield XO, Chiocca EA. Multimodal cancer treatment mediated by a replicating oncolytic virus that delivers the oxazaphosphorine/rat cytochrome P450 2B1 and ganciclovir/herpes simplex virus thymidine kinase gene therapies. Cancer Res 1999;59:3861–3865.

67. Andreansky S, He B, van Cott J, et al. Treatment of intracranial gliomas in immunocompetent mice using herpes simplex viruses that express murine interleukins. Gene Ther 1998'5:121–130.

68. Parker JN, Gillespie GY, Love,CE, Randall S, Whitley RJ, Markert JM. Engineered herpes simplex virus expressing IL-12 in the treatment of experimental murine brain tumors. Proc Natl Acad Sci USA 2000;97:2208–2213.

69. Carew JF, Kooby DA, Halterman MW, Kim SH, Federoff HJ, Fong Y. A novel approach to cancer therapy using an oncolytic herpes virus to package amplicons containing cytokine genes. Mol Ther 2001;4:250–256.

70. Wong RJ, Patel SG, Kim S, et al. Cytokine gene transfer enhances herpes oncolytic therapy in murine squamous cell carcinoma. Hum Gene Ther 2001;12:253–265.

71. Todo T, Martuza RL, Dallman MJ, Rabkin SD. In situ expression of soluble B7-1 in the context of oncolytic herpes simplex virus induces potent antitumor immunity. Cancer Res 2001;61:153–161.

72. Liu BL, Robinson M, Han ZQ, et al. ICP34.5 deleted herpes simplex virus with enhanced oncolytic, immune stimulating, and anti-tumour properties. Gene Ther 2003;10:292–303.

73. Kruyt FA, Curiel DT. Toward a new generation of conditionally replicating adenoviruses: pairing tumor selectivity with maximal oncolysis. Hum Gene Ther 2002;13:485–495.

74. van Beusechem VW, van den Doel PB, Grill J, Pinedo HM, Gerritsen WR. Conditionally replicative adenovirus expressing p53 exhibits enhanced oncolytic potency. Cancer Res 2002;62:6165–6171.

75. Mi J, Li ZY, Ni S, Steinwaerder D, Lieber A. Induced apoptosis supports spread of adenovirus vectors in tumors. Hum Gene Ther 2001;12:1343–1352.

76. Yu DC, Chen Y, Dilley J, et al. Antitumor synergy of CV787, a prostate cancer-specific adenovirus, and paclitaxel and docetaxel. Cancer Res 2001;61:517–525.

77. Toyoizumi T, Mick R, Abbas AE, Kang EH, Kaiser LR, Molnar-Kimber KL. Combined therapy with chemotherapeutic agents and herpes simplex virus type 1 ICP34.5 mutant (HSV-1716) in human non-small cell lung cancer. Hum Gene Ther 1999;10:3013–3029.

78. Cinatl J, Jr, Cinatl J, Michaelis M, et al. Patient oncolytic activity of multimutated herpes simplex virus G207 in combimation with vincristine against human rhabdomyosarcoma. Cancer Res 2003;63:1508–1514.

79. Rogulski KR, Freytag SO, Zhang K, et al. In vivo antitumor activity of ONYX-015 is influenced by p53 status and is augmented by radiotherapy. Cancer Res 2000;60:1193–1196.

80. DeWeese TL, van der Poel H, Li S, et al. A phase I trial of CV706, a replication-competent, PSA selective oncolytic adenovirus, for the treatment of locally recurrent prostate cancer following radiation therapy. Cancer Res 2001;61:7464–7472.

81. Chen Y, DeWeese T, Dilley J, et al. CV706, a prostate cancer-specific adenovirus variant, in combination with radiotherapy produces synergistic antitumor efficacy without increasing toxicity. Cancer Res 2001;61:5453–5460.

82. Geoerger B, Grill J, Opolon P, et al. Potentiation of radiation therapy by the oncolytic adenovirus dl1520 (ONYX-015) in human malignant glioma xenografts. Br J Cancer 2003;89:577–584.

83. Blank SV, Rubin SC, Coukos G, Amin KM, Albelda SM, Molnar-Kimber KL. Replication-selective herpes simplex virus type 1 mutant therapy of cervical cancer is enhanced by low-dose radiation. Hum Gene Ther 2002;13:627–639.

84. Stanziale SF, Petrowsky H, Joe JK, et al. Ionizing radiation potentiates the antitumor efficacy of oncolytic herpes simplex virus G207 by upregulating ribonucleotide reductase. Surgery 2002;132:353–359.

85. Jorgensen TJ, Katz S, Wittmack EK, et al. Ionizing radiation does not alter the antitumor activity of herpes simplex virus vector G207 in subcutaneous tumor models of human and murine prostate cancer. Neoplasia 2001;3:451–456.

86. Spear MA, Sun F, Eling DJ, et al. Cytotoxicity, apoptosis, and viral replication in tumor cells treated with oncolytic ribonucleotide reductase-defective herpes simplex type 1 virus (hrR3) combined with ionizing radiation. Cancer Gene Ther 2000;7:1051–1059.

87. Advani SJ, Sibley GS, Song PY, et al. Enhancement of replication of genetically engineered herpes simplex viruses by ionizing radiation: a new paradigm for destruction of therapeutically intractable tumors. Gene Ther 1998;5:160–165.

88. Bradley JD, Kataoka Y, Advani S, et al. Ionizing radiation improves survival in mice bearing intracranial high-grade gliomas injected with genetically modified herpes simplex virus. Clin Cancer Res 1999;5:1517–1522.

89. Rogulski KR, Wing MS, Paielli DL, Gilbert JD, Kim JH, Freytag SO. Double suicide gene therapy augments the antitumor activity of a replication-competent lytic adenovirus through enhanced cytotoxicity and radiosensitization. Hum Gene Ther 2000;11:67–76.

24 Biological Modifiers

Alexander Mason, Steven Toms, and Aleck Hercbergs

Summary

Conventional multimodailty therapies have not altered the dismal prognosis of glioblastoma which has prompted alternative investigational approaches utilising biological modifiers of response.We review here interferon alpha (IFN-α) and beta (IFN-β), interleukin-2 (IL-2), tumor necrosis factor-α TNF, interleukin 4 (IL-4) , monoclonal antibodies to EGFR, EGFRvIII and radio-labeled anti-tenascin monoclonal antibody. A current novel approach is exploitation of some of the biological consequences of thyroid hormone deprivation on tumor biology. In a preliminary Phase I/II trial significant improvement in survival and tumor regression rates in recurrent high grade glioma patients were observed following propylthiouracil induced mild (chemical) hypothyroidism combined with high dose tamoxifen.The background to this approach is reviewed.

Key Words: glioblastoma; biological modifiers; hypothyroidism; tamoxifen

INTRODUCTION

Despite advances in surgical resection, computer assisted radiation therapy, and novel chemotherapeutic agents, survival for malignant glioma remains poor. The 2-yr survival of glioblastoma multiforme (GBM), the most malignant form of glioma, remains less than 20%.

In light of poor outcomes with more traditional therapies, a number of alternatives have been explored. Immunotherapy has had some success against tumors such as melanoma and renal cell carcinoma. Cell-based immunotherapy and vaccine trials will be the subject of other chapters. In this chapter we will focus on the role of biological response modifiers in the treatment of malignant glioma

Biological response modifiers may be defined as any naturally occurring substance, such as cytokine or hormone, that may be used to influence tumor growth. These substances may directly induce cell death, alter growth rates, or augment the body's own immune response.

Malignant gliomas are the most common primary brain tumor in adults and the current prognosis for patients with glioma remains poor. Despite mainstay treatment options including surgery, radiation, and chemotherapy, the estimated 2-yr survival remains less than 20% (1). One strategy in the spectrum of treatment options involves activation of the host immunologic response to destroy malignant glioma cells. Cytokines have been extensively studied as a vehicle of in vitro and in vivo immunologic activation and will be the focus of this chapter.

TUMOR NECROSIS FACTOR FAMILY

The cytokine tumor necrosis factor-α (TNF- α) was discovered by Carswell et al. in 1975 and has been shown to have cytotoxic effects in vitro and in vivo on tumor cells (2). TNF- α

From: *Current Clinical Oncology: High-Grade Gliomas: Diagnosis and Treatment*
Edited by: G. H. Barnett © Humana Press Inc., Totowa, NJ

is produced by macrophages, monocytes and has also been shown to be produced by activated microglial and glioma cells *(3)*. It has been shown to inhibit lipoprotein lipase *(4)*, simulate granulocytes and the proliferation of fibroblasts, and has antiviral activity and endothelial cytotoxicity that varies by cell type *(5)*. Tumor response to TNF-α is quite variable in that it inhibits growth and causes apoptosis in several tumor cell lines, but can stimulate growth in others *(3,6–8)*. Additionally, this cytokine enhances major histocompatability complex (MHC) expression in glioma lines *(9)* and induces the production of intercellular adhesion molecule-1 in glioblastoma cell lines *(10)*.

In recent years, the TNF family of cytokines - α has been extensively studied in association with apoptosis in human malignant glioma cell. TNF-related apoptosis-inducing ligand (TRAIL) is a member of the TNF family that rapidly triggers apoptosis in various types of tumors *(11)*. TRAIL preferentially triggers apoptosis in glioma cell lines vs normal stromal/ endothelial cells *(12)*. TRAIL is characterized by activation of capase-8 caspase –3, DNA fragmentation and apoptosis in >50% of glioma cell lines *(13)*. Its selective induction of apoptosis in glioma but not in primary cultures of normal astrocytes suggests the possibility of tumor suppression in vivo. Unfortunately, TNF-α induces apoptosis in human hepatocyte cultures, implying that it may be a poor choice for systemic use. Local, intratumoral administration with convection-enhanced delivery *(12,14)* or with genetically modified stem cell delivery of TNF-α may play a role in the future.

Another member of the TNF-α family that exerts strong antiglial activity is the CD95 ligand. Certain human glioma cell lines express CD95, also known as Fas/APO-1, and using an endogenous pathway, undergo apoptosis when exposed to antibodies to this ligand *(15)*. The cytotoxicity of this endogenous pathway was shown to significantly increase when exposed to exogenous cytokines such as TNF-α, IFN-β, Il-1, and Il-8 *(15)*. Like TNF-α there is concern that CD95 ligand immunotherapy given systemically may lead to liver failure *(16)*. It has been proposed in the recent literature that Taxol works synergistically with CD95 to sensitize glioma cells to the CD95 ligand, and may reduce systemic toxic effects *(17)*.

Recombinant human TNF-α has been used systemically with mixed responses *(18,19)*. Yoshida administered the cytokine intra-arterially in 20 cases of malignant gliomas with a reported 20% response rate and minimal side effects *(5)*. Recent detailed examination of ultra-structural sequelae of intra-arterial TNF-α administrated in an experimental rat model demonstrated necrotizing effects on tumor vascular endothelium, thus suggesting another mechanism of the anti-tumoral effect of TNF-α *(20)*.

Interleukin-1 [IL-1], a key pro-inflammatory cytokine which initiates the production of a variety of other cytokines, has been found to increase the immune response to glioma *(21)*. Convection-enhanced delivery (CED) has been investigated as a means to overcome the problem of weak tumor response to systemically administered IL-1. The effect of intratumoral delivery of interleukin (IL)-1 and interferon (IFN)- (IFN-α) by CED on tumor immune cell invasion in a rat glioma model demonstrated that intratumoral cytokine infusion using CED leads to strong tumor invasion with macrophages and lymphocytes suggesting a tumor specific immune response. Survival ongoing studies are yet to be reported.

INTERLEUKIN-2

Interleukin-2 (IL-2), originally called T-cell growth factor, is a potent, well-studied 15.5 kDa cytokine that is important in the generation of anti-tumor immunity. When T-helper cells are exposed to tumor antigens, they release small quantities of IL-2. This acts locally to activate cytotoxic T-cells and natural killer (NK) cells that mediate systemic tumor cell destruction *(22)*. It has been shown that intravenous, intralymphatic, or intralesional administration of IL-2 has produced responses in several types of cancer such as renal cell carcinoma and melanoma, but that systemic routes of therapy can cause severe side effects such as hypotension, bradycardia, and extreme fatigue *(22)*. Additionally, long-term central administration of IL-2 in rat model has neurotoxic consequences associated with elevated IL-2 central nervous system (CNS) levels *(23)*. Nonetheless, IL-2 therapy by systemic, local, or genetic means has been an intriguing target of study because of its potent effect on the immune system and encouraging impact on gliomas in preclinical testing.

The immunoregulatory effects of IL-2 are complex and varied. IL-2 is a growth factor that stimulates the proliferation of cytotoxic T-cells, helper T-cells, NK cells, and LAK cells, all of which can participate in the host's response to tumor cells *(24,25)*. Although there is a decreased immune response in vivo to glioma cells because of poor antigen presentation and the release of suppressor factors *(26)*, effector cells such as cytotoxic T-cells or NK cells have been shown to be activated by IL-2, causing a more effective lytic process in certain glial-tumor lines *(27–29)*. Clinically, methods of combining tumor antigens and genetically modified cytokine-producing tumor cells (i.e., tumor vaccine) have had mixed successes *(30,31)*. Autologous dendritic cell (DC) vaccines have attracted attention for the treatment of gliomas with or without IL-2 or other cytokine activation *(32,33)*. DC vaccines have attracted attention for the treatment of gliomas, as survival time was elongated in patients with malignant gliomas and other brain tumors *(33,34)*. These will be covered in more detail in the chapter on cellular immunotherapy.

Because of the relative immunologic isolation of glial tumors within the CNS, blunted immune response and the systemic toxicity of IL-2, experiments using local and regional delivery of IL-2 by means of direct injection, polymer-based IL-2, or gene transfer has been examined. In small clinical studies using direct tumor bed injection of activated NK cells and IL-2, no significant effect on prognosis was seen *(35)*. A variety of genetically modified viruses have been examined as vectors for secreting IL-2 locally. In one approach, replication-deficient herpes simplex virus (HSV) with a mutated thymidine kinase produced tumor cell death locally *(36)*. In another study, IL-2 was secreted in low levels from cells with their tumorgenicity removed ("package cells"), and such cytokine release induced a long-lasting protective immune response against challenge with a tumorigenic dose of tumor cells *(38)*. Although there have been mixed results, the injection of cytokine secreting allogenic tumor cells into a tumor bed is hypothesized to induce an anti-tumor immune response capable of prolonging survival *(22,39)*. Although preclinical studies with IL-2 gene therapy have been promising *(21)*, there have been limited clinical trials *(22,39)*.

INTERLEUKIN-4

The cytokine interleukin 4 (IL-4) was first described in 1982 as a B-cell stimulator with activating and growth factor potential *(41)*. It also has been associated with T-cell activation, and can be inactivated by IFN-γ. In addition, recent studies have demonstrated that IL-4 modulates the proliferation and expression of cell surface antigens on several types of neoplastic cells, an effect that can be enhanced with other cytokines, including IFN-γ and TNF-α *(42,43)*. Iwasaki and colleagues initially studied the effects of IL-4 on cloned human glioblastoma in combination with IFN-β and TNF-α and confirmed the synergistic effects of these two cytokines. It has been postulated that enhancement of antigen presentation is responsible for the synergy *(41)*.

Gene transfer of IL-4 into tumor cell lines has been achieved with both adenovirus and HSV. In both cell culture and mouse xenograft tumor models, there was decreased tumor growth. Animal model effects of IL-4 include eosiniphilic infiltrate, tumor necrosis and improved survival vs control *(44,45)*. Glioma cell lines are characterized by the overexpression of a high-affinity receptor of IL-4 (IL-4R) *(46)*. The IL-4R was targeted with a chimeric molecule composed of an IL-4 molecule and a mutant *Pseudomonas* exotoxin that is cytotoxic towards human glioblastoma tumor cells in a dose-dependent manner *(46)*. Clinical efforts using this xotoxin have been conducted using stereotactically placed microcathethers in nine patients without systemic toxicity and demonstrating a preliminary antitumor response *(47–49)*.

INTERLEUKIN-12

IL-12 is a heterodimeric protein consisting of two subunits (p35 and p40) and is secreted by antigen presenting cells (APCs) such as DC and macrophages. IL-12 is an important immunoregulatory cytokine, which enhances the function of cytotoxic immune cells, including CTL and NK cells, and possesses potent IFN–γdependent therapeutic activity. Recombinant IL-12 treatment has shown a dramatic antitumor effect on mouse tumor models *(50)*. Immunohistochemistry demonstrated increased CD4+ and CD8+ T-cell infiltration of the tumor compared with controls. Animals treated with IL-12 had prolonged survival vs controls *(50)*. A phase I/II clinical study in adult patients with recurrent GBM is planned and aimed at evaluating safety and antitumor efficacy of a genetically modified replication-disabled Semliki forest virus vector (SFV) carrying the human IL-12 gene and encapsulated in cationic liposomes *(51)*.

INTERLEUKIN-13

IL-13 is predominantly produced by activated T cells and mast cells, and is intimately involved in immune modulation and differentiation *(47)*. Both IL-13 and IL-4 share a number of biological functions and are mediated by cell surface receptors *(46)*. It has been shown that human malignant glioma cell lines express a large number of intermediate-affinity IL-13 receptors (IL-13R), as compared with human immune cells (B and T cells) that have low or no levels of IL-13R *(47,52)*. To utilize this relative over-expression of IL-13R, a protein cytotoxin produced by *Pseudomonas aeruginosa* bacteria was bound to human IL-13 *(47,53)*. This complex is then translocated into cellular cytosol, eventually leading to cellular death *(48,49)*. Phase III clinical trials are currently underway with infusion via intratumoral microinfusion *(47)*.

INTERFERON

Interferons (IFN) have been used to treat malignant gliomas since the early 1980s with varying degrees of success. Interferon-α (IFN-α) and beta (IFN-β) have been the main focus of clinical trials, but promising results have also been shown with IFN-γ and IFN-α.

INTERFERON-α

Recombinant interferon-α (IFN-α) exhibits antiviral, immunomodulatory, antineoplastic, and antiangiogenesis properties. Preclinical studies suggested synergy between BCNU and

IFN-α *(7)*. The combination of BCNU and IFN-α produced responses in 29% of 35 patients with recurrent glioma *(54)*. IFN-α does not, however improve time to disease progression or overall survival in patients with high-grade glioma (HGG) and appears to add significantly to treatment toxicity.

INTERFERON-β

IΦN–β has been used as an anti-tumor drug against human glioma, melanoma, and medullo-blastoma since the 1980s. Because stimulation of the immune system is one mechanism of anti-tumor effect induced by IFN-β gene therapy, Saito et al. hypothesized of the effectiveness of immunotherapy IFN-β gene therapy with immunotherapy might increase its effectiveness *(55)*. They tested a combination therapy of IFN-βgene therapy and immunotherapy using tumor cell lysate-pulsed DCs in an experimental mouse intracranial glioma (GL261) (which cannot be cured by either IFN-β gene therapy or DC immunotherapy alone.) In this investigation, IFN-β gene therapy following DC immunotherapy resulted in a significant prolongation in survival of the mice *(50,53,56–58)*.

INTERFERON-γ

IFN-γis a multimodal cytokine with a number of different antiproliferative effects on cell lines, but is of crucial importance for the interaction of T cells with APCs such as macrophages and NK cells. One rationale for use of IFN-γ in glioma patients evokes the impaired cell-based immunity seen in glioma patients *(53)*. T-cell function is enhanced by IFN-γby up-regulation of antigen presentation and activation of NKcells. Increased MHC class I expression leads to higher cytotoxicity of certain glioma cell lines in vitro *(59)*. This IFN-γ mechanism may antagonize the TGF-β mediated down-regulation of MHC expression in certain cell lines *(43,60)*.

IFN-γ can inhibit growth of glioma cell lines in vitro by increasing levels of p21, a cyclin-dependent kinase inhibitor, which acts by inhibiting G_1/S phase transition *(61)*. Interferon-γ has also been shown to activate cytotoxic lymphocytes in the presence of IL-2, as well as increase the antigen presentation of glioma cells to the immune system *(22,59,60)*. Many models for protein or antibody mediated therapy have focused on the CD95 ligand (fas/APO-1), a proapoptotic receptor *(63)*. It has been theorized that resistance to Fas-mediated apoptosis is one manner in which malignant gliomas evade the immune system. IFN-γ has been shown to increase Fas-mediated apoptosis in human glioma lines *(64)*. There are several clinical studies of IFN-γ on patients with malignant glioma. Although patients have tolerated local and systemic IFN-γ without the toxicity of some other immunomodulators, clinical responses have not been dramatic *(53,65,66)*.

THYROID HORMONE

Thyroid hormones play important roles in normal brain maturation and normal brain function *(67)*. It has been demonstrated that thyroid hormones are required for malignant transformation of cultured cells by ionizing irradiation or chemical induction *(68,69)*. It has also been suggested that thyroid hormones may have a pathophysiological role in the development of brain tumors. Thyroid hormone receptors have been identified in brain tumors *(70)*, and thyroid hormones may be involved in the proliferation of brain tumor cells *(71)*.

Several convergent lines of evidence suggest that thyroid hormones are involved in tumorigenesis and tumor growth. Tri-iodothyronine (T3), the most biologically active of the thyroid hormones, has marked effects on the cell cycle, stimulating mitosis *(72,73)* and proliferation of both normal *(74)* and neoplastic cells *(71–73)*. These effects are caused, in part, by modulation of the autocrine, paracrine, and endocrine growth factor signaling systems such as insulin-like growth factor 1 [IGF-1] *(76,77)*, epidermal growth factor receptor [EGF-r] *(78–80)*, and cyclins *(73)*. In glioma cell lines, depletion of thyroid hormone has been shown to reduce cell proliferation and to induce cell–cycle arrest via p21 (WAF1/Cip1) *(71)*. Thyroid hormone depletion studies in cell culture and preclinical studies of thyroid gland suppression in experimental animal and human xenograft solid tumor systems have demonstrated that thyroid-ablated mice have decreased tumor proliferation/ growth rates and prolonged survival *(81–86)*. There are anecdotal reports of spontaneous remission of metastatic nonsmall cell lung cancer following myxedema coma *(87)*—a severe thyroid deficiency event—and, in contrast, accelerated progression of metastatic breast cancer has been observed shortly after initiating thyroid hormone supplementation in hypothyroid women *(88)*.

A body of data suggests that up regulation of the major growth factor systems/mechanisms such as IGF-1 and IGF- II and EGFR may in part mediate these pro-growth effects but there is also evidence for direct modulation of mitosis by tri-iodothyronine [T3] *(73,89)*. Thyroid hormones are also known to modulate microtubule assembly protein *(90)* and mitochondrial biogenesis *(91)*. In addition, they have been shown to up-regulate cathepsinD, which facilitates tumor invasion and metastasis *(92)*. Recent studies have demonstrated that L-thyroxine functions as a ligand for the cell membrane integrin α V β 3 and in a chorio-allantoic membrane model induces significant neoangiogenesis in endothelial and glioma cell lines *(93–95)*. Thyroid hormone promotes BCL-2 expression whereas hypothyroidism alters the expression of bcl-2 family genes to induce enhanced apoptosis in the developing cerebellum *(96,97)*.

Epidemiologic and clinical studies suggest that survival is improved in hypothyroid individuals across a variety of tumor types including breast, lung, and renal cancer *(98–105)*. In epidemiological studies, radio-iodine ablation of the thyroid for benign disease and hypothyroidism are associated with a significantly reduced incidence of cancer and lower mortality rate *(106)*. In clinical studies of patients with advanced solid tumor survival and treatment responses to a variety of modalities including cytokines (IL-2) correlated with a diagnosis of hypothyroidism *(96–106)*.

Until very recently endocrine therapy in the form of thyroid manipulation had not formally been studied as an anticancer modality. In a phase I/II clinical study *(107,108)* of patients with recurrent GBM an attempt was made to reduce thyroid hormone levels with propylthiouracil (PTU). In this study 38 patients with recurrent HGG were given high doses of tamoxifen and PTU in an effort to induce chemical hypothyroidism.

Of 36 evaluable patients, in the 19 that achieved chemical hypothyroidism, 5 (28%) had more than a 50% reduction in tumor size on magnetic resonance imaging (MRI), compared with 0 of 17 (0%) that remained euthyroid ($p < 0.037$). One patient had a partial response to PTU alone. Only one patient experienced clinically symptomatic hypothyroidism. Median survival for the hypothyroid group was 10.6 mo vs 3.1 mo for the group that remained euthyroid ($p < 0.002$). This study concluded that PTU-induced chemical hypothyroidism was associated with significantly improved survival in malignant glioma patients treated with tamoxifen. Failure to successfully induce and maintain chemical hypothyroidism was associated with significantly shorter survival.

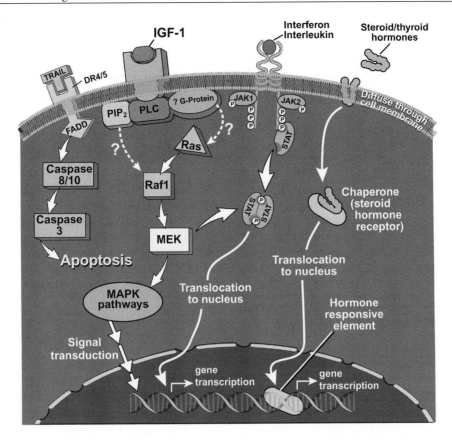

Fig. 1. Biological response modifiers alter cellular transcription and signaling in a variety of ways. This schematic highlights mitogen activated protein kinase (MAPK) and signal transduction and activator of transcription (STAT) pathways of signal-transduction inducing gene expression via interferons, interleukins, and autocrine growth factors such as IGF-1. Steroids and thyroid hormones are bound by chaperones (hormonal receptors) after they diffuse through the outer cell membrane. The chaperones transport the hormones to the nucleus where they induce gene transcription. A final method of biological response modification is illustrated in the schematic by TNF apoptosis-inducing ligand (TRAIL). TRAIL binds a cell surface death receptor (DR 4/5), directly inducing caspase activation and cellular death via apoptosis.

STEROIDS

Glucocorticoids are known anti-inflammatory agents that are frequently used in the management of glial tumors. Although results in the literature are contradictory, a number of researchers have examined the impact of glucocorticoids, or its commonly used synthetic form, dexamethasone, on tumor growth and proliferation. Dexamethasone has been used for several decades for the treatment of symptomatic vasogenic edema with most types of intracranial masses. Although the exact mechanism has not been elucidated, there is evidence that in one glial cell line, dexamethasone may have a therapeutic effect related to the inhibition of tumor-associated angiogenesis *(109,110)*. This effect occurs by several mechanisms, however it has been shown in vitro that dexamethasone decreases tumor-associated angiogenesis by decreasing vascular endothelial growth factor (VEGF) expression in several glial cell lines in vivo *(111,112)*.

The immunosuppressive function of dexamethasone in glial tumors is another area of interest. Steroids have been shown to significantly inhibit infiltration of both lymphocytes and microglia in a dose dependent manner in gliomas *(113)*. The clinical relevance of lymphocytes in the anti-tumor response is uncertain. However, as cellular immunotherapy approaches are developed any immunosuppressive factor may have deleterious effects on these treatment modalities *(113,114)*.

Glucocorticoids diffuse through the cellular membrane and are bound by intracytoplasmic steroid transporters. These receptors transport the steroid through the nuclear membrane, where they bind DNA and act at a transcriptional level *(115)*. It has been shown that gene expression may be inhibited by glucocorticoid receptors antagonists, and lead to decreased proliferation of some glial cell lines *(115,116)*. Dexamethasone may also inhibit a variety of genes involved in the inflammation process, including those activated by nuclear factor-κb *(117)*. The steroid receptor may act with NF-κB binding sites in the regulatory regions of an anti-apoptotic gene.This mechanism appears to synergistically enhance the ability of TNF-α to prevent apoptosis in some cell lines *(118)*. Other mechanisms have been elucidated, including the upregulation of anti-apoptotic proteins and the associated cellular-signaling cascade and the inhibition of apoptosis, with the clinical significance of potentially interfering with the efficacy of chemotherapeutic drugs *(119)*.

Although glucocorticoids are used widely in the clinical setting and their utility has been widely accepted, their effect in vivo on antitumor activity remains an area of interest. It has been shown that dexamethasone significantly enhances the antitumor activity of carboplatin and gemcitabine in mice models *(120)*. Frequently employed for their potent anti-inflammatory response, glucocorticoids have potential direct and synergistic antitumor activity.

CONCLUSIONS

Biological response modifiers are a group of naturally occurring substances that may be used to influence tumor response to therapy. These substances may have powerful roles working synergistically with immuno, radio-and chemotherapies in the treatment of malignant gliomas.

REFERENCES

1. Mahaley MS Jr, Mettlin C, Natarajan N, Laws ER Jr, Peace BB. National survey of patterns of care for in-tumor patients. J Neurosurg 1989;71(6):826–836.
2. Carswell EA, Old LJ, Kassel RL, Green S, Fiore N, Williamson B. An endotoxin-induced serum factor that causes necrosis of tumors. Proc Natl Acad Sci USA 1975;72(9):3666–3670.
3. Chen TC, Hinton DR, Apuzzo ML, Hofman FM. Differential effects of tumor necrosis factor-alpha on proliferation, cell surface antigen expression, and cytokine interactions in malignant gliomas. Neurosurgery 1993;32(1):85–94.
4. Beutler B, Cerami A. Cachectin: more than a tumor necrosis factor. N Engl J Med 1987;316(7):379–385.
5. Yoshida J, Wakabayashi T, Mizuno M, et al. Clinical effect of intra-arterial tumor necrosis factor-alpha for malignant glioma. J Neurosurg 1992;77(1):78–83.
6. Bethea JR, Gillespie GY, Chung IY, Benveniste EN. Tumor necrosis factor production and receptor expression by a human malignant glioma cell line, D54-MG. J Neuroimmunol 1990;30(1):1–13.
7. Rutka JT, Giblin JR, Berens ME, et al. The effects of human recombinant tumor necrosis factor on glioma-derived cell lines: cellular proliferation, cytotoxicity, morphological and radioreceptor studies. Int J Cancer 1988;41(4):573–582.
8. Toms SA, Hercbergs A, Liu J, et al. Antagonist effect of insulin-like growth factor I on protein kinase inhibitor-mediated apoptosis in human glioblastoma cells in association with bcl-2 and bcl-xL. J Neurosurg 1998;88(5):884–889.

9. Benveniste EN, Sparacio SM, Bethea JR.Related Articles, Links Tumor necrosis factor-alpha enhances interferon-gamma-mediated class II antigen expression on astrocytes. J Neuroimmunol 1989;25(2–3):209–219.

10. Kuppner MC, van Meir E, Hamou MF, de Tribolet N. Cytokine regulation of intercellular adhesion molecule-1 (ICAM-1) expression on human glioblastoma cells. Clin Exp Immunol 1990;81(1):142–148.

11. Wiley SR, Schooley K, Smolak PJ, et al. Identification and characterization of a new member of the TNF family that induces apoptosis. Immunity 1995;3(6):673–682.

12. Hao C, Beguinot F, Condorelli G, et al. Induction and intracellular regulation of tumor necrosis factor-related apoptosis-inducing ligand (TRAIL) mediated apotosis in human malignant glioma cells. Cancer Res 2001; 61(3):1162–1170.

13. Krishnamoorthy B, Darnay B, Aggarwal B, et al. Glioma cells deficient in urokinase plaminogen activator receptor expression are susceptible to tumor necrosis factor-alpha-related apoptosis-inducing ligand-induced apoptosis. Clin Cancer Res 2001;7(12):4195–201.

14. Jo M, Kim TH, Seol DW, et al. Apoptosis induced in normal human hepatocytes by tumor necrosis factor-related apoptosis-inducing ligand. Nat Med 2000;6(5):564–567.

15. Weller M, Frei K, Groscurth P, Krammer PH, Yonekawa Y, Fontana A.Anti-Fas/APO-1 antibody-mediated apoptosis of cultured human glioma cells. Induction and modulation of sensitivity by cytokines. J Clin Invest 1994;94(3):954–964.

16. Ogasawara J, Watanabe-Fukunaga R, Adachi M, et al. Lethal effect of the anti-Fas antibody in mice. Nature 1993 Aug 26;364(6440):806-9. Erratum in: Nature 1993;365(6446):568.

17. Roth W, Wagenknecht B, Grimmel C, Dichgans J, Weller M. Taxol-mediated augmentation of CD95 ligand-induced apoptosis of human malignant glioma cells: association with bcl-2 phosphorylation but neither activation of p53 nor G2/M cell cycle arrest. Br J Cancer 1998;77(3):404–411.

18. Creagan ET, Kovach JS, Moertel CG, Frytak S, Kvols LK. A phase I clinical trial of recombinant human tumor necrosis factor. Cancer 1988;62(12):2467–471.

19. Old LJ. Tumor necrosis factor (TNF). Science 1985;230(4726):630–632.

20. Isaka T, Maruno M, Muhammad AK, Kato A, Nakagawa H, Yoshimine T. Ultrastructural changes of the vascular endothelium after intra-arterial administration of tumor necrosis factor-alpha (TNFalpha) in rat gliomas. J Neurooncol 2000;46(2):145–150.

21. Lichtor T, Glick RP, Tarlock K, Moffett S, Mouw E, Cohen EP. Application of interleukin-2-secreting syngeneic/allogeneic fibroblasts in the treatment of primary and metastatic brain tumors. Cancer Gene Ther 2002;9(5):464–469.

22. Lichtor T, Glick RP. Cytokine immuno-gene therapy for treatment of brain tumors. J Neurooncol 2003;65(3): 247–259.

23. Hanisch UK, Neuhaus J, Rowe W, et al. Neurotoxic consequences of central long-term administration of interleukin-2 in rats. Neuroscience 1997;79(3):799–818.

24. Chen TC, Hinton DR, Apuzzo ML, Hofman FM. Differential effects of tumor necrosis factor-alpha on proliferation, cell surface antigen expression, and cytokine interactions in malignant gliomas. Neurosurgery 1993;32(1):85–94.

25. Erard F, Corthesy P, Nabholz M, et a l. Interleukin 2 is both necessary and sufficient for the growth and differentiation of lectin-stimulated cytolytic T lymphocyte precursors. J Immunol 1985; 134(3):1644–1652.

26. Tjuvajev J, Gansbacher B, Desai R, et al. RG-2 glioma growth attenuation and severe brain edema caused by local production of interleukin-2 and interferon-gamma. Cancer Res 1995;55(9):1902–1910.

27. Yamasaki T, Kikuchi H, Yamashita J, et al. Immunoregulatory effects of interleukin 2 and interferon on syngeneic murine malignant glioma-specific cytotoxic T-lymphocytes. Cancer Res 1988;48(11):2981–2987.

28. Jean WC, Spellman SR, Wallenfriedman MA, et al. Effects of combined granulocyte-macrophage colony-stimulating factor (GM-CSF), interleukin-2, and interleukin-12 based immunotherapy against intracranial glioma in the rat. J Neurooncol 2004;661–2):39–49.

29. Hayes RL, Koslow M, Hiesiger EM, et al. Improved long term survival after intracavitary interleukin-2 and lymphokine-activated killer cells for adults with recurrent malignant glioma. Cancer 1995;76(5):840–852.

30. Iwadate Y, Yamaura A, Sato Y, Sakiyama S, Tagawa M.Induction of immunity in peripheral tissues combined with intracerebral transplantation of interleukin-2-producing cells eliminates established brain tumors. Cancer Res 2001;61(24):8769–8774.

31. Yu JS, Liu G, Ying H, Yong WH, Black KL, Wheeler CJ. Vaccination with tumor lysate-pulsed dendritic cells elicits antigen-specific, cytotoxic T-cells in patients with malignant glioma. Cancer Res 2004;64(14):4973–4979.

32. Liau LM, Black KL, Prins RM, et al. Treatment of intracranial gliomas with bone marrow-derived dendritic cells pulsed with tumor antigens. J Neurosurg 1999;90(6):1115–1124.

33. Ishikawa E, Tsuboi K, Takano S, Uchimura E, Nose T, Ohno T. Intratumoral injection of IL-2-activated NK cells enhances the antitumor effect of intradermally injected paraformaldehyde-fixed tumor vaccine in a rat intracranial brain tumor model. Cancer Sci 2004;95(1):98–103.

34. Geiger JD, Hutchinson RJ, Hohenkirk LF, et al. Vaccination of pediatric solid tumor patients with tumor lysate-pulsed dendritic cells can expand specific T cells and mediate tumor regression. Cancer Res 2001;61(23):8513–8519.

35. Boiardi A, Silvani A, Ruffini PA, et al. Loco-regional immunotherapy with recombinant interleukin-2 and adherent lymphokine-activated killer cells (A-LAK) in recurrent glioblastoma patients. Cancer Immunol Immunother 1994;39(3):193–197.

36. Martuza RL, Malick A, Markert JM, Ruffner KL, Coen DM. Experimental therapy of human glioma by means of a genetically engineered virus mutant. Science 1991;252(5007):854–856.

37. Kaplitt MG, Tjuvajec JG, Leib DA, et al. Mutant herpes simplex virus induced regression of tumors growing in immunocompetent rats. J Neurooncol 1994;19(2):137–147.

38. Gansbacher B, Zier K, Daniels B, Cronin K, Bannerji R, Gilboa E. Interleukin 2 gene transfer into tumor cells abrogates tumorigenicity and induces protective immunity. J Exp Med 1990;172(4):1217–1224.

39. Ram Z, Walbridge S, Heiss JD, Culver KW, Blaese RM, Oldfield EH. In vivo transfer of the human interleukin-2 gene: negative tumoricidal results in experimental brain tumors. J Neurosurg 1994;80(3):535–540.

40. Sobol RE, Fakhrai H, Shawler D, et al. Interleukin-2 gene therapy in a patient with glioblastoma. Gene Ther 1995;2(2):164–167.

41. Roth W, Weller M. Chemotherapy and immunotherapy of malignant glioma: molecular mechanisms and clinical perspectives. Cell Mol Life Sci 1999;56(5-6):481–506.

42. Iwasaki K, Rogers LR, Estes ML, Barna BP. Modulation of proliferation and antigen expression of a cloned human glioblastoma by interleukin-4 alone and in combination with tumor necrosis factor-alpha and/or interferon-gamma. Neurosurgery 1993;33(3):489–493; discussion 493–494.

43. Hoon DS, Banez M, Okun E, Morton DL, Irie RF. Modulation of human melanoma cells by interleukin-4 and in combination with gamma-interferon or alpha-tumor necrosis factor. Cancer Res 1991;51(8):2002–2008.

44. Weber FW, Floeth F, Asher A, et al. Local convection enhanced delivery of IL4-Pseudomonas exotoxin (NBI-3001) for treatment of patients with recurrent malignant glioma. Acta Neurochir Suppl 2003;88:93–103.

45. Yu JS, Wei MX, Chiocca EA, Martuza RL, Tepper RI. Treatment of glioma by engineered interleukin 4-secreting cells. Cancer Res 1993;53(13):3125–128.

46. Puri RK, Leland P, Kreitman RJ, Pastan I. Human neurological cancer cells express interleukin-4 (IL-4) receptors which are targets for the toxic effects of IL4-Pseudomonas exotoxin chimeric protein. Int J Cancer 1994;58(4):574–581.

47. Husain SR, Puri RK. Interleukin-13 receptor-directed cytotoxin for malignant glioma therapy: from bench to bedside. J Neurooncol 2003;65(1):37–48.

48. Souweidane MM, Occhiogrosso G, Mark EB, Edgar MA. Interstitial infusion of IL13-PE38QQR in the rat brain stem. J Neurooncol 2004;67(3):287–293.

49. Wikstrand CJ, Cokgor I, Sampson JH, Bigner DD. Monoclonal antibody therapy of human gliomas: current status and future approaches. Cancer Metastasis Rev 1999;18(4):451–464.

50. Mahaley MS Jr, Gillespie GY. New therapeutic approaches to treatment of malignant gliomas: chemotherapy and immunotherapy. Clin Neurosurg 1983;31:456–469.

51. Ren H, Boulikas T, Lundstrom K, Soling A, Warnke PC, Rainov NG. Immunogene therapy of recurrent glioblastoma multiforme with a liposomally encapsulated replication-incompetent Semliki forest virus vector carrying the human interleukin-12 gene–a phase I/II clinical protocol. J Neurooncol 2003;64(1–2):147–154; erratum J Neurooncol 2003;65(2):191.

52. Husain SR, Obiri NI, Gill P, et al. Receptor for interleukin 13 on AIDS-associated Kaposi's sarcoma cells serves as a new target for a potent Pseudomonas exotoxin-based chimeric toxin protein.Clin Cancer Res 1997;3(2):151–156.

53. Farkkila M, Jaaskelainen J, Kallio M, et al. Randomised, controlled study of intratumoral recombinant gamma-interferon treatment in newly diagnosed glioblastoma. Br J Cancer 1994;70(1):138–141.

54. Brandes AA, Scelzi E, Zampieri P, et al. Phase II trial with BCNU plus alpha-interferon in patients with recurrent high-grade gliomas. Am J Clin Oncol 1997;20(4):364–367.

55. Saito R, Mizino M, Nakahara N, et al. Vaccination with Tumor Cell Lysate –Pulsed Dendritic Cells Augments the Effect of IFN-beta Gene Therapy for Malignant Glioma in an Experimental Mouse Intracranial Glioma Int J Cancer 2004;111:L777–782.

56. Yung WK, Prados M, Levin VA, et al. Intravenous recombinant interferon beta in patients with recurrent malignant gliomas: a phase I/II study. J Clin Oncol 1991;9(11):1945–1949.

57. Shitara N, Nakamura H, Genka S, Takakura K. Efficacy of interferon-beta and interleukin-2 as cytokines for malignant brain tumor treatment Gan To Kagaku Ryoho 1987;14(12):3235–3244; abstract only.

58. Allen J, Packer R, Bleyer A, Zeltzer P, Prados M, Nirenberg A. Recombinant interferon beta: a phase I-II trial in children with recurrent brain tumors. J Clin Oncol 1991;9(5):783–788.

59. Schiltz PM, Gomez GG, Read SB, Kulprathipanja NV, Kruse CA. Effects of IFN-gamma and interleukin-1beta on major histocompatibility complex antigen and intercellular adhesion molecule-1 expression by 9L gliosarcoma: relevance to its cytolysis by alloreactive cytotoxic T lymphocytes. J Interferon Cytokine Res 2002;22(12):1209–1216.

60. Hong LL, Johannsen L, Krueger JM. Modulation of human leukocyte antigenDR expression in glioblastoma cells by interferon gamma and other cytokines. J Neuroimmunol 1991;35(1–3):139–152.

61. Kominsky S, Johnson HM, Bryan G, et al. IFN gamma inhibition of cell growth in glioblastomas correlates with increased levels of the cyclin dependent kinase inhibitor p21WAF1/CIP1. Oncogene 1998;17(23):2973–2979.

62. Wen PY, Lampson MA, Lampson LA. Effects of gamma-interferon on major histocompatibility complex antigen expression and lymphocytic infiltration in the 9L gliosarcoma brain tumor model: implications for strategies of immunotherapy. J Neuroimmunol 1992;36(1):57–68.

63. Roth W, Fontana A, Trepel M, Reed JC, Dichgans J, Weller M. Immunochemotherapy of malignant glioma: synergistic activity of CD95 ligand and chemotherapeutics. Cancer Immunol Immunother 1997;44(1):55–63.

64. Choi C, Jeong E, Benveniste EN. Caspase-1 mediates Fas-induced apoptosis and is up-regulated by interferon-gamma in human astrocytoma cells. J Neurooncol 2004;67(1–2):167–176.

65. Jan C, Buckner JC, Schomberg PJ, et al. A Phase III Study of Radiation Therapy plus Carmustine with or without Recombinant Interferon-a in the Treatment of Patients with Newly Diagnosed High-Grade Glioma. Cancer 2001;92:420–433.

66. Mahaley MS Jr, Bertsch L, Cush S, Gillespie GY. Systemic gamma-interferon therapy for recurrent gliomas. J Neurosurg 1988;69(6):826–829.

67. Bernal J, Guadano-Ferraz A, Morte B. Perspectives in the study of thyroid hormone action on brain development and function. Thyroid 2003;13(11):1005–1012

68. Guernsey DL, Ong A, Borek C. Thyroid hormone modulation of x-ray induced in vitro neoplastic transformation. Nature 1980;288:591–592.

69. Borek C, Guernsey DL, Ong A, et al. Critical role played by thyroid hormone in induction of neoplastic transformation by chemical carcinogenesis Critical role played by thyroid hormone in induction of neoplastic transformation by chemical carcinogens in tissue culture. Proc Natl Acad Sci USA 1983;80(18):5749–5752.

70. Magrassi L, Butti G, Silini E, Bono F, Paoletti P, Milanesi G. The expression of genes of the steroid-thyroid hormone receptor superfamily in central nervous system tumors. Anticancer Res 1993;13:859–866.

71. Toms SA, Hercbergs A, Liu J, et al. Thyroid hormone depletion inhibits astrocytoma proliferation via a p53-independent induction of p21 (WAF/1CIP1). Anticancer Res 1998;18:289–294.

72. DeFesi CR, Fels ED, Surks MI. L-Triiodothyronine (T3) stimulates growth of cultured GC cells by action early in the G1 period: Evidence for mediation by the nuclear T3 receptor. Endocrinol 1985;116:2062–2069.

73. Barrera-Hernandez G, Soo Park K.,Dace A.,Zhan Q., Cheng S. :Thyroid Hormone –induced cell proliferation in GC Cells is mediated by changes in G1 cyclin/cyclin-dependent kinase levels and activity. Endocrinology 1999;140(11):5267–5274.

74. Humes HD, Cieslinski DA, Johnson L, et al. Triiodothyronine enhances renal tubule cell replication by stimulating EGF receptor gene expression. Am J Physiol 1992;262:F540–F545.

75. Yoshida S, Maruo T, Matsuo H, Mochizuki M. Effects of estrogen and thyroid hormone on EGF receptor expression, proliferative activity and SCC production in the CaSki cervical carcinoma cells]. Nippon Sanka Fujinka Gakkai Zasshi 1995;47(2):149–155.

76. Matsuo K,Yamashita S, Niwa M,et al. Thyroid hormone regulates rat pituitary insulin-like growth factor-1 receptors. Endocrinology 1990;126:550–554.

77. Binoux M, Fairvre-Bauman A, Lassarre C, Marret A, Tixier-Vidal A. Triiodothyronine stimulates the production of insulin-like growth factors IGF by fetal hypothalamus cells cultured in serum-free medium. Brain Res 1985;353:319–321.

78. Mukku VR: Regulation of epidermal growth factor receptor levels by thyroid hormone. J Biol Chem 1984;259:6543–6547.

79. Fernandes-Pol, JA: Modulation of EGF proto-oncogene expression by growth factors and hormones in human breast carcinoma cells, Crit Rev Oncogen 1991;2(2):173–185.

80. Fernandes-Pol, J.A., Modulation of transforming growth factor alpha-dependent expression of growth factor receptor gene by transforming growth factor-beta, triiodothyronine, and retinoic acid. J Cell Biochem 1989;41,[3]:159–170.

81. Theodossiou C, Skrepnik N, Robert EG, et al. Propylthiouracil-induced hypothyroidism reduces xenograft tumor growth in athymic nude mice. Cancer 1999;86(8):1596–1601.

82. Kinoshita, S., Effects of hyper- and hypothyroidism on natural defenses against Lewis lung carcinoma and its spontaneous pulmonary metastasis in C57BL/6 Mice. Tokushima I Exper Med 1991;38(2):25–35.

83. Mishkin SY. Inhibition of local and metastatic hepatoma growth and prolongation of survival after induction of hypothyroidism. Cancer Res 1981;41:3040–3045.

84. Shoemaker JP, Dagher RK. Remissions of mammary adenocarcinoma in hypothyroid mice given 5-fluorouracil and chloroquine phosphate. JNCI 1976;62:1575–1578.

85. Kumar MS, Chiang T, Deodhar SD. Enhancing effect of thyroxine on tumor growth and metastases in syngeneic mouse tumor . Cancer Res 1979;39:3515–3518.

86. Lin KH, Lin YW, Parkinson C, Cheng SY. Stimulation of proliferation by 3,3,5,-triiodothyronine in poorly differentiated human hepatocarcinoma cells over-expressing B01 thyroid hormone receptor. Cancer Let 1994;85;189–194.

87. Hercbergs A, Leith J. Spontaneous remission of metastatic lung cancer following myxedema coma—an apoptosis-related phenomenon? J Natl Cancer Inst 1993;85(16):1342–1343.

88. Hercbergs A. The thyroid gland as an intrinsic biologic response-modifier in advanced neoplasia—a novel paradigm. In Vivo 1996;2:245–247.

89. Hercbergs A. Spontaneous remission of cancer–a thyroid hormone dependent phenomenon? Anticancer Res 1999;19:4839–4844.

90. Nunez J, Gauchio D, Aniello F, Bridoux AM. Regulation by thyroid hormone of microtubule assembly and neuronal differentiation. Neurochem Res 1991;16:975–982.

91. Mulvei A, Anderson G, Nelson BD. Thyroid hormone and not growth hormone is the principal regulator of mammalian mitochondrial mitogenesis. Acta Endocrinol 1989;121:223–238.

92. Satav JG, Katyare SS. Thyroid hormones and cathepsin D activity in the rat liver, kidney, and brain. Experientia 1981;37:100–103.

93. Davis F B, Mousa S A, O'Connor L, et al. Proangiogenic Action of Thyroid Hormone Is Fibroblast Growth Factor–Dependent and Is Initiated at the Cell Surface. Circ Res 2004;94(11):1500–1506.

94. Bergh J, Lin HY, Mohamed SN, Mousa SA, Davis FB, Davis PJ. L-Thyroxine Induces Mitogen-Activated Protein Kinase Activation via Binding to Integrin aVb3. American Thyroid Association 76th Annual Meeting, Vancouver. Thyroid 2004;14(9)690; abstract no. 26.

95. Muller Y, Rocchi E, Lazaro JB, Clos J. Thyroid hormone promotes BCL-2 expression and prevents apoptosis of early differentiating cerebellar granule neurons. Int J Dev Neurosci 1995;13(8):871–885.

96. Goldman MB, Monson RR, Maloof P. Benign thyroid disease and the risk of death from breast cancer. Oncol 1992;49:461–466.

97. Hercbergs A. Does hypothyroidism favor the response to therapy in metastatic breast cancer? Proc ASCO 1988;7:20.

98. Hercbergs A, Mason J, Reddy C, Elson P. Thyroid hormones and Lung Cancer:Primary hypothyroidism is prognostically significant for survival in lung cancer: Abstract 4844. 95th Annual Meeting, The American Association for Cancer Research. Orlando, FL, March 30, 2004

99. Atkins MB, Mier JW, Parkinson DR, et al. Hypothyroidism after treatment with interleukin-2 and lymphokine activated killer cells. N Engl J Med 1988;318:1557–1563.

100. Reid I, Sharpe I, McDevitt J, et al. Thyroid dysfunction can predict response to immunotherapy with interleukin-2 and interferon-2a. Br J Cancer 1991;64:915–918.

101. Weijl NI, Van der Harst D, Brand A, Kooy Y, Van Luzemberg S. Hypothyroidism during immunotherapy with interleukin-2 is associated with antithyroid antibodies and response to treatment. J Clin Oncol 1993;11:1376–1383.

102. Franzke A, Prest D, Probst-Kopper M, et al. Autoimmunity resulting from cytokine treatment predicts long-term survival in patients with metastatic renal cell cancer. J Clin Oncol 1999; 17(2):529–533.

103. Franklyn JA, ,Maisonneuve P, Sheppard M, Bettenridge J, Boyle P. Cancer incidence and mortality after radioiodine treatment for hyperthyroidism: a population-based cohort study. Lancet 1999;353:2111–2115.

104. Hercbergs A, Brok-Simoni F, Holtzman F, Bar-Am J, Leith J, Brenner H: Erythrocyte glutathione and tumor response to chemotherapy. Lancet 1992;339: 1074–1076.

105. Hercbergs A. High tumor response rate to radiation therapy in biochemically hypothyroid patients. Proc Am Assoc Cancer Res 1997;248:1667.

106. Hercbergs, A. Hypothyroidism and tumor regression. N Engl J Med 1989;319:1351–1352.

107. Hercbergs AA, Goyal LK, Suh JH, et al. Propylthiouracil-induced chemical hypothyroidism with high-dose tamoxifen prolongs survival in recurrent high grade glioma: a phase I/II study. Anticancer Res 2003;23(1B): 617–626.

108. Hercbergs J, Suh C, Reddy B, et al. Propylthiouracil- Induced Chemical Hypothyroidism with High-Dose Tamoxifen Prolongs Survival with Increased Response Rate in Recurrent High Grade Glioma- Proceedings of the American Association for Cancer Research. 93rd Annual Meeting San Francisco, Abstract no. 2442, April 8, 2002;43:491.

109. Wolff JE, Guerin C, Laterra J; et al. Dexamethasone reduces vascular density and plasminogen activator activity in 9L rat brain tumors. Brain Res 1993;604(1–2):79–85.

110. Badruddoja MA, Krouwer HG, Rand SD, Rebro KJ, Pathak AP, Schmainda KM. Antiangiogenic effects of dexamethasone in 9L gliosarcoma assessed by MRI cerebral blood volume maps. Neurooncol 2003;5(4):235–243.

111. Machein MR, Kullmer J, Ronicke V, et al. Differential downregulation of vascular endothelial growth factor by dexamethasone in normoxic and hypoxic rat glioma cells. Neuropathol Appl Neurobiol 1999;25(2):104–112.

112. Proescholdt MA, Heiss JD, Walbridge S, et al..Vascular endothelial growth factor (VEGF) modulates vascular permeability and inflammation in rat brain. J Neuropathol Exp Neurol 1999;58(6):613–627.

113. Badie B, Schartner JM, Paul J, Bartley BA, Vorpahl J, Preston JK. Dexamethasone-induced abolition of the inflammatory response in an experimental glioma model: a flow cytometry study. J Neurosurg 2000;93(4): 634–639.

114. Koufali MM, Moutsatsou P, Sekeris CE, Breen KC. The dynamic localization of the glucocorticoid receptor in rat C6 glioma cell mitochondria. Mol Cell Endocrinol 2003;209(1–2):51–60.

115. Kawamura A, Tamaki N, Kokunai T. Effect of dexamethasone on cell proliferation of neuroepithelial tumor cell lines. Neurol Med Chir (Tokyo) 1998;38(10):633–638

116. Kaup B, Schindler I, Knupfer H, Schlenzka A, Preiss R, Knupfer MM. Time-dependent inhibition of glioblastoma cell proliferation by dexamethasone. J Neurooncol 2001;51(2):105–110.

117. McKay LI, Cidlowski JA. Cross-talk between nuclear factor-kappa B and the steroid hormone receptors: mechanisms of mutual antagonism. Mol Endocrinol 1998;12(1):45–56.

118. Webster JC, Huber RM, Hanson RL, et al.. Dexamethasone and tumor necrosis factor-alpha act together to induce the cellular inhibitor of apoptosis-2 gene and prevent apoptosis in a variety of cell types. Endocrinology 2002;143(10):3866–3874.

119. Gorman AM, Hirt UA, Orrenius S, Ceccatelli S.Dexamethasone pre-treatment interferes with apoptotic death in glioma cells. Neuroscience 2000;96(2):417–425.

120. Wang H, Li M, Rinehart JJ, Zhang R. Pretreatment with dexamethasone increases antitumor activity of carboplatin and gemcitabine in mice bearing human cancer xenografts: in vivo activity, pharmacokinetics, and clinical implications for cancer chemotherapy. Clin Cancer Res 2004;10(5):1633–1644.

25 Gene Therapy

Maciej S. Lesniak and Alessandro Olivi

Summary

High-grade gliomas (HGG) represent the most common primary malignant tumor of the adult central nervous system. Unfortunately, the median survival after surgical intervention alone is only 6 mo and the addition of radiotherapy can extend this time to 9 mo *(1,2)*. Consequently, efforts aimed at developing new therapies have focused on new treatment strategies that specifically target tumor cells and spare normal cells. One such modality, gene therapy, has shown promise in the spectrum of agents utilized against brain tumors. In this chapter, we review the principles of gene therapy and discuss results of recent clinical trials in which gene therapy was employed against HGG.

Key Words: Gene therapy; glioma; adenovirus; herpes virus; immunotherapy.

INTRODUCTION

The concept of gene therapy arose from the observation that certain human diseases are caused by the inheritance of a single nonfunctional gene *(3)*. The ability to replace the defective or missing gene with a normal, functional copy appeared as an alternative treatment strategy. Early work focused on diseases caused by these single-gene defects, such as subacute combined immunodeficiency disorder (SCID) *(4)* and cystic fibrosis *(5)*. However, more recent detection of common genetic alterations shared by a variety of human neoplasms has fostered interest in the application of gene transfer techniques to the development of novel therapies for cancer, including high-grade glioma (HGG). In fact, cancer gene therapy has become one of the most rapidly evolving areas in preclinical and clinical cancer research. The idea that human neoplasms might be the result of accumulated genetic lesions that culminate in a transformed phenotype has increased optimism that gene therapy techniques may provide a rational basis for intervention. In this setting, gene therapy is intended to broaden the spectrum of available therapies. However, with more than 200 cancer gene therapy trials approved worldwide since the early 1990s, it has become increasingly clear that several issues remain to be addressed before the full potential of gene therapy in the care of cancer patients can be realized.

The most important obstacles in gene therapy are the low efficiency of gene transfer achieved by currently available gene-delivery vectors and the lack of selectivity of these vectors to specifically target cancer cells *(5–10)*. As a consequence of these limitations, the delivery of DNA to target cells can be achieved through one of the following distinct modalities. In the first method, tumor cells are removed from a patient, manipulated in vitro, and subsequently transferred back to the patient. Alternatively, DNA can be delivered directly into

From: *Current Clinical Oncology: High-Grade Gliomas: Diagnosis and Treatment*
Edited by: G. H. Barnett © Humana Press Inc., Totowa, NJ

the target tissue (*in situ*), provided this tissue is localized and accessible to manipulation. Examples include injection of a tumor mass with a vector carrying a gene for a cytokine or toxin, or the infusion of adenoviral vectors into the trachea and bronchi of patients with cystic fibrosis. The third method is in vivo gene therapy, in which a vector is administered systemically yet the gene is delivered locally to cells of interest. The realization of such targeted vector therapies that can be safely administered intravenously will represent a major breakthrough in the field of gene therapy, given the systemic nature of most malignancies.

DELIVERY VEHICLES FOR LOCAL AND SYSTEMIC GENE THERAPY

Currently, targeted gene delivery can be achieved in one of two ways: by delivering the gene of interest selectively to target cells (vector targeting), or by creating vector constructs with tissue-specific promoters such that the delivered genes can only be expressed in certain cell types (cell- or tissue-specific gene expression). Moreover, viral vectors employed for gene therapy of human gliomas can be further divided into replication defective vectors and conditionally replicative vectors. A great deal of effort has been generated toward the use of viral agents as nonreplicating vectors for gene insertion in treating cancers. Renewed interest in the use of viruses as oncolytic therapy was sparked with the development of a herpes simplex virus (HSV) containing an inactivating mutation in the thymidine kinase gene *(11)*. With the demonstration of a replicating virus, capable of infecting neoplastic cells, producing progeny, and lysing the host cell, came excitement over the engineering of novel oncolytic viruses. Ideally, these viruses are constructed such that they possess several characteristics beyond those found in their counterparts that are used simply as delivery vectors. These characteristics include selectivity for neoplastic cells alone, minimal toxicity to normal tissues, proliferation within neoplastic cells with systematic killing of tumor tissue, the ability to disseminate throughout the tumor mass, and enduring efficacy *(12)*. As such, several oncolytic viruses have been developed that have exhibited antitumoral properties in both animal models and clinical studies.

In the following section, we will focus on specific viral vectors and discuss the clinical experience with these viruses against malignant brain tumors (Table 1).

RETROVIRUS

One of the first viral vectors utilized in gene therapy trials of HGG was the retroviral vector. The family *Retroviridae* comprise a variety of enveloped RNA viruses, such as endogenous retroviruses, leukemia viruses, or human immunodeficiency virus-1 (HIV-1), the replicative strategy of which includes as essential steps reverse transcription of the virion RNA into linear double-stranded DNA and the subsequent integration of this DNA into the genome of the cell. The RNA is 7 to 12 kb long, linear, and single-stranded. Retroviral vectors exhibit restricted cell tropism, which depends on cell-type division. This is an attractive aspect of retroviral based gene therapy for HGG. However, retroviruses exhibit low transduction efficiency and small capacity for transgene expression. Retroviral based gene therapy of HGG has been investigated since the 1980s.

Perhaps the best-known transgene/vector system is the herpes simplex virus thymidine kinase (HSV-tk) gene transferred by a replication-incompetent retrovirus vector, which is released *in situ* by fibroblast-derived retroviral vector-producing cells. Some of the first clinical studies of this vector involved either stereotactic intratumoral injection of the virus in patients with recurrent HGG or local administration of the virus during surgical resection of

Table 1
Examples of Viral Vectors Utilized Against HGG

Virus	Strain	Trials	Tumor type	Results/comments
HSV-1	G207	Preclinical animal studies (mice, nonhuman primates) (28,29)	U87 glioma cell line	I.C. treatment prolonged survival in murine brain tumor model, acceptable safety profile in nonhuman primates
		Phase I (30)	Glioma	No dose-limiting toxicities identified, therapeutic benefit suggested
		Phase Ib, II	Glioma	In progress
	HSV 1716	Preclinical animal studies (mice, SCID mice) (31–33)	Melanoma, human embryonal carcinoma	Low virulence in SCID mice following ic injection (31), antitumoral effects against ic injected tumors (32,33)
		Phase I (34,35)	Recurrent glioma	No dose-limiting toxicities, possible intratumoral replication (36)
		Phase II	Glioma	In progress
Adenovirus	ONYX-015	Phase I (27)	Glioma	No dose-limiting toxicities with injection into tumor resection cavity
		Phase I, II (24–26)	Head and neck cancers	Acceptable safety profile, potential therapeutic benefit
		Phase III		In progress
Newcastle Disease Virus (NVD)	73-T	Preclinical animal studies (mice) (42–44)	Fibrosarcoma, neuroblastoma and other solid human cancers	Effective tumor regression with systemic and intratumoral administration
	PV701	Phase I (46)	Variety of cancers	Some serious side-effects (including death) noted
	MTH-68/H	Phase II, case report and case series (44,45,47,48)	Variety of cancers, GBM	Case reports of progressive tumor shrinkage and long-term survival in GBM patients treated with iv NDV
Reovirus	Reolysin	Preclinical animal studies (SCID mice, immunocompetent rats, nonhuman primates) (38,39)	U87, 9L and RG2 glioma cell lines	Significant toxicities in SCID mice, no significant toxicities with ic injection into nonhuman primates
		Phase I (12,40)	Subcutaneous metastases from systemic cancers; recurrent glioma	No dose-limiting toxicities (40); in progress (12)

Abbr: ic, intracerebral; iv, intravenous.

the tumor. For instance, Ram et al. treated 15 patients with progressive growth of recurrent malignant brain tumors using a HSV-tk retroviral vector. Antitumor activity was detected in five of the smaller tumors. *In situ* hybridization for HSV-TK demonstrated survival of vector-producing cells at 7 d but indicated limited gene transfer to tumors, suggesting that indirect, "bystander," mechanisms provide local antitumor activity in human tumors *(13)*. Similarly, Shand et al. investigated the effects of HSV-tk gene transfer followed by ganciclovir (GCV) treatment as adjuvant gene therapy to surgical resection in patients with recurrent glioblastoma multiforme (GBM). The study was open and single-armed, and aimed at assessing the feasibility and safety of the technique and indications of antitumor activity. In 48 patients a suspension of retroviral vector-producing cells was administered by intracerebral injection immediately after tumor resection. Intravenous GCV was infused daily 14 to 27 d after surgery. Patients were monitored for adverse events and for life by regular biosafety assaying. Tumor changes were monitored by magnetic resonance imaging (MRI). Reflux during injection was a frequent occurrence but serious adverse events during the treatment period (days 1–27) were few and of a nature not unexpected in this population. One patient experienced transient neurological disorders associated with post-GCV MRI enhancement. There was no evidence of replication-competent retrovirus in peripheral blood leukocytes or in tissue samples of reresection or autopsy. Vector DNA was shown in the leukocytes of some patients but not in autopsy gonadal samples. The median survival time was 8.6 mo, and the 12-mo survival rate was 13 of 48 patients (27%). On MRI studies, tumor recurrence was absent in 7 patients for at least 6 mo and for at least 12 mo in 2 patients, 1 of whom remained recurrence free at more than 24 mo. Treatment-characteristic images of injection tracks and intracavitary hemoglobin were apparent. Based on these results, the authors concluded that gene therapy is feasible and appears to be satisfactorily safe as an adjuvant to the surgical resection of recurrent GBM *(14)*.

The positive results obtained in some of these phase I and II studies led to a phase III clinical evaluation of HSV-tk and GCV gene therapy as an adjuvant to surgical resection and radiation in adults with previously untreated GBM. A total of 248 patients with newly diagnosed, previously untreated GBM received, in equal numbers, either standard therapy (surgical resection and radiotherapy) or standard therapy plus adjuvant gene therapy during surgery. Progression-free median survival in the gene therapy group was 180 d compared with 183 d in control subjects. Median survival was 365 vs 354 d, and 12-m survival rates were 50 vs 55% in the gene therapy and control groups, respectively. These differences were not significant. Therefore, the adjuvant treatment improved neither time to tumor progression nor overall survival time, although the feasibility and good biosafety profile of this gene therapy strategy were further supported *(15)*.

The overall lack of success with HSV-tk/GCV retroviral therapy prompted a renewed interest in other forms of vector based gene therapy. Among them, adenoviruses, herpes viruses, reoviruses, and the Newcastle virus are prominent.

ADENOVIRUSES

Recombinant adenoviruses are an attractive alternative vehicles for gene therapy. A major advance over other viral vectors is the ability of recombinant adenoviruses to mediate a high-efficiency gene transfer to a wide variety of cell types, including nondividing cells. They are also able to host large transgenes (up to approx 30 Kb). The viral genome remains episomal and does not undergo rearrangement at a high rate. The virus is easily propagated and remains concentrated within permissive cells long after yields have reached maximum levels, and because the nonenveloped viral particles are relatively stable, they can be readily concentrated to high titers.

The majority of adenoviral vectors developed to date are derived from human serotypes 2 (Ad2) and 5 (Ad5), because the biology and genetics of these viruses have been intensively investigated. The first generation adenoviral vectors were rendered replication-incompetent though the ablation of the E1 viral sequence, which was replaced with transgenes of about 5 to 8 Kb. Subsequently, other adenoviral vectors were produced with the elimination of the E2 and E3 sequences, allowing the insertion of larger transgenes while reducing the host's immune response to viral infection, thus increasing the duration of therapeutic gene expression.

One of the major historical limitations of adenoviral vectors has been efficient gene delivery into target cells. Whereas adenoviral vectors exhibit superior levels of in vivo gene transfer compared to available alternative vector systems, the present generation of adenoviral vectors used for in vivo gene therapy has demonstrated limited efficacy *(16)*. Two explanations for these suboptimal responses have been proposed. First, in several reported human clinical trials based on in vivo gene delivery, variable clinical responses have been observed in patients. Several studies have found that the relative resistance of HGG to the adenoviral vector is based on the lack of cell-surface expression by the tumor cells of the primary adenoviral receptor, the coxsackie adenovirus receptor (CAR). Thus, variability of adenovirus receptor density expressed by tumors may influence gene transfer efficiency and the ultimate therapeutic response observed in patients. Second, whereas tumor expression of the adenoviral receptor may be low, there is widespread distribution of this cellular receptor in normal human tissues, thus precluding the targeting to tumor specific cell types and making dose-rated vector toxicities limit the overall therapeutic index achievable with adenoviral vectors. Several groups have attempted and continue to generate rational strategies to overcome these limitations as the understanding of the biology and life-cycle of adenoviruses becomes further elucidated.

Trask et al. *(22)*, treated 13 patients with advanced recurrent malignant brain tumors (9 with GBM, 1 with gliosarcoma, and 3 with anaplastic astrocytoma [AA]) with a single intratumoral injection of a replication-defective adenoviral vector bearing the HSV-tk gene driven by the Rous sarcoma virus promoter (Adv.RSVtk), followed by GCV treatment. The primary objective of the study was to determine the safety of this treatment. Injection of Adv.RSVtk in doses up to 2×10^{11} viral particles (vp), followed by GCV, was safely tolerated. Patients treated with the highest dose, 2×10^{12} vp, exhibited central nervous system (CNS) toxicity with confusion, hyponatremia, and seizures. One patient was living and stable 29.2 mo after treatment. Two patients survived for more than 25 mo before succumbing to tumor progression. Ten patients died within 10 mo of treatment, 9 from tumor progression and 1 from sepsis and endocarditis. Neuropathologic examination of postmortem tissue demonstrated cavitation at the injection site, intratumoral foci of coagulative necrosis, and variable infiltration of the residual tumor with macrophages and lymphocytes.

Most recently, the adenovirus ONYX-015, an oncolytic, replication-competent virus has been investigated for the treatment of HGG in human clinical trials. This virus selectively replicates within and lyses cells with defects in p53 or the p53 pathway *(23)*. ONYX-015 has demonstrated effective anti-tumor activity in animal studies and phase I and II trials for treatment of head and neck cancers have shown safety and potential efficacy as well *(24–26)*. Additionally, the recently-published results of a phase I trial for the treatment of glioma have demonstrated safety with injection of ONYX-015 within resection cavities *(27)*. The NABTT CNS Consortium conducted a dose-escalation trial of intracerebral injections of ONYX-015. Cohorts of 6 patients at each dose level received doses of vector from 10^7 plaque-forming units (pfu) to 10^{10} pfu into a total of 10 sites within the resected glioma cavity. Adverse events were identified on physical exams and testing of hematologic, renal, and liver functions. Efficacy data were obtained from serial MRI scans. None of the 24 patients experienced serious adverse events. The maximum tolerated dose was not reached. The median time to progression after treatment with ONYX-015 was 46 d (ranging from 13 to 452 + d). The median survival time was 6.2 mo (ranging from 1.3 to 28.0+ mo). One patient did not progress and 1 patient showed regression of interval-increased enhancement. After more than 19 mo of follow-up, one-sixth of the recipients at a dose of 10^9 and two-sixths at a dose of 10^{10} pfu remained alive. In 2 patients who underwent a second resection 3 mo after ONYX-015 injection, a lymphocytic and plasmacytoid cell infiltrate was observed. This study confirmed that injection of the virus are well tolerated and not associated with any dose-limiting toxicities.

HERPES SIMPLEX VIRUS

HSV has a number of advantages as a gene delivery vector. First, the virus has a propensity to infect only neurons. Moreover, it is readily grown in culture to high-titre. As a result of its large genome, the virus accommodates large transgenes. Considerable progress has been made in effectively disabling the virus so that it does not damage the cells it infects but can still deliver an inserted gene effectively. In addition, it is now possible to obtain long-term expression of the transgene in the CNS, using regulatory elements derived from the latency-associated transcript of the virus.

The HSV-1 mutant G207 (a replication-competent virus whose life cycle is dependent upon proliferating cells) was shown to effectively reduce the growth of subcutaneous U87 glioma cells and prolong survival of mice injected with these cells intracranially *(28)*. Subsequent neurotoxicity studies with intracerebral injection in nonhuman primates demonstrated acceptable safety profiles despite the use of doses far greater than those shown to be efficacious in mouse tumor studies *(29)*. These results led to a phase I G207 clinical trial in humans with recurrent or progressive HGG. The safety of intratumoral injection was demonstrated over a range of viral concentrations such that no maximally tolerated dose (MTD) or dose-limiting toxicities could be established *(30)*. Additionally, whereas the goal of this study was to ascertain a safety profile for this treatment, a therapeutic benefit was suggested. Currently, phase Ib/II trials have begun in hopes of verifying safety and tolerability of intratumoral G207 injections for HGG.

The HSV 1716 (an HSV-1 mutant attenuated in its ability to replicate in neurons of the CNS) is another herpes-virus strain that has made its way from animal studies to early clinical trials. In addition to avirulence in SCID mice, efficacy studies showed anti-neoplastic effects against intracranially injected melanoma and human embryonal carcinoma (NT2) tumors *(31–33)*. The virus was also found to be unable to replicate within neuronally differentiated counterparts of NT2 cells underscoring the selectivity of this virus for tumor cells *(33)*. These results have lead to early trials to assess the safety and toxicity profiles of HSV1716 as an innovative anti-glioma agent in humans *(34)*. As with G207, HSV1716 was well tolerated and an MTD could not be established as no patient exhibited signs of encephalitis postinjection—even with the highest dose administered. Additionally, further studies have suggested that HSV 1716 replicates in at least some of the HGG treated with intratumoral injection and there has been no toxicity after viral injection into the surrounding brain tissue following surgical resection of the tumor *(35,36)*. Survival data from these studies has generated excitement over clinical trials designed to evaluate the therapeutic benefit of intratumoral HSV1716 treatment.

REOVIRUS

Reovirus, a nonenveloped virus associated with mild respiratory and gastrointestinal tract symptoms in humans, is known to infect and proliferate in cells with unregulated *Ras* pathway activity. Because *Ras* pathway dysregulation is common in gliomas (coupled with the cytolytic activity of reovirus at the end of its replication cycle) the use of this virus for oncolytic therapy has become attractive. SCID mice implanted in the flank with the glioblastoma cell line U87 had significantly decreased tumor growth compared to control following intratumoral injection of reovirus *(37)*. Furthermore, the virus was found to remain confined to the tumor mass and did not proliferate into normal tissues. Intratumoral/intracerebral injection of reovirus into glioma-bearing SCID mice resulted in significant tumor regression—however, significant virus-related toxicities were noted in these immunodeficient hosts *(38)*. Similarly, significant effectiveness upon tumor regression (without the aforementioned toxicities) was later demonstrated with immunocompetent rats and nonhuman primates *(39)*. Phase I trials injecting reovirus into subcutaneous metastases from systemic cancers have shown no dose-limiting toxicities *(40)*. Meanwhile, phase I dose-escalation trials with intratumoral/intracranial injection in patients with recurrent high-grade glioma are in progress *(12)*.

NEWCASTLE VIRUS

Newcastle disease virus (NDV) is an enveloped paramyxovirus that has been found to have selectively increased replication in neoplastic cells, prompting interest in its use as an oncolytic virus *(41)*. Several animal studies have demonstrated effective tumor regression in fibrosarcoma and neuroblastoma cells using the 73-T strain administered intratumorally and systemically *(42–44)*. Additionally, phase I and II trials using PV701 and MTH-68/H NDV strains respectively, have been performed for the treatment of various cancers *(45,46)*. Whereas fever and flu-like symptoms were the most common troublesome effects associated with virus administration, some serious side-effects—including one possible treatment-associated death—were also noted. Interestingly, the literature also reveals case reports of patients with GBM treated with intravenous NDV resulting in progressive tumor shrinkage and long-term survival *(47,48)*. Finally, NDV has also displayed significant potential when delivered as a cancer vaccine (rather than an oncolytic virus) as NDV-infected cancer cells exhibit enhanced recruitment and activation of CTLs and NK cells *(49)*.

IMMUNOTHERAPY

With the exception of the HSV-tk/ganciclovir gene therapy, viral vectors have been also extensively used to delivery immunomodulatory genes against HGG. Although a complete discussion of the rationale involving the use of immunotherapy is beyond the scope of this chapter, there is compelling data that local augmentation of the immune response may offer a potential benefit to brain tumor patients *(50,51)*. As a result, several vectors have been used to deliver cytokines to brain tumors. This work, while still in preclinical stages, is likely to be evaluated in the context of a clinical trial in the nearby future.

To date, the efficacy of several immunomodulatory genes has been examined in the context of HGG (Table 2). For instance, HSV has been used to deliver IL-4, IL-10, and IL-12 against experimental glioma *(52–54)*. Miyatake et al. predicted that if an immune response plays a role in survival following intratumoral treatment of tumor-bearing animals with HSV, expression of IL-4 should prolong survival whereas expression of IL-10 should reduce it. The results showed that: (1) these cytokines can be expressed by HSV in productively infected cells both

Table 2
Viral Delivery of Immunomodulatory Genes Against HGG

Virus	Gene delivered	Tumor type	Results/comments
Adenovirus (replication incompetent)	IL-4	sc C6 rat glioma model (69)	Adenovirally-delivered IL-4 significantly inhibited tumor growth
	IL-12	ic. GL-26 glioma-bearing mice (55)	Results in Table 1
	TNF-α	ic U87 glioblastoma-bearing mice (57)	Adenovirally-delivered TNF-α coupled with temozolomide prolonged survival
HSV (replication competent)	IL-4, IL-10	ic GL-261 GBM-bearing mice (54)	HSV/IL-4 treatment augmented the oncolytic effect of HSV and improved survival alone or coupled with virally-mediated IL-10 delivery
	IL-12	Murine neuro-blastoma model (53)	Results in Table 1
	Thymidine kinase	sc GL-261 tumors in mice (52)	HSV-TK infection (with aid of HSV helper virus) resulted in significantly reduced tumor size
Vaccinia Virus (replication competent)	IL-2, IL-12	C6 glioma model in mice (58)	Virally-delivered IL-2 and IL-12 augmented the antitumor effect of vaccinia virus alone

Abbr: ic, intracerebral; sc, subcutaneous.

in vitro and in vivo; (2) HSV-expressing IL-4 or IL-10 genes were able to infect and destroy glioma cells in vitro; and, (3) intracerebral inoculation of HSV expressing either IL-4 or IL-10 into syngeneic murine glioma GL-261 cells implanted in the brains of immunocompetent C57BL/6 mice produced dramatically opposite physiologic responses. The IL-4 HSV significantly prolonged survival of tumor bearers, whereas tumor-bearing mice that received the IL-10 HSV had a median survival that was identical to that of saline treated controls. In fact, the combination of HSV/IL-4 was shown to augment the oncolytic effect of HSV alone and improve the survival of mice with experimental brain tumors. Likewise, local expression of IL-12 via HSV was shown to increase Th1 response and significantly increase the survival of mice with intracranial tumors.

The effects observed with HSV have been documented with adenoviral vectors for the delivery of IL-4, IL-12 and tumor necrosis factor (TNF)-α (55–57) and vaccinia-mediated delivery of IL-2 and IL-12 (58). For example, mice bearing GL-26 gliomas in the right corpus striatum were treated with direct intratumoral administration of AdmIL-12, AdLacZ, or normal saline to determine the effect of local adenoviral delivery of IL-12 on glioma immunogenicity. Survival was significantly prolonged in AdmIL-12-treated animals and immunohistochemistry demonstrated robust CD4+ and CD8+ T-cell infiltration in these mice compared with the two control groups. Glioma-infiltrating T lymphocytes from mice that received AdmIL-12 also demonstrated relatively increased, albeit statistically nonsignificant tumor killing. Similarly, attenuated recombinant vaccinia virus (rVV) carrying murine cytokine genes interleukin IL-2 and IL-12 was shown to inhibit pre-established subcutaneously implanted C6 glioma. An antitumor effect did not depend on the dose of the viruses and all viruses induced a high level of cytokine expression in vitro and in vivo. The antitumor activity of rVV-mIL-12 was associated with increases in both the percentage and number of natural killer T cells in the spleen. Local detection of interferon-γ and TNF-α was also correlated with tumor growth arrest induced by the treatment. High-dose VV control vector *per se* induced tumor inhibition by activating Mac-1+ cells in blood, but the antitumor effect was less pronounced compared with rVV-carrying cytokine genes ($p < 0.05$). Taken together, these results suggest that mice intracerebrally implanted with viral vectors producing IL-2, IL-4, IL-12 or TNF-α survive significantly longer than those implanted with noncytokine-secreting vectors. Furthermore, these results confirm the use of local cytokine delivery against brain tumors and when used in combination with oncolytic therapy, suggest a powerful means for targeted brain tumor therapy.

TARGETED BIOLOGIC THERAPIES

Although the focus of this review has been on currently available viral-based gene therapies, recent advances in the understanding of molecular changes that occur in HGG have yielded important information for design of targeted therapies. For instance, gliomas frequently exhibit increased activation of growth factor receptor pathways. Among them, the epidermal growth factor receptor (EGFR) is an attractive therapeutic target which is amplified in up to 40% of primary GBMs *(59–61)*. Likewise, the platelet-derived growth factor receptor (PDGFR) appears to be an important factor contributing to the transformed phenotype of malignant brain tumors *(61–63)*. Agents, which target these receptor as well their downstream activation pathways represent an area of active development. These include tyrosinase kinase inhibitors, farnesyltransferase inhibitors, as well as mammalian target of rapamycin inhibitors. Other potential targets for therapy of HGG include proteosomes, heat shock protein 90 (Hsp90), chemokine receptor 4 (CXCR4), proto-oncogene RAF, histone deacetylases, and cell-cycle components such as CDK4. The ability of viral vectors to modulate these regulatory pathways via gene therapy may hold important implication for glioma therapy.

An excellent example of a potential targeted biologic therapy involves the Sonic Hedgehog (Shh) pathway. Recent studies have suggested that the Shh signaling pathway plays a critical role in regulating the proliferation of cerebellar granule cell precursors and is also a major target of mutation in the cerebellar tumor medulloblastoma *(64–67)*. Romer et al. used a mouse model of medulloblastoma to show that inhibition of the Shh pathway provides a novel therapy for medulloblastoma. By using an inhibitor of the Shh pathway the authors observed suppression of several genes highly expressed in medulloblastoma, inhibition of cell proliferation, increase in cell death and, at the highest dose, complete eradication of tumors. Long-term treatment prolonged medulloblastoma-free survival *(68)*. These findings support the development of Shh antagonists for the treatment of medulloblastoma and suggest that the delivery of targeted gene therapy may improve the survival of patients with these highly aggressive tumors.

CONCLUSIONS

The promise of gene therapy continues to stimulate interest in the field of neuro-oncology. However, despite over a decade of experience in this arena, the field of gene therapy in neuro-oncology is in its early stages of testing and development.

The first viral vectors utilized in gene therapy studies consisted of replication defective vectors. Although well tolerated with an acceptable safety profile, these vectors lacked specificity and exhibited poor transgene expression. In this setting, newer and more complex oncolytic vectors have been designed to selectively replicate within tumor cells. The goal of these vectors is to not only to deliver the gene of interest but also to destroy the tumor cells. Whereas the preliminary data is encouraging, these viruses await testing within the clinical setting. Finally, nonviral vectors, including polymers and nanoparticles, are likely to be used in for the delivery of gene therapy.

In the future, combination of gene therapy along with currently available anti-neoplastic treatments is likely to make an impact on patients with HGG. In the meantime, however, the challenge remains to design vectors which spare normal and healthy brain and selectively target the tumor. Only then will the ability to selectively deliver an appropriate gene to a defective or cancerous cell become a reality, which ultimately may impact on the course of one of the most devastating of human disease.

REFERENCES

1. Black PM. Brain tumor, part 1. N Engl J Med 1991;324(21):1471–1476.
2. Black PM. Brain tumor, part 2. N Engl J Med 1991;324(22):1555–1564.
3. Mavilio F, Bordignon C. Gene therapy. Nature 1993;362(6418):284.
4. Blaese RM, et al., T lymphocyte-directed gene therapy for ADA- SCID: initial trial results after 4 years. Science 1995;270(5235):475–480.
5. Crystal RG. Transfer of genes to humans: early lessons and obstacles to success. Science 1995;270(5235): 404–410.
6. Verma IM, Somia N. Gene therapy—promises, problems and prospects. Nature 1997;389(6648):239–242.
7. Miller N, Vile R. Targeted vectors for gene therapy. FASEBJ 1995;9(2):190–199.
8. Marchisone C, et al. Progress towards gene therapy for cancer. J Exp Clin Cancer Res 2000;19(3):261–270.
9. Galanis E, Vile R, Russell SJ. Delivery systems intended for in vivo gene therapy of cancer: targeting and replication competent viral vectors. Crit Rev Oncol Hematol 2001;38(3):177–192.
10. Anderson WF. Human gene therapy. Nature 1998;392(6679 Suppl):25–30.
11. Martuza RL, et al. Experimental therapy of human glioma by means of a genetically engineered virus mutant. Science 1991;252(5007):854–856.
12. Shah AC, et al. Oncolytic viruses: clinical applications as vectors for the treatment of malignant gliomas. J Neurooncol 2003;65(3):203–226.
13. Ram Z, et al. Therapy of malignant brain tumors by intratumoral implantation of retroviral vector-producing cells. Nat Med 1997;3(12):1354–1361.
14. Shand N, et al. A phase 1-2 clinical trial of gene therapy for recurrent glioblastoma multiforme by tumor transduction with the herpes simplex thymidine kinase gene followed by ganciclovir. GLI328 European-Canadian Study Group. Hum Gene Ther 1999;10(14):2325–2335.
15. Rainov NG. A phase III clinical evaluation of herpes simplex virus type 1 thymidine kinase and ganciclovir gene therapy as an adjuvant to surgical resection and radiation in adults with previously untreated glioblastoma multiforme. Hum Gene Ther 2000;11(17):2389–2401.
16. Goebel EA, et al. Adenovirus-mediated gene therapy for head and neck squamous cell carcinomas. Ann Otol Rhinol Laryngol 1996;105(7)562–567.
17. Miller CR, et al. Differential susceptibility of primary and established human glioma cells to adenovirus infection: targeting via the epidermal growth factor receptor achieves fiber receptor-independent gene transfer. Cancer Res 1998;58(24):5738–5748.
18. Li,Y, et al. Loss of adenoviral receptor expression in human bladder cancer cells: a potential impact on the efficacy of gene therapy. Cancer Res 1999;59(2):325–330.
19. Li D, et al. Variability of adenovirus receptor density influences gene transfer efficiency and therapeutic response in head and neck cancer. Clin Cancer Res 1999;5(12):4175–4181.
20. Hemmi S, et al. The presence of human coxsackievirus and adenovirus receptor is associated with efficient adenovirus-mediated transgene expression in human melanoma cell cultures. Hum Gene Ther 1998;9(16): 2363–2373.

21. Asaoka K, et al. Dependence of efficient adenoviral gene delivery in malignant glioma cells on the expression levels of the Coxsackievirus and adenovirus receptor. J Neurosurg 2000;92(6):1002–1008.

22. Trask TW, et al. Phase I study of adenoviral delivery of the HSV-tk gene and ganciclovir administration in patients with current malignant brain tumors. Mol Ther 2000;1(2):195–203.

23. Bischoff JR, et al. An adenovirus mutant that replicates selectively in p53-deficient human tumor cells. Science 1996;274(5286):373–376.

24. Nemunaitis J, et al. Selective replication and oncolysis in p53 mutant tumors with ONYX-015, an E1B-55kD gene-deleted adenovirus, in patients with advanced head and neck cancer: a phase II trial. Cancer Res 2000; 60(22):6359–6366.

25. Heise C, et al. ONYX-015, an E1B gene-attenuated adenovirus, causes tumor-specific cytolysis and antitumoral efficacy that can be augmented by standard chemotherapeutic agents. Nat Med 1997;3(6):639–645.

26. Khuri FR, et al. A controlled trial of intratumoral ONYX-015, a selectively-replicating adenovirus, in combination with cisplatin and 5-fluorouracil in patients with recurrent head and neck cancer. Nat Med 2000; 6(8):879–885.

27. Chiocca EA, et al. A phase I open-label, dose-escalation, multi-institutional trial of injection with an E1B-Attenuated adenovirus, ONYX-015, into the peritumoral region of recurrent malignant gliomas, in the adjuvant setting. Mol Ther 2004;10(5):958–966.

28. Mineta T, et al. Attenuated multi-mutated herpes simplex virus-1 for the treatment of malignant gliomas. Nat Med 1995;1(9):938–943.

29. Hunter WD, et al. Attenuated, replication-competent herpes simplex virus type 1 mutant G207: safety evaluation of intracerebral injection in nonhuman primates. J Virol 1999;73(8):6319–6326.

30. Markert JM, et al. Conditionally replicating herpes simplex virus mutant, G207 for the treatment of malignant glioma: results of a phase I trial. Gene Ther 2000;7(10):867–874.

31. Valyi-Nagy T, et al. The herpes simplex virus type 1 strain 17+ gamma 34.5 deletion mutant 1716 is avirulent in SCID mice. J Gen Virol 1994;75(Pt 8):2059–2063.

32. Randazzo BP, et al. Treatment of experimental intracranial murine melanoma with a neuroattenuated herpes simplex virus 1 mutant. Virology 1995;211(1):94–101.

33. Kesari S, et al. Therapy of experimental human brain tumors using a neuroattenuated herpes simplex virus mutant. Lab Invest 1995;73(5):636–648.

34. Rampling R, et al. Toxicity evaluation of replication-competent herpes simplex virus (ICP 34.5 null mutant 1716) in patients with recurrent malignant glioma. Gene Ther 2000;7(10):859–66.

35. Harrow S, et al. HSV1716 injection into the brain adjacent to tumour following surgical resection of high-grade glioma: safety data and long-term survival. Gene Ther 2004;11(22):1648–1658.

36. Papanastassiou V, et al. The potential for efficacy of the modified (ICP 34.5(-)) herpes simplex virus HSV1716 following intratumoural injection into human malignant glioma: a proof of principle study. Gene Ther 2002; 9(6):398–406.

37. Coffey MC, et al. Reovirus therapy of tumors with activated Ras pathway. Science 1998;282(5392):1332–1334.

38. Wilcox ME, et al. Reovirus as an oncolytic agent against experimental human malignant gliomas. J Natl Cancer Inst 2001;93(12):903–912.

39. Yang WQ, et al. Efficacy and safety evaluation of human reovirus type 3 in immunocompetent animals: racine and nonhuman primates. Clin Cancer Res 2004;10(24):8561–8576.

40. Oncolytics Biotech releases REOLYSIN phase I clinical trial results. Expert Rev Anticancer Ther 2002;2 (2):139.

41. Reichard KW, et al. Newcastle disease virus selectively kills human tumor cells. J Surg Res 1992;52(5):448–453.

42. Phuangsab A, et al. Newcastle disease virus therapy of human tumor xenografts: antitumor effects of local or systemic administration. Cancer Letter 2001;172(1):27–36.

43. Lorence RM, et al. Complete regression of human fibrosarcoma xenografts after local Newcastle disease virus therapy. Cancer Res 1994;54(23):6017–6021.

44. Lorence RM, et al. Complete regression of human neuroblastoma xenografts in athymic mice after local Newcastle disease virus therapy. J Natl Cancer Inst 1994;86(16):1228–1233.

45. Csatary LK, et al. Attenuated veterinary virus vaccine for the treatment of cancer. Cancer Detect Prev 1993; 17(6):619–627.

46. Lorence RM, et al. Overview of phase I studies of intravenous administration of PV701, an oncolytic virus. Curr Opin Mol Ther 2003;5(6):618–624.

47. Csatary LK, Bakacs T. Use of Newcastle disease virus vaccine (MTH-68/H) in a patient with high-grade glioblastoma. JAMA 1999;281(17):1588–1589.

48. Csatary LK, et al. MTH-68/H oncolytic viral treatment in human high-grade gliomas. J Neurooncol 2004;67 (1–2):83–93.

49. Haas C, et al. Introduction of adhesive and costimulatory immune functions into tumor cells by infection with Newcastle Disease Virus. Int J Oncol 1998;13(6):1105–1115.

50. Liau LM, et al. Tumor immunity within the central nervous system stimulated by recombinant Listeria monocytogenes vaccination. Cancer Res 2002;62(8):2287–2293.

51. Prins RM, Liau LM. Cellular immunity and immunotherapy of brain tumors. Front Biosci 2004;9:124–136.

52. Miyatake S, Martuza RL, Rabkin SD. Defective herpes simplex virus vectors expressing thymidine kinase for the treatment of malignant glioma. Cancer Gene Ther 1997;4(4):222–228.

53. Parker JN, et al. Engineered herpes simplex virus expressing IL-12 in the treatment of experimental murine brain tumors. Proc Natl Acad Sci USA 2000;97(5):2208–2213.

54. Andreansky S, et al. Treatment of intracranial gliomas in immunocompetent mice using herpes simplex viruses that express murine interleukins. Gene Ther 1998;5(1):121–130.

55. Liu Y, et al. *In situ* adenoviral interleukin 12 gene transfer confers potent and long-lasting cytotoxic immunity in glioma. Cancer Gene Ther 2002;9(1):9–15.

56. Yoshikawa K, et al. Immune gene therapy of experimental mouse brain tumor with adenovirus-mediated gene transfer of murine interleukin-4. Cancer Immunol Immunother 2000;49(1):23–33.

57. Yamini B, et al. Transcriptional targeting of adenovirally delivered tumor necrosis factor alpha by temozolomide in experimental glioblastoma. Cancer Res 2004;64(18):6381–6384.

58. Chen B, et al. Low-dose vaccinia virus-mediated cytokine gene therapy of glioma. J Immunother 2001;24(1):46–57.

59. Newton HB. Molecular neuro-oncology and development of targeted therapeutic strategies for brain tumors. Part 1: Growth factor and Ras signaling pathways. Expert Rev Anticancer Ther 2003;3(5):595–614.

60. Rich JN, Bigner DD. Development of novel targeted therapies in the treatment of malignant glioma. Nat Rev Drug Discov 2004;3(5):430–446.

61. Maher EA, et al. Malignant glioma: genetics and biology of a grave matter. Genes Dev 2001;15(11):311–333.

62. Ostman A. PDGF receptors-mediators of autocrine tumor growth and regulators of tumor vasculature and stroma. Cytokine Growth Factor Rev 2004;15(4):275–286.

63. Guha A, et al. Expression of PDGF and PDGF receptors in human astrocytoma operation specimens supports the existence of an autocrine loop. Int J Cancer 1995;60(2):168–173.

64. Newton HB. Molecular neuro-oncology and development of targeted therapeutic strategies for brain tumors. Part 2: PI3K/Akt/PTEN, mTOR, SHH/PTCH and angiogenesis. Expert Rev Anticancer Ther 2004;4(1):105–128.

65. Wechsler-Reya RJ. Analysis of gene expression in the normal and malignant cerebellum. Recent Prog Horm Res 2003;58:227–248.

66. Wechsler-Reya R, Scott MP. The developmental biology of brain tumors. Annu Rev Neurosci 2001;24:385–428.

67. Pomeroy SL, et al. Prediction of central nervous system embryonal tumour outcome based on gene expression. Nature 2002;415(6870):436–442.

68. Romer JT, et al. Suppression of the Shh pathway using a small molecule inhibitor eliminates medulloblastoma in Ptc1(+/–)p53(–/–) mice. Cancer Cell 2004;6(3):229–240.

69. Wei MX, et al. Effects on brain tumor cell proliferation by an adenovirus vector that bears the interleukin-4 gene. J Neurovirol 1998;4(2):237–241.

26 Boron Neutron Capture Therapy of Brain Tumors

Current Status and Future Prospects

Rolf F. Barth, Jeffrey A. Coderre, M. Graça H. Vicente, Thomas E. Blue, and Shin-Ichi Miyatake

Summary

Boron neutron capture therapy (BNCT) is based on the nuclear reaction that occurs when non-radioactive boron-10 is irradiated with low-energy thermal neutrons to yield high-linear energy transfer α particles and recoiling lithium-7 nuclei. Clinical interest in BNCT has focused primarily on the treatment of high-grade gliomas (HGG), and either cutaneous primaries or cerebral metastases of melanoma. Neutron sources for BNCT currently are limited to nuclear reactors and these are available in the United States, Japan, and several European countries. Accelerators also can be used to produce epithermal neutrons and these are being developed in a number of countries, but at this time none are being used for BNCT. Two boron drugs have been used clinically, sodium borocaptate (BSH) ($Na_2B_{12}H_{11}SH$), and a dihydroxyboryl derivative of phenylalanine, referred to as boronophenylalanine (BPA). The major challenge in the development of boron delivery agents has been the requirement for selective tumor-targeting in order to achieve boron concentrations sufficient to deliver therapeutic doses of radiation to the tumor with minimal normal tissue toxicity. Over the past 20 yr, a wide variety of boron-containing compounds have been designed and synthesized. These include boron containing amino acids, biochemical precursors of nucleic acids, DNA binding molecules, and porphyrin derivatives. In addition, high-molecular-weight delivery agents have been developed, including liposomes and monoclonal antibodies (MAbs) and their fragments, which can recognize a tumor-associated epitope, such as epidermal growth factor. However, it is unlikely that any single agent will target all or even most of cells of brain tumors, and that combinations of agents will be required and their dosage and delivery will have to be optimized. Current or recently completed clinical trials have been carried out in Japan, Europe, and the United States. The vast majority of patients have had HGG. Treatment has consisted, first, of "debulking" surgery to remove as much of the tumor as possible, followed by BNCT at varying times after surgery. BSH and BPA have been used as the boron delivery agents, administered either intravenously or intra-arterially as was the case in the early studies with BSH. The best survival data from these studies are at least comparable to those obtained with surgery and external beam photon irradiation, and the safety of the procedure has been established. Critical issues that must be addressed include the need for more selective and effective boron delivery agents, the development of methods to provide semiquantitative estimates of tumor boron content prior to treatment, improvements in clinical implementation of BNCT, and finally, a need for randomized clinical trials with an unequivocal demonstration of therapeutic efficacy. If these issues are adequately addressed, then BNCT could move forward as a treatment modality.

Key Words: BNCT; delivery agents; HGG; GBM.

From: *Current Clinical Oncology: High-Grade Gliomas: Diagnosis and Treatment*
Edited by: G. H. Barnett © Humana Press Inc., Totowa, NJ

INTRODUCTION

After decades of intensive research, high-grade gliomas (HGG), and specifically glioblastoma multiforme (GBM), are still extremely resistant to all current forms of therapy, including surgery, chemotherapy, radiotherapy, immunotherapy, and gene therapy *(1–5)*. The 5-yr survival rate of patients diagnosed with GBM in the United States is less than a few percent, despite aggressive treatment using combinations of therapeutic modalities *(6,7)*. The failure of surgery to cure patients with HGG in part results from the fact that by the time they have had surgical resection of their tumors, malignant cells have infiltrated beyond the margins of resection and have spread into both gray and white matter *(8,9)*. Therefore, high-grade supratentorial gliomas must be regarded as a whole brain disease *(10)*. Glioma cells and their neoplastic precursors have biochemical properties that allow them to invade the unique extracellular environment of the brain *(11,12)*, and biologic properties that allow them to evade a tumor-associated host immune response *(13)*. The inability of chemo- and radiotherapy to cure patients with HGG results from their failure to eradicate microinvasive tumor cells within the brain. However, as recent molecular genetic studies of glioma suggest *(14)*, it may be much more complicated than this, and the challenge facing us is to develop molecular strategies that can selectively target malignant cells with little or no effect on normal cells and tissues adjacent to the tumor.

Boron neutron capture therapy (BNCT), in theory, provides a way to selectively destroy malignant cells and spare normal cells. It is based on the nuclear capture and fission reactions that occur when boron-10, which is a nonradioactive constituent of natural elemental boron, is irradiated with low-energy thermal neutrons to yield high-linear energy transfer (LET) α particles (^{4}He) and recoiling lithium -7 (^{7}Li) nuclei, as shown below.

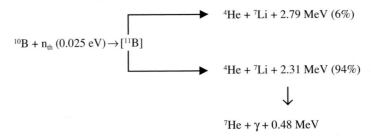

In order for BNCT to be successful, a sufficient amount of ^{10}B must be selectively delivered to the tumor (~20 µg/g weight or ~10^9 atoms/cell), and enough thermal neutrons must be absorbed by them to sustain a lethal ^{10}B(n,α) ^{7}Li capture reaction. Because the high LET particles have limited pathlengths in tissue (5–9 µm), the destructive effects of these high-energy particles is limited to boron containing cells. Clinical interest in BNCT has focused primarily on the treatment of HGG *(15)*, and either cutaneous primaries *(16)*, or cerebral metastases of melanoma *(17)*, and most recently head and neck and liver cancer. Because BNCT is a biologically rather than physically targeted type of radiation treatment, the potential exists to destroy tumor cells dispersed in the normal tissue parenchyma, if sufficient amounts of ^{10}B and thermal neutrons are delivered to the target volume. This review will cover radiobiological considerations upon which BNCT is based, boron agents and optimization of their delivery, neutron sources, which at this time are exclusively nuclear reactors, past and ongoing clinical studies, and critical issues that must be addressed if BNCT is to be successful. Readers interested in more in depth coverage of these and other topics related to BNCT are referred to several recent reviews and monographs *(18–20)*.

RADIOBIOLOGICAL CONSIDERATIONS

Types of Radiation Delivered

The radiation doses delivered to tumor and normal tissues during BNCT result from energy deposition from three types of directly ionizing radiation that differ in their LET characteristics: (1) low-LET γ rays, resulting primarily from the capture of thermal neutrons by normal tissue hydrogen atoms [$^1H(n,\gamma)^2H$]; (2) high-LET protons, produced by the scattering of fast neutrons and from the capture of thermal neutrons by nitrogen atoms [$^{10}N(n,p)^{14}C$]; and (3) high-LET, heavier charged alpha particles (stripped down ^4He nuclei) and lithium-7 ions. These are released as products of the thermal neutron capture and fission reactions with ^{10}B [$^{10}B(n,\alpha)^7Li$]. The greater density of ionizations along tracks of high-LET particles results in an increased biological effect compared to the same physical dose of low-LET radiation. This usually is referred to as relative biological effectiveness (RBE), which is the ratio of the absorbed dose from a reference source of radiation (e.g., X-rays) to that of the test radiation that produces the same biological effect. Because both tumor and surrounding normal tissues are present in the radiation field, even with an ideal epithermal neutron beam, there will be an unavoidable, nonspecific background dose, consisting of both high- and low-LET radiation. However, a higher concentration of ^{10}B in the tumor will result in it receiving a higher total dose than that of adjacent normal tissues, which is the basis for the therapeutic gain in BNCT *(21)*. As recently reviewed *(18)*, the total radiation dose delivered to any tissue can be expressed in photon-equivalent units as the sum of each of the high-LET dose components multiplied by weighting factors, which depend on the increased radiobiological effectiveness of each of these components.

Biological Effectiveness Factors

The dependence of the biological effect on the microdistribution of ^{10}B requires the use of a more appropriate term than RBE to define the biological effects of the $^{10}B(n, \alpha)^7Li$ reaction. Measured biological effectiveness factors for the components of the dose from this reaction have been termed compound biological effectiveness (CBE) factors and are drug-dependent *(21–23)*. The mode and route of drug administration, the boron distribution within the tumor, normal tissues, and even more specifically within cells, and even the size of the nucleus within the target cell population all can influence the experimental determination of the CBE factor. CBE factors, therefore, are fundamentally different from the classically defined RBE, which primarily is dependent on the quality (i.e., LET) of the radiation administered. CBE factors are strongly influenced by the distribution of the specific boron delivery agent, and can differ substantially, although they all describe the combined effects of α particles and ^7Li ions. The CBE factors for the boron component of the dose are specific for both the boron-10 delivery agent and the tissue. A weighted Gray (Gy) unit (Gy[w]) has been used to express the summation of all BNCT dose components and indicates that the appropriate RBE and CBE factors have been applied to the high-LET dose components. However, for clinical BNCT the overall calculation of photon-equivalent (Gy(w)) doses requires a number of assumptions about RBEs, CBE factors and the boron concentrations in various tissues, which have been based on the currently available human or experimental data *(24,25)*.

Clinical Dosimetry

Biological weighting factors, summarized in Table 1, have been used in all of the recent clinical trials in patients with HGG, using BPA in combination with an epithermal neutron

Table 1
Assumptions Used in the Clinical Trials of BPA-Based BNCT for Calculation
of the $^{10}B(n,\alpha)^7Li$ Component of the Gy(w) Dose in Various Tissues

Tissue	Boron concentration [a]	CBE factor
Tumor	3.5 × blood (163)	3.8 (29)
Brain	1.0 × blood (27,28)	1.3 (22)
Scalp/skin	1.5 × blood (27,28)	2.5 (26)
Blood	Measured directly	

[a] An RBE of 3.2 was used for the high-LET component of the beam dose: protons from the $^{14}N(n,n)^{14}C$ reaction, and the recoil protons from fast neutron collisions with hydrogen. Literature references are given in parentheses.

beam. The $^{10}B(n,\alpha)^7Li$ component of the radiation dose to the scalp has been based on the measured boron concentration in the blood at the time of BNCT, assuming a blood:scalp boron concentration ratio of 1.5:1 (26–28) and a CBE factor for BPA in skin of 2.5 (26). An RBE of 3.2 has been used in all tissues for the high-LET components of the beam: protons resulting from the capture reaction with nitrogen, and recoil protons resulting from the collision of fast neutrons with hydrogen (27–29). It must be emphasized that the tissue distribution of the boron delivery agent in humans should be similar to that in the experimental animal model in order to use the experimentally derived values for estimation of Gy(w) doses in clinical radiations.

Dose calculations become much more complicated when combinations of agents are used. At its simplest, this could be the two low-molecular-weight drugs BPA and BSH. These have been shown to be highly effective when used in combination to treat F98 glioma bearing rats (30,31), and currently are being used in combination in a clinical study in Japan (32). Because it currently is impossible to know the true biodistribution of each drug, dosimetric calculations in experimental animals have been based on independent boron determinations in other tumor bearing animals that have received the same doses of drugs but not BNCT. More recently, the radiation delivered has been expressed as a physical or absorbed dose rather than using CBE factors to calculate an RBE equivalent dose (33). The calculations are further complicated if low and high molecular weight delivery agents are used in combination with one another. Tumor radiation dose calculations, therefore, are based on multiple assumptions regarding boron biodistribution, which may vary from patient to patient, as well as within different regions of the tumor and among tumor cells. However, normal brain boron concentrations are much more predictable and uniform, and therefore, it has been shown to be both safe and reliable to base dose calculations on normal brain tolerance.

BORON DELIVERY AGENTS

General Requirements

The development of boron delivery agents for BNCT began approx 50 yr ago and is an ongoing and difficult task of the highest priority. The most important requirements for a successful boron delivery agent are: (1) low systemic toxicity and normal tissue uptake with high tumor uptake and concomitantly high tumor:brain (T:Br) and tumor:blood (T:Bl) concentration ratios (>3–4:1); (2) tumor concentrations in the range of about 20 μg ^{10}B/g tumor; and (3) rapid clearance from blood and normal tissues and persistence in tumor during BNCT.

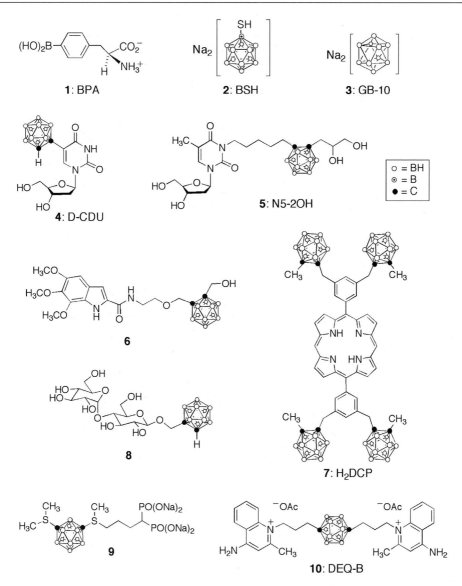

Fig. 1. Some low-molecular-weight BNCT agents under investigation. The nucleosides BPA (**cpd 1**) and BSH (**cpd 2**) are currently in clinical use in the United States, Japan, and Europe. GB-10 (**cpd 3**) has shown promise in animal models. The nucleoside derivatives D-CDU (**cpd 4**) and N5-2OH (**cpd 5**) are tumor-selective and can be phosphorylated into the corresponding nucleotides. The trimethoxyindole derivative **cpd 6** has shown promise in vitro and the porphyrin derivative **cpd 7** was shown to be tumor-selective. The maltose derivative **8** has shown low cytotoxicity and tumor cell uptake in vitro, the bisphosphorate **cpd 9** has tumor targating ability and the dequalinium derivative DEQ-B (**cpd 10**) has shown promise in in vitro studies.

However, it should be noted that at this time no single boron delivery agent fulfills all of these criteria. With the development of new chemical synthetic techniques and increased knowledge of the biological and biochemical requirements needed for an effective agent and their modes of delivery, a number of promising new boron agents has emerged (Fig. 1).

The major challenge in their development has been the requirement for selective tumor targeting in order to achieve boron concentrations sufficient to deliver therapeutic doses of radiation to the tumor with minimal normal tissue toxicity. The selective destruction of GBM cells in the presence of normal cells represents an even greater challenge compared with malignancies at other anatomic sites, because they are highly infiltrative of normal brain, histologically complex and heterogeneous in their cellular composition.

First and Second Generation Boron Delivery Agents

The clinical trials of BNCT in the 1950s and early 1960s used boric acid and some of its derivatives as delivery agents, but these simple chemical compounds were nonselective, had poor tumor retention, and attained low-T:Br ratios (34,35). In the 1960s, two other boron compounds emerged from investigations of hundreds of low-molecular-weight boron-containing chemicals, one, (L)-4-dihydroxy-borylphenylalanine, referred to as boronophenyl-alanine (BPA) (**cpd 1**) was based on arylboronic acids (36), and the other was based on a newly discovered polyhedral borane anion, sodium mercaptoundecahydro-*closo*-dodecaborate (37), referred to as sodium borocaptate (BSH) (**cpd 2**). These "second" generation compounds had low toxicity, persisted longer in animal tumors compared with related molecules, and had T:Br and T:Bl boron ratios greater than 1. As will be described later, ^{10}B enriched BSH and BPA, complexed with fructose to improve its water solubility, have been used clinically in Japan, the United States, and Europe. Although these drugs are not ideal, their safety following intravenous administration has been established. Over the past 20 yr, several other classes of boron-containing compounds have been designed and synthesized in order to fulfill the requirements indicated at the beginning of this section. Detailed reviews of the state-of-the-art in compound development for BNCT have been published (38–41), and in this overview, we will only summarize the main classes of compounds with an emphasis on recently published work in the area, and we will discuss the general biochemical requirements for an effective boron delivery agent.

Third Generation Boron Delivery Agents

So-called "third" generation compounds mainly consist of a stable boron group or cluster attached via a hydrolytically stable linkage to a tumor-targeting moiety, such biomolecules or monoclonal antibodies (MAbs). For example, the targeting of the epidermal growth factor receptor (EGFR) and its mutant isoform EGFRvIII, which are over-expressed in gliomas and squamous cell carcinomas of the head and neck, has been one such approach (42). Low-molecular-weight biomolecules, such as porphyrins, have been shown to have selective targeting properties and many are at various stages of development for cancer chemo-therapy, photodynamic therapy (PDT), or antiviral therapy. The tumor cell nucleus and DNA are especially attractive targets because the amount of boron required to produce a lethal effect may be substantially reduced, if it is localized within or near the nucleus (43). Other potential subcellular targets are mitochondria, lysosomes, endoplasmic reticulum, and the Golgi apparatus. Water solubility is an important factor for a boron agent that is to be administered systemically, whereas lipophilicity is necessary for it to cross the blood–brain barrier (BBB) and diffuse within the brain and tumor. Therefore, amphiphilic compounds possessing a suitable balance between hydrophilicity and lipophilicity have been of primary interest because they should provide the most favorable differential boron concentrations between tumor and normal brain, thereby enhancing tumor specificity. However, for low-molecular-weight molecules that target specific biological transport systems and/or are incorporated into a delivery vehicle, such as liposomes, the amphiphilic character is not as crucial. The molecular weight of the boron-containing delivery agent also is an important factor, since it determines the rate of diffusion both within the brain and the tumor.

LOW-MOLECULAR-WEIGHT AGENTS

Boron Containing Amino Acids and Polyhedral Boranes

Recognizing that BPA and BSH are not ideal boron delivery agents, considerable effort has been directed toward the design and synthesis of third generation, boron-containing amino acids and functionalized polyhedral borane clusters. Examples include various derivatives of BPA and other boron-containing amino acids such as glycine, alanine, aspartic acid, tyrosine, cysteine, methionine, as well as non-naturally occurring amino acids (44–49). The most recently reported delivery agents contain one or more boron clusters and concomitantly larger amounts of boron by weight compared with BPA. The advantages of such compounds are that they can potentially deliver higher concentrations of boron to tumors without increased toxicity. The polyhedral borane dianions, $closo$-$B_{10}H_{10}^{2-}$ and $closo$-$B_{12}H_{12}^{2-}$ and the icosahedral carboranes $closo$-$C_2B_{10}H_{12}$ and $nido$-$C_2B_9H_{12}^-$, have been the most attractive boron clusters for linkage to targeting moieties as a result of their relatively easy incorporation into organic molecules, high boron content, chemical and hydrolytic stability, hydrophobic character and, in most cases, their negative charge. The simple sodium salt of $closo$-$B_{10}H_{10}^{2-}$ (GB-10, **cpd 3**) has been shown to have tumor-targeting ability and low systemic toxicity in animal models (41) and it has been considered as a candidate for clinical evaluation (50). Other polyhedral borane anions with high boron content include derivatives of $B_{20}H_{18}^{2-}$, although these compounds have shown little tumor specificity and therefore may be better candidates for encapsulation into either targeted or nontargeted liposomes (51,52) and folate receptor targeting, boron containing polyamidoamino (PAMAM) dendrimers (53), and liposomes (54). Boron-containing dipeptides also have shown low toxicity and good tumor-localizing properties (55,56).

Biochemical Precursors and DNA Binding Agents

Several boron-containing analogues of the biochemical precursors of nucleic acids, including purines, pyrimidines, nucleosides and nucleotides, have been synthesized and evaluated in cellular and animal studies (57–61). Some of these compounds, such as β-5-o-carboranyl-2'-deoxyuridine (D-CDU, **cpd 4**) and the 3-(dihydroxypropyl-carboranyl-pentyl)thymidine derivative N5-2OH (**cpd 5**), have shown low toxicities, selective tumor cell uptake and significant rates of phosphorylation into the corresponding nucleotides (62–64). Intracellular nucleotide formation potentially can lead to enhanced tumor uptake and retention of these types of compounds (63,64).

Another class of low-molecular-weight delivery agents are boron-containing DNA binding molecules, such as alkylating agents, intercalators, groove binders, and polyamines. Some examples are derivatives of aziridines, acridines, phenanthridines (e.g., **cpd 6**), trimethoxyindoles, carboranylpolyamines, Pt(II)-amine complexes, and di- and tri-benzimidazoles (65–68). A limitation of boron-containing polyamines is their frequently observed in vitro and in vivo toxicity, although promising derivatives with low cytotoxicity have been synthesized (69–72). Other nuclear-targeting molecules are $nido$-carboranyl oligomeric phosphate diesters (OPDs). Despite their multiple negative charges, OPDs have been shown to target the nuclei of TC7 cells following microinjection (73), suggesting that the combination of OPDs with a cell-targeting molecule capable of crossing the plasma membrane could provide both selectivity and nuclear binding. Such a conjugate has been designed and synthesized *(74)*, although its biological evaluation has yet to be reported.

Boron Containing Porphyrins and Related Structures

Several boron-containing fluorescent dyes, including porphyrin, tetrabenzoporphyrin and phthalocyanine derivatives, have been synthesized and evaluated *(75–78)*. These have the advantage of being easily detected and quantified by fluorescence microscopy, and they have the potential for interacting with DNA because of their planar aromatic structures. Among these macrocycles, boron-containing porphyrins (e.g., **cpd 7**: H_2DCP) have attracted special attention because of their low systemic toxicity compared with other dyes, easy synthesis with high boron content, and their remarkable stability *(78–81)*. Porphyrin derivatives have been synthesized that contain up to 44% boron by weight using *closo-* or *nido-*carborane clusters linked to the porphyrin macrocycle via ester, amide, ether, methylene or aromatic linkages *(75–84)*. The nature of these linkages is believed to influence their stability and systemic toxicity. Therefore, with these and other boron delivery agents, chemically stable carbon–carbon linkages have been preferred over ester and amide linkages that potentially can be cleaved in vivo. Boron-containing porphyrins have excellent tumor-localizing properties *(75–81)* and have been proposed for dual application as boron delivery agents and photosensitizers for PDT of brain tumors *(84–90)*. Our own preliminary data with H_2TCP (tetra[*nido-*carboranylphenyl]porphyrin), administered intracerebrally by means of convection enhanced delivery (CED) to F98 glioma bearing rats, showed tumor boron concentrations of 150 µg/g tumor with concomitantly low normal brain and blood concentrations *(91)*. Ozawa et al. recently described a newly synthesized polyboronated porphyrin, designated TABP-1, which was administered by CED to nude rats bearing intracerebral implants of the human glioblastoma cell line U-87 MG *(92)*. High tumor and low blood boron concentrations were observed and both we and Ozawa have concluded that direct intracerebral administration of the carboranyl porphyrins by CED is superior to systemic administration. Furthermore, despite the bulkiness of the carborane cages, carboranylporphyrins have been shown to interact with DNA and thereby produce in vitro DNA damage following light activation *(93,94)*. Boronated phthalocyanines have been synthesized, although these compounds usually have had decreased water-solubility and an increased tendency to aggregate, compared to the corresponding porphyrins *(75,76,85,86)*. Boron-containing acridine molecules also have been reported to selectively deliver boron to tumors with high T:Br and T:Bl ratios, whereas phenanthridine derivatives were found to have poor specificity for tumor cells *(93–95)*.

Other Low-Molecular-Weight Boron Delivery Agents

Carbohydrate derivatives of BSH and other boron-containing glucose, mannose, ribose, gulose, fucose, galactose, maltose (e.g., **cpd 8**), and lactose molecules have been synthesized, and some of these compounds have been evaluated in both in vitro and in vivo studies *(98–104)*. These compounds usually are highly water-soluble and, as a possible consequence of this, they have shown both low toxicity and uptake in tumor cells. It has been suggested that these hydrophilic low-molecular-weight derivatives have poor ability to cross tumor cell membranes. However, they might selectively accumulate within the glycerophospholipid membrane bilayer and in other areas of the tumor, such as the vasculature.

Low-molecular-weight boron-containing receptor-binding molecules have been designed and synthesized. These have been mainly steroid hormone antagonists, such as derivatives of tamoxifen, 17β-estradiol, cholesterol, and retinoic acid *(105–109)*. The biological properties of these agents depend upon the density of the targeted receptor sites, although to date very little biological data have been reported. Other low-molecular-weight boron-containing compounds that have been synthesized include phosphates, phosphonates, (e.g. **cpd 9**), phenylureas, thioureas, nitroimidazoles, amines, benzamides, isocyanates, nicotinamides, azulenes, and dequalinium derivatives (e.g., dequalinium-B, **cpd 10**) *(110–112)*. Because no single chemical compound, as yet synthesized, has the requisite properties, the use of multiple boron delivery agents is probably essential for targeting different subpopulations of tumor cells and subcellular sites. Furthermore, lower doses of each individual agent would be needed, which could reduce systemic toxicity while at the same time enhancing tumor boron levels to achieve a therapeutic effect.

HIGH-MOLECULAR-WEIGHT AGENTS

Monoclonal Antibodies, Other Receptors Targeting Agents and Liposomes

High-molecular-weight boron delivery agents such as MAbs and their fragments, which can recognize a tumor-associated epitope, have been *(113–115)* and continue to be of interest to us *(116,117)* and are the subject of a recent review *(118)*. Although they can be highly specific, only very small quantities reach the brain and tumor following systemic administration as a result of their rapid clearance by the reticuloendothelial system and the BBB, which effectively limits their ability to cross capillary vascular endothelial cells. Boron-containing bioconjugates of EGF *(119,120)*, the receptor for which is overexpressed on a variety of tumors, including GBM *(121,122)*, also have been investigated as potential delivery agents to target brain tumors. However, it is unlikely that either boronated antibodies or other bioconjugates would attain sufficiently high concentrations in the brain following systemic administration, but, as described later in this section, direct intracerebral delivery could solve this problem. Another approach would be to directly target the vascular endothelium of brain tumors using either boronated MAbs or VEGF, which would recognize amplified VEGF receptors. The use of boron containing VEGF bioconjugates would obviate the problem of passage of a high-molecular-weight agent across the BBB, but their use most likely would require repeated applications of BNCT because tumor neovasculature can continuously regenerate. Backer et al. have reported that targeting a Shiga-like toxin-VEGF fusion protein was selectively toxic to vascular endothelial cells overexpressing VEGFR-2 *(123)*. Recently, a bioconjugate has been produced by chemically linking a heavily boronated polyaminoamido (PAMAM) dendrimer to VEGF *(124)*. This selectively targeted tumor blood vessels overexpressing VEGFR-2 in mice bearing 4T1 breast carcinoma. There also has been a longstanding interest on the use of boron-containing liposomes as delivery agents *(51,52, 125,126)*, but their size has limited their usefulness as brain tumor targeting agents, because they are incapable of traversing the BBB unless they have diameters <50 nm *(127)*. If, on the other hand, they were administered intracerebrally or were linked to an actively transported carrier molecule such as transferin, or alternatively, if the BBB was transiently opened, these could be very useful delivery agents, especially for extra-cranial tumors such as liver cancer.

Recent work has focused on the use of a chemeric MoAb, cetuximab (IMC-C225 also known as Erbitux®), produced by ImClone Systems, Inc. *(117)*. This antibody recognizes both wildtype EGFR and its mutant isoform, EGFRvIII *(128)*, and now is in use for the treatment of EGFR(+) recurrent colon cancer *(129)* and head and neck cancer. Using previously developed methodology *(113)*, a PAMAM or "starburst" dendrimer was heavily boronated and then linked by means of heterobifunctional reagents to EGF *(120)*, cetuximab *(117)*, or another MAb, L8A4 *(130)*, which is specifically directed against EGFRvIII *(131)*. In order to completely bypass the BBB, the bioconjugates were administered by either direct intratumoral (it) injection *(132)* or CED *(130,133)* to rats bearing intracerebral implants of the F98 glioma that had been genetically engineered *(132)* to express either wildtype EGFR *(133)* or EGFRvIII *(130)*. Administration by either of these methods resulted in tumor boron concentrations that were in the therapeutic range (i.e., ~20 µg/g tumor weight). Based on the favorable uptake of these bioconjugates, therapy studies were initiated at the Massachusetts Institute of Technology nuclear reactor (MITR). The mean survival times (MST) of animals that received either boronated cetuximab *(134)* or EGF *(135)* were significantly prolonged compared to those of animals bearing receptor negative tumors. A further improvement in MSTs was seen if the animals received BPA, administered intravenously (iv) in combination with the boronated bioconjugates, thereby validating our hypothesis that combinations of agents may be superior to any single agent *(31)*. As can be seen from the preceding discussion, the design and synthesis of low- and high-molecular-weight boron agents have been the subject of intensive investigation. However, optimization of their delivery has not received enough attention, but nevertheless it is of critical importance.

OPTIMIZING DELIVERY OF BORON CONTAINING AGENTS

General Considerations

Delivery of boron agents to brain tumors is dependent on: (1) the plasma concentration profile of the drug, which depends upon the amount and route of administration, (2) the ability of the agent to traverse the BBB, (3) blood flow within the tumor, and (4) the lipophilicity of the drug. In general, a high steady-state blood concentration will maximize brain uptake, whereas rapid clearance will reduce it, except in the case of intra-arterial (ia) drug administration. Although the iv route currently is being used clinically to administer both BSH and BPA, this may not be ideal and other strategies may be needed to improve their delivery. Delivery of boron-containing drugs to extracranial tumors, such as head, neck, and liver cancer, presents a different set of problems, including non-specific uptake and retention in adjacent normal tissues.

Intra-arterial Administration With or Without Blood–Brain Barrier Disruption

As shown in experimental animal studies *(30,31,134–136)*, enhancing the delivery of BPA and BSH can have a dramatic effect both on increasing tumor boron uptake and the efficacy of BNCT. This has been demonstrated in the F98 rat glioma model where intracarotid (ic) injection of either BPA or BSH doubled the tumor boron uptake compared to that obtained by iv injection *(30)*. This was increased fourfold by disrupting the BBB by infusing a hyperosmotic (25%) solution of mannitol via the internal carotid artery. MST of animals that received either BPA or BSH ic with BBB-D were increased 295 and 117%, respectively, compared with irradiated controls *(30)*. The best survival data were obtained using both BPA and BSH in combination, administered by ic injection with BBB-D. The MST was 140 d with a cure rate of 25%, compared with 41 d following iv injection with no longterm surviving animals *(31)*. Similar data have been obtained using a rat model for melanoma metastatic to the brain. BPA was administered ic to nude rats bearing intracerebral implants of the human MRA 27 melanoma with or without BBB-D. The MSTs were 104 to 115 d with 30% long-term survivors compared with a MST of 42 d following iv administration *(134)*. A similar enhancement in tumor boron uptake and survival was observed in F98 glioma bearing rats following ic infusion of the bradykinin agonist, RMP-7 (receptor mediated permeabilizer-7), and more recently called Cereport™ *(136)*. In contrast to the increased tumor uptake, normal brain boron values at 2.5 h following ic injection were very similar for the iv and ic routes with or without BBB-D. Because BNCT is a binary system, normal brain boron levels only are of significance at the time of irradiation and high values at earlier time points are inconsequential. These studies have shown that a significant therapeutic gain can be achieved by optimizing boron drug delivery, and this should be important for both ongoing and future clinical trials using BPA and/or BSH.

Direct Intracerebral Delivery

Different strategies may be required for other low-molecular-weight boron containing compounds whose uptake is cell cycle dependent, such as boron containing nucleosides, where continuous administration over a period of days may be required. We recently have reported that direct it injection or CED of the borononucleoside N5-2OH (**cpd 5**) were both effective in selectively delivering potentially therapeutic amounts of boron to rats bearing intracerebral implants of the F98 glioma *(60)*. Direct it injection or CED most likely will be necessary for a variety of high-molecular-weight delivery agents such as boronated MAbs and ligands such as EGF *(129,134)*, as well as for low-molecular-weight agents such as nucleosides and porphyrins *(134)*. Recent studies have shown that CED of a boronated porphyrin derivative similar to **cpd 7**, designated H_2DCP, resulted in the highest tumor boron values and T:Br and T:Bl ratios that we have seen with any of the boron agents that we have ever studied *(135)*.

NEUTRON SOURCES FOR BNCT

Nuclear Reactors

Neutron sources for BNCT currently are limited to nuclear reactors and in the present section we will only summarize information that is described in more detail in a recently published review *(138)*. Reactor derived neutrons are classified according to their energies as thermal ($E_n < 0.5$ eV), epithermal (0.5 eV $< E_n < 10$ keV), or fast ($E_n > 10$ keV). Thermal neutrons are the most important for BNCT because they usually initiate the $^{10}B(n, \alpha)^7Li$ capture reaction. However, because thermal neutrons have a limited depth of penetration, epithermal neutrons, which lose energy and fall into the thermal range as they penetrate tissues, are now preferred for clinical therapy. A number of reactors with very good neutron beam quality have been developed and currently are being used clinically. These include: (1) Massachusetts Institute of Technology Research Reactor, shown schematically in Fig. 2 *(139)*; (2) the FiR1 clinical reactor in Helsinki, Finland *(140)*; (3) R2-0 High Flux Reactor (HFR) at Petten in the Netherlands *(141)*; (4) LVR-15 reactor at the Nuclear Research Institute (NRI) in Rez, Czech Republic *(142)*; (5). Kyoto University Research Reactor (KURR) in Kumatori, Japan *(143)*; (6) JRR4 at the Japan Atomic Energy Research Institute (JAERI) *(144)*; (7) the RA-6 CNEA reactor in Bariloche, Argentina *(145)*; and (8) until June 2005, the R2-0 clinical reactor, operated by a private company Studsvik Medical AB in Sweden *(146)*. Other reactor facilities are being designed, notably the TAPIRO reactor *(147)* at the Ente Nazionale Energia Atomica (ENEA) Casaccia Center near Rome, Italy, which is unique in that it will be a low-power fast-flux reactor, and a facility in Beijing, China, which will be used exclusively for BNCT *(148)*. This reactor will have a power of 30 kW and currently is under construction adjacent to the "401" hospital in a southwestern suburb of Beijing. Two reactors that have been used in the

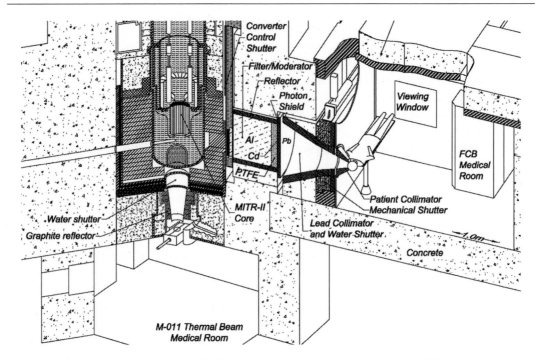

Fig. 2. Schematic diagram of the Massachusetts Institute of Technology Reactor (MITR). The fission converter based epithermal neutron irradiation (FCB) facility is housed in the experimental hall of the MITR and operates in parallel with other user applications. The FCB contains an array of 10 spent MITR-II fuel elements cooled by forced convection of heavy water coolant. A shielded horizontal beam line contains an aluminum and Teflon® filter-moderator to tailor the neutron energy spectrum into the desired epithermal energy range. A patient collimator defines the beam aperture and extends into the shielded medical room to provide circular apertures ranging from 16 to 8 cm in diameter. The in-air epithermal flux for the available field sizes ranges from 3.2 to 4.6×10^9 n /cm^2 s at the patient position. The measured specific absorbed doses are constant for all field sizes and are well below the inherent background of 2.8×10^{-12} RBE Gy cm^2/n produced by epithermal neutrons in tissue. The dose distributions achieved with the FCB approach the theoretical optimum for BNCT.

past for clinical BNCT are the Musashi Institute of Technology (MuITR) reactor in Japan *(149)* and the Brookhaven Medical Research Reactor (BMRR) at the Brookhaven National Laboratory (BNL) in Upton, Long Island, New York *(150)*. The MuITR was used by Hatanaka *(149)* and later by Hatanaka and Nakagawa *(151)*. The BMRR was used for the clinical trial that was conducted at the Brookhaven National Laboratory between 1994 and 1999 *(28,152)* and the results are described in detail later in this section. For many reasons reasons, including the cost of maintaining the BMRR, it has been deactivated and is no longer available for use.

Reactor Modifications

Two approaches are being used to modify reactors for BNCT. The first or direct approach, is to moderate and filter neutrons that are produced in the reactor core. The second, the fission converter-plate approach, is indirect in that neutrons from the reactor core create fissions within a converter-plate that is adjacent to the moderator assembly, and these moderated neutrons produce a neutron beam at the patient port. The MITR (Fig. 2), which utilizes a fission converter-plate, currently sets the standard in the world for the combination of high neutron beam quality and short treatment time *(153)*. It operates at a power of 5 megawatts (MW) and has been used for clinical as well as experimental studies for BNCT. Although the power is high compared with the majority of other reactors that are being used, the treatment time is unusually short because it utilizes a fission converter-plate to create the neutron beam. All other reactors use the direct approach to produce neutron beams for BNCT. Three examples are the FiR1 reactor in Finland *(140)*, the Studsvik reactor in Sweden *(146)*, and the Washington State University (WSU) reactor in the United States *(154)*, which was built for the treatment of both small and large experimental animals.

Accelerators

Accelerators also can be used to produce epithermal neutrons and accelerator based neutron sources (ABNSs) are being developed in a number of countries *(155–161)*, and interested readers are referred to a recently published detailed review on this subject *(162)*. For ABNSs, one of the more promising nuclear reactions involves bombarding a ^{7}Li target with 2.5 MeV protons. The average energy of the neutrons that are produced is 0.4 MeV and the maximum energy is 0.8 MeV. Reactor derived fission neutrons have greater average and maximum energies than those resulting from the ^{7}Li(p,n)^{7}Be reaction. Consequently, the thickness of the moderator material that is necessary to reduce the energy of the neutrons from the fast to the epithermal range is less for an ABNS than it is for a reactor. This is important because the probability that a neutron will be successfully transported from the entrance of the moderator assembly to the treatment port decreases as the moderator assembly thickness increases. As a result of lower and less widely distributed neutron source energies, ABNSs potentially can produce neutron beams with an energy distribution that is equal to or better than that of a reactor. However, reactor derived neutrons can be easily collimated, while on the other hand, it may not be possible to achieve good collimation of ABNSs neutrons at reasonable proton beam currents. The necessity of good collimation for the effective treatment of GBM is an important and unresolved issue that may affect usefulness of ABNSs for BNCT. ABNSs also are compact enough to be sited in hospitals, thereby allowing for more effective, but technically more complicated, procedures to carry out BNCT. However, to date, no ABNSs have been constructed which can be sited in a hospital and that provide a current of sufficient magnitude to treat patients in less than 30 min with a beam quality comparable to that of the MITR. Furthermore, issues relating to target manufacture and cooling must be solved before ABNS become a reality. The ABNS that is being developed at the University of Birmingham in England, by modifying a Dynamitron linear electrostatic accelerator *(155)*, may be the first facility where patients will be treated, although progress has been slow. Another ABNSs is being constructed by LINAC Systems, Inc. in Albuquerque, New Mexico *(163)*, and this could be easily sited in a hospital and produce an epithermal neutron beam.

Beam Optimization

For both reactors and ABNSs, a moderator assembly is necessary to reduce the energy of the neutrons to the epithermal range. The neutrons comprising the neutron beam have a distribution of energies and are accompanied by unwanted X-rays and γ photons. A basic tenet of BNCT is that the dose of neutrons delivered to the target volume should not exceed the tolerance of normal tissues, and this applies to neutron beam design, as well as to treatment planning *(25)*. The implications of this for beam design is that the negative consequences of increased normal tissue damage for more energetic neutron beams at shallow depths outweighs the benefits of more deeply penetrating energetic neutrons. For fission reactors, the average energy of the neutrons produced is approx 2 MeV, but small numbers have energies as high as 10 MeV. There is generally a trade off between treatment time and the optimum beam for patient treatment in terms of the energy distribution of the neutrons and the contamination of the neutron beam with X-rays and γ photons. Not surprisingly, reactors with the shortest treatment time (i.e., the highest normal tissue dose rate) operate at the highest power, because the number of neutrons that is produced per unit time is proportional to the power, measured in MW. Furthermore, high beam quality is most easily achieved using reactors with high power, because a larger fraction of the neutrons can be filtered, as the neutrons traverse the moderator assembly without making the treatment time exceedingly long.

CLINICAL STUDIES OF BNCT FOR BRAIN TUMORS

Early Trials

Although the clinical potential of BNCT was recognized in the 1930s (164), it was not until the 1950s that the first clinical trials were initiated by Farr at the BNL (34) and by Sweet and Brownell at the Massachusetts General Hospital (MGH) using the MIT reactor (35,165, 166). The disappointing outcomes of these trials, which ended in 1961, were carefully analyzed by Slatkin (167). These were primarily attributable to: (1) inadequate tumor specificity of the inorganic boron chemicals that had been used as capture agents, (2) insufficient tissue penetrating properties of the thermal neutron beams, and (3) high blood–boron concentrations that resulted in excessive damage to normal brain vasculature and to the scalp (35,165,166).

Japanese Clinical Trials

Clinical studies were resumed by Hatanaka in Japan in 1967, following a 2-yr fellowship in Sweet's laboratory at the MGH, using a thermal neutron beam and BSH, which had been developed as a boron delivery agent by Soloway at the MGH (37). In Hatanaka's procedure (149,151), as much of the tumor was surgically removed as possible ("debulking"), and at some time thereafter, BSH was administered by a slow infusion, usually intra-arterially (149), but later intravenously (151). Twelve to 14 h later, BNCT was carried out at one or another of several different nuclear reactors. Because thermal neutrons have a limited depth of penetration in tissue, this necessitated reflecting the skin and raising the bone flap in order to directly irradiate the exposed brain. This eliminated radiation damage to the scalp and permitted treatment of more deep-seated residual tumors. As the procedure evolved over time, a ping-pong ball or silastic sphere was inserted into the resection cavity to create a void space in order to improve neutron penetration into deeper regions of the tumor bed and adjacent brain (149,151,168,169). This is a major difference between the procedure carried out by Hatanaka, Nakagawa, and other Japanese neurosurgeons and the BNCT protocols that have been carried out in the United States and Europe. The latter have utilized epithermal neutron beams that have not required reflecting the scalp and raising the bone flap at the time of irradiation. This has made it difficult to directly compare the Japanese clinical results with those obtained elsewhere. This continued until very recently, when the Japanese started using epithermal neutron beams. Most recently, Miyatake et al. have initiated a clinical study utilizing the combination of BSH and BPA, both of which were administered iv at 12 h and 1 h, respectively, prior to irradiation with an epithermal neutron beam (32). A series of 11 patients with HGG have been treated, and irrespective of the initial tumor volume, magnetic resonance imaging (MRI) and computed tomography (CT) images showed a 17 to 51% reduction in tumor volume and this reached a maximum of 30 to 88% (Fig. 3). However, the survival times

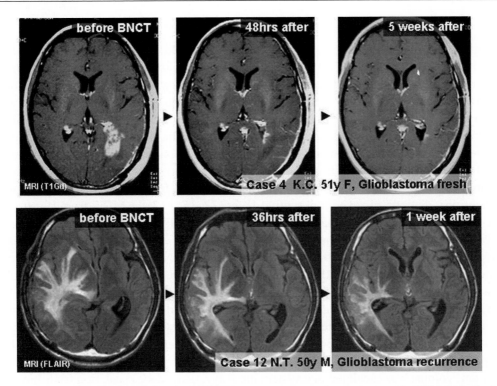

Fig. 3. Radiographic changes following BNCT in two representative patients with GBM. In both, there was a reduction in both mass and peritumoral edema without the administration of corticosteroids or mannitol within a few days. This is also shown in the FLAIR image of Case no. 12.

of these patients were not improved over historical controls and further studies are planned to optimize the dosing and delivery of BPA and BSH.

Analysis of the Japanese Clinical Results

Retrospective analysis of subgroups of patients treated in Japan by Hatanaka and Nakagawa *(168,169)* have described 2-, 5-, and 10-yr survival rates (11.4, 10.4, and 5.7%, respectively) that were significantly better than those observed among patients treated with conventional, fractionated, external beam photon therapy. However, a cautionary note was sounded by Laramore and Spence *(170)* who analyzed the survival data of a subset of 12 patients from the United States who had been treated by Hatanaka between 1987 and 1994. They concluded that there were no differences in their survival times compared with those of age matched controls, analyzed according to the stratification criteria utilized by Curran et al. *(6)*. In a recent review of Hatanaka's clinical studies, Nakagawa reported that the physical dose from the $^{10}B(n, \alpha)^7Li$ reaction, delivered to a target point 2 cm beyond the surgical margin, correlated with survival *(169)*. For 66 patients with GBMs, those who survived less than 3 yr ($n = 60$) had a minimum target point dose of 9.5 ± 5.9 Gy, whereas those who survived for more than 3 yr ($n = 6$) had a minimum target point dose of 15.6 ± 3.1 Gy from the $^{10}B(n, \alpha)^7Li$ reaction *(169)*. The boron concentrations in brain tissue at the target point, which are required to calculate the physical radiation dose attributable to the $^{10}B(n, \alpha)^7Li$ capture reaction, were estimated to be 1.2 times that of the patient's blood–boron concentration *(171)*.

Other Recent and Ongoing Clinical Trials

Beginning in 1994 a number of clinical trials, summarized in Table 2, were initiated in the United States and Europe. These marked a transition from low energy thermal neutron irradiation to the use of higher energy epithermal neutron beams with improved tissue penetrating properties, which obviated the need to reflect skin and bone flaps prior to irradiation. Until recently, the procedure carried out in Japan required neurosurgical intervention immediately prior to irradiation, whereas the current epithermal neutron-based clinical protocols are radiotherapeutic procedures, performed several weeks after debulking surgery and without the need for this. Clinical trials for patients with brain tumors were initiated at a number of locations including: (1) the BMR at BNL from 1994 to 1999 for GBM using BPA with one or two neutron radiations, given on consecutive days *(172–174)*; (2) the MITR from 1996 to 1999 for GBM and intracerebral melanoma *(175,176)*; (3) the HFR, Petten, The Netherlands and the University of Essen in Germany in 1997 using BSH *(177)*; (4) the FiR1 at the Helsinki University Central Hospital *(140)* from 1999 to the present; (5) the Studsvik reactor facility in Sweden from 2001 to June 2005, carried out by the Swedish National Neuro-Oncology Group *(146)* and finally, (6) the NRI reactor in Rez, Czech Republic by Tovarys using BSH *(178)*. The number of patients treated in this study is small and the followup is still rather short.

Initially clinical studies using epithermal neutron beams were primarily phase I safety and dose-ranging trials and a BNCT dose to a specific volume or critical region of the normal brain was prescribed. In both the BNL and the Harvard/MIT clinical trials, the peak dose delivered to a 1 cm^3 volume was escalated in a systematic way. As the dose escalation trials have progressed, the treatments have changed from single-field irradiations or parallel opposed irradiations, to multiple non-coplanar irradiation fields, arranged in order to maximize the dose delivered to the tumor. A consequence of this approach has been a concomitant increase in the average doses delivered to normal brain. The clinical trials at BNL and Harvard/MIT using BPA and an epithermal neutron beam in the USA have now been completed.

Analysis of the Brookhaven and MIT Clinical Results

The BNL and Harvard/MIT studies have provided the most detailed data relating to normal brain tolerance following BNCT. A residual tumor volume of 60 cm^3 or greater lead to a greater incidence of acute CNS toxicity. This primarily was related to increased intracranial pressure, resulting from tumor necrosis and the associated cerebral edema *(179)*. The most frequently observed neurological side effect associated with the higher radiation doses, other than the residual tumor volume-related effects, was radiation related somnolence. This is a well recognized effect following whole brain photon irradiation, especially in children with leukemia or lymphoma, who have received CNS irradiation. However, somnolence is not a very well-defined radiation related endpoint because it frequently is diagnosed after tumor recurrence has been excluded. Therefore, it is not particularly well suited as a surrogate marker for normal tissue tolerance. In the dose escalation studies carried out at BNL *(152,174)*, the occurrence of somnolence in the absence of a measurable tumor dose response was clinically taken as the maximum tolerated normal brain dose. The volume-averaged whole brain dose and the incidence of somnolence increased significantly as the BNL and Harvard/MIT trials progressed. The volume of tissue irradiated has been shown to be a determining factor in the development of side effects *(180,181)*. Average whole brain doses greater than 5.5 Gy(w) were associated with somnolence in the trial carried out at BNL, but not in all of the patients in the Harvard/ MIT study *(175,182)*. The BNL and Harvard/MIT trials were completed in 1999. Both pro-

Table 2
Summary of Current or Recently Completed Clinical Trials of BNCT for the Treatment of GBM

Facility	No. of patients	Duration of administration	Drug	Dose (µg/kg)	Boron concentration[a] (µg ^{10}B/g)	Estimated peak normal brain dose [Gy(w)]	Average normal brain dose [Gy(w)][h]	Ref.
HTR, MuITR, JRR, KURR, Japan (1968–2003)	>200	1 h	BSH	100	~20–30	15 Gy[b] ^{10}B component	ND	157,158
HFR, Petten, The Netherlands (1997–2001)	26	100 mg/kg/min	BSH	100	30[c]	8.6–11.4 Gy[d] ^{10}B component	ND	166
LVR-15, Rez, Czech Republic (2001–pres)	5	1 h	BSH	100	~20–30	<14.2 ^{10}B component	<2	167
BMRR Brookhaven, USA (1994–1999)	53	2 h	BPA	250–330	12–16	8.4–14.8	1.8–8.5	141,168
MITR-II, M67 MIT, USA (1996–1999)	20[e]	1–1.5 h	BPA	250–350	10–12	8.7–16.4	3.0–7.4	165
MITR-II, FCB MIT, USA (2001)	6	1.5 h	BPA	350	~15			Unpublished
Fir 1, Helsinki Finland (1999–pres) protocol P-01	18	2 h	BPA	290–400	12–15	8–13.5	3–6	130
Fir 1, Helsinki Finland (2001–pres)[g] protocol P-03	3	2 h	BPA	290	12–15	<8	2–3	130
R2-0 Studsvik AB Sweden (2001–2005)	17(30)[f]	6 h	BPA	900	24 (range: 15–34)	7.3–15.5	3.6–6.1	136

Notes: [a] During the irradiation.

[b] ^{10}B physical dose component dose to a point 2-cm deeper than the air-filled tumor cavity.

[c] 4 fractions, each with a BSH infusion, 100 mg/kg the first day, enough to keep the average blood concentration at 30 µg ^{10}B/g during treatment on days 2–4.

[d] ^{10}B physical dose component at the depth of the thermal neutron fluence maximum.

[e] Includes 2 intracranial melanomas.

[f] J. Capala, unpublished, personal communication.

[g] Retreatment protocol for recurrent GBM.

[h] ND, not determined

447

duced median and 1-yr survival times that were comparable to conventional external beam photon therapy *(6)*. Although both were primarily phase I trials to evaluate the safety of dose escalation as the primary endpoint for radiation related toxicity, the secondary endpoints were quality-of-life, time to progression, and overall survival. The MST for 53 patients from the BNL trial and the 18 GBM patients from the Harvard/MIT trial were 13 and 12 mo, respectively. Following recurrence, most patients received some form of salvage therapy, which may have further prolonged overall survival. Time to progression, which would eliminate salvage therapy as a contributing factor, probably would be a better indicator of the efficacy of BNCT, although absolute survival time is still the "gold standard" for any clinical trial. The quality-of-life for most of the BNL patients was very good, especially considering that treatment was given in one or two consecutive daily fraction(s).

Clinical Trials Carried out in Sweden and Finland

The clinical team at the Helsinki University Central Hospital and VTT (Technical Research Center of Finland) have reported on 18 patients, using BPA as the capture agent (290 mg/kg infused over 2-h), with 2 irradiation fields and whole brain average doses in the range of 3 to 6 Gy(w) *(140)*. The estimated 1-yr survival was 61%, which was very similar to the BNL data. This trial is continuing and the dose of BPA has been escalated to 450 mg/kg and will be increased to 500 mg/kg, infused over 2 h (H. Joensuu, personal communication). Because BNCT can deliver a significant dose to tumor with a relatively low average brain dose, this group also has initiated a clinical trial for patients who have recurrent GBM after having received full-dose photon therapy. In this protocol, at least 6 mo must have elapsed from the end of photon therapy to the time of BNCT and the peak brain dose should be less than 8 Gy(w) and the whole brain average dose less than 6 Gy(w). As of June 2005, 30 patients with primary GBM had been treated under protocol I and 10 patients with recurrent GBM have been treated under protocol II. In addition, approx 12 patients with head and neck cancer also had also been treated.

Investigators in Sweden have carried out a phase 2 BPA-based trial using an epithermal neutron beam at the Studsvik Medical AB reactor *(146)*. This study differed significantly from all previous clinical trials in that the total amount of BPA administered was increased to 900 mg/kg, infused iv over 6 h. This approach was based on the following preclinical data: (1) the in vitro observation that several hours were required to fully load cells with BPA *(182)*; (2) long-term iv infusions of BPA in rats increased the absolute tumor boron concentrations in the 9L gliosarcoma model, although the T:Bl ratio remained constant *(183,184)*, and (3) most importantly, long-term iv infusions of BPA appeared to improve the uptake of boron in infiltrating tumor cells at some distance from the main tumor mass in rats bearing intracerebral 9L gliosarcomas *(185,186)*. The longer infusion time of BPA was well tolerated *(187,188)* by the 30 patients who were enrolled in this study. All patients were treated with 2 fields, and the average weighted whole brain dose was 3.2 to 6.1 Gy(w), which was lower than the higher end of the doses used in the Brookhaven trial, and the minimum dose to the tumor ranged from 15.4 to 54.3 Gy(w). At 10 mo following BNCT, 23 of 29 evaluable patients had died with a median time to progression following BNCT of 5.8 mo and a MST of 14.2 mo. These results are comparable but not better than those obtained with external beam radiation therapy. Furthermore, they emphasize the need to improve the delivery of BPA, as well as BSH. As part of a broader plan to restructure the company, a decision was made by Studsvik AB in June 2005 to terminate operation of both the R2-0 reactor, which was used for this clinical trial, and the R2 reactor as part of a broader plan to restructure the company.

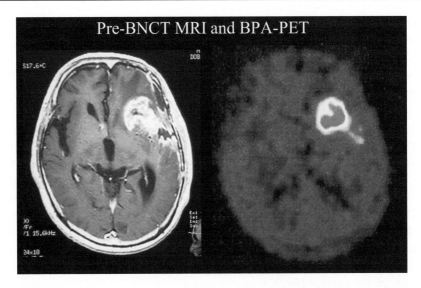

Fig. 4. Fluorine-18 boronophenylalanine images. Contrast-enhanced T1-weighted MRI of representative GBM patient and ^{18}F-labeled BPA-PET image, almost the same axial level. Patients received ^{18}F-BPA-PET to assess the distribution of BPA and to estimate boron concentrations in tumors before BNCT and without direct sampling of tumor tissue. The L/N ratio of the core of the tumor was 7.8. Note even the peripheral of the main mass (i.e., the infiltrative portion of the tumor) showed BPA uptake. The L/N ratio of BPA uptake can be estimated from this study and dose planning was done according to this L/N ratio. If the L/N ratio was more than 2.5 then BNCT was initiated. ^{18}F-BPA-PET readily gave us an accurate BPA accumulation and distribution as previously reported *(180–182)*.

Critical Issues

There are a number of critical issues that must be addressed if BNCT is to become a useful modality for the treatment of brain tumors. *First* and foremost, there is a need for more selective and effective boron agents, which when used either alone or in combination, could deliver the requisite amounts (~20 µg/g) of boron to the tumor. The superiority of the combination of BPA and BSH over either alone has been demonstrated in experimental animal studies *(31,192)*, this combination was recently used clinically by Miyatake and his co-workers in Japan *(32,193)*. Because a number of studies have shown that there is considerable patient-to-patient, as well intratumoral variability in the uptake of both BSH *(189)* and BPA *(173)*, their delivery must be optimized in order to improve both tumor uptake and cellular microdistribution, especially to different subpopulations of tumor cells. At this point in time the dose and delivery of these drugs have yet to be optimized, but based on experimental animal data *(30,31,33,132–135)*, improvement in dosing and delivery could have a significant impact on increasing tumor uptake and microdistribution.

Second, because the radiation dosimetry for BNCT is based on the microdistribution of [10]B *(192)*, which is indeterminable on a real time basis, methods are needed to provide semi-quantatative estimates of the boron content in the residual tumor. Imahori and his co-workers *(193–195)* in Japan and Kabalka *(196)* in the United States have carried out imaging studies with ^{18}F-labeled BPA. An example of such a patient treated by Miyatake, et al. *(32)* is shown in Fig. 4. ^{18}F-PET imaging also has been used as a prognostic indicator for patients with GBM who may or may not have received BNCT *(194,195)*. In the former group, it has been used to establish the feasibility of carrying out BNCT, based on the uptake and distribution of ^{18}F-BPA within the tumor, and in the latter, to monitor the response to therapy. The possibility of using MRI for either ^{10}B or ^{11}B has been under investigation *(197)*, and this may prove to be useful for real time localization of boron in residual tumor prior to BNCT. Magnetic resonance spectroscopy (MRS) and magnetic resonance spectroscopic imaging (MRSI) also may be useful for monitoring the response to therapy *(198)*. Kojimoto and Miyatake et al. recently have used MRS to analyze the target specificity of BPA and the effects of BNCT in a group of 6 patients using multivoxel proton MRS *(199)*. There was a reduction in the choline/creatine ratio without a reduction of the N-acetlylaspartate/creatine ratio at 14 d following BNCT, strongly suggesting that there was selective destruction of tumor cells and a sparing of normal neurons *(199)*. Noninvasive procedures such as MRSI may be a powerful way to follow the clinical response to BCNT in addition to MRI. However, in the absence of real time tumor boron uptake data, the dosimetry for BNCT is very problematic. This is evident from the discordance of estimated doses of radiation delivered to the tumor and the therapeutic responses, which would have been greater than that which was seen if the tumor dose estimates were correct *(152)*.

Third, there is a discrepancy between the theory behind BNCT, which is based on a very sophisticated concept of selective cellular and molecular targeting of high-LET radiation, and the implementation of clinical protocols, which are based on very simple approaches to drug administration, dosimetry, and patient irradiation. This in part results from the fact that BNCT has not been carried out in advanced medical settings with a highly multidisciplinary clinical team in attendance. At this time BNCT has been totally dependent upon nuclear reactors as neutron sources. These are a medically unfriendly environment and are located at sites at varying distances from tertiary care medical facilities, which has made it difficult to attract patients, and the highly specialized medical team that ideally should be involved in clinical BNCT. Therefore, there is an urgent need for either very compact medical reactors, such as one that is being constructed in Beijing, China or ABNS that could be easily sited at selected centers that treat large numbers of patients with brain tumors.

Fourth, there is a need for randomized clinical trials. This is especially important because almost all major advances in clinical cancer therapy have come from these, and up until this time no randomized trials of BNCT have been conducted. The pitfalls of nonrandomized clinical trials for the treatment of brain tumors have been well documented *(200,201)*. It may be somewhat wishful thinking to believe that the clinical results with BNCT will be so clearcut that a clear determination of efficacy could be made without such trials. These will require a reasonably large number of patients in order to provide unequivocal evidence of efficacy with survival times significantly better than those obtainable with promising currently available therapy for both GBMs *(202,203)* and metastatic brain tumors *(204)*. The best hope for randomized trials are those that are in the planning stage at the Beijing Neurosurgical Institute/Tiantan Hospital (BNI) in China, The BNI is the largest neurosurgical center in the world and sees in excess of 300 new patients with HGG per year. This phase II trial initially will compare surgery followed by either BNCT, using BPA as the delivery agent, plus temozolomide or external beam X-irradiation plus temozolomide. This approach is based on recent reports from Stupp et al. showing a significant improvement (3.5 mo) in overall median survival compared with patients that had surgery followed by radiation therapy alone *(202,203)*. In the United States and Europe, such trials might best be accomplished through cooperative groups such as the Radiation Therapy Oncology Group (RTOG) or the European Organization for Research Treatment of Cancer (EORTC). Such trials will require a reasonably large number of patients in order to provide unequivocal evidence of efficacy with survival times significantly better than those obtainable with promising currently available therapy for both GBM and metastatic brain tumors.

Finally, there are several promising leads that could be pursued. The upfront combination of BNCT with external beam photon radiation has not been explored, although recently published experimental data suggest that there may be a significant gain if BNCT is combined with photon irradiation *(33)*. The extension of animal studies showing enhanced survival of brain tumor bearing rats following the use of BSH and BPA in combination administered intra-arterially with or without BBB-D has not been evaluated clinically. This is a promising approach that would require the skills and expertise of interventional neuroradiologists.

As is evident from this review, BNCT represents an extraordinary joining together of nuclear technology, chemistry, biology, and medicine to treat HGG. Sadly, the lack of progress in developing more effective treatments for GBM has been part of the driving force that continues to propel research in this field. BNCT may be best suited as an adjunctive treatment, used in combination with other modalities, including surgery, chemotherapy, and external beam radiation therapy, which, when used together, may result in an improvement in survival of patients with both primary and metastatic brain tumors. Clinical studies have demonstrated the safety of BNCT. The challenge facing clinicians and researchers in the field of BNCT is how to move beyond the current impasse. This final section has provided a road map to move forward, but its implementation is a challenge, that, if successful, could significantly improve treatment of brain tumors *(205)*.

ACKNOWLEDGMENTS

We thank Mrs. Michelle Smith for secretarial assistance in the preparation of this manuscript. Text and several figures, which appear in this article, have been published in *Clinical Cancer Research* with copyright release from the American Association of Cancer Research, Inc.

Experimental studies described in this article have been supported by the National Institutes of Health grants 1R01 CA098945 (to R.F.B.) and 1R01 CA098902 to (M.G.H.V.) and Department of Energy Grants DE-FG02-93ER61612 (to T.E.B.) and DE-FG02-01ER63194 (to J.A.C.) and the Royal G. and Mae H. Westaway Family Memorial Fund at the Massachusetts Institute of Technology (to J.A.C.).

REFERENCES

1. Berger MS. Malignant astrocytomas: surgical aspects. Seminars in Oncology 1994;21:172–185.
2. Gutin PH, Posner JB. Neuro-oncology: diagnosis and management of cerebral gliomas – past, present, and future. Neurosurgery 2000;47:1–8.
3. Parney IF, Chang SM. Current chemotherapy for glioblastoma. In: Market J, DeVita VT, Rosenberg SA, Hellman S, eds. Glioblastoma Multiforme, 1st Ed., Sudbury: Jones and Bartlett Publishers, 2005;161–177.
4. Paul DB, Kruse CA. Immunologic approaches to therapy for brain tumors. Current Neurology and Neuroscience Reports 2001;1:238–244.
5. Rainov NG. Gene therapy for human malignant brain tumors. In: Market J, DeVita VT, Rosenberg SA, Hellman S, eds. Glioblastoma Multiforme, 1st Ed., Sudbury: Jones and Bartlett Publishers, 2005;249–265.
6. Curran WJ, Scott CB, Horton J, et al. Recursive partitioning analysis of prognostic factors in three radiation oncology group malignant glioma trials. J Nat Canc Inst 1993;85:704–710.
7. Lacroix M, Abi-Said D, Fourney DR, et al. A multivariate analysis of 416 patients with glioblastoma multiforme: prognosis, extent of resection, and survival. J Neurosurgery 2001;95:190–198.
8. Hentschel SJ, Lang FF. Current surgical management of glioblastoma. In: Market J, DeVita VT, Rosenberg SA, Hellman S, eds. Glioblastoma Multiforme, 1st Ed., Sudbury: Jones and Bartlett Publishers, 2005;108–130.

9. Laws ER, Shaffrey ME. The inherent invasiveness of cerebral gliomas: implications for clinical management. Intl J Devl Neuroscience 1999;17:413–420.

10. Parsa AT, Wachhorst S, Lamborn KR, et al. Prognostic significance of intracranial dissemination of glioblastoma multiforme in adults. J Neurosurgery 2005;102:622–628.

11. Kaczarek E, Zapf S, Bouterfa H, Tonn JC, Westphal M, Giese A. Dissecting glioma invasion: interrelation of adhesion, migration and intercellular contacts determine the invasive phenotype. Intl J Devl Neuroscience 1999;17:625–641.

12. Huang S, Prabhu S, Sawaya R. Molecular and biological determinants of invasiveness and angiogenesis in central nervous system tumors. In: Zhang W, Fuller GN (eds). Genomic and Molecular Neuro-Oncology, Sudbury, MA: Jones and Bartlette Publishers, 2004;97–118.

13. Parney IF, Hao C, Petruk K. Glioma immunology and immunotherapy. Neurosurgery 2000;46:778–792.

14. Ware ML, Berger MS, Binder DK. Molecular biology of glioma tumorigenesis. Histology and Histopathology 2003;18:207–216.

15. Barth RF. A critical assessment of boron neutron capture therapy: An overview. J Neuro-Oncology 2003;62: 1–5.

16. Mishima Y. Selective thermal neutron capture therapy of cancer cells using their specific metabolic activities – melanoma as prototype. In: Mishima Y, ed. Cancer Neutron Capture Therapy. Plenum Press, New York, 1996;1–26.

17. Busse PM, Harling OK, Palmer MR, et al. A critical examination of the results from the Harvard-MIT NCT program phase I clinical trial of neutron capture therapy for intracranial disease. J Neuro-Oncology 2003; 62:111–121

18. Coderre JA, Turcotte JC, Riley KJ, Binns PJ, Harling OK, Kiger III WS. Boron neutron capture therapy: cellular targeting of high linear energy transfer radiation. Technol Caner Res Treat 2003;2:1–21.

19. Sauerwein W, Moss R, Wittig A, eds, Research and Development in Neutron Capture Therapy. Bologna, Italy: Monduzzi Editore S.p.A., International Proceedings Division; 2002.

20. Coderre JA, Rward MJ, Patel H, Zamenhof RG. Proc 11th World Congress on Neutron Capture Therapy. App Radiat Isotopes 2004;61s.

21. Coderre JA, Morris GM. The radiation biology of boron neutron capture therapy. Radiat Res 1999;151: 1–18.

22. Morris GM, Coderre JA, Hopewell JW, et al. Response of the central nervous system to boron neutron capture irradiation: Evaluation using rat spinal cord model. Radiother Oncol 1994;32:249–255.

23. Morris GM, Coderre JA, Hopewell JW, Micca PL, Rezvani M. Response of rat skin to boron neutron capture therapy with p-boronophenylalanine or borocaptate sodium. Radiother Oncol 1994;32:144–153.

24. Gupta N, Gahbauer RA, Blue TE, Albertson B. Common challenges and problems in clinical trials of boron neutron capture therapy of brain tumors. J Neuro-Oncology 2003;62:197–210.

25. Nigg DW. Computational dosimetry and treatment planning considerations for neutron capture therapy. J Neuro-Oncology 2003;62:75–86.

26. Fukuda H, Hiratsuka J, Honda C, et al. Boron neutron capture therapy of malignant melanoma using [10]B-paraboronophenylalanine with special reference to evaluation of radiation dose and damage to the skin. Radiat Res 1994;138:435–442.

27. Coderre JA, Elowitz EH, Chadha M, et al. Boron neutron capture therapy for glioblastoma multiforme using p-boronophenylalanine and epithermal neutrons: Trial design and early clinical results. J Neuro-Oncology 1997;33:141–152.

28. Elowitz EH, Bergland RM, Coderre JA, Joel DD, Chadha M, Chanana AD. Biodistribution of p-boronophenylalanine in patients with glioblastoma multiforme for use in boron neutron capture therapy. Neurosurgery 1998;42:463–469.

29. Coderre JA, Makar MS, Micca PL, et al. Derivations of relative biological effectiveness for the high-LET radiations produced during boron neutron capture irradiations of the 9L rat gliosarcoma in vitro and in vivo. Intl J Radiat Oncol Biol Phys 1993;27:1121–1129.

30. Barth RF, Yang W, Rotaru JH, et al. Boron neutron capture therapy of brain tumors: enhanced survival following intracarotid injection of either sodium borocaptate or boronophenylalanine with or without blood-brain barrier disruption. Cancer Research 1997;57:1129–1136.

31. Barth RF, Yang W, Rotaru JH, et al. Boron neutron capture therapy of brain tumors: enhanced survival and cure following blood-brain barrier disruption and intracarotid injection of sodium borocaptate and boronophenylalanine. Intl J Radiat Oncol Biol Physics 2000;47:209–218.

32. Miyatake S-I, Kawabata S, Kajimoto Y, et al. Modified boron neutron capture therapy (BNCT) for malignant glioma using epithermal neutrons and two boron compounds with different accumulation mechanisms: effectiveness of BNCT on radiographic images. J Neurosurgery 2005;103:1000–1009.

33. Barth RF, Grecula JC, Yang W, et al. Combination of boron neutron capture therapy and external beam X-irradiation for the treatment of brain tumors. Intl J Radiat Oncol Biol Physics 2004;58:267–277.

34. Farr LE, Sweet WH, Robertson JS, et al. Neutron capture therapy with boron in the treatment of glioblastoma multiforme. Amer J Roentgenology 1954;71:279–291.

35. Godwin JT, Farr LE, Sweet WH, Robertson JS. Pathological study of eight patients with glioblastoma multiforme treated by neutron-capture therapy using boron 10. Cancer 1955;8:601–615.

36. Snyder HR, Reedy AJ, Lennarz WJ. Synthesis of aromatic boronic acids, aldehydo boronic acids and a boronic acid analog of tyrosine. J Am Chem Soc 1958;80:835–838.

37. Soloway AH, Hatanaka H, Davis MA. Penetration of brain and brain tumor. VII. Tumor-binding sulfhydryl boron compounds. J Med Chem 1967;10:714.

38. Hawthorne MF. The role of chemistry in the development of boron neutron capture therapy of cancer. Angew Chem Int Ed Engl 1993;32:950–984.

39. Morin C. The chemistry of boron analogues of biomolecules. Tetrahedron 1994;50:12,521–12,569.

40. Soloway AH, Tjarks W, Barnum BA, Rong F-G, Barth RF, Codogni IM, Wilson JG. The chemistry of neutron capture therapy. Chemical Rev 1998;98:1515–1562.

41. Hawthorne MF, Lee MW. A critical assessment of boron target compounds for boron neutron capture therapy. J Neuro-oncology 2003;62:33–45.

42. Olsson P, Gedda L, Goike H, et al. Uptake of a boronated epidermal growth factor-dextran conjugate in CHO xenografts with and without human EGF-receptor expression. Anticancer Drug Des 1998;13:279–289.

43. Gabel D, Foster S, Fairchild RG. The Monte Carlo simulation of the biological effect of the $^{10}B(n, \alpha)^7L$ reaction in cells and tissue and its implication for boron neutron capture therapy. Radiat Res 1987;111:14–25.

44. Srivastava RR, Singhaus RR, Kabalka GW. 4-Dihydroxyborylphenyl analogues of 1-aminocyclobutanecarboxylic acids: potential boron neutron capture therapy agents. J Org Chem 1999;64:8495–8450.

45. Das BC, Das S, Li G, Bao W, Kabalka GW. Synthesis of a water soluble carborane containing amino acid as a potential therapeutic agent. Syn Letters 2001;9:1419–1420.

46. Kabalka GW, Yao M-L. Synthesis of a novel boronated 1-amino-cyclobutanecarboxylic acid as a potential boron neutron capture therapy agent. Applied Organomet Chem 2003;17:398–402.

47. Diaz S, Gonzalez A, De Riancho SG, Rodriguez A. Boron complexes of S-trityl-L-cysteine and S-tritylglutathione. J Organomet Chem 2000;610:25–30.

48. Lindström P, Naeslund C, Sjöberg S. Enantioselective synthesis and absolute configurations of the enantiomers of o-carboranylalanine. Tetrahedron Lett 2000;41:751–754.

49. Masunaga S-I, Ono K, Kirihata M, et al. Potential of α-amino alcohol p-boronophenylalaninol as a boron carrier in boron neutron capture therapy, regarding its enantiomers. J Cancer Research and Clin Oncol 2003; 129:21–28.

50. Diaz A, Stelzer K, Laramore G, Wiersema R. Pharmacology studies of $Na_2{}^{10}B_{10}H_{10}$ (GB-10) in human tumor patients. In: W. Sauerwein, R. Moss and A. Wittig, eds. Research and Development in Neutron Capture Therapy, Bologna: Monduzzi Editore, International Proceedings Division, 2002;993–999.

51. Hawthorne MF, Feakes DA, Shelly K. Recent results with liposomes as boron delivery vehicles from boron neutron capture therapy. In: Mishima Y, ed. Cancer Neutron Capture Therapy. Plenum Press, New York, 1996;27–36.

52. Feakes DA, Waller RC, Hathaway DK, Morton VS. Synthesis and in vivo murine evaluation of $Na_4[1-(1'-B_{10}H_9)-6-SHB_{10}H_8]$ as a potential agent for boron neutron capture therapy. Proc Natl Acad Sci USA 1999; 96:6406–6410.

53. Shukla S, Wu G, Chatterjee M, et al. Evaluation of folate receptor targeted boronated starburst dendrimer as a potential targeting agent for boron neutron capture therapy. Bioconj Chem 2003;14:158–167.

54. Sudimack J, Adams DM, Shukla S, Sekido M, Tjarks W, Barth RF, Lee RJ. Intracellular delivery of lipophilic boron compound using folate receptor-targeted liposomes, Pharm Res 2002;19:1502–1508.

55. Takagaki M, Powell W, Sood A, et al. Boronated dipeptide borotrimethylglycylphenylalanine as a potential boron carrier in boron neutron capture therapy for malignant brain tumors. Radiat Res 2001;156:118–122.

56. Wakamiya T, Yamashita T, Fujii T, Yamaguchi Y, Nakano T, Kirihata M. Synthesis of 4-boronophenylalanine-containing peptides for boron neutron capture therapy of cancer cells. Peptide Science 1999;36:209–212.

57. Lesnikowski ZJ and Schinazi RF. Boron containing oligonucleotides. Nucleosides Nucleotides 1998;17:635–647.

58. Soloway AH, Zhuo J-C, Rong F-G, et al. Identification, development, synthesis and evaluation of boron-containing nucleosides for neutron capture therapy. J Organometallic Chemistry 1999;581:150–155.

59. Lesnikowski ZJ, Shi J, Schinazi RF. Nucleic acids and nucleosides containing carboranes. J Organo-metallic Chemistry 1999;581:156–169.

60. Lunato AJ, Wang J, Woollard JE, et al. Synthesis of 5-(carboranylalkylmercapto)-2'-deoxyuridines and 3-(carboranylalkyl)thymidines and their evaluation as substrates for human thymidine kinases 1 and 2. J Med Chem 1999;42:3378–3389.

61. Al-Madhoun AS, Johnsamuel J, Yan J, et al. Synthesis of a small library of 3-(carboranylalkyl)thymidines and their biological evaluation as substrates for human thymidine kinases 1 and 2. J Med Chem 2002;45:4018–4028.

62. Schinazi RF, Hurwitz SJ, Liberman I, et al. Treatment of isografted 9L rat brain tumors with b-5-o-carboranyl-2'-deoxyuridine neutron capture therapy. Clinical Cancer Research 2000;6:725–730.

63. Al-Madhoun AS, Johnsamuel J, Barth RF, Tjarks W, Eriksson S. Evaluation of human thymidine kinase 1 substrates as new candidates for boron neutron capture therapy. Cancer Research 2004;64:6280–6286.

64. Barth RF, Yang W, Al-Madhoun AS, et al. Boron containing nucleosides as potential delivery agents for neutron capture therapy of brain tumors. Cancer Research 2004;64:6287–6295.

65. Sjöberg S, Carlsson J, Ghaneolhosseini H, et al. Chemistry and biology of some low molecular weight boron compounds for boron neutron capture therapy. J Neuro-oncology 1997;33:41–52.

66. Tietze LF, Griesbach U, Bothe U, Nakamura H, Yamamoto Y. Novel carboranes with a DNA binding unit for the treatment of cancer by boron neutron capture therapy. Chem Bio Chem 2002;3:219–225.

67. Bateman SA, Kelly DP, Martin RF, White JM. DNA binding compounds. VII. Synthesis, characterization and DNA binding capacity of 1,2-dicarba-closo-dodecaborane bibenzimidazoles related to the DNA minor groove binder Hoechst 33258. Aust J Chem 1999;52:291–301.

68. Woodhouse SL, Rendina LM. Synthesis and DNA-binding properties of dinuclear platinum(II)-amine complexes of 1,7-dicarba-closo-dodecaborane(12). Chem Commun 2001;2464–2465.

69. Cai J, Soloway AH, Barth RF, et al. Boron-containing polyamines as DNA-targeting agents for neutron capture therapy of brain tumors: synthesis and biological evaluation. J Med Chem 1997;40:3887–3896.

70. Zhuo J-C, Cai J, Soloway AH, et al. Synthesis and biological evaluation of boron-containing polyamines as potential agents for neutron capture therapy of brain tumors. J Med Chem 1999;42:1281–1292.

71. Martin B, Posseme F, Le Barbier C, et al. N-Benzylpolyamines as vectors of boron and fluorine for cancer therapy and imaging: synthesis and biological evaluation. J Med Chem 2001;44:3653–3664.

72. El-Zaria ME, Doerfler U, Gabel D. Synthesis of [(aminoalkylamine)-N-amino-alkyl]azanonaborane(11) derivatives for boron neutron capture therapy. J Med Chem 2002;45:5817–5819.

73. Nakanishi A, Guan L, Kane RR, Kasamatsu H, Hawthorne MF. Toward a cancer therapy with boron-rich oligomeric phosphate diesters that target the cell nucleus. Proc Natl Acad Sci USA 1999;96:238–241.

74. Maderna A, Huertas R, Hawthorne MF, Luguya R, Vicente MGH. Synthesis of a porphyrin-labelled carboranyl phosphate diester: a potential new drug for boron neutron capture therapy of Cancer. Chem Commun 2002; 1784–1785.

75. Vicente MGH. Porphyrin-based sensitizers in the detection and treatment of cancer: recent progress. Current Medicinal Chemistry, Anti-Cancer Agents 2001;1:175–194.

76. Bregadze VI, Sivaev IB, Gabel D, Wöhrle D. Polyhedral boron derivatives of porphyrins and phthalocyanines. J Porphyrins and Phthalocyanines 2001;5:767–781.

77. Evstigneeva RP, Zaitsev AV, Luzgina VN, Ol'shevskaya VA, Shtil AA. Carboranylporphyrins for boron neutron capture therapy of cancer. Current Medicinal Chemistry: Anti-Cancer Agents 2003;3:383–392.

78. Vicente MGH, Wickramasighe A, Nurco DJ, et al. Syntheses, toxicity and biodistribution of two 5,15-di[3,5-(nido-carboranyl-methyl)phenyl]porphyrin in EMT-6 tumor bearing mice. Bioorg Med Chem 2003;11:3101–3108.

79. Miura M, Micca PL, Fisher CD, Gordon CR, Heinrichs JC, Slatkin DN. Evaluation of carborane-containing prophyrins as tumour agents for boron neutron capture therapy. Brit J Radiol 1998;71:773–781.

80. Miura M, Joel DD, Smilowitz HM, et al. Biodistribution of copper carboranyltetraphenylporphyrins in rodents bearing an isogeneic or human neoplasm. J Neuro-oncology 2001;52:111–117.

81. Miura M, Morris GM, Micca PL, et al. Boron neutron capture therapy of a murine mammary carcinoma using a lipophilic carboranyltetraphenylporphyrin. Radiat Res 2001;155:603–610.

82. Gottumukkala V, Luguya R, Fronczek FR, Vicente MGH. Synthesis and cellular studies of an octa-anionic 5,10,15,20-tetra[3,5-(nido-carboranylmethyl)phenyl]porphyrin (H$_2$OCP) for application in BNCT. Bioorg Med Chem 2005;13:1633–1640

83. Hao E, Vicente MGH. Expeditious synthesis of porphyrin-cobaltacarborane vonjugates. Chem Commun 2005;1306–1308

84. Ongayi O, Gottumukkala V, Fronczek FR, Vicente MGH. Synthesis and characterization of a carboranyl-tetrabenzoporphyrin. Bioorg Med Chem Lett 2005;15:1665–1668

85. Fabris C, Jori G, Giuntini F, Roncucci G. Photosensitizing properties of a boronated phthalocyanine: studies at the molecular and cellular level. J Photochem Photobiol B Biol. 2001;64:1–7.

86. Giuntini F, Raoul Y, Dei D, et al. Synthesis of tetrasubstitited Zn(II)-phthalocyanines carrying four carboranyl-units as potential BNCT and PDT agents. Tetrahedron Lett 2005;46:2979–2982.

87. Luguya R, Fronckzek FR, Smith KM, Vicente MGH. Synthesis of novel carboranylchlorins with dual application in boron neutron capture therapy (BNCT) and photodynamic therapy (PDT). Appl Rad Isotopes 2004; 61:1117–1123

88. Rosenthal MA, Kavar B, Uren S, Kaye AH. Promising survival in patients with high-grade gliomas following therapy with a novel boronated porphyrin. J Clin Neurosci 2003;10:425–427.

89. Rosenthal MA, Kavar B, Hill JS, et al. Phase I and pharmacokinetic study of photodynamic therapy for high-grade gliomas using a novel boronated porphyrin. J Clin Oncol 2001;19:519–524.

90. Hill JS, Kahl SB, Stylli SS, Nakamura Y, Koo M-S, Kaye AH. Selective tumor kill of cerebral glioma by photodynamic therapy using a boronated phorhyrin photosensitizer. Proc Natl Acad Sci USA 1995;92: 12126–12130.

91. Kawabata S, Barth RF, Yang W, et al. Evaluation of the carboranyl porphyrin H_2TCP as a delivery agent for boron neutron capture therapy (BNCT). Proceeding from the 13th World Congress of Neurological Surgery, Marakesh, Morocca, June 19–24, 2005.

92. Ozawa T, Santos RA, Lamborn KR, et al. In vivo evaluation of the boronated porphyrins TABP-1 in U-87 MG intracerebral human glioblastoma xenografts. Molecular Pharmaceutics 2004;5:368–374.

93. Lauceri R, Purrello R, Shetty SJ, Vicente MGH. Interactions of anionic carborylated porphyrins with DNA. J Am Chem Soc 2001;123:5835–5836.

94. Vicente MGH, Nurco DJ, Shetty SJ, Osterloh J, Ventre E, Hedge V, Deutch WA. Synthesis, dark toxicity and induction of in vitro DNA photodamage by a tetra(4-nido-carboranylphenyl)porphyrin. J Photochem Photobiol B: Biol 2002;68:123–132.

95. Ghaneolhosseini H, Tjarks W, Sjöberg S. Synthesis of novel boronated acridines and spermidines as possible agents for BNCT. Tetrahedron 1998;54:3877–3884.

96. Gedda L, Silvander M, Sjöberg S, Tjarks W, Carlsson J. Cytotoxicity and subcellular localization of boronated phenanthridinium analogs. Anti-Cancer Drug Design 1997; 12:671–685.

97. Gedda L, Ghaneolhosseini H, Nilsson P, Nyholm K, Pettersson J, Sjöberg S, Carlsson J. The influence of lipophilicity on binding of boronated DNA-intercalating compounds in human glioma spheroids. Anti-Cancer Drug Design 2000;15:277–286.

98. Giovenzana GB, Lay L, Monti D, Palmisano G, Panza L. Synthesis of carboranyl derivatives of alkynyl glycosides as potential BNCT agents. Tetrahedron 1999;55: 14,123–14,136.

99. Tietze LF, Bothe U, Griesbach U, et al. ortho-carboranyl glycosides for the treatment of cancer by boron neutron capture therapy. Bioorg Med Chem 2001;9:1747–1752.

100. Orlova AV, Zinin AI, Malysheva NN, Kononov LO, Sivaev IB, Bregadze VI. Conjugates of polyhedral boron compounds with carbohydrates. 1. New approach to the design of selective agents for boron neutron capture therapy of cancer. Russ Chem Bull 2003;52:2766–2768.

101. Tietze LF, Bothe U. Ortho-carboranyl glycosides of glucose, mannose, maltose and lactose for cancer treatment by boron neutron-capture therapy. Chem Eur J 1998;4:1179–1183.

102. Raddatz S, Marcello M, Kliem H-C, et al. Synthesis of new boron-rich building blocks for boron neutron capture therapy or energy-filtering transmission electron microscopy. Chem Bio Chem 2004;5:474–482.

103. Tietze LF, Griesbach U, Schuberth I, Bothe U, Marra A, Dondoni A. Novel carboranyl C-glycosides for the treatment of cancer by boron neutron capture therapy. Chem Eur J 2003;9:1296–1302.

104. Basak P, Lowary TL. Synthesis of conjugates of L-fucose and ortho-carborane as potential agents for boron neutron capture therapy. Can J Chem 2002;80:943–948.

105. Endo Y, Iijima T, Yamakoshi Y, Kubo A, Itai A. Structure-activity study of estrogenic agonists bearing dicarba-closo-dodecaborane. Effect of geometry and separation distance of hydroxyl groups at the ends of molecules. Bioorg Med Chem Lett 1999;9:3313–3318.

106. Lee J-D, Lee C-H, Nakamura H, Ko J, Kang SO. A convenient synthesis of the novel carboranyl-substituted tetrahydroisoquinolines: application to the biologically active agent for BNCT. Tetrahedron Lett 2002;43: 5483–5486.

107. Valliant JF, Schaffer P, Stephenson KA, Britten JF. Synthesis of Boroxifen, a nido-carborane analogue of tamoxifen. J Org Chem 2002;67:383–387.

108. Feakes DA, Spinler JK, Harris FR. Synthesis of boron-containing cholesterol derivatives for incorporation into unilamellar liposomes and evaluation as potential agents for BNCT. Tetrahedron 1999;55:11,177–11,186.

109. Endo Y, Iijima T, Yamakoshi Y, et al. Potent estrogen agonists based on carborane as a hydrophobic skeletal structure: a new medicinal application of boron clusters. Chem Biol 2001;8:341–355.

110. Tjarks W, Barth RF, Rotaru JH, et al. In vivo evaluation of phosphorous-containing derivatives of dodecahydro-closo-dodecaborate for boron neutron capture therapy of gliomas and sarcomas. Anticancer Res 2001;21:841–846.

111. Adams DM, Ji W, Barth RF, Tjarks W. Comparative in vitro evaluation of dequalinium B, a new boron carrier for neutron capture therapy (NCT). Anticancer Research 2000;20:3395–3402.

112. Zakharkin LI, Ol'shevskaya VA, Spryshkova RA, Grigorieva EY, Ryabkova VI, Borisov GI. Synthesis of bis(dialkylaminomethyl)-o- and m-carboranes and study of these compounds as potential preparations for boron neutron capture therapy. Pharm Chem J 2000;34:301–304.

113. Barth RF, Adams DM, Soloway AH, Alam F, Darby MV. Boronated starburst dendrimer-monoclonal antibody immunoconjugates: evaluation as a potential delivery system for neutron capture therapy. Bioconjug Chem 1994;5:58–66.

114. Liu L, Barth RF, Adams DM, Soloway AH, Reisfeld RA. Critical evaluation of bispecific antibodies as targeting agents for boron neutron capture therapy of brain tumors. Anticancer Res 1996;16:2581–2588.

115. Liu L, Barth RF, Adams D, Soloway AH, Reisfeld RA. Bispecific antibodies as targeting agents for boron neutron capture therapy of brain tumors. J Hematother 1995;4:477–483.

116. Novick S, Quastel MR, Marcus S, et al. Linkage of boronated polylysine to glycoside moieties of polyclonal antibody; Boronated antibodies as potential delivery agents for neutron capture therapy. Nucl Med Biol 2002;29:93–101.

117. Wu G, Barth RF, Yang W, et al. Site-specific conjugation of boron containing dendrimers to anti-EGF receptor monoclonal antibody cetuximab (IMC-C225) and its evaluation as a potential delivery agent for neutron capture therapy. Bioconjugate Chemistry 2004;15:185–194.

118. Wu G, Barth RF, Yang W, et al. Boron containing macromolecules and nanovehicales as delivery agents for neutron capture therapy. Anti-Cancer Agents in Medicinal Chemistry 2006;6:167–184

119. Carlsson J, Gedda L, Grönvik C, et al. Strategy for boron neutron capture therapy against tumor cells with over-expression of the epidermal growth factor receptor. Intl J Radiat Oncol Biol Phys 1994;30:105–115.

120. Capala J, Barth RF, Bendayan M, et al. Boronated epidermal growth factor as a potential targeting agent for boron neutron capture therapy of brain tumors. Bioconjugate Chem 1996;7:7–15.

121. Sauter G, Maeda T, Waldman FM, Davis RL, Feuerstein BG. Patterns of epidermal growth factor receptor amplification in malignant gliomas. Amer J Pathology 1996;148:1047–1053.

122. Schwechheimer K, Huang S, Cavenee WK. EGFR gene amplification-rearrangement in human glioblastoma. Intl J Cancer 1995;62:145–148.

123. Backer MV, Backer JM. Targeting endothelial cells overexpressing VEGFR-2: selective toxicity of Shiga-like toxin-VEGF fusion proteins. Bioconjugate Chem 2001;12:1066–1073.

124. Backer MV, Gaynutdinov TI, Patel V, et al. Vascular endothelial growth factor selectively targets boronated dendrimers to tumor vasculature. Mol Cancer Ther 2005;4:1423–1429.

125. Feakes DA, Shelly K, Hawthorne M. Selective boron delivery to murine tumors by lipophilic species incorporated in the membranes of unilamellar liposomes. Proc Natl Acad Sci USA 1995;92:1367–1370.

126. Carlsson J, Kullberg EB, Capala J, Sjöberg S, Edwards K, Gedda L. Ligand liposomes and boron neutron capture therapy. J Neuro-Oncology 2003;62:47–59,

127. Pardridge WM. Drug delivery to the brain. J Cerebral Blood Flow Metabol 1997;17:713–731.

128. Mendelsohn, J. Targeting the epidermal growth factor receptor for cancer therapy. J Clin Oncol 2002;20:1s–13s.

129. Nygren P, Sorbye H, Osterland P, Pfeiffer P. Targeted drugs in metastatic colorectal cancer with emphasis on guidelines for the use of bevacizumab and cetuximab. An Acta Oncologic expert report. Acta Oncologica 2005;44:203–218.

130. Yang W, Barth RF, Wu G, et al. Development of a syngeneic rat brain tumor model expressing EGFRvIII and its use for molecular targeting studies with monoclonal antibody L8A4. Clin Cancer Res 2005;11:341–350.

131. Wikstrand CJ, Cokgor I, Sampson JH, Bigner DD. Monoclonal antibody therapy of human gliomas: current status and future approaches. Cancer Metastasis Rev 1999;18:451–64.

132. Barth RF, Yang W, Adams DM, et al. Molecular targeting of the epidermal growth factor receptor for neutron capture therapy of gliomas. Cancer Res 2002;62:3159–3166.

133. Yang W, Barth RF, Adams DM, et al. Convection enhanced delivery of boronated epidermal growth factor for molecular targeting of EGFR positive gliomas. Cancer Res 2002;62:6552–6558.

134. Barth RF, Wu G, Yang W, et al. Neutron capture therapy of epidermal growth factor positive gliomas using boronated cetuximab (IMC-C225) as a delivery agent. App Radiat Isotopes 2004;61:899–903.

135. Yang W, Barth RF, Wu G, et al. Boronated epidermal growth factor as a delivery agent for neutron capture therapy of EGFR positive gliomas. App Radiat Isotopes 2004;61:981–985.

136. Barth RF, Yang W, Moeschberger ML, Goodman JH, Bartus RT. Enhanced delivery of boronophenylalanine for neutron capture therapy of brain tumors using the bradykinin analogue, Cereport. Neurosurgery 1999; 44:350–359.

137. Barth RF, Yang W, Bartus RT, et al. Neutron capture therapy of intracerebral melanoma: Enhanced survival and cure following blood-brain barrier opening to improve delivery of boronophenylalanine. Intl J Radiat Oncol Biol Phys 2002;52:858–868.

138. Harling O, Riley K. Fission reactor neutron sources for neutron capture therapy—a critical review. J Neuro-oncology 2003;2:7–17.

139. Harling O, Riley K, Newton T, et al. The fission converter-based epithermal neutron irradiation facility at the Massachusetts Institute of Technology Reactor. Nucl Sci Eng 2002;140:223–240.

140. Joensuu H, Kankaanranta L, Seppälä T, et al. Boron neutron capture therapy of brain tumors: clinical trials at the Finnish Facility using boronophenylalanine. J Neuro-oncology 2003;62:123–134.

141. Moss RL, Stecher-Rasmussen F, Ravensberg K, Constantine G, Watkins P. Design, construction and installation of an epithermal neutron beam for BNCT at the High Flux Reactor Petten. In: B.J. Allen, et al., eds. Progress in Neutron Capture Therapy for Cancer, New York: Plenum Press, 1992;63–66.

142. Marek M, Viererbl M, Burian J, Jansky B. Determination of the geometric and spectral characteristics of BNCT beam (neutron and gamma-ray). In: Hawthorne MF, Shelly K, Wiersema RJ, eds. Neutron Capture Therapy, Vol. I, New York: Kluwer Academic/Plenum Publishers, 2001; 381–389.

143. Kobayashi T, Sakurai Y, Kanda K, Fujita Y, Ono K. The remodeling and basic characteristics of the heavy water neutron irradiation facility of the Kyoto University Research Reactor, Mainly for Neutron Capture Therapy. Nucl Technol 2000;131:354–378.

144. Yamamoto K, Kumada H, Torii Y, Hori N, Kishi T, Takada J, Ohtake S. Characteristics of neutron beams for BNCT. Proceedings of the 9th Symposium on Neutron Capture Therapy, Osaka, Japan, October 2–6, 2000; 243–244.

145. Blaumann HR, Larrieu OC, Longhino JM, Albornoz AF. NCT facility development and beam characterisation at the RA-6 Reactor. In Hawthorne MF, Shelly K, Wiersema RJ, eds. Frontiers in Neutron Capture Therapy, Vol I, New York: Kluwer Academic/Plenum Publishers, 2001; 313–317.

146. Capala J, H.-Stenstam B, Sköld K, et al. Boron neutron capture therapy for glioblastoma multiforme: clinical studies in Sweden. J Neuro-oncology 2003;62:135–144.

147. Agosteo S, Foglio Para A, et al. Design of neutron beams for boron neutron capture therapy in a fast reactor. IAEA Technical Committee Meeting about the Current Issues Relating to Neutron Capture Therapy, Vienna, Austria, June 14–18, 1999.

148. Zhou Y, Gao Z, Zhu J. In hospital neutron irradiation. In: Sauerwein W, Moss R, Wittig A, eds. Research and Development in Neutron Capture Therapy. Monduzzi Editore, 2002;181–184.

149. Hatanaka H. Boron neutron capture therapy for brain tumors. In: Karin ABMF, Laws E, eds. Glioma. Berlin: Springer-Verlag, 1991;233–249.

150. Fairchild RG, Kalef-Ezra JK, Saraf SK, et al. Installation and testing of an optimized epithermal neutron beam at the Brookhaven Medical Research Reactor (BMRR). Proceedings of the Workshop on Neutron Beam Design, Development and Performance for Neutron Capture Therapy. MIT, Cambridge, MA, March 29–31, 1989.

151. Hatanaka H, Nakagawa Y. Clinical results of long-surviving brain tumor patients who underwent boron neutron capture therapy. Intl J Radiat Oncol Biol Phys 1994;28:1061–1066.

152. Diaz AZ. Assessment of the results from the phase I/II boron neutron capture therapy trials at the Brookhaven National Laboratory from a clinician's point of view. J Neuro-oncology 2003;62:101–109.

153. Riley K, Binns P, Harling O. Performance characteristics of the MIT fission converter based epithermal neutron beam. Phy Med Biol 2003;48:943–958.

154. Nigg D, et al. Initial neutronic performance assessment of an epithermal neutron beam for neutron capture therapy research at Washington State University. Research and Development in Neutron Capture Therapy. Proceedings of the 10th International Congress on Neutron Capture Therapy, 2002;135–139.

155. Beynon T, Forcey KS, Green S, Cruickshank G, James N. Status of the Birmingham accelerator-based BNCT facility. Research and Development in Neutron Capture Therapy, Proceedings of the 10th International Congress on Neutron Capture Therapy, 2002;225–228.

156. Burlon A, Kreiner A, Valda A, et al. Optimization of a neutron production target and beam shaping assembly based on the $^7Li(p,n)^7Be$ reaction. In: Sauerwein W, Moss R, Wittig A, eds. Research and Development in Neutron Capture Therapy. Monduzzi Editore 2002;229–234.

157. Kononov O, Kononov V, Korobeynikov V, et al. Investigations of using near-threshold $^7Li(p,n)^7Be$ reaction for NCT based on in-phantom dose distribution. In: Sauerwein W, Moss R, Wittig A, eds. Research and Development in Neutron Capture Therapy. Monduzzi Editore 2002;241–246.

158. Blackburn B, Yanch J, Klinkowstein R. Development of a high-power water cooled beryllium target for use in accelerator-based boron neutron capture therapy. Med Phys 1998;25:1967–1974.

159. Hawk A, Blue T, Woollard J, Gupta N. Effects of target thickness on neutron field quality for an ABNS. Research and Development in Neutron Capture Therapy, Proceedings of the 10th International Congress on Neutron Capture Therapy, 2002;253–257.

160. Sakurai Y, Kobayashi T, Ono K. Study on accelerator-base neutron irradiation field aiming for wider application in BNCT - spectrum shift and regional filtering. Research and Development in Neutron Capture Therapy, Proceedings of the 10th International Congress on Neutron Capture Therapy, 2002;259–263.

161. Giusti V, Esposito J. Neutronic feasibility study of an accelerator-based thermal neutron irradiation cavity. Research and Development in Neutron Capture Therapy, Proceedings of the 10th International Congress on Neutron Capture Therapy, 2002;305–308.

162. Blue TE, Yanch JC. Accelerator-based epithermal neutron sources for boron neutron capture therapy of brain tumors. J Neuro-Oncology 2003;62:19–31.

163. Starling WJ. RFI Linac for accelerator-based neutrons. Abstracts of the 11th World Congress on Neutron Capture Therapy. Boston, MA, October 11–15, 2004.

164. Locher GL. Biological effects and therapeutic possibilities of neutrons. Am J Roetgenol Radium Ther 1936; 36:1–13.

165. Asbury AK, Ojemann, Nielson SL, Sweet WH. Neuropathologic study of fourteen cases of malignant brain tumor treated by boron-10 slow neutron capture therapy. J Neuropathol Exp Neurol 1972;31:278–303.

166. Sweet WH. Practical problems in the past in the use of boron-slow neutron capture therapy in the treatment of glioblastoma multiforme. Proceedings of the First International Symposium on Neutron Capture Therapy 1983;376–378.

167. Slatkin DN. A history of boron neutron capture therapy of brain tumours. Postulation of a brain radiation dose tolerance limit. Brain 1991;114:1609–1629.

168. Nakagawa Y, Hatanaka H. Boron neutron capture therapy: Clinical brain tumor studies. J Neuro-Oncology 1997;33:105–115.

169. Nakagawa Y, Pooh K, Kobayashi T, Kageji T, Uyama S, Matsumura A, Kumada H. Clinical review of the Japanese experience with boron neutron capture therapy and a proposed strategy using epithermal neutron beams. J Neuro-oncology 2003;62: 87–99.

170. Laramore GE, Wootton P, Livesey JC, et al. Boron neutron capture therapy: a mechanism for achieving a concomitant tumor boost in fast neutron radiotherapy. Intl J Radiat Oncol Biol Phys 1994;28:1135–1142.

171. Kageji T, Nakagawa Y, Kitamura K, Matsumoto K, Hatanaka H. Pharmacokinetics and boron uptake of BSH ($Na_2B_{12}H_{11}SH$) in patients with intracranial tumors. J Neuro-oncology 1997;33:117–130.

172. Bergland R, Elowitz E, Coderre JA, Joel D, Chadha M. A Phase 1 trial of intravenous boronophenylalanine-fructose complex in patients with glioblastoma multiforme. In: Mishima Y, ed. Cancer Neutron Capture Therapy. Y. New York: Plenum Press, 1996;739–746.

173. Coderre JA, Chanana AD, Joel DD, et al. Biodistribution of boronophenylalanine in patients with glioblastoma multiforme: Boron concentration correlates with tumor cellularity. Radiat Res 1998;149:163–170.

174. Chanana AD, Capala J, Chadha M, et al. Boron neutron capture therapy for glioblastoma multiforme: interim results from the phase I/II dose-escalation studies. Neurosurgery 1999;44:1182–1193.

175. Busse P, Zamenhof R, Harling O, et al. The Harvard-MIT BNCT program: overview of the clinical trials and translational research. In: Hawthorne MF, Shelly K, Wiersema RJ eds. Frontiers in Neutron Capture Therapy, Vol. 1. New York: Kluwer Academic/Plenum Publishers, 2001;37–60.

176. Palmer MR, Goorley JT, Kiger WS, et al. Treatment planning and dosimetry for the Harvard-MIT phase I clinical trial of cranial neutron capture therapy. Intl J Radiat Oncol Biol Phys 2002;53:1361–1379.

177. Wittig A , Hideghety K, Paquis P, et al. Current clinical results of the EORTC-study 11961, In: Sauerwein W, Moss R and Wittig A, eds. Research and Development in Neutron Capture Therapy. Bologna: Monduzzi Editore 2002; 1117–1122.

178. Burian J, Marek M, Rataj J, et al. Report on the first patient group of the Phase I BNCT trial at the LVR-15 reactor. IIn: Sauerwein W, Moss R and Wittig A, eds. Research and Development in Neutron Capture Therapy. Bologna: Monduzzi Editore, 2002;1107–1112.

179. Coderre JA, Hopewell JW, Turcotte JC, et al. Tolerance of normal human brain to boron neutron capture therapy. Applied Radiat and Isotopes 2004;61:1084–1087.

180. Emami B, Lyman J, Brown A, Coia L, Goitein M, Munzenrider JE, Shank B, Solin LJ, Wesson M. Tolerance of normal tissue to therapeutic irradiation. Int J Radiat Oncol Biol Phys 1991;21:109–122.

181. Flickinger JC, Kondziolka D, Lunsford LD, et al. Development of a model to predict permanent symptomatic postradiosurgery injury for arteriovenous malformation. Arteriovenous Malformation Radiosurgery Study Group. Int J Radiat Oncol Biol Phys 2000;46:1143–1148.

182. Wittig A, Sauerwein WA, Coderre JA. Mechanisms of transport of p-borono-phenylalanine through the cell membrane in vitro. Radiat Res 2000;153:173–180.

183. Joel DD, Coderre JA, Micca PL, Nawrocky MM. Effect of dose and infusion time on the delivery of p-boronophenylalanine for neutron capture therapy. J Neuro-oncology 1999;41:213–221.

184. Morris GM, Micca PL, Nawrocky MM, Weissfloch LE, Coderre JA. Long-term infusions of p-boronophenyl-alanine for boron neutron capture therapy: evaluation using rat brain tumor and spinal cord models. Radiat Res 2002;158:743–752.

185. Smith D, Chandra S, Barth R, Yang W, Joel D, Coderre J. Quantitative imaging and microlocalization of boron-10 in brain tumors and infiltrating tumor cells by SIMS ion microscopy: Relevance to neutron capture therapy. Cancer Research 2001;61:8179—8187.

186. Dahlström M, Capala J, Lindström P, Wasseson A, Lindström A. Accumulation of boron in human malignant glioma cells in vitro is cell type dependent. J Neuro-oncology 2004;68:199–205.

187. Bergenheim AT, Capala J, Roslin M, Henriksson R. Distribution of BPA and metabolic assessment in glio-blastoma patients during BNCT treatment: a microdialysis study. J Neuro-oncology 2005;71:287–293.

188. H-Stenstam B, Henriksson R, Capala J, et al. Boron neutron capture therapy (BNCT) for glioblastoma multiforme: a phase 2 study evaluating a prolonged high dose of boronophenylalanine (BPA) at the Studsvik facility in Sweden. Presented at Eleventh World Congress on Neutron Capture Therapy, Boston, MA, October 11–15, 2004.

189. Goodman JH, Yang W, Barth RF, et al. Boron neutron capture therapy of brain tumors: biodistribution, pharmacokinetics, and radiation dosimetry of sodium borocaptate in glioma patients. Neurosurgery 2000; 47:608–622.

190. Hideghéty K, Sauerwein W, Wittig A, et al. Tissue uptake of BSH in patients with glioblastoma in the EORTC 11961 phase I BNCT trial. J Neuro-Oncology 2003;62;145–156.

191. Coderre JA, Chanana AD, Joel DD, et al. Biodistribution of boronophenylalanine in patients with glioblas-toma multiforme: boron concentration correlates with tumor cellularity. Radiat Res 1998;149:163–170.

192. Santa Cruz GA, Zamenhof RG. The microdosimetry of the ^{10}B reaction in boron neutron capture therapy: a new generalized theory. Radiat Res 2004;162:702–710.

193. Imahori Y, Ueda S, Ohmori Y, et al. Positron emission tomography-based boron neutron capture therapy using boronophenylalanine for high-grade gliomas: part 1. Clinical Cancer Res 1998;4:1825–1832.

194. Imahori Y, Ueda S, Ohmori Y, et al. Positron emission tomography-based boron neutron capture therapy using boronophenylalanine for high-grade gliomas: part 1. ClinCancer Res 1998;4:1833–1841.

195. Takahasi Y, Imahori Y, Mineura K. Prognostic and therapeutic indicator of fluoroboronophenylalanine positron emission tomography in patients with gliomas. Clin Cancer Res 2003;9:5888–5895.

196. Kabalka GW, Nichols TL, Smith GT, Miller LF, Khan MK, Busse PM. The use of positron emission tomog-raphy to develop boron neutron capture therapy treatment plans for metastatic malignant melanoma. J Neuro-oncology 2003;62:187–195.

197. Bendel P. Biomedical applications of ^{10}B and ^{11}B NMR. NMR Biomed 2005;18:74–82.

198. Bendel P, Margalit R, Salomon Y. Optimized ^{1}H MRS and MRSI methods for the in vivo detection of boronophenylalanine. Magnet Res Med 2005;53:1166–1171.

199. Kajimoto Y, Mitatake S-I, Kawabata S, et al. Unpublished data.

200. Perry JR, DeAngelis LM, Schold SC, et al. Challenges in the design and conduct of phase III brain tumor therapy trials. Neurology 1997;49:912–917.

201. Shapiro W. Bias in uncontrolled brain tumor trials. Can J Neurol Sci 1997;24:269–270.

202. Stupp R, Dietrich P-Y, Kraljevic SO, et al. Promising survival for patients with newly diagnosed glioblastoma multiforme treated with concomitant radiation plus temozolomide followed by adjuvant temozolomide. J Clin Oncol 2002;20:1375–1382.

203. Stupp R, Mason WP, Van Den Bent MJ, et al. Radiotherapy plus concomitant and adjuvant temozolomide for gliomblastomas. N Engl J Med 2005;325:987–996.

204. Agarwala SS, Kirkwood JM, Gore M, et al. Temozolomide for the treatment of brain metastases associated with metastatic melanoma: a phase II study. J Clin Oncol 2004;22:2101–2107.

205. Barth RF, Joensuu H. Boron neutron capture therapy in the treatment of glioblastoma: as effective, more effective or less effective than photon irradiation? Radiother Oncol 2006 (In press).

Photodynamic Therapy

Bhadrakant Kavar and Andrew H. Kaye

Summary

Cerebral gliomas are inherently invasive tumors, and the vast majority of tumors recur locally despite optimal conventional therapies. Photodynamic therapy has been used as an adjuvant therapy to help control the tumor locally. Photodynamic therapy is a binary treatment involving the selective uptake of a sensitizer by the cancer cell followed by irradiation of the tumor to activate the retained photosensitizer, thereby causing selective tumor destruction. Laboratory investigations have confirmed the selective uptake of sensitizers as well as determining the optimal therapeutic index dose of sensitizer and irradiated light. Clinical studies have shown that when photodynamic therapy is used as an adjuvant it may have significant benefit in not only controlling local disease but also prolonging tumor-free survival.

Key Words: Glioma; glioblastoma multiforme; photodynamic therapy; laser therapy; local glioma therapy; adjuvant glioma therapy.

INTRODUCTION

The biological hallmark of cerebral glioma is their extensive invasion through the brain. The tumors inevitably recur, as conventional treatments are unable to destroy the invading tumor cells with most tumors recurring within or adjacent to the original tumor bed (1,2).

Photodynamic therapy (PDT) is a form of localized adjuvant treatment. It involves a selective uptake of a sensitiser by the cancer cell, followed by irradiation of the tumor to activate the retained sensitizer causing selective tumor destruction. Laboratory studies have demonstrated the selective uptake and retention of porphyrin photosensitizers such as hematoporphyrin derivative (HpD) by cerebral glioma. The initial clinical studies of PDT were disappointing (Table 1), but these studies often utilized treatment regimes involving end-stage gliomas and doses of light irradiation that were 100-fold lower than those used in systemic tumors.

Animal studies have demonstrated both tumor selectivity of porphyrin sensitizers such as HpD and selective destruction of tumors. We have reported the results of adjuvant PDT in the treatment of high-grade gliomas (HGG) using HpD photosensitizers (3,4). There are numerous variables in the administration of photodynamic therapy, including the type of composition of sensitizer use, the dose of photosensitizer administered, the relative uptake of the sensitizer into the tumor, and the symmetry of the light used to activate the sensitizer. In this chapter we will briefly discuss the relative laboratory and clinical studies as a background for the use of PDT to treat cerebral glioma.

From: *Current Clinical Oncology: High-Grade Gliomas: Diagnosis and Treatment*
Edited by: G. H. Barnett © Humana Press Inc., Totowa, NJ

Table 1
Various Series Reporting Photodynamic Therapy of Cerebral Tumors

Study	No. of patients	Power (watts)	Total dose to tumor (J)	Dose per unit surface area (J/cm²)
Perria et al. (5)	9	0.025	—[a]	0.9–9
Perria et al. (76)	8	0.06–0.4	720–2400	—[a]
McCulloch et al. (74)	16	0.280–0.460	1620–2520	—[a]
Laws et al. (75)	5	0.250–0.400	540–1440	—[a]
Wharen et al. (77)	3	—[a]	—[a]	180 [b]
Muller & Wilson (73)	50	0.175–1.00	439–3888	8–175
Kostron et al. (78)	20	—[a]	—[a]	25–200
Powers et al. (30)	7	—[a]	658–2028	400 J/cm [c]
Laws et al. (67,75)	23	<0.200	500–1000 [d]	150–200 [e] 24–180 [f]
Laws et al.[g] (79)	31	<0.200	500–1000 [d]	150–200 [e] 24–180[f]
Origitano & Reichman (29)	15	1.0–4.0 [h]	1400–14300[i]	50[j]
Kaye et al. (3,15,16)	116	0.75–5.0	3360–12613	72–260

[a] Information not available.
[b] Derived from 100 mW/cm² for 30 min delivered by xenon arc lamp.
[c] Refers to J/cm of length of interstitial stereotactic fibers.
[d] Insterstitial stereotactic therapy.
[e] To supratentorial resection cavities.
[f] To infratentorial resection cavities.
[g] Includes patients from Laws et al.
[h] 1 W/cm for interstitial stereotactic fibers.
[i] 100 J/cm of fiber for interstitial stereotactic delivery.
[j] Based on reported 2.5 cm depth of implantation of interstitial fibers.

HISTORY

Photodynamic therapy (PDT) research has been aimed at finding the combination of ideal wavelength of light that will penetrate tissue to activate a photosensitizer that is selectively localized into the tumor. PDT was first introduced into clinical neurology by Perria et al. in 1980 with a series of nine patients with cerebral glioma who were treated with hematoporphyrin derivative and a helium neon laser (5). A brief historic account of PDT is summarized in Table 2 and a colorful yet detailed history of PDT has been reported by Daniell and Hill (6).

LABORATORY MODELS OF CEREBRAL GLIOMA

PDT has been used to kill glioma cells in vitro and in vivo. The in vitro models have included monolayer cell cultures, single-cell suspensions, and multicellular spheroids (7–9). Numerous animal models have been used to study PDT on cerebral glioma, however no animal model completely represents the human situation. Our laboratory has used the C6 glioma cell line implanted intracerebrally into rats or mice (8,10).

GLIOMAS AND THE BLOOD–BRAIN BARRIER

The uptake of a photosensitizer into glioma is at least partially dependent on the disruption of the barrier between blood and the tumor, but there are also other active processes that are,

Table 2
The History of Photodynamic Therapy

1841	Scherer	Hematoporphyrin extracted from blood.
1900	Raab	Light essential for antimalarial activity of acridine dye.
1903	Jesionek & von Tappeiner	Eosin and light used to treat human skin cancer.
1904	von Tappeiner & Jodlbauer	Oxygen necessary for photosensitization.
1913	Meyer-Betz	Self injection of hematoporphyrin causes prolonged skin photosensitization.
1924	Policard	Florescence of animal tumors due to endogenous porphyrin accumulation.
1942	Auler & Banzer	Necrosis of animal tumors using hematoporphyrin and quartz lamp.
1957	Wise & Taxdal	Exogenous hematoporphyrin concentrated in human brain tumors.
1966	Lipson	First use of photodynamic therapy in human breast cancer.
1972	Diamond	First use of photodynamic therapy in experimental glioma.
1978	Dougherty	First human trial of photodynamic therapy for systemic tumors.
1980	Perria	First human trial of photodynamic therapy for glioma.
1986	Kay	Introduction of gold metal vapour laser.
1993		Use of KTP dye module.
2001		Introduction of solid state laser.

as yet, not fully understood. The selective uptake of the photosensitizer into the tumor and not the normal brain depends on an intact blood–brain barrier (BBB). Gliomas of increasing grade are associated with increasing disruption of the BBB and destruction of the normal brain parenchyma.

High-grade cerebral glioma consists of a number of different regions, ranging from a necrotic centre to a peripheral vascular rim of proliferating tumor cells with high mitotic activity and more peripheral cells invading into the adjacent brain. The BBB is most disrupted in the peripheral rim and the oedematous brain-adjacent-to-tumor (BAT) region. It is progressively less disrupted in the less oedematous and more peripheral areas of the tumor cell invasion. The selective uptake of the photosensitizer depends upon both the disruption of the brain–tumor barrier (BTB) as well as the relative preservation of the BBB.

PHOTOSENSITIZERS

Photosensitizers are molecules that absorb and re-emit light of a specific wavelength that is unique to the individual compound. Porphyrins are naturally occurring photosensitizers whose chemical structure is based on the tetrapyrrole ring (Fig. 1). The best-known examples of porphyrin are the iron-containing molecule protoporphyrin, which binds oxygen in hemoglobin; the series of cytochromes in the mitochondrial respiratory chain of enzymes; and the plant pigment chlorophyll.

The photosensitizers most studied clinically in cerebral glioma are the first-generation agents—hematoporphyrin derivative and Photofrin® (a derivative of hematoporphyrin). Numerous other sensitizers have been investigated in laboratory studies (11). Hematoporphyrin is a complex mixture of porphyrins, the composition of which can vary depending on the method of synthesis and storage (12). The term hematoporphyrin derivative is confusing as

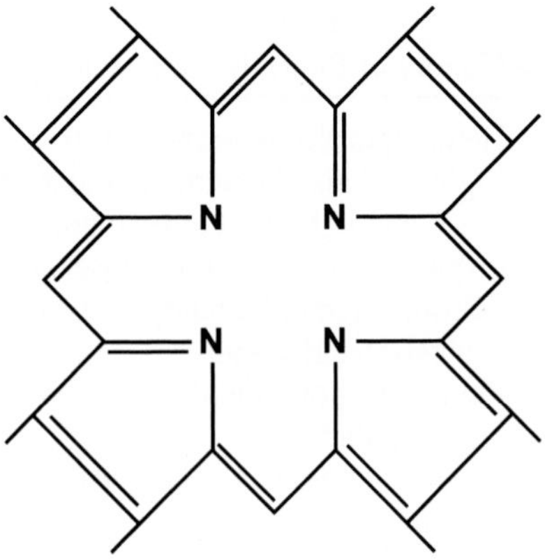

Fig. 1. A 20 sided tetrapyrrole ring that forms the basic structure of porphyrins

the compound is not a single "derivative," but rather a series of structurally related porphyrins *(13)*. Photofrin is as complex a mixture as hematoporphyrin derivative but is enriched in the tumor-localizing fraction. The names Photofrin II (Quadralogics, Vancouver, British Columbia, Canada), dihematoporphyrin ether (DHE), and porfimer sodium (Lederle, Pearl River, New York) are synonymous, but Photofrin is now the accepted term. It is highly likely that no single component of hematoporphyrin derivative is active by itself, but a series of related compounds may all be active or may act in synergy to induce a photochemical effect. A description of the chemistry of hematoporphyrin derivative and Photofrin is given by Kessell *(14)*, and outlined in Fig. 2.

The existence of multiple active compounds in hematoporphyrin derivative and Photofrin has greatly complicated scientific research because of the difficulty in identifying specific molecules with respect to their activity and site of action. The other major disadvantage of hematoporphyrin derivative and other porphyrins is that an activating wavelength of 628 nm must be used to achieve adequate tissue penetration. However, a wavelength of 628 nm is not ideal to achieve optimal absorbance by a sensitizer; 400 nm is better, but this wavelength penetrates tissue very poorly (Fig. 3). A sensitizer with an absorbance maximum in the 650- to 800-nm region would be desirable because light of these wavelengths penetrates tissue better than does light of 628-nm wavelength.

An ideal photosensitizer for PDT of cerebral tumors should have the following characteristics: systemically non-toxic, single compound, has maximal tumor-brain selectivity, is able to cross an intact BBB to reach infiltrating cells but does not enter normal brain cells, is able to undergo peak activation by light of a wavelength capable of maximal tissue penetration (650- to 800- nm), is able to accomplish maximal cytotoxic injury to tumor cells and minimal "bystander" injury, and is rapidly excreted from systemic tissue to diminish photosensitivity.

Numerous second-generation photosensitizers exist, and although all possess desirable photochemical and spectroscopic properties, not enough studies have been performed for them to displace hematoporphyrin derivative and Photofrin from clinical use (Table 3) *(7,15–23)*.

Two-second generation photosensitizers are of particular interest. Foscan (Biolitec Pharma Ltd, Edinburgh, UK) consists of only one type of molecule, temoporfin, and its pharmacology

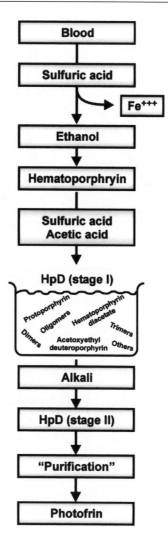

Fig. 2. A brief schematic presentation of the synthesis of first generation photosensitizer: hematopor-phyrin derivative (HpD) and Photofrin.

is better understood than Photofrin's. It is injected systemically and can cause severe photo-sensitivity, but it clears in 2 to 3 wk. Foscan however, is activated at 652 nm and is said to accumulate more selectively in tumor and absorbs light more efficiently *(24)* . The second photosensitizer, Metvix (Photocure), has met with success in Europe for skin lesions. Metvix's active ingredient is methyl aminolevulinate, a derivative of aminolevulinic acid. To-date Metvix has not been used for human intracranial tumors. Bourre et al. reported the synthesis of a new diphenylchlorin photosensitizer, 2,3-dihydro-5,15-di(3,5-digydroxyphenyl) por-phyrin (SIM01). The photodynamic properties, cell uptake, and localization of SIM01 were compared with those of structurally related meso-tetra(hydroxyphenyl)chlorin (m-THPC). Their study suggested that SIM01 would be a more powerful sensitizer than m-THPC *(25)*. There are no human trials yet to determine its efficacy.

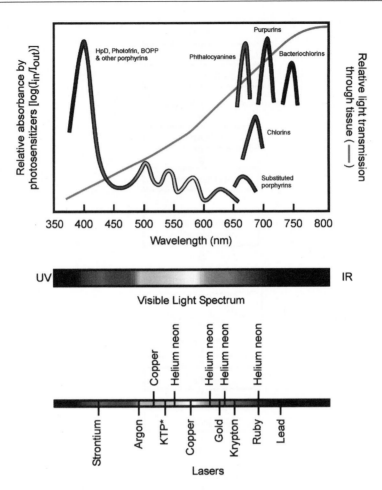

Fig. 3. Schematic relationships of absorption spectra of photosensitizers to visible light spectrum and laser wavelength. Relative light transmission through brain parenchyma is indicated by the gray line. Potassium-titanium-phosphate (KTP) laser produces light at 532 or 1064 nm: light can be transduced from 532 to 628 nm by a dye module. Reprinter with permission from ref. *97*.

TUMOR SELECTIVITY FOR PHOTOSENSITIZERS

Tumor selectivity for hematoporphyrin derivative has been demonstrated in various human tumors, and a good correlation has been noted between fluorescence and biopsy-proven cancer (Fig. 3) *(26)*. Florescence microscopy is the most direct method used to determine intracellular localization of photosensitizer, and it has been revolutionized by confocal laser scanning microscopy *(17,27)*. Microscopy and subcellular fractionation studies have generally shown exclusion of the sensitizer from the nucleus with concentration in lysosomes, mitochondria, microsomes and cytoplasm (Fig. 4).

A study of biopsy material from patients undergoing PDT for cerebral glioma in a phase I-II trial at the Royal Melbourne Hospital showed that hematoporphyrin derivative was selectively localized into all glioma grades, with a correlation between the grade of the glioma and the hematoporphyrin derivative level in the tumor (Fig. 4) *(28)*.

Table 3
Characteristics of the First– and Second–Generation Photsensitizers Used in Photodynamic Therapy of Brain Tumors

Photosensitizer	Generation	Porphyrin	Pure Compound	Clinical studies	Laboratory studies	Glioma:brain uptake ratio	Reactions and benefits	Refs.
Heamtoporphyrin derivative	1st	+	−	+	+	30:1		
Photofrin	1st	+	−	+	+	?		
Porphyrin C	2nd	+	+	−	+	1000:1	Low skin photosensitivity	15,16
Boronated protoporphyrin (BOPP)	2nd	+	+	+[a]	+	400:1	Potential for combined use of BNCT+ with photodynamic therapy	17
Purpurins	2nd	−	+	−	+		Better absorption spectra than 1st–generation agents	16
Phthalocyanines Aluminum Chloraluminum	2nd	−	+	−	+			7
Rhodamine 123	2nd	−	+	−	+	Potentially very high	A lipophilic cationic dye that localizes to mitochondria: major disadvantage is blue–green peak absorption (490–515 nm)	18
Merocyanine 540	2nd	−	+	−	+		Phase I trials done in hematologic malignancies	19
Pheophorbide	2nd	−	+	−	+		Minimal skin photosensitization	20
mTHPP	2nd	−	+	−	+		More efficacious at 100% O_2	21
TPP	2nd	−	+	−	+		A lipophilic cationic dye	22
Chlorins	2nd	−	+	−	−		Desirable photochemical and spectroscopic properties as noted in Fig. 3[b]	23
Bacteriochlorins	2nd	−	+	−	−			23
Porphycenes	2nd	−	+	−	−			23
Verdins	2nd	−	+	−	−			23
Hypericin	2nd	−	+	−	+			

[a] Studied with boron neutron capture therapy (BNCT), but not photodynamic therapy.
[b] Figure 3 reflects the relationship between absorption of sensitizer and wavelength.

467

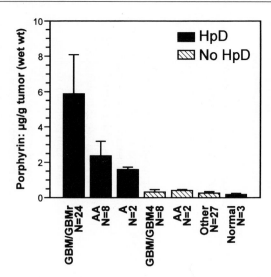

Fig. 4. Graph of hematoporphyrin derivative (HpD) concentration in human tissue samples of various grades of astrocytoma. A, diffuse (WHO grade II) astrocytoma; AA, anaplastic (WHO grade III) astrocytoma; GBM, glioblastoma multiforme; GBMr, recurrent glioblastoma multiforme. Reprinted with permission from ref. *28*.

The levels were highest in glioblastoma multiforme (GBM) (hematoporphyrin derivative tumor to brain ratio 30:1) and lower in anaplastic astrocytoma (AA) (12:1), and astrocytoma (8:1). Origitano and co-workers *(29)* have reported a clinical study investigating radioactively labeled Photofrin monitored by single photon emission computed tomography (SPECT) and also found that the concentration of sensitizer correlates with glioma grade. A separate finding in the Royal Melbourne Hospital study was that hematoporphyrin derivative was selectively localized into tumor cells in the BAT region, in some cases at higher levels than in the tumor bulk *(28)*; this has also been confirmed by others *(30)*.

At the Royal Melbourne Hospital we performed a phase I *(31)* and phase II trial with a novel boronated porphyrin (BOPP) *(32)*. We found it was tolerated well and had high specificity for the tumor. Early data appeared favorable, however a phase III trial is required.

Metronomic photodynamic therapy has been suggested as a new paradigm for PDT *(33)*. The concept is to deliver both the photosensitizer and light continuously at low rates for extended periods to increase selective tumor kill through apoptosis. Bisland et al. used rat models with 5-aminolevulinic acid (ALA) and prototype light sources and delivery devices to prove metronomic photodynamic therapy produces apoptosis in tumor periphery and microinvading colonies *(33)*.

Stylli et al. studied the uptake of photosensitizer into the tumor specimens in 104 of the 358 patients who had PDT at the Royal Melbourne Hospital. They analyzed the tumor uptake of HpD (hematoporphyrin derivative) vs the clinical outcome as confirmed by the Victoria cancer registry. Fifty-eight patients were diagnosed with GBM with the remaining 46 having AA. They found the HpD uptake was significantly higher in GBM as compared with AA. Recurrent tumors had a higher uptake than primary tumors for equivalent tumors grades *(34)*. This confirms the significant concentration of the sensitizer in tumor tissue. There was a correlation between sensitizer uptake and survival in each of the tumor grades.

Sarissky and his group showed that the photocytotoxic effect of hypericin (a second-generation photosensitizer) in glioma cells can be potentiated by diazepam. Diazepam is a nonselective ligand of peripheral benzodiazepine receptor and is said to have a role in apoptosis regulation. This combination may improve the effectiveness of photodynamic therapy *(35)*.

An in vitro study by Hirschberg and his group assessed the anti-tumor effect of concurrent ALA-mediated PDT and hyperthermia in human and rat glioma spheroids. They found PDT and hyperthermia had a synergistic effect and the degree of synergism increased with increasing temperature and light fluence *(36)*.

BLOOD–BRAIN BARRIER

Impairment of the BBB around a tumor (BTB) almost certainly has a major role in the uptake of photosensitizer. Malignant cerebral tumor in various animal models have demonstrated selective uptake of hematoporphyrin and hematoporphyrin derivative with exclusion of sensitizer from the normal brain and with accumulation in regions known to be outside of the BBB, such as the pituitary gland and area postrema *(28,37,38)*.

Photofrin, however, has been reported to cross the BBB in photoirradiated but otherwise normal brain to enter astrocytes, neurons, and endothelial cells *(39)*. These results may be encouraging because photosensitizers are likely to be more effective if they can cross normal BBB to reach the more peripheral infiltrating tumor cells, provided that the sensitizer retains the selectivity for tumor cells. In our C6 glioma model, the photosensitizers hematoporphyrin derivative and boronated protoporphyrin (BOPP) were detected within isolated tumor cells infiltrating the BAT region *(28,40)* and confocal microscopy has identified similar uptake of hematoporphyrin derivative into these nests of cells in human biopsy specimens (Hill, JS, Kaye AH: Unpublished results, 1986). This is a critical finding because it is the first unequivocal evidence that the photosensitizer is taken up into the very cells that are thought to be responsible for tumor recurrence after surgery *(2)*.

Experimental data by Ito and his team have demonstrated an increase in oedema following 5-aminolaevulinic acid PDT. This, however, was only partly counteracted by steroid therapy in the rat model they used. This raises the possibility of steroid resistant oedema as a concern to be considered during human treatment.*(41)*

SERUM PROTEIN-MEDIATED UPTAKE

Several investigators have suggested that serum proteins play a vital role in photosensitizer transport and cellular uptake. Hematoporphyrin derivative has been shown to bind to serum albumin and to lipoproteins (particularly low-density lipoprotein [LDL], which is the major serum carrier of cholesterol) *(42)*. Cholesterol is in increased demand by proliferating cells, and it is perhaps teleologically understandable that cancer cells should have elevated numbers of LDL receptors compared to those of their normal counterparts *(43)*. It has been suggested that the intracellular localization of sensitizer is mediated at least in part by LDL receptors, whereas complexes of hematoporphyrin derivative with albumin or high-density lipoprotein enter tumor by nonreceptor-mediated processes to localize in the interstitial stroma *(44)*.

EXTRACELLULAR PH

Extracellular pH is known to be lower in tumors than in normal tissue and correlates with a tissue's nutrient supply and rate of metabolism. Extracellular acidosis causes an increase in the passive diffusion of porphyrins into cells and may contribute to selective photosensitizer localization *(45)*.

MITOCHONDRIA-RELATED FACTORS

Mitochondria appear to be a major target for phototoxic damage, and their selective targeting by photosensitizers may be mediated by benzodiazepine receptor binding *(46)*. The class of lipophilic cationic dyes, of which rhodamine 123 is an example, appears to have selective mitochondrial localization related to the internal negative membrane potential of the mitochondria *(47)*.

LIGHT AND LASERS

Light

Light output is measured in watts (joules/s) and recorded at the tip of the delivery fiber. Light dose delivered to a surface is measured as energy delivered per unit area of irradiated surface (joules/cm^2). For implanted fibers, light dose is measured as joules per centimeter of length along the delivery fiber.

The penetration depth of light into tissue is defined as the depth at which the incident irradiance is reduced to $1/e$ (where e is the Euler number equaling 2.718281828), or 37%. In more practical terms, the effective depth of PDT-induced necrosis is approximately three times the penetration depth *(48)*. Direct tumor cell phototoxicity is not the sole mechanism for necrosis, and PDT-induced vascular ischemic damage certainly plays an additional role *(16,39)*.

Light penetration determines the extent of tissue damage, and both increase as a function of the following variables: (1) wavelength, increasing from 350 mm to above 800 mm (Fig. 3); (2) light dose, increasing above a threshold to a maximum value that causes damage to normal BBB and cellular elements, with or without preadminstered photosensitizer *(8,49–51)*; and (3) cellularity of tissue, increasing with the grade of tumor, up to twofold the penetration depth of normal brain *(52)*.

If a tumor contains sufficient sensitizer to mediate a photochemical reaction, the depth of tumor necrosis should largely be related to the penetration of light. However, some sensitizers are more effective than others in producing a photochemical reaction; increased doses of photosensitizer may not result in greater depth of necrosis, but they could increase the degree of cerebral edema *(8)*. The optimal wavelength for photoactivation of hematoporphyrin derivative and Photofrin is red light at 628 mm, but the penetration depth is approx 1.5 mm for normal brain and 2.9 mm for tumor *(53)*. The therapeutic depth of activity of 638-mm light is therefore only about 9 mm, 3 times the penetration depth in tumor, which is a major limitation of PDT in its current form *(54)*. Our own laboratory studies have shown a selective tumor destruction of up to 1 cm with hematoporphyrin derivative and red light in the rat model *(8)*. As assessed on computed tomography (CT) and magnetic resonance imaging (MRI) scans, the crude estimated depth of therapeutic effect of PDT has been up to 18 mm *(30)*.

Heating of cerebral tissue by microwave light could potentially occur with PDT, but this can be avoided by irrigation with normal saline at body temperature *(8)*. It has been suggested that hyperthermia is a significant component of PDT's efficacy *(55)*, but tumor destruction has clearly been shown to occur without significant heating of tissue *(8)*. Our laboratory has endeavored to study the pure effects of PDT, but in the future it is possible that hyperthermia could be used advantageously to produce a synergistic effect.

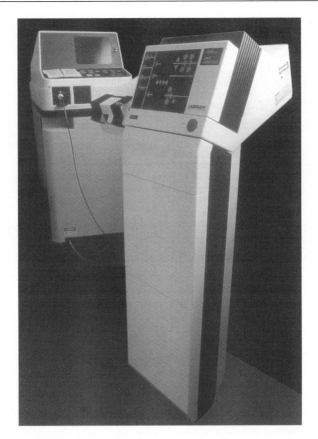

Fig. 5. The neodymium-yttrium-aluminum-garnet (YAG) potassium-titanium-phosphate (KTP) laser (background). The dye module (foreground) transduces KTP light into red 628 nm light, which is delivered through an optical diffusion fiber.

Lasers

Lasers produce high doses of light of a single known wavelength and are the most efficient method of light delivery. The power output can be accurately measured and the light can be delivered by a fiber optic cable to a tumor, either stereotactically or under direct vision *(3,30, 56)*. The laser systems used have included the helium neon, argon-ion pumped dye, and gold metal vapor lasers *(3,57,58)*. The argon pumped dye laser produces continuous light but is relatively immobile and has an ineffective coupling mechanism, which results in a significant loss of light during delivery. The gold metal vapor laser is easier to transport, produces a much higher intensity light at 627.8 mm and has the theoretical advantage of producing a pulsed rather than a continuous beam. Pulsed light may improve sensitizer activation and increase the depth of penetration, but its benefit compared with continuous laser light has not yet been proved experimentally. We have used a frequency-doubled Nd-YAG-KTP (neodymium-yttrium-aluminum-garnet-potassium-titanium-phosphate) laser to pump a tunable dye laser (Fig. 5). The KTP laser has the advantage of delivering high doses of light, the wavelength can be varied for use with different photosensitizers in the laboratory, it requires minimal maintenance, and it is easily moved from the laboratory to the operating room.

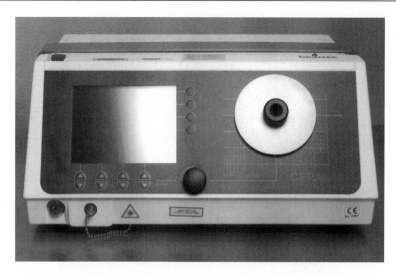

Fig. 6. The new smaller, lighter and portable Ceralas PDT 630 Diode Laser (CeramOptec GmbH, Germany)

Schmidt et al. evaluated the toxicity of PDT (using Photofrin) and a new light delivery devise based on light-emitting diode (LED) technology and tunable dye laser. Though they only treated 20 patients, all had tumor responses with mean time to tumor progression after PDT at 67 wk with minimal toxicity *(59)*.

Madsen et al. *(60)* sensitized human glioma spheroids with 5-aminolevulinic acid and subjected them to multiple treatments of sub-threshold light fluences. In all cases, suppression of tumor growth was observed for the duration of treatment and it was found that low fluence rates (≤ 5 mW/cm^2) to be more effective than high fluence rates (25 mW/cm^2)

There has been significant improvement in diode lasers making them smaller, lighter and cheaper. This provides a more stable light source for PDT. Recently, we have started using the Ceralas PDT 630 Diode Laser (Fig. 6) with a wavelength of 630 nm $\pm$ 5 nm, and a maximum optical output of 4 W (manufactured by CeramOptec GmbH, Germany); with a weight of 20 kg and dimensions of 190 mm $\times$ 430 mm $\times$ 380 mm, it is a far more mobile laser than the previous machines. The light is delivered via a flat cut 600 micron quartz fiber with SMA 905 connection. It is important that the laser has an efficient fiber delivery system that is robust, reliable, and accurate.

PHYSIOCHEMICAL BASIS OF PHOTODYNAMIC THERAPY

The photophysical and photochemical properties of photosensitizers vary markedly, but the processes leading to a photosensitizing effect are similar for all of these compounds. Following the absorption of activating light of an appropriate wavelength, the sensitizer is converted from ground state to an excited singlet state, in which no unpaired electrons are present (Fig. 7) *(61)*. The sensitizer may de-excite and lose its energy by a variety of competing pathways. From the singlet state the sensitizer can decay back to ground state and emit energy in the form of fluorescence, or it may decay down to an intermediate state from which level the sensitizer can transfer to the metastable triplet state, in which two unpaired electrons are

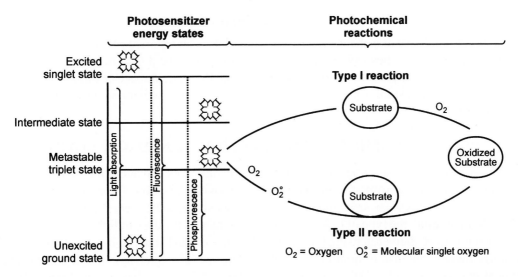

Fig. 7. Schematic presentation of photosensitizer activation by light. Energy level diagram (*left*) shows activation of the photosensitizer's electron shell from ground state and the various possible pathways of decay. A photosensitizer in its metastable triplet state (*right*) may undergo release of energy as phosphorescence or it may become involved is a type I or type II (molecular singlet oxygen formation) reaction.

present. From the metastable triplet state the sensitizer can either decay back to ground state, with the emission of energy in the form of long-lived phosphorescence, or it can participate in a series of photochemical reactions, which are designated as type I or II *(11)*. In a type I reaction, the sensitizer in its metastable triplet state reacts directly with a cellular substrate to yield a radical ion pair. In a type II reaction, the sensitizer reacts directly with oxygen to produce the highly reactive molecular singlet oxygen ($^1O_2$), and this reaction is thought to be the major mechanism of damage to biomolecules and cells following PDT. The type I and II reactions are competitive, with increases in oxygen concentration pushing the equilibrium in favor of the type II reaction; but both cause oxidation of target molecules and have an absolute requirement for oxygen.

PATHOLOGIC EFFECTS OF PHOTODYNAMIC THERAPY

Damage to sensitized tumor and brain parenchyma by PDT is observed experimentally and clinically within 48 h of photoirradiation *(30,49,50,56)*. The controversy surrounding the precise site of action of PDT has yet to be resolved. This confusion results partly from PDT's powerful ability to induce numerous cellular changes and the fact that hematoporphyrin derivative's heterogeneous nature results in variable localization and subsequent phototoxic damage due to its accumulation in numerous intracellular and extracellular sites.

Cytotoxic Damage

Experimental models of photosensitized but otherwise normal rat brain have revealed lethal injury to astrocytes, and later to neurons, occurring within 24 to 48 h of photoirradiation when high doses of sensitizer and light are used *(49,50)*. CT and MRI studies in patients treated with PDT have likewise shown the development of radiologic changes in a similar time frame *(30,56)*.

Vascular Injury

Histologic evidence of ischemic necrosis by PDT has been reported consistently in experimental and clinical studies *(39,50,57)*. Vascular injury may be a significant component of PDT and appears to explain tissue damage beyond the theoretical reach of phototoxic injury *per se*. Experimental studies have demonstrated evidence of vascular damage as early as 15 min after PDT *(62)*.

PHOTODYNAMIC THERAPY IN CLINICAL NEUROSURGERY

The use of PDT to treat gliomas in clinical practice involves consideration of a number of practical and technical problems; this has resulted in a wide variation of treatment techniques used in different series. These include the choice of sensitizer to be used, the dose and timing of its administration, the type of light irradiation system, and the dose of light and mechanism by which it is to be delivered to the tumor. The delivery of PDT must be balanced not only to optimize therapy but also to minimize possible complications, such as cerebral edema. The clinical experience with PDT at the Royal Melbourne Hospital has evolved since 1985 *(3,16,57,63)*. Our current practice is described below and is discussed with reference to other management regimens.

Preoperative Management

Patients are given routine preparation for surgery, which includes administration of dexamethasone, 16 mg/d. Hematoporphyrin derivative is administered intravenously 24 h preoperatively *(3,57)*, as our laboratory data have indicated this to be the optimal time *(38)*. The principles of hematoporphyrin derivative administration are that it should be well diluted (5 mg/kg in 200 mL of normal saline), protected from light, and given slowly over 30 to 60 min through a well-running intravenous cannula. Skin contamination and subcutaneous extravasation must be avoided, because local photosensitivity would persist for months; consequently, hematoporphyrin derivative should never be given in a dorsal hand vein. Patients are considered to be immediately photosensitive and must avoid direct or indirect sunlight for 3 to 4 wk followed by gradual desensitization, but no restriction is placed on exposure to normal indoor lighting.

Other groups have reported the use of hematoporphyrin derivative in doses from 2.5 to 5.0 mg/kg. Photofrin is usually administered at 2.0 to 2.5 mg/kg. A recent SPECT study of labeled Photofrin has reported that photosensitizer uptake into tumor varies between patients and that the timing of PDT may need to be tailored *(29)*.

INTRAOPERATIVE MANAGEMENT

Surgery

The patient is positioned as for a routine craniotomy, but additional attention is paid to the orientation of the anticipated resection cavity so that it may maximally retain the solution used for light dispersion. The tumor is approached and resected as for any craniotomy. A maximal tumor excision has been performed in all patients, usually with the aid of the CUSA (Cavitron Ultrasonic Surgical Aspirator, Cooper Laboratories, Stanford, Calif) *(3,57)*. It has been suggested that entry into the ventricular system should be avoided, but no theoretical grounds have been established for this practice, and our experience with ventricular entry has not proved to be a problem. After hemostasis is achieved, the resection bed is left in a raw state, without any haemostatic agents in situ that could potentially retard light delivery to tissue.

The surface area to be irradiated is measured, the laser power output at the optical diffusion fiber tip is calibrated and light from the fiber is directed onto the resection bed by attachment to a fixed retractor arm. The aim is to deliver between 220 and 240 J/cm² of light to the exposed tumor bed. An inspired oxygen concentration of 100% may be of value for the duration of photoirradiation (21), which has been between 12 and 94 min (median 50 min). The fiber is moved at regular intervals to cover the tumor bed and to ensure even distribution of the hot-spot emanating from the tip. The optical diffusion fiber used usually has a "flat cut" delivery end, but more recently we have used cylindrical or spherical ends. Diffuse delivery of light to the resection bed is greatly improved if resection results, as is usually the case, in a cavity that allows use of Intralipid (Tuta Laboratories, Braeside, Melbourne, Australia), diluted to 0.5%, as a light dispersion agent (58). We no longer measure brain temperature routinely, but this was monitored in the first 40 cases by a thermal diffusion cerebral blood, flow monitor on the irradiated surface (Flowtronics Inc., Phoenix, Ariz) and by a thermocouple at 2-mm depth (model RFG-3B Lesion Generator System, Radionics Inc., Burlington, Mass). Our experimental studies have shown a temperature rise within brain/tumor parenchyma of 5 to 7°C within 1 min of irradiation with a laser emitting from 800 to 1200 mW from the fiber tip (8,64). Brain temperature can easily be kept below 37.5°C by irrigation with Intralipid or with physiologic saline solutions at room temperature.

In all cases, surgical closure has involved complete dural closure and replacement of the bone flap. The total time for surgery, including PDT, has varied from 2 to 5.5 h, with a median time of 3 h (3).

Surgical Issues

STEREOTAXIS

Direct intratumoral injection of photosensitizer has been advocated for the treatment of glioma (61) but this would seem to be inappropriate, as the basis of PDT is its selectivity for tumor cells, especially those infiltrating beyond the margins of the proposed resection. The sensitizer is most likely to be effective if it can localize into infiltrating cells beyond surgical reach, and it is unlikely to do so if injected intratumorally. However, stereotactic delivery of light is particularly suitable for deeper lesions and may be effective when administered to gliomas without resection (30). Computer-assisted stereotaxy can be applied to guide resection of lesions at all depths (65) and has been reported to predict the theoretical volume of gross phototoxic damage in PDT using implanted fibers (30,56). Delayed phototoxic injury to eloquent neural structures, such as has been reported with the optic apparatus, may be reduced with this technology (30).

EXTENT OF DECOMPRESSION

Cytoreductive issues aside, we believe that a radical decompression minimizes the effects of postoperative cerebral edema that are caused by the effects of PDT on residual tumor. It is probable that PDT-induced cerebral edema increases in proportion to the amount of residual tumor bulk, because more photoirradiated tissue is available to undergo necrosis. Maximal tumor resection should therefore diminish the amount of tissue that undergoes phototoxic reactions and allow more room into which edematous brain may expand. We therefore do not advocate PDT without tumor decompression. The benefits of maximal tumor resection have been shown in a controlled animal study (66) and by Origitano and Reichman (56), who monitored postoperative and intracranial pressure in 15 patients following PDT. Powers and colleagues (30) reported clinically significant cerebral edema in their patients following stereotactic administration of light; steroids were not used and tumor mass was not resected. The use of PDT in eloquent regions of the central nervous system (CNS) would require greater selectivity of the sensitizer-light combination *(67)*. PDT of posterior fossa tumors would require careful dosimetry and has been reported in pediatric patients, including those with ependymona *(68)*. An animal study reported the use of PDT in the treatment of posterior fossa tumors *(69)*. These authors advocated lower light doses than have been used conventionally and recommended the use of intratumoral rather than intracavitary photoradiation. Being cognizant of the need to modify both surgery and photoradiation in eloquent CNS, we recommend maximal tumor resection and agree with the approach of Wharen and co-workers *(68)*, who performed gross total resections of posterior fossa neoplasms and obtained "their most encouraging results" in this small group of patients. Although not yet described in clinical practice, PDT could also potentially be used to treat spinal cord gliomas, but this would require exquisite sensitizer-light selectivity *(67)*.

LASER-TUMOR INTERFACE TECHNIQUES

Apart from Intralipid instillation into resection cavities, various surgical techniques have been used to interface light and tumor, including light shone directly onto the resection bed *(3,57)* and illumination through an inflatable balloon *(53)*. The inflatable balloon applicator adopts the shape of the resection cavity to produce a uniform distribution of light, but it is not particularly suited to irradiation of a tumor bed with a flat surface (e.g., such as occurs after a lobectomy). Interstitial laser light has been administered by stereotactic implantation of single *(30)* or multiple *(56)* optical diffusion fibers.

Light Irradiation Systems

An argo-rhodamine pumped dye laser (Spectra-Physics, model 164-05, argon laser: Spectra-Physics, model 375 dye laser; Spectra-Physics, Mountain View, Calif) was used to treat our first 18 patients. A gold metal vapor laser (Quentron, Adelaide, South Australia, Australia) was used to treat most of the remaining patients, but more recently a KTP laser (KTP/532 Laserscope Surgical Laser Systems, San Jose, Calif) has been used. A 16-W light of 532-nm wavelength is delivered from the KTP laser and transduced to 628nm by a dye module, which produces light up to 3.2 W at the fiber tip (Dye Module 600 series, Laserscope Surgical Systems). A flat-cut quartz fiber (600-µm diameter early in the series, and 1 mm in the remainder) has been used as our optical diffusion fiber, but it is unsuitable for stereotactic implantation because of excessive heating and local charring at the tip. This major technical problem has been overcome by the development of a new fiber, which allows safe use of PDT in stereotaxy *(30)*.

At present we are using a diode laser that produces a maximum of 4 W of 630 nm light at the fiber tip.

Light Dosimetry

The accuracy of light dosimetry requires further improvement and standardization so that results can be optimally compared between study groups. Output from the laser needs to be calibrated prior to every use, because minor fluctuations in power output occur. Determination of the exact dose of laser light delivered can be difficult because of inaccuracies in the measurement of the surface area, loss of light from the tumor cavity, and lack of uniformity of light distribution.

Our initial laboratory studies *(8)* showed that higher light doses could be tolerated than had been used in earlier clinical series (Table 1), and we have therefore used a light output up to 5 W *(3,63)*. In our initial experience, treatment commenced with 70 J/cm^2, and the dose has been elevated to 260 J/cm^2 without increased toxic effects. We now regularly use from 220 to 240 J/cm^2, which is considerably higher than doses reported in other published series.

Postoperative

The patient requires standard post craniotomy care with an emphasis on avoiding direct sunlight and closely monitoring not any neurologic deficit that may arise from cerebral swelling. The steroids are to be tapered far more gradually as edema is likely to be a greater problem.

Radiotherapy

There were initial concerns present about the possible interaction of postoperative radiotherapy with photosensitizer that might remain in the normal brain tissue *(70,71)*. Wharen and others *(72)* studied the in vitro interaction between X-irradiation and hematoporphyrin derivative in a rat glioma model and found potentiation of radiosensitivity only at high intracellular hematoporphyrin derivative concentrations and at large X-irradiation fraction sizes. Although hematoporphyrin derivative does not cross an intact BBB, it may remain in small vessels for some time; consequently, it has been our policy not to commence radiotherapy until 4 wk after PDT. In patients treated with conventional radiotherapy, no increase in radiation-related complications was observed *(3)*. Muller and Wilson *(73)* also reported no increased toxic effects in 17 patients treated with higher doses of postoperative radiotherapy.

Side Effects

Cerebral Edema

Cerebral edema has been reported as a clinical complication of PDT despite perioperative steroid administration *(73,74)*, although, in our experience, this can be easily controlled with steroid therapy *(3,63)*. Our patients receive 16 mg/d of dexamethasone preoperatively (32 mg the first postoperative day and then a slowly tapering dose over 2 wk). It has been suggested that more than 12 mg of dexamethasone/d may affect the BTB and may result in diminished photosensitizer uptake *(29)*, but in studies of the rat C6 glioma model we have noted no effect of steroids on hematoporphyrin derivative uptake except at very high doses of steroid (Megison PD, Hill JS, Kaye AH: Unpublished observations, 1985). Laws and co-workers *(75)* suggested that the avoidance of tissue heating during PDT prevented post-therapy cerebral edema, but this has not been confirmed by others *(53,73)*.

Skin Photosensitization

Hematoporphyrin derivative and Photofrin both accumulate in the skin to cause photosensitization. Our initial instructions to patients are to remain out of direct sunlight for 4 to 6 wk, depending on the time of year. Skin testing is then performed to determine if direct sunlight can be tolerated, and the patients are instructed to gradually increase their daily exposure to the sun.

The longest period of significant sensitization has lasted 18 wk with a median period of 7 wk. Various strategies have been suggested to reduce skin photosensitivity from the currently available drugs, including administration of lower doses of sensitizer and co-administration of carotene-containing substances. It is likely that the second-generation photosensitizers will produce less skin photosensitization.

Imaging Studies

Radiologic testimony to the efficacy of PDT in malignant glioma has been reported by Powers and co-workers *(30)*. In this series, light was delivered stereotactically without tumor resection and produced CT and MRI evidence of tumor destruction at 24 h, evidenced by loss of contrast enhancement of the treated volume. New contrast enhancement appeared peripherally, presumably corresponding to phototoxic damage to the BAT region, and has been reported to persist for up to 3 mo on MRI *(56)*. Of note is that when the tumor recurred, it did so outside the stereotactically targeted volume of treatment *(30, 56)*.

CLINICAL SERIES

PDT has been evaluated as a form of adjuvant treatment for malignant cerebral tumors by a number of investigators; these series are summarized in Table 1 and include updates of the Royal Melbourne Hospital series *(3,5,30,56,63,68,73–79)*. Overall assessment of the reported series is difficult because of the wide variation of techniques, extent of resection, doses of photosensitizer and light, and types of cerebral tumor. Most of the series have been small, and length of follow-up has been short. The majority of tumors have been high-grade or recurrent gliomas, but most reports have included small numbers of metastatic tumors, and, more recently, our group has been treating patients with low-grade gliomas. The clinical results in the initial series were disappointing because recurrent HGG were the predominant tumors treated, and the doses of light used were up to 100 times lower than were used in systemic tumors *(5,66,74,75)*. Lower light doses were used because of the lack of availability of powerful light-producing sources and also because of the fear of side effects of PDT in high doses, particularly when combined with X-ray therapy *(71)*.

In the Royal Melbourne Hospital series, a total of 358 patients with cerebral glioma have been treated with 5 mg/kg of hematoporphyrin derivative and up to 260 J/cm^2 of red light at 628 nm. Initially only patients with glioblastoma multiforme were selected for treatment, but patients with lower grade tumors have more recently been included following the observation that sensitizer was also selectively retained in astrocytoma and AA *(28)*. Twenty-eight patients have had re-treatment with PDT when the tumor recurred. In our most recent analysis of patients resident in the State of Victoria and followed up through the Victorian Cancer register, the median survival for patients with GBM was 14.3 mo, and 25% of patients survived beyond 3 yr. The median survival for patients with recurrent GBM was 14 mo, and 37% survived 3 yr. A historically matched control group of 100 patients with GBM at the Royal Melbourne Hospital had a median survival of 8 mo, and no patient survived longer than 3 yr. Median survival with AA is 76.5 mo *(4)*. One serious complication directly from PDT occurred in the Royal Melbourne Hospital study, involving severe cerebral swelling after PDT for recurrent GBM resulting in death of the patient. In addition, one patient died from an acute myocardial infarction and another suffered hemiplegia after resection of a medial temporal lobe GBM.

Schmidt et al. *(59)* used Photofrin as a sensitizer with direct LED exposure or LED with a balloon adapter. They found the treatment was tolerated well near the eloquent area and in the posterior fossa.

In the series of Muller and Wilson *(73)* of patients with malignant supratentorial tumors, median survival time was 6.3 mo for 50 patients with newly diagnosed GBM *(73)*. This median survival was shorter than that of the Royal Melbourne Hospital series, and may have resulted from the lower doses of light used (8 to 175 J/cm^2; median 27 J/cm^2 at the other centers. Muller and Wilson noted no significant difference in median survival between the group of patients who received a total dose greater than 1400 J and those who received less than 1400 J, but the higher light dose group did have a greater proportion of 1- and 2-yr survivors.

In 18 patients (12 with GBM, 5 with AA, and 1 with malignant ependymoma) the light dose was delivered in 3 groups of 6 patients each: 1500 to 700 J, 3700 to 5500 J, and 4400 to 5900 J *(80)*. Krishnamurthy et al. found that increasing the light dose increased the neruologic deficit but did not improve survival or time to tumor recurrence *(80)*.

Wharen and colleagues *(68)* reported a median survival of 10 mo for 6 patients with recurrent malignant glioma treated with interstitial PDT. Sixteen other patients with recurrent malignant glioma had a mean survival of 11 mo after resection and intracavitary PDT, but it should be noted that this figure was quoted with respect to 8 patients who died. This group also described posterior fossa tumors, including ependymoma, that have been treated with lower doses of light than had been used for supratentorial tumors (68,79). No complications were noted following gross total resection of tumor, and the therapy was well tolerated.

The initial results of the larger clinical studies of PDT for the treatment of glioma do show a favorable trend, particularly in the percentage of patients with long-term survival. However, no phase III clinical trials have yet been undertaken, and it is therefore not possible to draw absolute conclusions concerning the efficacy of PDT *(81)*.

THERAPY FOR BRAIN TUMORS OTHER THAN GLIOMA

Little experience is available regarding the role of PDT and non-glioma cerebral tumors. Theoretically PDT would be suitable for cerebral metastases as local recurrence can be controlled with surgery and adjuvant radiotherapy *(79)*.

Unresected metastatic malignant melanoma has been reported to be more resistant to intratumoral PDT than gliomas *(30)*, although we recommend that PDT should be delivered after gross tumor resection is possible.

PDT has been advocated for recurrent meningioma involving posterior sagittal sinus where they cannot be resected completely *(68)*. Stereotactic PDT has been used to manage cystic craniopharyngioma over the instillation of radionuclide because light can be effectively attenuated by the cyst wall *(68,79)*.

PDT for brain stem gliomas has not been described clinically but could potentially be used. This would require exquisite selectivity *(82)*.

FUTURE APPLICATIONS

The clinical application of PDT for the treatment of gliomas is still in its infancy. Improvements in PDT will depend on obtaining an understanding of tumor biology and of the basic sciences (i.e., physics, chemistry), and it is critical that the development of photosensitizers and lasers proceed together rather than in isolation. It is probable that laser and sensitizer development will focus on wavelengths of less than 900 mm, as the absorption of incident energy by water at longer wavelengths becomes significant, with subsequent decreases in penetration depth of light *(83)*. The titanium-dopes sapphire crystal (Ti:sapphire) and alexandrite lasers are solid-state lasers that operate at 700 to 900 nm and 720 to 800 nm, respectively *(84)*.

A problem with testing PDT as an adjuvant treatment is that the tumor responses are difficult to measure. Because the depth of tumor kill of PDT is probably only 0.5 to 1.0 cm, it could be expected that PDT has little to offer as a sole treatment of large tumors. At surgery, most GBM consist of approx 10^{11} cells. Resection and radiotherapy can result in three orders of magnitude of cellular reduction, with the remaining tumor burden still being of the order of 10^8 tumor cells. Further adjuvant therapies need to reduce the tumor burden to at least 10^4 to 10^5 tumor cells, at which level the body's immune system may be able to eliminate the residual tumor cells (85). In the foreseeable future, the strategies for treating gliomas should be aimed at using multiple adjuvant therapies that have been optimized so as to achieve the maximal reduction of residual tumor cells. This multimodal therapy will also overcome the inherent problems of the state of tumor cell heterogeneity in which subpopulations of resistant cells may remain following a particular therapy, resulting in tumor recurrence.

The possibility of combining binary treatment systems, such as PDT and boron neutron capture therapy (BNCT) (86), is an exciting development made possible by the synthesis of boronated porphyrins such as BOPP (17,87–89), which may act as a dual sensitizer for both PDT and BNCT. BOPP has the same spectral properties as hematoporphyrin derivative, and it is possible to envisage a treatment protocol of surgery with adjuvant PDT followed several days later by BNCT. BOPP has a long duration of retention in tumor tissue, and the several centimeter penetration capacity of an epithermal neutron beam would overcome the limited penetration of red light.

The PDT process is now being investigated by molecular biology techniques at the protein and genetic level. Porphyrin photosensitivity has been examined in tumor cell lines that express the multidrug resistance (MDR) phenotype, and tumor cells with high expression of MDR genes have shown decreased uptake of hematoporphyrin derivative and subsequent resistance to PDT-induced damage (90). Increasing our understanding of the PDT reaction at the molecular level and the interaction of the process with intracellular signaling pathways may allow for improvement in the overall effectiveness of the treatment in the future (91–96).

Techniques in molecular biology involving gene therapies appear to be the most likely avenue to produce the "cure" for gliomas, but in the foreseeable future the strategies for treating gliomas should be aimed at using multiple adjuvant therapies to achieve the maximal reduction of residual tumor and overcoming the inherent problems of tumor cell heterogeneity of subpopulations of resistant cells. Until biologic control of neoplasia is developed, PDT is likely to become one of a number of adjuvant therapies in the treatment armamentarium for cerebral glioma.

ACKNOWLEDGMENTS

The laboratory studies mentioned in this chapter as being performed by the authors were undertaken with the aid of grants from the National Health and Medical Research Council, The Royal Melbourne Neuroscience Foundation, the Anti-Cancer Council of Victoria, the Royal Australasian College of Surgeons, the Royal Melbourne Hospital Victor Hurley Medical Research Fund, and the Stroke Research Foundation.

REFERENCES

1. Bashir R, Hochberg F, Oot R. Regrowth patterns of glioblastoma multiforme related to planning of interstitial brachytherapy radiation fields. Neurosurgery 1988;23(1):27–30.
2. Choucair A, Levin V, Gutin P, et al. Development of multiple lesions during radiation therapy and chemotherapy in patients with gliomas. J Neurosurg 1986;65(5):654–658.
3. Kaye AH, Morstyn G, Brownbill D. Adjuvant high-dose photoradiation therapy in the treatment of cerebral glioma: a phase 1–2 study. J Neurosurg 1987;67(4):500–505.
4. Stylli S, Kaye A, MacGregor L, et al. Photodynamic therapy of high grade glioma—long term survival. J Clin Neurosci 2005;12(4):389–398.
5. Perria C, Capuzzo T, Cavagnaro G, et al. First attempts at the photodynamic treatment of human gliomas. J Neurosurg Sci 1980:24(3–4):119–29.

6. Daniell MD, Hill JS. A history of photodynamic therapy. Aust N Z J Surg 1991;61(5):340–348.

7. Abernathey CD, Anderson RE, Kooistra KL, et al. Activity of phthalocyanine photosensitizers against human glioblastoma in vitro. Neurosurgery 1987;21(4):468–473.

8. Kaye AH, Morstyn G. Photoradiation therapy causing selective tumor kill in a rat glioma model. Neurosurgery 1987;20(3):408–415.

9. Christensen T, Moan J, Sandquist T, et al. Multicellular spheroids as an in vitro model system for photoradiation therapy in the presence of Hpd. Prog Clin Biol Res 1984;170:381–390.

10. Kaye AH, Morstyn G, Gardner I. Development of a xenograft glioma model in mouse brain. Cancer Res 1986; 46:1367–1373.

11. Mitchell JB, Cook JA, Russo A. Biological basis for phototherapy. In: Morstyn KAG, ed. Phototherapy of Cancer, Harwood Academic Publishers: London, 1990;1–22.

12. Kessel D, Thompson P, Musselman B, et al. Probing the structure and stability of the tumor-localizing derivative of hematoporphyrin by reductive cleavage with LiAlH4. Cancer Res 1987;47(17):4642–4545.

13. Berenbaum MC, Bonnett R, Scourides PA. In vivo biological activity of the components of haematoporphyrin derivative. Br J Cancer 1982;45(4):571–81.

14. Kessel D. Chemistry of photosensitizing products derived from hematoporphyrin. In: Morstyn KAG, ed., Phototherapy of Cancer, Harwood Academic Publishers: London, 1990;23–35.

15. Kaye AH. Photoradiation therapy of brain tumours. Ciba Found Symp 1989;146:209–221; discussion 221–224.

16. Kaye AH. Photodynamic therapy of cerebral tumors. Neurosurg Q 1992;1:233–358.

17. Hill JS, Kahl SB, Kaye AH, et al. Selective tumor uptake of a boronated porphyrin in an animal model of cerebral glioma. Proc Natl Acad Sci USA, 1992;89(5):1785–1789.

18. Powers SK, Pribil S, Gillespie GY 3rd., et al. Laser photochemotherapy of rhodamine–123 sensitized human glioma cells in vitro. J Neurosurg 1986;64(6):918–923.

19. Whelan HT, Traul DL, Przybylski C, et al. Interactions of merocyanine 540 with human brain tumor cells. Pediatr Neurol 1992;8(2):117–120.

20. Fujishima I, Sakai T, Tanaka T, et al. Photodynamic therapy using pheophorbide and Nd:YAG laser. Neurol Med Chir (Tokyo) 1991;31(5):257–263.

21. Lindsay EA, Berenbaum MC, Bonnett R, et al. Photodynamic therapy of a mouse glioma: intracranial tumours are resistant while subcutaneous tumours are sensitive. Br J Cancer 1991;63(2):242–246.

22. Steichen JD, Weiss MJ, Elmaleh DR, et al. Enhanced in vitro uptake and retention of 3H-tetraphenylphosphonium by nervous system tumor cells. J Neurosurg 1991;74(1):116–122.

23. Van Lier J. New sensitizers for photodynamic therapy of cancer.Photodynamic Therapy. In: Douglas MJ, Dall'Acqua RH, eds., Light in Biology and Medicine. Plenum: New York 1988;133–140.

24. Butkus B. Europe Takes the Lead in Photodynamic Cancer Therapy. Biophotonics International, July 2003; 40–47.

25. Bourre L, Simonneaux G, Ferrand Y, et al. Synthesis, and in vitro and in vivo evaluation of a diphenylchlorin sensitizer for photodynamic therapy. J Photochem Photobiol B 2003;69(3):179–192.

26. Benson, R., Phototherapy of bladder cancer. In: Morstyn KAG, ed., Phototherapy of Cancer. Harwood Academic Publishers: London, 1990;199–214.

27. Woodburn KW, Vardaxis NJ, Hill JS, et al. Subcellular localization of porphyrins using confocal laser scanning microscopy. Photochem Photobiol 1991;54(5):725–732.

28. Hill JS, Kaye AH, Sawyer WH, et al. Selective uptake of hematoporphyrin derivative into human cerebral glioma. Neurosurgery 1990;26(2):248–254.

29. Origitano TC, Karesh SM, Henkin RE, et al. Photodynamic therapy for intracranial neoplasms: investigations of photosensitizer uptake and distribution using indium-111 Photofrin-II single photon emission computed tomography scans in humans with intracranial neoplasms. Neurosurgery 1993;32(3):357–363; discussion 363–364.

30. Powers SK, Cush SS, Walstad DL, et al. Stereotactic intratumoral photodynamic therapy for recurrent malignant brain tumors. Neurosurgery 1991;29(5):688–695; discussion 695–696.

31. Rosenthal MA, Kavar B, Hill JS, et al. Phase I and pharmacokinetic study of photodynamic therapy for high-grade gliomas using a novel boronated porphyrin. J Clin Oncol 2001;19(2):519–524.

32. Rosenthal MA, Kavar B, Uren S, et al. Promising survival in patients with high-grade gliomas following therapy with a noval boronated porphyrin. J Clin Neurosci 2003;10(4):425–427.

33. Bisland SK, Lilge L, Lin A, et al. Metronomic photodynamic therapy as a new paradigm for photodynamic therapy: rationale and preclinical evaluation of technical feasibility for treating malignant brain tumors. Photochem Photobiol 2004;80:22–30.

34. Stylli SS, Howes M, MacGregor L, et al. Photodynamic therapy of brain tumours: evaluation of porphyrin uptake versus clinical outcome. J Clin Neurosci 2004;11(6):584–596.

35. Sarissky M, Lavicka J, Kocanova S, et al. Diazepam enhances hypericin-induced photocytotoxicity and apoptosis in human glioblastoma cells. Neoplasma 2005;52(4):352–359.
36. Hirschberg H, Sun CH, Tromberg BJ, et al. Enhanced cytotoxic effects of 5-aminolevulinic acid-mediated photodynamic therapy by concurrent hyperthermia in glioma spheroids. J Neurooncol 2004;70(3):289–299.
37. Goldacre RJ, Sylven B. On the access of blood–borne dyes to various tumour regions. Br J Cancer 1962;16:306–322.
38. Kaye AH, Morstyn G, Ashcroft RG. Uptake and retention of hematoporphyrin derivative in an in vivo/in vitro model of cerebral glioma. Neurosurgery 1985;17(6):883–890.
39. Yoshida Y, Dereski MO, Garcia JH, et al. Photoactivated Photofrin II: astrocytic swelling precedes endothelial injury in rat brain. J Neuropathol Exp Neurol 1992;51(1):91–100.
40. Hill JS, Kahl SB, Stylli SS, et al. Selective tumor kill of cerebral glioma by photodynamic therapy using a boronated porphyrin photosensitizer. Proc Natl Acad Sci USA 1995;92(26):12126–12130.
41. Ito S, Rachinger W, Stepp H, et al. Oedema formation in experimental photo–irradiation therapy of brain tumours using 5-ALA. Acta Neurochir (Wien) 2005;147(1):57–65.
42. Kongshaug M, Moan J, Brown SB. The distribution of porphyrins with different tumour localising ability among human plasma proteins. Br J Cancer 1989;59(2):184–188.
43. Gal D, MacDonald PC, Porter JC, et al. Cholesterol metabolism in cancer cells in monolayer culture. III. Low-density lipoprotein metabolism. Int J Cancer 1981;28(3):315–319.
44. Jori G. Transport and tissue delivery of photosensitizers. In: C.F.S.N. 146, ed. Photosensitizing Compounds: Their Chemistry, Biology and Clinical Use. John Whiley & Sons: Chichester, UK, 1980;78–94.
45. Evenson JF, Moan J, Hindar A, et al. Tissue distribution of 3H–hematoporphyrin derivative and its main components, 67Ga and 131I-albumin in mice bearing Lewis lung carcinoma. In: Doiron GC DR, ed., Porphyrin Localization and Treatment of Tumours. Alan R Liss: New York, 1984;541–562.
46. Verma A, Nye JS, Snyder SH. Porphyrins are endogenous ligands for the mitochondrial (peripheral–type) benzodiazepine receptor. Proc Natl Acad Sci USA 1987;84(8):2256–2260.
47. Oseroff AR, Ohuoha D, Ara G, et al. Intramitochondrial dyes allow selective in vitro photolysis of carcinoma cells. Proc Natl Acad Sci USA 1986;83(24):9729–9733.
48. Dougherty TJ, Weishaupt KR, Boyle DG. Photodynamic sensitizers. In: DeVita VT Jr, Rosenberg SA, eds., Cancer: Principles and Practice of Oncology. JB Lippincott: Philadelphia, 1985;2272–2279.
49. Leach MW, Khoshyomn S, Bringus J, et al. Normal brain tissue response to photodynamic therapy using aluminum phthalocyanine tetrasulfonate in the rat. Photochem Photobiol 1993;57(5):842–845.
50. Yoshida Y, Dereski MO, Garcia JH, et al. Neuronal injury after photoactivation of photofrin II. Am J Pathol 1992;141(4):989–997.
51. Ji Y, Walstad D, Brown JT, et al. Interstitial photoradiation injury of normal brain. Lasers Surg Med 1992;12(4):425–431.
52. Svaasand LO, Ellingsen R. Optical penetration in human intracranial tumors. Photochem Photobiol 1985;41(1):73–76.
53. Muller PJ, Wilson BC. Photodynamic therapy: cavitary photoillumination of malignant cerebral tumours using a laser coupled inflatable balloon. Can J Neurol Sci 1985;12(4):371–373.
54. Muller PJ, Wilson BC. An update on the penetration depth of 630 nm light in normal and malignant human brain tissue in vivo. Phys Med Biol 1986;31(11):1295–1297.
55. Waldow SM, Dougherty TJ. Interaction of hyperthermia and photoradiation therapy. Radiat Res 1984;97(2):380–385.
56. Origitano TC, Reichman OH. Photodynamic therapy for intracranial neoplasms: development of an image-based computer-assisted protocol for photodynamic therapy of intracranial neoplasms. Neurosurgery 1993;32(4):587–595; discussion 595–596.
57. Berenbaum MC, Hall GW, Hoyes AD. Cerebral photosensitisation by haematoporphyrin derivative. Evidence for an endothelial site of action. Br J Cancer 1986;53(1):81–89.
58. Allardice JT, Abulafi AM, Webb DG, et al. Standardization of intralipid for light scattering in clinical photodynamic therapy. Lasers Med Sci 1992;7:461–465.
59. Schmidt MH, Meyer GA, Reichert KW, et al. Evaluation of photodynamic therapy near functional brain tissue in patients with recurrent brain tumors. J Neurooncol 2004;67(1–2):201–207.
60. Madsen SJ, Sun CH, Tromberg BJ, et al. Repetitive 5-aminolevulinic acid–mediated photodynamic therapy on human glioma spheroids. J Neurooncol 2003;62(3):243–250.
61. Doiron D. Photophysics of an instrumentation for porphyrin detection and activation. In Doiron GCDR, ed., Porphyrin localization and treatment of tumors. Alan R Liss: New York, 1984;41–73.
62. Bugelski PJ, Porter CW, Dougherty TJ. Autoradiographic distribution of hematoporphyrin derivative in normal and tumor tissue of the mouse. Cancer Res 1981;41(11 Pt 1):4606–4612.

63. Kaye A.H. Photoradiation therapy of brain tumours. In C.F.S.N. 146, ed., Photosensitising Compounds:Their Chemistry, Biology and Clinical Use. John Wiley & Sons: Chichester, United Kingdom. 1989;209–221.

64. Kaye AH, Hill JS. A review of photoradiation therapy in the management of central nervous system tumours. Aust N Z J Surg 1988;58(10):767–780.

65. Kelly PJ, Kall BA, Goerss S, et al. Computer-assisted stereotaxic laser resection of intra-axial brain neoplasms. J Neurosurg 1986;64(3):427–439.

66. Ji Y, Walstad D, Brown JT, et al. Improved survival from intracavitary photodynamic therapy of rat glioma. Photochem Photobiol 1992;56(3):385–390.

67. Laws Jr ER, Wharen Jr RE, Anderson RE. Photoradiation therapy for malignant glioma. In Wlikins RSRH, ed., Neurosurgery Update I. McGraw–Hill: New York, 1990;260–265.

68. Wharen RE, Anderson RE, Laws E Jr. Photoradiationtherapy of brain tumours. In: Salcman M, ed., Neurobiology of Brain Tumours. Williams & Wilkins: Baltimore, 1991;341–357.

69. Whelan HT, Schmidt MH, Segura AD, et al. The role of photodynamic therapy in posterior fossa brain tumors. A preclinical study in a canine glioma model. J Neurosurg 1993;79(4):562–568.

70. Schwatrz SK, Absolon K, Vermund H. Some relationships of porphyrins, x-rays and tumours. U Minn Med Bull 1955;27:7–13.

71. Forbes IJ, Ward AD, Jacka FJ, et al. A multi–disciplinary approach to phototherapy of human cancers. In: Doiron DR, Gomer CJ, eds., Porphyrin Localisation and Treatment of Tumors. Alan R Liss: New York, 1984; 693–708.

72. Wharen Jr RE, So S, Anderson RE, et al. Hematoporphyrin derivative photocytotoxicity of human glioblastoma in cell culture. Neurosurgery 1986;19(4):495–501.

73. Muller PJ, Wilson BC. Photodynamic therapy of malignant brain tumours. Can J Neurol Sci 1990;17(2): 193–198.

74. McCulloch GAJ, Forbes IJ, Lee See K, et al. Phototherapy in malignant brain tumours. In: Doiron GCDR, ed., Porphyrin Localisation and Treatment of Tumors. Alan R Liss: New York, 1984;709–717.

75. Laws ER Jr, Cortese DA, Kinsey JH, et al. Photoradiation therapy in the treatment of malignant brain tumors: a phase I (feasibility) study. Neurosurgery 1981;9(6):672–678.

76. Perria C, Carai M, Falzoi A, et al. Photodynamic therapy of malignant brain tumors: clinical results of, difficulties with, questions about, and future prospects for the neurosurgical applications. Neurosurgery 1988; 23(5):557–563.

77. Wharen RE Jr, Anderson RE, Laws ER Jr. Quantitation of hematoporphyrin derivative in human gliomas, experimental central nervous system tumors, and normal tissues. Neurosurgery 1983;12(4):446–450.

78. Kostron H, Fritsch E, Grunert V. Photodynamic therapy of malignant brain tumours: a phase I/II trial. Br J Neurosurg 1988;2(2):241–248.

79. Laws ER Jr, Wharen RE Jr, Anderson R.E. The treatment of brain tumors by photoradiation. In: Pluchino BGF, ed., Advanced Technology in Neurosurgery. Springer-Verlag: Berlin, 1988;46–60.

80. Krishnamurthy S, Powers SK, Witmer P, et al. Optimal light dose for interstitial photodynamic therapy in treatment for malignant brain tumors. Lasers Surg Med 2000;27(3):224–234.

81. Noske DP, Wolbers JG, Sterenborg HJ. Photodynamic therapy of malignant glioma. A review of literature. Clin Neurol Neurosurg 1991;93(4):293–307.

82. Popovic EA, Kaye AH, Hill JS. Photodynamic therapy of brain tumors. Semin Surg Oncol 1995;11(5):335–345.

83. Wilson B. Photodynamic therapy: Light delivary and dosage for second generation sensitizers. In: C.F.S.N. 146 ed., Photosensitising Compounds: Their Chemistry, Biology and Clinical Use. John Wiley & Sons: Chichester, United Kingdom, 1989;60–77.

84. Aimsworth MD, Piper JA. Laser systems for photodynamic therapy. In: Morstyn G, Kaye AH, eds., Phototherapy of Cancer. Harwood Academic Publishers: London, 1990;37–72.

85. Kaye AH. Adjuvant treatment of malignant brain tumours. Aust N Z J Surg 1989;59(11):831–833.

86. Barth RF, Soloway AH, Fairchild RG. Boron neutron capture therapy for cancer. Sci Am 1990;263(4):100–103,106–107.

87. Ozawa T, Afzal J, Lamborn KR, et al. Toxicity, biodistribution, and convection–enhanced delivery of the boronated porphyrin BOPP in the 9L intracerebral rat glioma model. Int J Radiat Oncol Biol Phys 2005;63 (1):247–252.

88. Ozawa T, Santos RA, Lamborn KR, et al. In vivo evaluation of the boronated porphyrin TABP-1 in U-87 MG intracerebral human glioblastoma xenografts. Mol Pharm 2004;1(5):368–374.

89. Dozzo P, Koo MS, Berger S, et al. Synthesis, characterization, and plasma lipoprotein association of a nucleus–targeted boronated porphyrin. J Med Chem 2005;48(2):357–359.

90. Gomer CJ, Rucker N, Ferrario A, et al. Properties and applications of photodynamic therapy. Radiat Res 1989; 120(1):1–18.

91. Almeida RD, Manadas BJ, Carvalho AP, et al. Intracellular signaling mechanisms in photodynamic therapy. Biochim Biophys Acta 2004;1704(2):59–86.
92. Plaetzer K, Kiesslich T, Oberdanner CB, et al. Apoptosis following photodynamic tumor therapy: induction, mechanisms and detection. Curr Pharm Des 2005;11(9):1151–1165.
93. Agostinis P, Buytaert E, Breyssens H, et al. Regulatory pathways in photodynamic therapy induced apoptosis. Photochem Photobiol Sci 2004;3(8): 721–729.
94. Korbelik M, Sun J, Cecic I. Photodynamic therapy–induced cell surface expression and release of heat shock proteins: relevance for tumor response. Cancer Res 2005;65(3):1018–1026.
95. Schieke SM, von Montfort C, Buchczyk DP, et al. Singlet oxygen–induced attenuation of growth factor signaling: possible role of ceramides. Free Radic Res 2004;38(7):729–737.
96. Wong TW, Tracy E, Oseroff AR, et al. Photodynamic therapy mediates immediate loss of cellular responsiveness to cytokines and growth factors. Cancer Res 2003;63(13):3812–3818.
97. Popovic EA, Kaye AH, Hill JS. Current status of photodynamic therapy for brain tumors. In: Salcman M, ed., Current Techniques in Neurosurgery. Current Medicine: Philadelphia, 1994;124–140.

Index